*Springer Texts in Statistics*

**Springer**
*New York*
*Berlin*
*Heidelberg*
*Barcelona*
*Hong Kong*
*London*
*Milan*
*Paris*
*Singapore*
*Tokyo*

## Springer Texts in Statistics

*Alfred:* Elements of Statistics for the Life and Social Sciences
*Berger:* An Introduction to Probability and Stochastic Processes
*Bilodeau and Brenner:* Theory of Multivariate Statistics
*Blom:* Probability and Statistics: Theory and Applications
*Brockwell and Davis:* An Introduction to Times Series and Forecasting
*Chow and Teicher:* Probability Theory: Independence, Interchangeability, Martingales, Third Edition
*Christensen:* Plane Answers to Complex Questions: The Theory of Linear Models, Second Edition
*Christensen:* Linear Models for Multivariate, Time Series, and Spatial Data
*Christensen:* Log-Linear Models and Logistic Regression, Second Edition
*Creighton:* A First Course in Probability Models and Statistical Inference
*Dean and Voss:* Design and Analysis of Experiments
*du Toit, Steyn, and Stumpf:* Graphical Exploratory Data Analysis
*Durrett:* Essentials of Stochastic Processes
*Edwards:* Introduction to Graphical Modelling
*Finkelstein and Levin:* Statistics for Lawyers
*Flury:* A First Course in Multivariate Statistics
*Jobson:* Applied Multivariate Data Analysis, Volume I: Regression and Experimental Design
*Jobson:* Applied Multivariate Data Analysis, Volume II: Categorical and Multivariate Methods
*Kalbfleisch:* Probability and Statistical Inference, Volume I: Probability, Second Edition
*Kalbfleisch:* Probability and Statistical Inference, Volume II: Statistical Inference, Second Edition
*Karr:* Probability
*Keyfitz:* Applied Mathematical Demography, Second Edition
*Kiefer:* Introduction to Statistical Inference
*Kokoska and Nevison:* Statistical Tables and Formulae
*Kulkarni:* Modeling, Analysis, Design, and Control of Stochastic Systems
*Lehmann:* Elements of Large-Sample Theory
*Lehmann:* Testing Statistical Hypotheses, Second Edition
*Lehmann and Casella:* Theory of Point Estimation, Second Edition
*Lindman:* Analysis of Variance in Experimental Design
*Lindsey:* Applying Generalized Linear Models
*Madansky:* Prescriptions for Working Statisticians
*McPherson:* Statistics in Scientific Investigation: Its Basis, Application, and Interpretation
*Mueller:* Basic Principles of Structural Equation Modeling: An Introduction to LISREL and EQS

*(continued after index)*

Robert H. Shumway David S. Stoffer

# Time Series Analysis and Its Applications

With 152 Figures

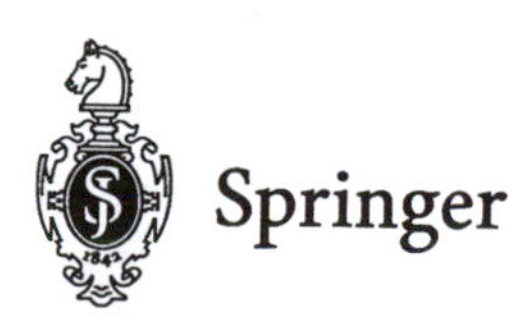


Springer

Robert H. Shumway
Division of Statistics
University of California, Davis
Davis, CA 95616
USA

David S. Stoffer
Department of Statistics
University of Pittsburgh
Pittsburg, PA 15260
USA



Library of Congress Cataloging-in-Publication Data
Shumway, Robert H.
Time series analysis and its applications / Robert H. Shumway, David S. Stoffer.
p. cm. — (Springer texts in statistics)
Includes bibliographical references and index.
ISBN 0-387-98950-1 (hc. : alk. paper)
1. Time-series analysis. I. Stoffer, David S. II. Title. III. Series.
QA280.S585 2000
519.5′5—dc21 99-046583

Printed on acid-free paper.



Production coordinated by Robert Wexler and managed by MaryAnn Brickner; manufacturing supervised by Jacqui Ashri.
Photocomposed copy prepared from the authors' LaTex files.
Printed and bound by R.R. Donnelley and Sons, Harrisonburg, VA.
Printed in the United States of America.

9 8 7 6 5 4 3 2 1

ISBN 0-387-98950-1 Springer-Verlag New York Berlin Heidelberg SPIN 10746200

*To my wife, Ruth, for her good-humored support and encouragement, and to my teacher, Solomon Kullback, for his guidance and enduring wisdom.*
*R.H.S.*

*To my family, Janice, Matthew and Lauren for laughing when I walked into walls, and to my parents, Benjamin and Rose for not laughing when I walked into walls.*
*D.S.S.*

# PREFACE

The goals of this book are to develop an appreciation for the richness and versatility of modern time series analysis as a tool for analyzing data, and still maintain a commitment to theoretical integrity, as exemplified by the seminal works of Brillinger (1981) and Hannan (1970) and the texts by Brockwell and Davis (1991) and Fuller (1995). The advent of more powerful computing, especially in the last three years, has provided both real data and new software that can take one considerably beyond the fitting of simple time domain models, such as have been elegantly described in the landmark work of Box and Jenkins (1970). The present book is designed to be useful as a text for courses in time series on several different levels and as a reference work for practitioners facing the analysis of time-correlated data in the physical, biological, and social sciences.

We believe the book will be useful as a text at both the undergraduate and graduate levels. An undergraduate course can be accessible to students with a background in regression analysis and might include Sections 1.1–1.8, 2.1–2.9, and 3.1–3.8. Similar courses have been taught at the University of California (Berkeley and Davis) in the past using the earlier book on applied time series analysis by Shumway (1988). Such a course is taken by undergraduate students in mathematics, economics, and statistics and attracts graduate students from the agricultural, biological, and environmental sciences. At the masters' degree level, it can be useful to students in mathematics, environmental science, economics, statistics, and engineering by adding Sections 1.9, 2.10–2.14, 3.9, 3.10, and 4.1–4.5, to those proposed above. Finally, a two-semester upper-level graduate course for mathematics, statistics and engineering graduate students can be crafted by adding selected theoretical sections from the last sections of Chapters 1, 2, and 3 for mathematics and statistics students and some advanced applications from Chapters 4 and 5. For the upper-level graduate course, we should mention that we are striving for a less rigorous level of coverage than that which is attained by Brockwell and Davis (1991), the classic entry at this level.

A useful feature of the presentation is the inclusion of data illustrating the richness of potential applications to medicine and in the biological, physical, and social sciences. We include data analysis in both the text examples and in the problem sets. All data sets are posted on the World Wide Web at the following URLs: `http://www.stat.ucdavis.edu/~shumway/tsa.html` and `http://www.stat.pitt.edu/~stoffer/tsa.html`, making them easily accessible to students and general researchers. In addition, an exploratory data analysis program written by McQuarrie and Shumway (1994) can be downloaded (as Freeware) from these websites to provide easy access to all of the techniques required for courses through the masters' level.

Advances in modern computing have made multivariate techniques in the time and frequency domain, anticipated by the theoretical developments in Brillinger (1981) and Hannan (1970), routinely accessible using higher level languages, such as MATLAB and S-PLUS. Extremely large data sets driven by periodic phenomena, such as the functional magnetic resonance imaging series or the earthquake and explosion data, can now be handled using extensions to time series of classical methods, like multivariate regression, analysis of variance, principal components, factor analysis, and discriminant or cluster analysis. Chapters 4 and 5 illustrate some of the immense potential that methods have for analyzing high-dimensional data sets.

The many practical data sets are the results of collaborations with research workers in the medical, physical, and biological sciences. Some deserve special mention as a result of the pervasive use we have made of them in the text. The predominance of applications in seismology and geophysics is a result of joint work of the first author with Dr. Robert R. Blandford of the Center for Monitoring Research and Dr. Zoltan Der of Ensco, Inc. We have also made extensive use of the El Niño and Recruitment series contributed by Dr. Roy Mendelssohn of the Pacific Fisheries Environmental Group of the National Marine Fisheries. In addition, Professor Nancy Day of the University of Pittsburgh provided the data used in Chapter 4 in a longitudinal analysis of the effects of prenatal smoking on growth, as well as some of the categorical sleep-state data posted on the World Wide Web. A large magnetic imaging data set that was developed during joint research on pain perception with Dr. Elizabeth Disbrow of the University of San Francisco Medical Center forms the basis for illustrating a number of multivariate techniques in Chapter 5. We are especially indebted to Professor Allan D.R. McQuarrie of North Dakota State University, who incorporated subroutines in Shumway (1988) into ASTSA for Windows.

Finally, we are grateful to John Kimmel, Executive Editor, Statistics, for his patience, enthusiasm, and encouragement in guiding the preparation and production of this book. Three anonymous reviewers made numerous helpful comments, and Dr. Rahman Azari and Dr. Mitchell Watnik of the University of California, Davis, Division of Statistics, read portions of the draft. Any remaining errors are solely our responsibility.

Robert H. Shumway
Davis, CA
David S. Stoffer
Pittsburgh, PA
August, 1999

# Contents

# CHAPTER 1

# Characteristics of Time Series

## 1.1 Introduction

The analysis of experimental data that have been observed at different points in time leads to new and unique problems in statistical modeling and inference. The obvious correlation introduced by the sampling of adjacent points in time can severely restrict the applicability of the many conventional statistical methods traditionally dependent on the assumption that these adjacent observations are independent and identically distributed. The systematic approach by which one goes about answering the mathematical and statistical questions posed by these time correlations is commonly referred to as ***time series analysis***.

The impact of time series analysis on scientific applications can be partially documented by producing an abbreviated listing of the diverse fields in which important time series problems may arise. For example, many familiar time series occur in the field of economics, where we are continually exposed to daily stock market quotations or monthly unemployment figures. Social scientists follow populations series, such as birthrates or school enrollments. An epidemiologist might be interested in the number of influenza cases observed over some time period. In medicine, blood pressure measurements traced over time could be useful for evaluating drugs used in treating hypertension. Functional magnetic resonance imaging of brain-wave time series patterns might be used to study how the brain reacts to certain stimuli under various experimental conditions.

Many of the most intensive and sophisticated applications of time series methods have been to problems in the physical and environmental sciences. This fact accounts for the basic engineering flavor permeating the language of time series analysis. One of the earliest recorded series is the monthly sunspot numbers studied by Schuster (1906). More modern investigations may center on whether a warming trend is present in global temperature measurements or whether levels of pollution may influence daily mortality in Los Angeles. The modeling of speech series is an important problem related to the efficient transmission of voice recordings. Common features in a time series characteristic known as the ***power spectrum*** are used to help computers recognize and translate speech. Geophysical time series such those produced by yearly depositions of various kinds can provide long-range proxies for temperature and rainfall. Seismic recordings can aid in mapping fault lines or in distinguishing between earthquakes and nuclear explosions.

The above series are only examples of experimental databases that can be used to illustrate the process by which classical statistical methodology can be applied in the correlated time series framework. It is extremely important to gain experience working with real data because, for the most part, statistical analyses tend to be used for quantifying observed relations or attaching a measure of uncertainty to a conclusion that might be visually evident from inspecting the data. In our view, the first step in any time series investigation always involves careful scrutiny of the recorded data plotted over time. This scrutiny often suggests the method of analysis as well as statistics that will be of use in summarizing the information in the data. Before looking more closely at the particular statistical methods, it is appropriate to mention that two separate, but not necessarily mutually exclusive, approaches to time series analysis exist, commonly identified as the ***time domain approach*** and the ***frequency domain approach***.

The time domain approach is generally motivated by the presumption that correlation between adjacent points in time is best explained in terms of a dependence of the current value on past values. The time domain approach focuses on modeling some future value of a time series as a parametric function of the current and past values. In this scenario, we begin with ***linear regressions*** of the present value of a time series on its own past values and on the past values of other series. This modeling leads one to use the results of the time domain approach as a forecasting tool and is particularly popular with economists for this reason.

One approach, advocated in the landmark work of see Box and Jenkins (1970), develops a systematic class of models called ***autoregressive integrated moving average*** (ARIMA) models to handle time-correlated modeling and forecasting. The approach includes a provision for treating more than one input series through multivariate ARIMA or through ***transfer function modeling***. The defining feature of these models is that they are ***multiplicative models***, meaning that the observed data are assumed to result from products of factors involving differential or difference equation operators responding to a white noise input.

A more recent approach to the same problem uses ***additive models*** more familiar to statisticians. In this approach, the observed data are assumed to result from sums of series, each with a specified time series structure; for example, in economics, assume a series is generated as the sum of trend, a seasonal effect and error. The ***state-space model*** that results is then treated by making judicious use of the celebrated ***Kalman filters and smoothers***, developed originally for estimation and control in space applications. Two recent and relatively complete presentations from this point of view are in Harvey (1989) and Kitagawa and Gersch (1996). Time series regression is introduced in this chapter, and ARIMA and related time domain models are studied in Chapter 2, with the emphasis on classical, statistical, univariate linear regression. The state-space model, Kalman filtering and smoothing, multivariate regression, and multivariate ARMA models are developed in Chapter 4.

Conversely, the frequency domain approach assumes the primary characteristics of interest in time series analyses relate to periodic or systematic sinusoidal variations found naturally in most data. These periodic variations are often caused by biological, physical, or environmental phenomena of interest. A series of periodic shocks may influence certain areas of the brain; wind may affect vibrations on an airplane wing; sea surface temperatures caused by El Niño oscillations may affect the number of fish in the ocean. The study of periodicity extends to economics and social sciences, where one may be interested in yearly periodicities in such series as monthly unemployment or monthly birth rates.

In ***spectral analysis***, the partition of the various kinds of periodic variation in a time series is accomplished by evaluating separately the variance associated with each periodicity of interest. This variance profile over ***frequency*** is called the ***power spectrum***. In our view, no schism divides time domain and frequency domain methodology, although cliques are often formed that advocate primarily one or the other of the approaches to analyzing data. In many cases, the two approaches may produce similar answers for long series, but the comparative performance over short samples is better done in the time domain. In some cases, the frequency domain formulation simply provides a convenient means for carrying out what is conceptually a time domain calculation. Hopefully, this book will demonstrate that the best path to analyzing many data sets is to use the two approaches in a complementary fashion. Expositions emphasizing primarily the frequency domain approach can be found in Bloomfield (1976), Priestley (1981) or Jenkins and Watts (1968). On a more advanced level, Hannan (1970), Brillinger (1981), Brockwell and Davis (1991) and Fuller (1995) are available as theoretical sources. Our coverage of the frequency domain is given in Chapters 3 and 5.

The objective of this book is to provide a unified and reasonably complete exposition of statistical methods used in time series analysis, giving serious consideration to both the time and frequency domain approaches. Because a myriad of possible methods for analyzing any particular experimental series can exist, we have integrated real data from a number of subject fields into the exposition and have suggested methods for analyzing these data.

## 1.2 The Nature of Time Series Data

Some of the problems and questions of interest to the prospective time series analyst can best be exposed by considering real experimental data taken from different subject areas. The following cases illustrate some of the common kinds of experimental time series data as well as some of the statistical questions that might be asked about such data.

**Example 1.1 Johnson & Johnson Quarterly Earnings**

Figure 1.1 shows quarterly earnings per share for the U.S. company Johnson & Johnson, furnished by Professor Paul Griffin (personal communication) of the Graduate School of Management, University of California, Davis. There are 84 quarters (21 years) measured from the first quarter of 1960 to the last quarter of 1980 (a quarter is 3 months). Modeling such series begins by observing the primary patterns in the time history. In this case, note the gradually increasing underlying trend and the rather regular variation superimposed on the trend that seems to repeat over quarters. Methods for analyzing data such as these are explored in Section 1.8 (see Problem 1.25) using regression techniques, and in Chapter 4, Section 4.5, using structural equation modeling.

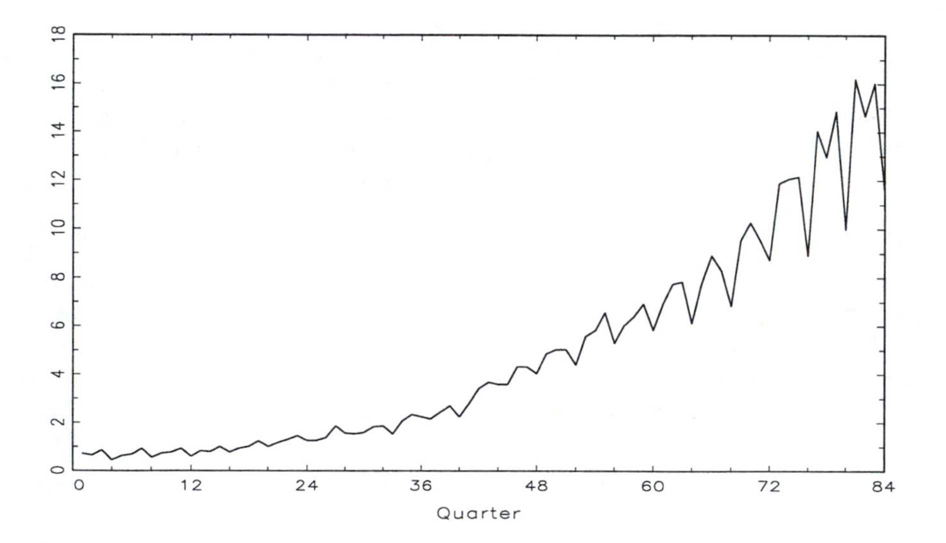


**Figure 1.1:** Johnson & Johnson quarterly earnings per share, 84 quarters, 1960-I to 1980-IV.

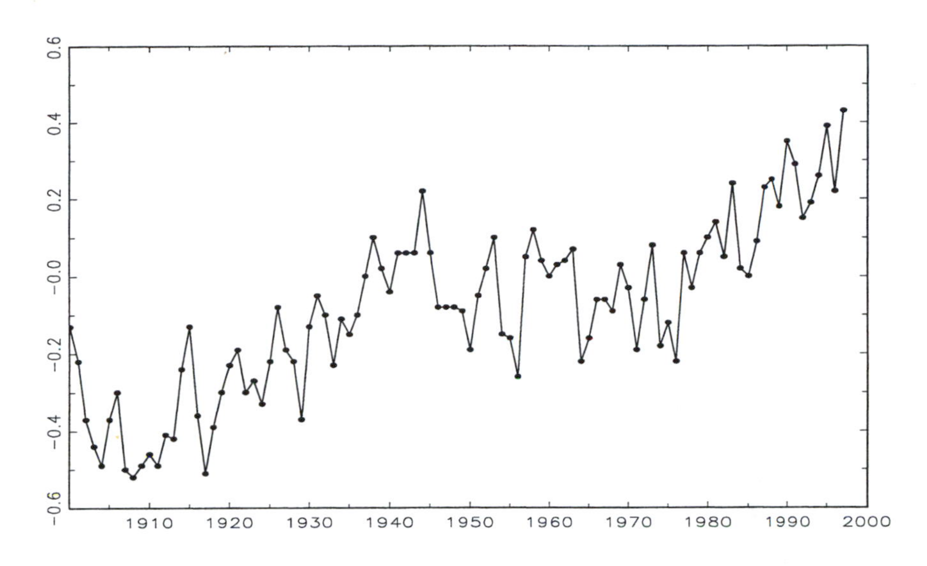


**Figure 1.2:** Yearly average global temperature deviations (1900-1997) in degrees Centigrade.

### Example 1.2 Global Warming

Consider a global temperature series record, discussed in Jones (1994) and Parker et al (1994, 1995). The data in Figure 1.2 are a combination of land-air average temperature anomalies (from 1961-1990 average), measured in degrees Centigrade, for the years 1900-1997. We note an apparent upward trend in the series that has been used as an argument for the global warming hypothesis. Note also the leveling off at about 1935 and then another rather sharp upward trend at about 1970. The question of interest for global warming proponents and opponents is whether the overall trend is natural or whether it is caused by some human-induced interface. Problem 1.23 examines 634 years of glacial sediment data that might be taken as a long-term temperature proxy. Such percentage changes in temperature do not seem to be unusual over a time period of 100 years. Again, the question of trend is of more interest than particular periodicities.

### Example 1.3 Speech Data

More involved questions develop in applications to the physical sciences. Figure 1.3 shows a small .1 second (1000 point) sample of recorded speech

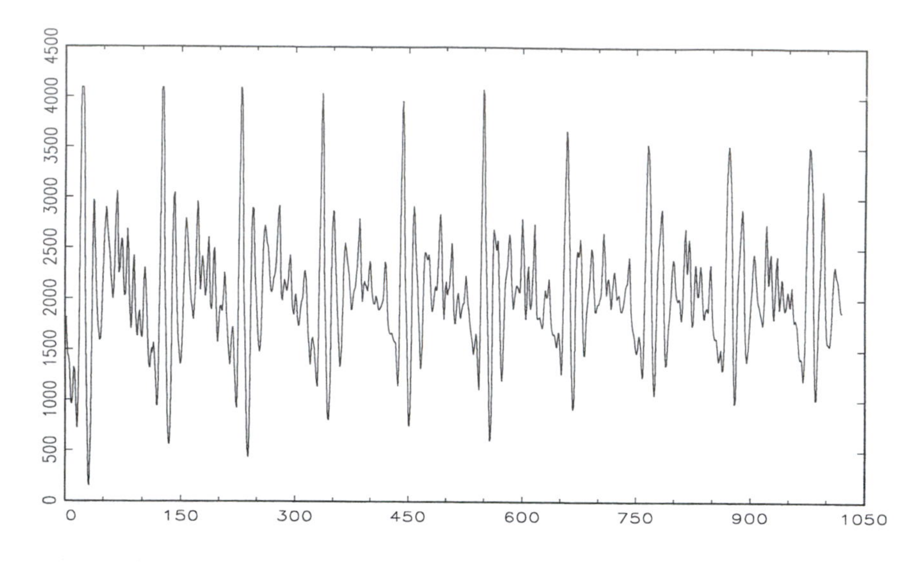


**Figure 1.3:** Speech recording of the syllable $aaa \cdots hhh$ sampled at 10,000 points per second with $n = 1020$ points.

for the phrase $aaa \cdots hhh$, and we note the repetitive nature of the signal and the rather regular periodicities. One current problem of great interest is computer recognition of speech, which would require converting this particular signal into the recorded phrase $aaa \cdots hhh$. Spectral analysis can be used in this context to produce a signature of this phrase that can be compared with signatures of various library syllables to look for a match. One can immediately notice the rather regular repetition of small wavelets. The separation between the packets is known as the ***pitch period*** and represents the response of the vocal tract ***filter*** to a periodic sequence of pulses stimulated by the opening and closing of the glottis.

### Example 1.4 El Niño and Fish Population

We may also be interested in analyzing several time series at once. Figure 1.4 shows monthly values of an environmental series called the ***Southern Oscillation Index*** (SOI) and associated ***Recruitment*** (number of new fish) furnished by Dr. Roy Mendelssohn of the Pacific Environmental Fisheries Group (personal communication). Both series are for a period of 453 months ranging over the years 1950-1987. The SOI measures changes in air pressure, related to sea surface temperatures in the central Pacific. The central Pacific Ocean warms every three to seven

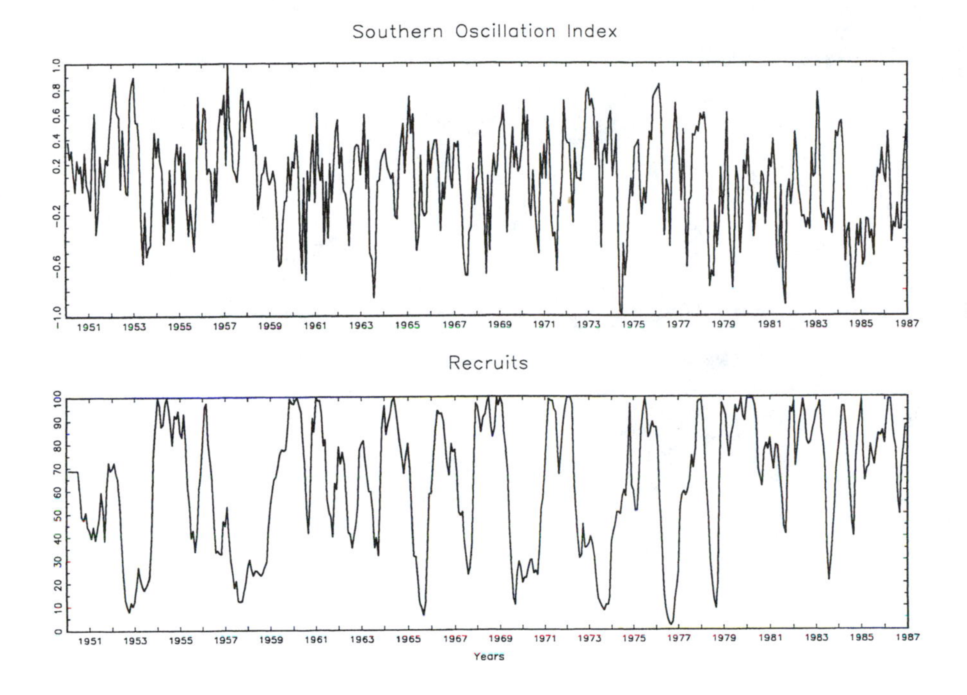


**Figure 1.4:** Monthly SOI and Recruitment (Estimated new fish), 1950-1987.

years due to the El Niño effect, which has been blamed, in particular, for the 1997 floods in the midwestern portions of the U.S. Both series in Figure 1.4 tend to exhibit repetitive behavior, with regularly repeating ***cycles*** that are easily visible. This periodic behavior is of interest because underlying processes of interest may be regular and the rate or ***frequency*** of oscillation characterizing the behavior of the underlying series would help to identify them. One can also remark that the cycles of the SOI are repeating at a faster rate than those of the Recruitment series. The Recruitment series also shows several kinds of oscillations, a faster frequency that seems to repeat about every 12 months and a slower frequency that seems to repeat about every 50 months. The study of the kinds of cycles and their strengths is the subject of Chapter 3. The two series also tend to be somewhat related; it is easy to imagine that somehow the fish population is dependent on the SOI. Perhaps, even a lagged relation exists, with the SOI signaling changes in the fish population. This possibility suggests trying some version of ***regression analysis*** as

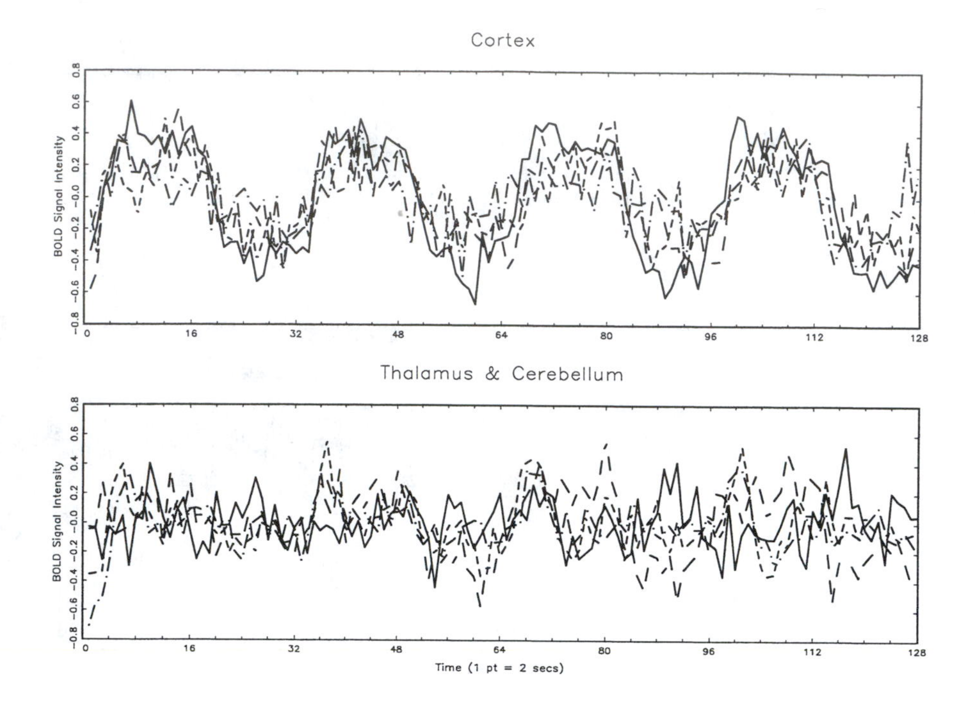


**Figure 1.5:** fMRI data from various location in the cortex, thalamus, and cerebellum; $n = 128$ points, one observation taken every 2 seconds.

a procedure for relating the two series. ***Transfer function modeling***, as considered in Chapter 2, can be applied in this case to obtain a model relating Recruitment to its own past and the past values of the SOI Index.

### Example 1.5 fMRI Imaging

A fundamental problem in classical statistics occurs when we are given a collection of independent series or vectors of series, generated under varying experimental conditions or treatment configurations. Such a set of series is shown in Figure 1.5, where we observe data collected from various locations in the brain via functional magnetic resonance imaging (fMRI). In this example, five subjects were given periodic brushing on the hand. The stimulus was applied for 32 seconds and then stopped for 32 seconds; thus, the signal period is 64 seconds. The sampling rate was one observation every two seconds for 256 seconds ($n = 128$). For this example, we averaged the results over subjects (these were evoked responses, and all subjects were in phase). The series shown in Figure 1.5 are consecutive measures of blood oxygenation-level dependent (BOLD) signal intensity, which measures areas of activation in the brain. Notice that the periodicities appear strongly in the motor cortex series and less strongly in the thalamus and cerebellum. The fact that one has series from different areas of the brain suggests testing whether the areas are responding differently to the brush stimulus. ***Analysis of variance*** techniques accomplish this in classical statistics and we show in Chapter 5 how these classical techniques extend to the time series case, leading to a ***spectral analysis of variance.***

**Example 1.6 Earthquakes and Explosions**

As a final example, the series in Figure 1.6, represent two phases or arrivals along the surface, denoted by P ($t = 1, \ldots, 1024$) and S ($t = 1025, \ldots, 2048$), at a seismic recording station. The recording instruments in Scandinavia are observing earthquakes and mining explosions with one of each shown in Figure 1.6. The general problem of interest is in distinguishing or discriminating between waveforms generated by earthquakes and those generated by explosions. Features that may be important are the rough amplitude ratios of the first phase P to the second phase S, which tend to be smaller for earthquakes than for explosions. In the case of the two events in Figure 1.6, the ratio of maximum amplitudes appears to be somewhat less than .5 for the earthquake and about 1 for the explosion. Otherwise, note a subtle difference exists in the periodic nature of the S phase for the earthquake. We can again think about spectral analysis of variance as a technique for testing the equality of the periodic components of earthquakes and explosions. We would also like to be able to classify future P and S components from events of unknown origin, leading to the ***time series discriminant functions*** developed in Chapter 5.

## 1.3 Time Series Statistical Models

The primary objective of time series analysis is to develop mathematical models that provide plausible descriptions for sample data, like that encountered in the previous section. In order to provide a statistical setting for describing the character of data that seemingly fluctuate in a random fashion over time, we assume a ***time series*** can be defined as a collection of random variables indexed according to the order they are obtained in time. For example, we may consider a time series as a sequence of random variables, $x_1, x_2, x_3, \ldots$, where the random variable $x_1$ denotes the value taken by the series at the first time point, the variable $x_2$ denotes the value for the second time period, $x_3$ denotes

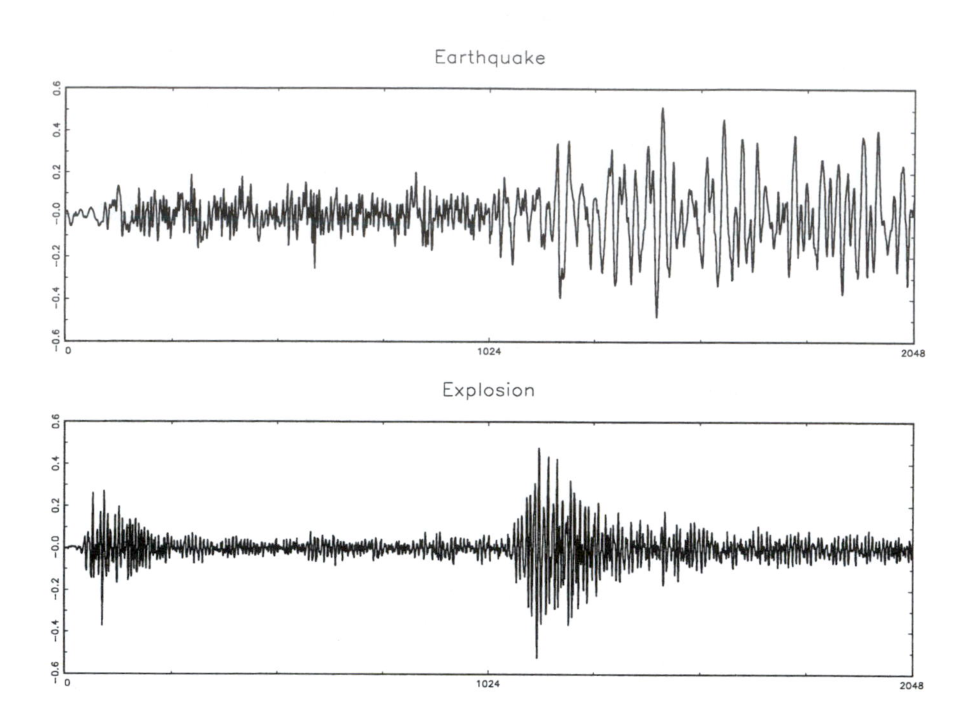


**Figure 1.6:** Arrival phases from an earthquake (top) and explosion (bottom) at 40 points per second.

the value for the third time period, and so on. In general, a collection of random variables, $\{x_t\}$, indexed by $t$ is referred to as a ***stochastic process***. In this text, $t$ will typically be discrete and vary over the integers $t = 0, \pm1, \pm2, ...$, or some subset of the integers. The observed values of a stochastic process are referred to as a ***realization*** of the stochastic process. Because it will be clear from the context of our discussions, we use the term ***time series*** whether we are referring generically to the process or to a particular realization and make no notational distinction between the two concepts.

It is conventional to display a sample time series graphically by plotting the values of the random variables on the vertical axis, or ordinate, with the time scale as the abscissa. It is usually convenient to connect the values at adjacent time periods to reconstruct visually some original hypothetical continuous time series that might have produced these values as a discrete sample. All series discussed in the previous section, for example, could have been observed at any continuous point in time and are conceptually more properly treated as ***continuous time series***. The approximation of these series by ***discrete time***

***parameter series*** sampled at equally spaced points in time is simply an acknowledgement that sampled data will, for the most part, be discrete because of restrictions inherent in the method of collection. Furthermore, the analysis techniques are then feasible using computers, which are limited to digital computations. Theoretical developments also rest on the idea that a continuous parameter time series should be specified in terms of finite-dimensional ***distribution functions*** defined over a finite number of points in time. This is not to say that the selection of the sampling interval or rate is not an extremely important consideration. The appearance of data can be changed completely by adopting an insufficient sampling rate. We have all seen wagon wheels in movies appear to be turning backwards because of the insufficient number of frames sampled by the camera. This phenomenon leads to a distortion called ***aliasing***.

The fundamental visual characteristic distinguishing the different series shown in Examples 1.1–1.6 is their differing degrees of smoothness. One possible explanation for this smoothness is that it is being induced by the supposition that adjacent points in time are ***correlated***, so the value of the series at time $t$, say, $x_t$, depends in some way on the past values $x_{t-1}, x_{t-2}, \ldots$. This model expresses a fundamental way in which we might think about generating realistic-looking time series. To begin to develop an approach to using collections of random variables to model time series, consider Example 1.7.

**Example 1.7 White Noise**

A simple kind of generated series might be a collection of uncorrelated random variables, $w_t$, with mean 0 and finite variance $\sigma_w^2$. The time series generated from uncorrelated variables is used as a model for noise in engineering applications, where it is called ***white noise***. The designation *white* originates from the analogy with white light and indicates that all possible periodic oscillations are present with equal strength. A particularly useful white noise series is ***Gaussian white noise***, wherein the $w_t$ are ***independent and identically distributed (iid) normal random variables***, with mean 0 and variance $\sigma_w^2$. Figure 1.7 shows in the upper panel a collection of 500 such random variables, with $\sigma_w^2 = 1$, plotted in the order in which they were drawn. The resulting series bears a slight resemblance the explosion in Figure 1.6 but is not smooth enough to serve as a plausible model for any of the other experimental series. The plot tends to show visually a mixture of many different kinds of oscillations in the white noise series.

As seen in Example 1.7, one problem with white noise as a model for time series is that the series is still quite choppy, which is caused because adjacent points are uncorrelated. If the stochastic behavior of all time series could be explained in terms of the white noise model, classical statistical methods developed for iid random variables would suffice.

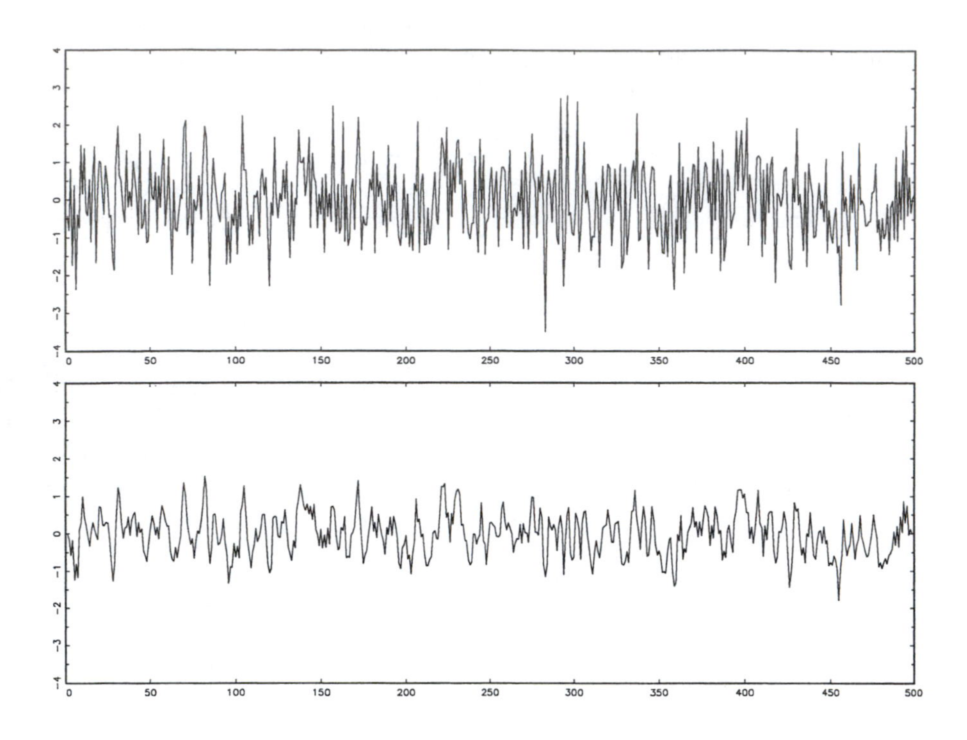


**Figure 1.7:** Gaussian white noise series (top) and three-point moving average of the Gaussian white noise series (bottom).

Two ways of introducing time series correlation and more smoothness into observed time series data are given in Examples 1.8 and 1.9.

### Example 1.8 Moving Averages

We might replace the white noise series $w_t$ by a ***moving average*** that smoothes the series. For example, consider replacing $w_t$ in Example 1.7 by an average of its current value and its immediate neighbors in the past and future. That is, let

$$v_t = \frac{1}{3}\big(w_{t-1} + w_t + w_{t+1}\big), \tag{1.1}$$

which leads to the series shown in the lower panel of Figure 1.7. Inspecting the series shows a smoother version of the first series, reflecting the fact that the slower oscillations are enhanced and some of the faster oscillations are taken out. We begin to notice a similarity to the SOI in Figure 1.4, or perhaps, to some of the fMRI series in Figure 1.5.

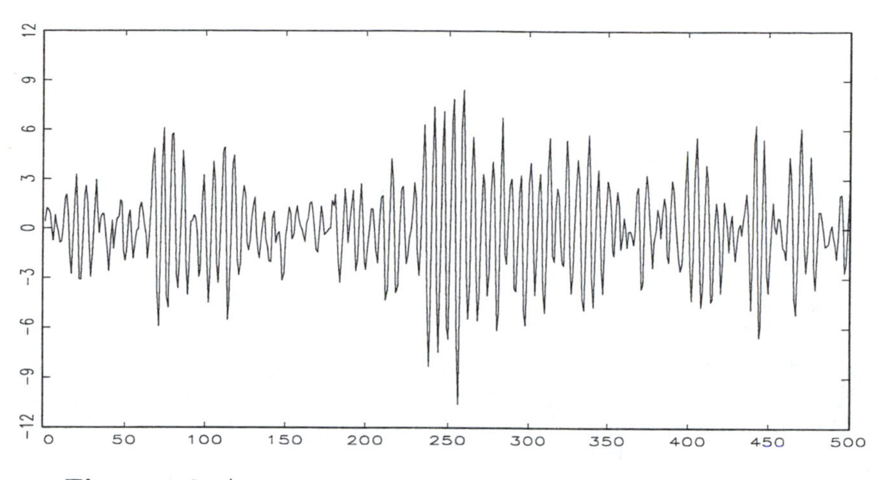


**Figure 1.8:** Autoregressive series generated from model (1.2).

The speech series in Figure 1.3 and the Recruitment series in Figure 1.4, as well as some of the MRI series in Figure 1.5, differ from the moving average series because one particular kind of oscillatory behavior seems to predominate, producing a sinusoidal type of behavior. A number of methods exist for generating series with this quasi-periodic behavior; we illustrate a popular one based on the autoregressive model considered in Chapter 2.

**Example 1.9 Autoregressions**

Suppose we consider the white noise series $w_t$ of Example 1.7 as input and calculate the output using the second-order equation

$$x_t = x_{t-1} - .90x_{t-2} + w_t \tag{1.2}$$

successively for $t = 1, 2, \ldots, 500$. Equation (1.2) represents a regression or prediction of the current value $x_t$ of a time series as a function of the past two values of the series, and, hence, the term ***autoregression*** is suggested for this model. A problem with startup values exists here because (1.2) also depends on the initial conditions $x_0$ and $x_{-1}$, but, for now, we assume that we are given these values and generate the succeeding values by substituting into (1.2). The resulting output series is shown in Figure 1.8, and we note the periodic behavior of the series, which is similar to that displayed by the speech series in Figure 1.3. The autoregressive model above and its generalizations can be used as an underlying model for many observed series and will be studied in detail in Chapter 2.

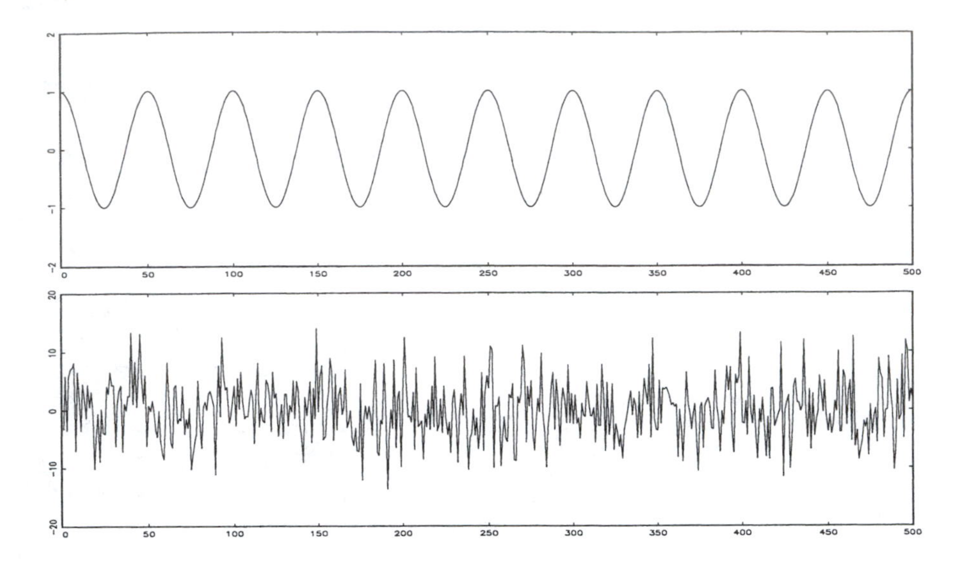


**Figure 1.9:** Cosine wave with period 50 points (top panel) compared with the cosine wave contaminated with additive white Gaussian noise (bottom panel).

**Example 1.10 Signal in Noise**

Many realistic models for generating time series assume an underlying signal with some consistent periodic variation, contaminated by adding a random noise. For example, consider the model

$$y_t = \cos\left(\frac{2\pi t}{50}\right) + w_t \tag{1.3}$$

for $t = 1, 2, ..., 500$, where the first term is regarded as the signal, shown in the upper panel of Figure 1.9. An additive noise term was taken to be white noise with $\sigma_w = 5$, drawn from a normal distribution. Adding the two together obscures the signal, as shown in the lower panel of Figure 1.9. Typically, we will only observe a signal contaminated with noise, and not the unobscured signal. In Chapter 3, we will study the use of ***spectral analysis*** as a possible technique for detecting regular or periodic signals, such as the one described above.

In general, we would emphasize the importance of simple additive models such as given above in the form

$$y_t = x_t + v_t, \tag{1.4}$$

where $x_t$ denotes some unknown signal and $v_t$ denotes a time series that may be white or correlated over time. The problems of detecting a signal and then in estimating or extracting the waveform of $x_t$ are of great interest in many areas of engineering and the physical and biological sciences. In economics, the underlying signal may be a trend or it may be a seasonal component of a series. Models such as (1.4), where the signal has an autoregressive structure, form the motivation for the state-space model of Chapter 4.

In the above examples, we have tried to motivate the use of various combinations of random variables emulating real time series data. Smoothness characteristics of observed time series were introduced by combining the random variables in various ways. Averaging independent random variables over adjacent time points, as in Example 1.8, or looking at the output of difference equations that respond to white noise inputs, as in Example 1.9 are common ways of generating correlated data. In the next section, we introduce various theoretical measures used for describing how time series behave. As is usual in statistics, the complete description involves the multivariate distribution function of the jointly sampled values $x_1, x_2, \ldots, x_n$, whereas more economical descriptions can be had in terms of the mean value and autocorrelation functions. Because correlation is an essential feature of time series analysis, the most useful descriptive measures are those expressed in terms of covariance and correlation functions.

## 1.4 Measures of Dependence: Autocorrelation and Cross-Correlation

A complete description of a time series, observed as a collection of $n$ random variables at arbitrary integer time points $t_1, t_2, \ldots, t_n$, for any positive integer $n$, is provided by the ***joint distribution function***, evaluated as the probability that the values of the series are jointly less than the $n$ constants, $c_1, c_2, \ldots, c_n$, i.e.,

$$F(c_1, c_2, \cdots, c_n) = P\big(x_{t_1} \leq c_1, x_{t_2} \leq c_2, \cdots, x_{t_n} \leq c_n\big). \tag{1.5}$$

Unfortunately, the multidimensional distribution function cannot usually be written easily unless the random variables are jointly normal, in which case, expression (1.5) comes from the usual multivariate normal distribution (see Anderson, 1984, or Johnson and Wichern, 1992). A particular case in which the multidimensional distribution function is easy would be for independent and identically distributed standard normal random variables, for which the joint distribution function can be expressed as the product of the marginals, say,

$$F(c_1, c_2, \cdots, c_n) = \prod_{t=1}^{n} \Phi(c_t), \tag{1.6}$$

where

$$\Phi(x) = \frac{1}{\sqrt{2\pi}} \int_{-\infty}^{x} \exp\{-\frac{z^2}{2}\}\, dz \tag{1.7}$$

is the cumulative distribution function of the standard normal.

Although the multidimensional distribution function describes the data completely, it is an unwieldy tool for displaying and analyzing time series data. The distribution function (1.5) must be evaluated as a function of $n$ arguments, so any plotting of the corresponding multivariate density functions is virtually impossible. The one-dimensional distribution functions

$$F_t(x) = P\{x_t \le x\}$$

or the corresponding ***one-dimensional density functions***

$$f_t(x) = \frac{\partial F_t(x)}{\partial x},$$

when they exist, are often informative for determining whether a particular coordinate of the time series has a well-known density function, like the normal (Gaussian) distribution. Similarly, the ***mean value function*** is defined as

$$\mu_{xt} = E(x_t) = \int_{-\infty}^{\infty} x f_t(x)\, dx, \tag{1.8}$$

provided it exists, where $E$ denotes the usual expected value operator. When no confusion exists about which time series we are referring to, we will drop a subscript and write $\mu_{xt}$ as $\mu_t$. The important thing to realize about $\mu_t$ is that it is a theoretical mean value for the series at one particular time point, where the mean is taken over all possible events that could have produced $x_t$.

**Example 1.11 Mean of a Moving Average Series**

If $w_t, t = 1, 2, \ldots$ denotes a white noise series, $\mu_t = E(w_t) = 0$ for all $t$. The top series in Figure 1.7 reflects this, as the series clearly fluctuates around a mean value of zero. Smoothing the series as in Example 1.8 does not change the mean because we can write

$$E(v_t) = \frac{1}{3}[Ew_{t-1} + Ew_t + Ew_{t+1}] = 0.$$

**Example 1.12 Mean of Signal Plus Noise**

A great many practical applications depend on assuming the observed data have been generated by a fixed signal waveform superimposed on a zero-mean noise process, leading to an additive signal model of the form

(1.3). It is clear, because the signal in (1.3) is a fixed function of time, we will have

$$\begin{aligned} E(y_t) &= E\big[\cos(2\pi t/50) + w_t\big] \\ &= \cos(2\pi t/50) + Ew_t \\ &= \cos(2\pi t/50), \end{aligned}$$

and the mean value is just the cosine wave.

The lack of independence between two adjacent values $x_s$ and $x_t$ can be assessed numerically, as in classical statistics, using the notions of covariance and correlation. Assuming these two values at time points $s$ and $t$, as shown in Figure 1.10, are jointly distributed random variables with distribution function $F(x_s, x_t)$, leads to an expression for the probability that any two points on the series are less than or equal to specified values. The ***autocovariance function*** is defined as the second moment product

$$\gamma_x(s,t) = E[(x_s - \mu_s)(x_t - \mu_t)], \tag{1.9}$$

for all $s$ and $t$. The autocovariance measures the *linear* dependence between two points on the same series observed at different times, as in Figure 1.10. Very smooth series exhibit autocovariance functions that stay large even when the $t$ and $s$ are far apart, whereas choppy series tend to have autocovariance functions that are nearly zero for large separations. The autocovariance (1.9) is the average cross product relative to the joint density $F(x_s, x_t)$. Recall from classical statistics that if $\gamma_x(s,t) = 0$, $x_s$ and $x_t$ are not linearly related, but there still may be some dependence structure between them. If, however, $x_s$ and $x_t$ are bivariate normal, $\gamma_x(s,t) = 0$ ensures their independence. It is clear that, for $s = t$, the autocovariance reduces to the variance, since

$$\gamma_x(t,t) = E[(x_t - \mu_t)^2]. \tag{1.10}$$

When no possible confusion exists about which time series we are referring to, we will drop the subscript and write $\gamma_x(s,t)$ as $\gamma(s,t)$.

### Example 1.13 Autocovariance of White Noise

The white noise series $w_t$, shown in the top panel of Figure 1.7, has $Es_t = 0$ and

$$\gamma(s,t) = E(w_s w_t) = \begin{cases} \sigma_w^2, & s = t \\ 0, & s \neq t \end{cases}$$

where, in this example, $\sigma_w^2 = 1$. Noting the independence of $w_s$ and $w_t$ for $s \neq t$, we would have $E(w_s w_t) = E(w_s)E(w_t) = 0$ because the mean values of the white noise variates are zero.

**Example 1.14 Autocovariance of a Moving Average**

Consider applying a three-point moving average to the white noise series $w_t$ of the previous example, as in Example 1.8 ($\sigma_w^2 = 1$). Because $v_t$ in (1.1) has mean zero, we have

$$\begin{aligned}
\gamma(s,t) &= E[(v_s - 0)(v_t - 0)] \\
&= \frac{1}{9}E[(w_{s-1} + w_s + w_{s+1})(w_{t-1} + w_t + w_{t+1})].
\end{aligned}$$

It is convenient to calculate it as a function of the separation, $s - t = h$, say, for $h = 0, \pm 1, \pm 2, \ldots$. For example, with $h = 0$,

$$\begin{aligned}
\gamma(t,t) &= \frac{1}{9}E[(w_{t-1} + w_t + w_{t+1})(w_{t-1} + w_t + w_{t+1})] \\
&= \frac{1}{9}[E(w_{t-1}w_{t-1}) + E(w_t w_t) + E(w_{t+1}w_{t+1})] \\
&= \frac{3}{9}.
\end{aligned}$$

When $h = 1$,

$$\begin{aligned}
\gamma(t+1,t) &= \frac{1}{9}E[(w_t + w_{t+1} + w_{t+2})(w_{t-1} + w_t + w_{t+1})] \\
&= \frac{1}{9}[E(w_t w_t) + E(w_{t+1}w_{t+1})] \\
&= \frac{2}{9},
\end{aligned}$$

using the fact that we may drop terms with unequal subscripts. Similar computations give $\gamma(t-1,t) = 2/9$, $\gamma(t+2,t) = \gamma(t-2,t) = 1/9$, and 0 for larger separations. We summarize the values for all $s$ and $t$ as

$$\gamma(s,t) = \begin{cases} 3/9, & s = t \\ 2/9, & |s-t| = 1 \\ 1/9, & |s-t| = 2 \\ 0, & |s-t| \geq 3. \end{cases} \tag{1.11}$$

Example 1.14 shows clearly that the smoothing operation introduces a covariance function that decreases as the separation between the two time points increases and disappears completely when the time points are separated by three or more time points. This particular autocovariance is interesting because it only depends on the time separation or ***lag*** and not on the absolute location of the points along the series. We shall see later that this dependence suggests a mathematical model for the concept of ***weak stationarity***.

As in classical statistics, it is more convenient to deal with a measure of association between $-1$ and 1 and this leads to a definition of the ***autocorrelation function (ACF)*** as

$$\rho(s,t) = \frac{\gamma(s,t)}{\sqrt{\gamma(s,s)\gamma(t,t)}}, \tag{1.12}$$

which measures the linear predictability of the series at time $t$, say, $x_t$, using only the value $x_s$. We can show easily that $-1 \leq \rho(s,t) \leq 1$ using the Cauchy–Schwarz inequality.[1] If we can predict $x_t$ *perfectly* from $x_s$ through a linear relationship, $x_t = \beta_0 + \beta_1 x_s$, then the correlation will be 1 when $\beta_1 > 0$, $-1$ when $\beta_1 < 0$, and 0 when $\beta_1 = 0$. Hence, we have a rough measure of the ability to forecast the series at time $t$ from the value at time $s$.

Often, we would like to measure the predictability of another series $y_t$ from the series $x_s$, leading to the notion of a ***cross-covariance function***

$$\gamma_{xy}(s,t) = E[(x_s - \mu_{xs})(y_t - \mu_{yt})], \tag{1.13}$$

where $\mu_{yt} = E(y_t)$ is the mean of the new series. The scaled version of the above, called the ***cross-correlation function (CCF)***, is defined as

$$\rho_{xy}(s,t) = \frac{\gamma_{xy}(s,t)}{\sqrt{\gamma_x(s,s)\gamma_y(t,t)}}, \tag{1.14}$$

where $\gamma_y(s,t)$ denotes the autocovariance function of the new series. An extension of the idea to more than two series, say, $x_{t1}, x_{t2}, \ldots, x_{tr}$, shows that the definition can be extended to include a ***multivariate time series*** with $r$ components. We note the extension of (1.9) in this case to

$$\gamma_{jk}(s,t) = E[(x_{sj} - \mu_{sj})(x_{tk} - \mu_{tk})] \tag{1.15}$$

for $j, k = 1, 2, \ldots, r$.

In the definitions above, the autocovariance and cross-covariance functions may change as one moves along the series because the values depend on both $s$ and $t$, the locations of the points in time. In Example 1.14, the autocovariance function depends on the separation of $x_s$ and $x_t$, say, $h = |s - t|$, and not on where the points are located in time. As long as the points are separated by $h$ units, the location of the two points doesn't matter. This notion, called ***weak stationarity***, when the mean is constant, is fundamental in allowing us to analyze sample time series data when only a single series is available.

## 1.5 Stationary Time Series

The preceding definitions of the mean and autocovariance functions are completely general. Although we have not made any special assumptions about the behavior of the time series, many of the preceding examples have hinted that a sort of regularity may exist over time in the behavior of a time series. We introduce the notion of regularity using a concept called ***stationarity***.

[1] The Cauchy–Schwarz inequality is given in (1.126) and applies with $x = x_s - \mu_s$ and $y = x_t - \mu_t$, so

$$|\gamma(s,t)| \leq \sqrt{\gamma(s,s)\gamma(t,t)}.$$

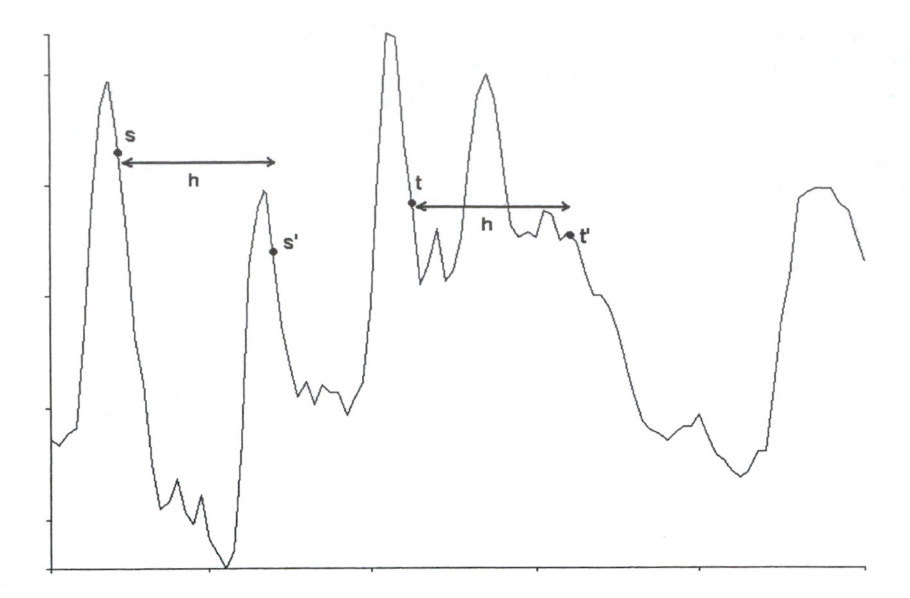


**Figure 1.10:** Time series with values at $s, t$ and $s' = s + h, t' = t + h$.

Suppose we let the value of the time series at some time point $t$ be denoted by $x_t$. A ***strictly stationary time series*** is one for which the probabilistic behavior of

$$x_{t_1}, x_{t_2}, \ldots, x_{t_k}$$

is identical to that of the shifted set

$$x_{t_1+h}, x_{t_2+h}, \ldots, x_{t_k+h}$$

for any collection of time points $t_1, t_2, \ldots, t_k$, for any number $k = 1, 2, \ldots$, and for any shift $h = 0, \pm 1, \pm 2, \ldots$ . This means that all of the multivariate distribution functions for subsets of variables must agree with their counterparts in the shifted set for all values of the shift parameter $h$. For the distribution functions, we would have

$$P\{x_{t_1} \leq c_{t_1}, \ldots, x_{t_k} \leq c_k\} = P\{x_{t_1+h} \leq c_1, \ldots, x_{t_k+h} \leq c_k\}. \tag{1.16}$$

For example, Figure 1.10 shows the series and the values at the time points $s, t$ and $s', t'$, where both sets of points are separated by a lag of $h$ units, and we must have, in this case,

$$\begin{aligned} P\{x_s \leq c_1, x_t \leq c_2\} &= P\{x_{s+h} \leq c_1, x_{t+h} \leq c_2\} \\ &= F(c_1, c_2). \end{aligned}$$

The version of stationarity in (1.16) is too strong for most applications, and we will use a milder version and define a ***weakly stationary*** time series as one which imposes conditions only on the first two moments of a time series. These conditions are that (i) the mean value function, $\mu_t$, defined in (1.8) is constant and does not depend on time $t$, and (ii) the covariance function, $\gamma(s,t)$, defined in (1.9) depends on $s$ and $t$ only through their difference $|s-t|$. In other words, letting $s = t+h$, where $h$ represents the time shift or ***lag***, then

$$\begin{aligned} \gamma(t+h,t) &= E[(x_{t+h}-\mu)(x_t-\mu)] \\ &= E[(x_h-\mu)(x_0-\mu)] \\ &= \gamma(h,0) \end{aligned}$$

does not depend on the time argument $t$. Implicit in this condition is the assumption that $\text{var}(x_t) = \gamma(0,0) < \infty$. We summarize by defining the mean value and autocovariance functions of the ***weakly stationary series*** as

$$E(x_t) = \mu \tag{1.17}$$

and

$$\gamma(h) = E[(x_{t+h}-\mu)(x_t-\mu)] \tag{1.18}$$

for all time $t$, where, for convenience, we write $\gamma(h) \equiv \gamma(h,0)$ because the autocovariance function of a weakly stationary process is only a function of time separation or lag $h$. Often, it is convenient to rewrite (1.18) as

$$\gamma(s-t) = E[(x_s-\mu)(x_t-\mu)], \tag{1.19}$$

which exhibits the autocovariance function in terms of two arbitrarily located points $x_s$ and $x_t$. The above equations constitute the definition of a weakly stationary series. Series satisfying both (1.17) and (1.18) will be referred to in the sequel as weakly stationary or just as stationary, for short. The ***autocorrelation function*** for a stationary time series can be written using (1.12) as

$$\rho(h) = \frac{\gamma(t+h,t)}{\sqrt{\gamma(t+h,t+h)\gamma(t,t)}} = \frac{\gamma(h)}{\gamma(0)}. \tag{1.20}$$

The Cauchy–Schwarz inequality shows again that $-1 \le \rho(h) \le 1$ for all $h$, enabling one to assess the relative importance of a given autocorrelation value by comparing with the extreme values $-1$ and 1.

**Example 1.15 Stationarity of White Noise**

The autocovariance function of the white noise series of Examples 1.7 and 1.13 is easily evaluated as

$$\gamma_w(h) = E(w_{t+h}w_t) = \begin{cases} \sigma_w^2, & h = 0 \\ 0, & h \neq 0, \end{cases}$$

where, in these examples, $\sigma_w^2 = 1$. This means that the series is weakly stationary or stationary. If the white noise variates are also normally distributed or Gaussian, the series is also strictly stationary, as can be seen by evaluating (1.16) using the relationship (1.6).

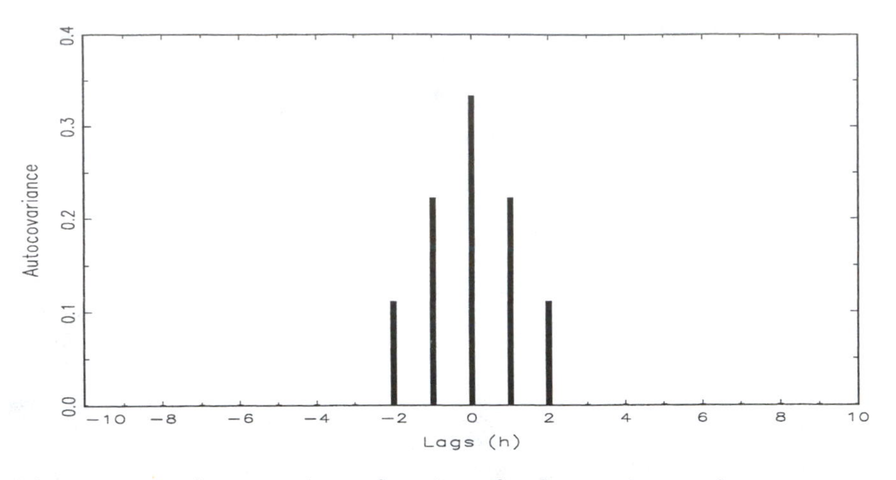


**Figure 1.11:** Autocovariance function of a three-point moving average.

**Example 1.16 Stationarity of a Moving Average**

The three-point moving average process used in Examples 1.8 and 1.14 is stationary because we may write the autocovariance function obtained in (1.11) as

$$\gamma_v(h) = \begin{cases} 3/9, & h = 0 \\ 2/9, & h = \pm 1 \\ 1/9, & h = \pm 2 \\ 0, & |h| \geq 3. \end{cases}$$

Figure 1.11 shows a plot of the autocovariance as a function of lag $h$. Interestingly, the autocovariance is symmetric and decays as a function of lag.

The autocovariance function of a stationary process has several useful properties. First, the value at $h = 0$, say

$$\gamma(0) = E[(x_t - \mu)^2] \tag{1.21}$$

is just the mean square error or ***variance*** of the time series and that the function $\gamma(h)$ takes its maximum value at $h = 0$. This property follows from the Cauchy–Schwarz inequality by an argument similar to that used earlier. A final useful property, noted for the examples above, is that autocovariance functions of stationary series are symmetric around the origin, that is,

$$\gamma(h) = \gamma(-h) \tag{1.22}$$

for all $h$. This property follows because shifting the series by $h$ means that

$$\gamma(h) \quad = \quad \gamma(t + h - t)$$

$$
\begin{aligned}
&= E[(x_{t+h} - \mu)(x_t - \mu)] \\
&= E[(x_t - \mu)(x_{t+h} - \mu)] \\
&= \gamma(t - (t+h)) \\
&= \gamma(-h),
\end{aligned}
$$

which shows how to use the notation as well as proving the result.

When several series are available, say, $x_t$ and $y_t$, the notion of stationarity still applies except that we need both means $\mu_x$, $\mu_y$ to be constant and both autocovariance functions $\gamma_x(h), \gamma_y(h)$ and the cross-covariance function

$$\gamma_{xy}(h) = E[(x_{t+h} - \mu_x)(y_t - \mu_y)] \tag{1.23}$$

to be functions only of lag $h$. The ***cross-correlation function***, defined as

$$\rho_{xy}(h) = \frac{\gamma_{xy}(h)}{\sqrt{\gamma_x(0)\gamma_y(0)}}, \tag{1.24}$$

expresses the relation between two series. Again, we have the result $-1 \leq \rho_{xy}(h) \leq 1$ which enables comparison with the extreme values $-1$ and 1 when looking at the relation between $x_{t+h}$ and $y_t$. The cross-covariance function satisfies

$$\gamma_{xy}(h) = \gamma_{yx}(-h), \tag{1.25}$$

which can be shown by manipulations similar to those used to show (1.22). Series with constant means and autocovariance and cross-covariance functions depending only on the separation $h$ are said to be ***jointly stationary***.

**Example 1.17 Joint Stationarity**

Consider the two series, $x_t$ and $y_t$, formed from the sum and difference of two successive values of a white noise process, say,

$$x_t = w_t + w_{t-1}$$

and

$$y_t = w_t - w_{t-1},$$

where $w_t$ are independent random variables with zero means and variance $\sigma_w^2$. It is easy to show that $\gamma_x(0) = \gamma_y(0) = 2\sigma_w^2$ and $\gamma_x(1) = \gamma_x(-1) = \sigma_w^2, \gamma_y(1) = \gamma_y(-1) = -\sigma_w^2$. Also,

$$
\begin{aligned}
\gamma_{xy}(1) &= E[(x_{t+1} - 0)(y_t - 0)] \\
&= E[(w_{t+1} + w_t)(w_t - w_{t-1})] \\
&= \sigma_w^2
\end{aligned}
$$

because only one product is nonzero. Similarly, $\gamma_{xy}(0) = 0, \gamma_{xy}(-1) = -\sigma_w^2$. We obtain, using (1.24),

$$
\rho_{xy}(h) = \begin{cases} 0, & h = 0 \\ 1/2, & h = 1 \\ -1/2, & h = -1 \\ 0, & |h| \geq 2. \end{cases}
$$

Clearly, the autocovariance and cross-covariance functions depend only on the lag separation, $h$, so the series are jointly stationary.

**Example 1.18 Prediction Using Cross-Correlation**

As a simple example of cross-correlation, consider the problem of determining possible leading or lagging relations between two series $x_t$ and $y_t$. If the model

$$y_t = Ax_{t-\ell} + w_t$$

holds, the series $x_t$ is said to lead $y_t$ for $\ell > 0$ and is said to lag $y_t$ for $\ell < 0$. Hence, the analysis of leading and lagging relations might be important in predicting the value of $y_t$ from $x_t$. Assuming, for convenience, that $x_t$ and $y_t$ have zero means, and the noise $w_t$ is uncorrelated with the $x_t$ series, the cross-covariance function can be computed as

$$\begin{aligned}\gamma_{yx}(h) &= E(y_{t+h}x_t) \\ &= AE(x_{t+h-\ell}x_t) + E(w_{t+h}x_t) \\ &= A\gamma_x(h-\ell).\end{aligned}$$

The cross-covariance function will look like the autocovariance of the input series $x_t$, with a peak on the positive side if $x_t$ leads $y_t$ and a peak on the negative side if $x_t$ lags $y_t$.

The concept of weak stationarity forms the basis for much of the analysis performed with time series. The fundamental properties of the mean and autocovariance functions (1.17) and (1.18) are satisfied by many theoretical models that appear to generate plausible sample realizations. In Examples 1.8 and 1.9, two series were generated that produced stationary looking realizations, and in Example 1.16, we showed that the series in Example 1.8 was, in fact, weakly stationary. Both examples are special cases of the so-called ***linear process***, defined in terms of linear combinations of an underlying sequence of white noise variates $w_t$. Suppose we define

$$\begin{aligned}x_t &= \mu + \psi_0 w_t + \psi_1 w_{t-1} + \psi_{-1} w_{t+1} + \dots \\ &= \mu + \sum_{j=-\infty}^{\infty} \psi_j w_{t-j}\end{aligned} \tag{1.26}$$

with the coefficients satisfying

$$\sum_{j=-\infty}^{\infty} |\psi_j| < \infty. \tag{1.27}$$

For this process (see Problem 1.12), we may show that the autocovariance function is given by

$$\gamma(h) = \sigma_w^2 \sum_{j=-\infty}^{\infty} \psi_{j+h}\psi_j \tag{1.28}$$

for $h \geq 0$ and $\gamma(-h) = \gamma(h)$. This method exhibits the autocovariance function of the process in terms of the lagged products of the coefficients. Note that, for Example 1.8, we have $\psi_0 = \psi_{-1} = \psi_1 = 1/3$ and the result in Example 1.16 comes out immediately. The autoregressive series in Example 1.9 can also be put in this form, as can the general autoregressive moving average processes considered in Chapter 2.

An important case in which a weakly stationary series is also strictly stationary is the ***normal*** or ***Gaussian*** series, in which the multivariate normal distribution is assigned to the $n$-dimensional vector $\boldsymbol{x} = (x_1, x_2, \ldots, x_n)'$. Then, defining the mean vector $\boldsymbol{\mu} = (\mu_1, \mu_2, \ldots, \mu_n)'$ and the $n \times n$ covariance matrix as $\Gamma = \{\gamma(s,t), s, t = 0, 1, \ldots, n-1\}$, the multivariate density function can be written as

$$f(\boldsymbol{x}) = (2\pi)^{-n/2}|\Gamma|^{-1/2} \exp\Big\{-\frac{1}{2}(\boldsymbol{x}-\boldsymbol{\mu})'\Gamma^{-1}(\boldsymbol{x}-\boldsymbol{\mu})\Big\}, \tag{1.29}$$

where $|\cdot|$ denotes the determinant. This assumption forms the basis for solving problems involving statistical inference for time series. If the time series is weakly stationary, $\gamma(s,t)$ is a function only of the time lag $\ell = s - t$, so the multivariate density $f(\boldsymbol{x})$ is a function only of that same time lag $\ell$. Because marginal density functions for jointly normal variates are jointly normal, with covariance functions chosen from the appropriate submatrices of $\Gamma$, all densities associated with the subvectors depend only on the time difference $h$. In the case in which all joint distributions depend only on the time shifts, the process is strictly stationary. We use the multivariate normal density in the form given above as well as in a modified version, applicable to complex random variables in the sequel.

## 1.6 Estimation of Correlation

Although the theoretical autocorrelation and cross-correlation functions are useful for describing the properties of certain hypothesized models, most of the analyses must be performed using sampled data. This limitation means the sampled points $x_1, x_2, \ldots, x_n$ only are available for estimating the mean value, autocovariance, and autocorrelation functions. From the point of view of classical statistics, this poses a probem because there will not be a number of iid copies of $x_t$, say, $x_{1t}, x_{2t}, \ldots, x_{Nt}$ might usually be available for estimating the covariance and correlation functions. In the usual situation with only one realization, however, the assumption of stationarity becomes critical. Somehow, we must use averages over this single realization to estimate the population means and covariance functions.

Accordingly, we estimate the mean value function (1.17) when it is constant by replacing the averaging over the population, denoted by $E$, with an average over the sample, say,

$$\overline{x} = \frac{1}{n}\sum_{t=1}^{n} x_t, \tag{1.30}$$

and the theoretical autocovariance (1.18) by the ***sample autocovariance function***

$$\widehat{\gamma}(h) = n^{-1}\sum_{t=1}^{n-h}(x_{t+h} - \bar{x})(x_t - \bar{x}), \tag{1.31}$$

for $h = 0, 1, 2, \ldots$ with $\widehat{\gamma}(-h) = \widehat{\gamma}(h)$. The sum in (1.31) runs over a restricted range, becauase $x_{t+h}$ is not available for $t + h > n$. The estimator in (1.31) is generally preferred to the one that would be obtained by dividing by $n - h$ because (1.31) is a non-negative definite function. The non-negative definite property ensures sample variances of linear combinations of the variates $x_t$ will always be non-negative. Note that neither dividing by $n$ or $n - h$ in (1.31) yields an unbiased estimate of $\gamma(h)$.

The ***sample autocorrelation function*** is defined, analogously to (1.20), as

$$\widehat{\rho}(h) = \frac{\hat{\gamma}(h)}{\widehat{\gamma}(0)}. \tag{1.32}$$

The sample autocorrelation function has a sampling distribution, under complete independence, which allows us to assess whether the data comes from a completely random or white series or whether correlations are statistically signficant at some lags. We have

***Property 1.1: Large Sample Distribution of the ACF***
*If $x_t$ is a stationary linear process of the form (1.26) with $Ew_t^4 < \infty$, for each $h = 1, 2, \ldots$, and large $n$, $\widehat{\rho}_x(h)$ will be approximately normal with mean $\rho_x(h)$ and variance depending on the true autocorrelation function $\rho_x(h)$, as shown in Theorem 1.7 at the end of this chapter. If the series $x_t$ is a white noise process, then $\rho(h) = 0$ for all $h \neq 0$, and the standard deviation reduces to*

$$\sigma_{\hat{\rho}(h)} = \frac{1}{\sqrt{n}}. \tag{1.33}$$

Based on the above result, we obtain a rough method of assessing whether peaks in $\widehat{\rho}(h)$ are significant by determining whether the observed peak is outside the interval $\pm z_{\alpha/2}/\sqrt{n}$, where $z_{\alpha/2}$ denotes the value of the standard normal variable $z$ with $P(|z| > z_{\alpha/2}) = \alpha$. The applications of this property develop because many statistical modeling procedures depend on reducing a time series to a white noise series by various kinds of transformations. After such a procedure is applied, the plotted ACF's of the residuals should then lie roughly within the limits given above.

The estimators for the cross-covariance function, $\gamma_{xy}(h)$, as given in (1.23) and the cross-correlation, $\rho_{xy}(h)$, in (1.24), are given, respectively, by the

***sample cross-covariance function***

$$\widehat{\gamma}_{xy}(h) = n^{-1} \sum_{t=1}^{n-h} (x_{t+h} - \bar{x})(y_t - \bar{y}), \tag{1.34}$$

where $\widehat{\gamma}_{xy}(-h) = \widehat{\gamma}_{yx}(h)$ determines the function for negative lags, and the ***sample cross-correlation function***

$$\widehat{\rho}_{xy}(h) = \frac{\widehat{\gamma}_{xy}(h)}{\sqrt{\widehat{\gamma}_x(0)\widehat{\gamma}_y(0)}}. \tag{1.35}$$

The sample cross-correlation function can be examined graphically as a function of lag $h$ to search for leading or lagging relations in the data using the property mentioned in Example 1.18 for the theoretical cross-covariance function. Because $-1 \leq \widehat{\rho}_{xy}(h) \leq 1$, the practical importance of peaks can be assessed by comparing their magnitudes with their theoretical maximum values. Furthermore, for $x_t$ and $y_t$ independent linear processes of the form (1.26), we have

***Property 1.2: Large Sample Distribution of the Cross-Correlation Under Independence***
*The large sample distribution of $\widehat{\rho}_{xy}(h)$ is normal with mean zero and*

$$\sigma_{\hat{\rho}_{xy}} = \frac{1}{\sqrt{n}} \tag{1.36}$$

*if at least one of the processes is white noise (see Theorem 1.8 at the end of the chapter).*

**Example 1.19 A Simulated Time Series**

To give an example of the procedure for calculating numerically the autocovariance and cross-covariance functions, consider a contrived set of data generated by tossing a fair coin, letting $x_t = 1$ when a head is obtained and $x_t = -1$ when a tail is obtained. Construct $y_t$ as

$$y_t = 5 + x_t - .7x_{t-1}. \tag{1.37}$$

Table 1.1 shows sample realizations of the appropriate processes with $n = 10$.

**Table 1.1** Sample Realization of the Contrived Series $y_t$

| t | 1 | 2 | 3 | 4 | 5 | 6 | 7 | 8 | 9 | 10 |
|---|---|---|---|---|---|---|---|---|---|---|
| Coin | H | H | T | H | T | T | T | H | T | H |
| $x_t$ | 1 | 1 | -1 | 1 | -1 | -1 | -1 | 1 | -1 | 1 |
| $y_t$ | 6.7 | 5.3 | 3.3 | 6.7 | 3.3 | 4.7 | 4.7 | 6.7 | 3.3 | 6.7 |
| $y_t - \bar{y}$ | 1.56 | .16 | -1.84 | 1.56 | -1.84 | -.44 | -.44 | 1.56 | -1.84 | 1.56 |

**Table 1.2** Theoretical and Sample ACF's for $n = 10$ and $n = 100$

| $h$ | $\rho_y(h)$ | $\widehat{\rho}_y(h)$ $n = 10$ | $\widehat{\rho}_y(h)$ $n = 10$ |
|---|---|---|---|
| 0 | 1.00 | 1.00 | 1.00 |
| $\pm 1$ | -.47 | -.55 | -.45 |
| $\pm 2$ | .00 | .17 | -.12 |
| $\pm 3$ | .00 | -.02 | .14 |
| $\pm 4$ | .00 | .15 | .01 |
| $\pm 5$ | .00 | -.46 | -.01 |

The sample autocorrelation for the series $y_t$ can be calculated using (1.31) and (1.32) for $h = 0, 1, 2, \ldots$ It is not necessary to calculate for negative values because of the symmetry. For example, for $h = 3$, the autocorrelation becomes the ratio of

$$\begin{aligned}
\widehat{\gamma}_y(3) &= 10^{-1} \sum_{t=1}^{7} (y_{t+3} - \bar{y})(y_t - \bar{y}) \\
&= 10^{-1} \Big[(1.56)(1.56) + (-1.84)(.16) + (-.44)(-1.84) \\
&\quad +(-.44)(1.56) + (1.56)(-1.84) + (-1.84)(-.44) \\
&\quad +(1.56)(-.44)\Big] \\
&= -.04848
\end{aligned}$$

to

$$\widehat{\gamma}_y(0) = \frac{1}{10}[(1.56)^2 + (.16)^2 + \cdots + (1.56)^2] = 2.0304$$

so that

$$\widehat{\rho}_y(3) = \frac{-.04848}{2.0304} = -.02388.$$

The theoretical ACF can be obtained from the model (1.37) using the fact that the mean of $x_t$ is zero and the variance of $x_t$ is one. From Problem 1.23 (d), it follows that

$$\rho_y(1) = \frac{-.7}{1 + .7^2} = -.47.$$

Furthermore $\rho_y(h) = 0$ for $|h| > 1$. Table 1.2 compares the theoretical ACF with sample ACF's for $n = 10$ and $n = 100$, and we note the increased variability in the smaller size sample.

**Example 1.20 ACF of Speech Signal**

Computing the sample ACF as in the previous example can be thought of matching the time series $h$ units in the future, say, $x_{t+h}$ against itself, $x_t$. Figure 1.12 shows the ACF of the speech series of Figure 1.3. The original series appears to contain a sequence of repeating short signals. The ACF confirms this behavior, showing repeating peaks spaced at about 106-109 points. Autocorrelation functions of the short signals appear, spaced at the intervals mentioned above. The distance between the repeating signals is known as the ***pitch period*** and is a fundamental parameter of interest in systems that encode and decipher speech. Because the series is sampled at 10,000 points per second, the pitch period appears to be between .0106 and .0109 seconds.

**Example 1.21 Correlation Analysis of SOI and Recruitment Data**

The autocorrelation and cross-correlation functions are also useful for analyzing the joint behavior of two stationary series whose behavior may be related in some unspecified way. In Example 1.4 (see Figure 1.4), we have considered simultaneous monthly readings of the SOI and the number of new fish (Recruitment) computed from a model. Figure 1.13 shows the autocorrelation and cross-correlation functions (ACF's and CCF) for these two series. Both of the ACF's exhibit periodicities corresponding to the correlation between values separated by 12 units. Observations 12

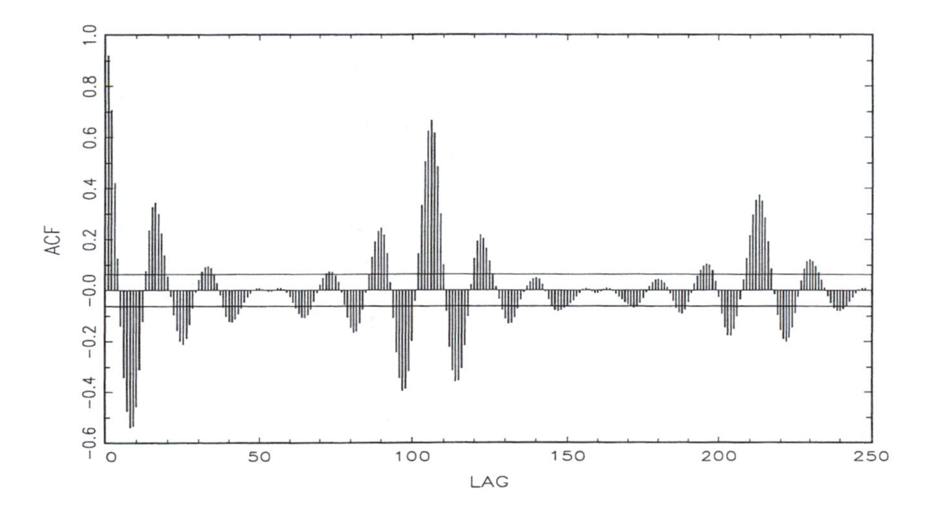


**Figure 1.12:** ACF of the speech series.

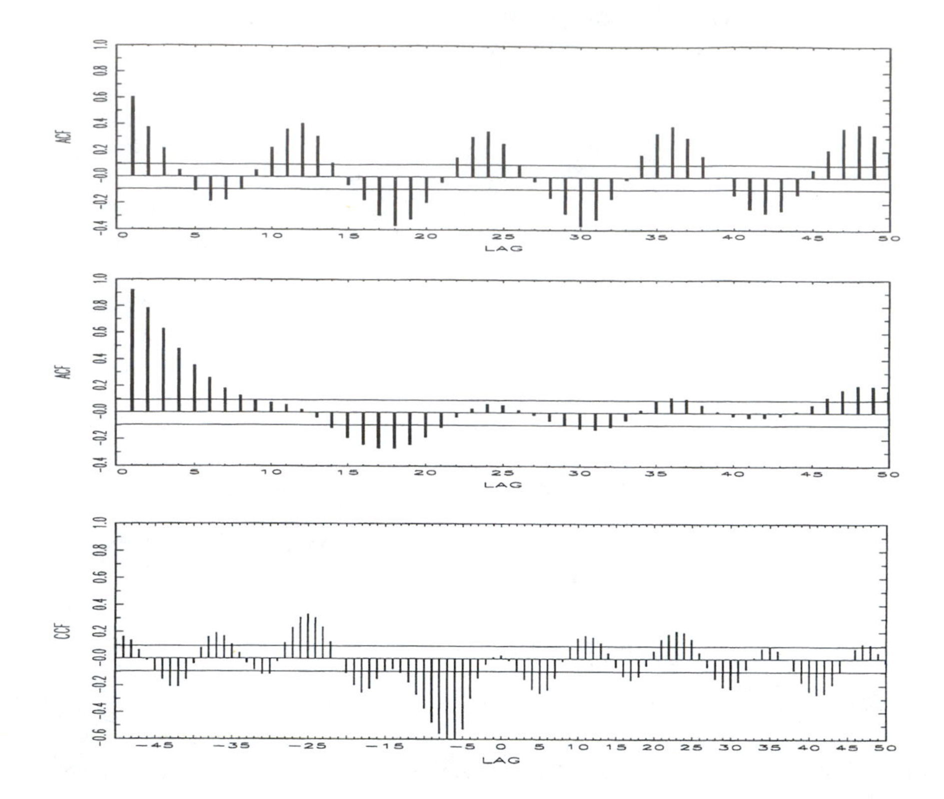


**Figure 1.13:** Sample ACF's of the SOI series (top) and of the Recruitment series (middle), and the sample CCF of the two series (bottom); negative lags indicate SOI leads Recruitment.

months or one year apart are strongly positively correlated, as are observations at multiples such as $24, 36, 48, \dots$ Observations separated by six months are negatively correlated, showing that positive excursions tend to be associated with negative excursions six months removed. This appearance is rather characteristic of the pattern that would be produced by a sinusoidal component with a period of 12 months. The cross-correlation function peaks at $h = -6$, showing that the SOI measured at time $t - 6$ months is associated with the Recruitment series at time $t$. We could say the SOI leads the Recruitment series by six months. The sign of the ACF is negative, leading to the conclusion that the two series move in different directions, i.e., increases in SOI lead to decreases in Recruitment and vice-versa. Again, note the periodicity of 12 months in the CCF. Upper and lower lines shown on the plots indicate $\pm 1.96/\sqrt{453}$, so that upper values would be exceeded about 2.5% of the time if the noise were white [see (1.33) and (1.36)].

## 1.7 Exploratory Data Analysis

In general, it is necessary for time series data to be stationary, so averaging lagged products over time, as in the previous section, will be a sensible thing to do. Hence, it is necessary that the stationarity assumptions (1.17) on the mean and (1.18) on the covariance functions be satisfied. Often, this is not the case, and we will mention some methods in this section for playing down the effects of nonstationarity so the stationary properties of the series may be studied.

A number of our examples came from clearly nonstationary series. The Johnson & Johnson series in Figure 1.1 has a mean that increases exponentially over time, and the increase in the magnitude of the fluctuations around this trend causes changes in the covariance function; $\gamma(0)$, for example, clearly increases as one progresses over the length of the series. The global temperature series, shown in Figure 1.2, contains some evidence of a trend over time; global warming advocates seize on this as empirical evidence to advance their hypothesis that temperatures are increasing. When the cosine wave in Figure 1.9 is added, the mean of the series is not constant, as was pointed out in Example 1.12. Such departures from stationarity cause distortions in the sample autocorrelation function (1.32) and sample cross-correlation function (1.35). To see this, one might only need to consider how the autocorrelation might behave if all points tend to be randomly distributed around a straight line, which makes adjacent products positive and produces an ACF that decays very slowly away from lag 0.

A natural way of limiting the effects on stationarity caused by a linear trend is to fit a straight line of the form $\beta_0 + \beta_1 t$ for $t = 1, ..., n$, through the data, $x_1, ..., x_n$, using ***simple linear regression***. In this case, one is proposing the model

$$x_t = \beta_0 + \beta_1 t + w_t \tag{1.38}$$

where $w_t$ is white noise; see Figure 1.14. The ***least squares*** estimates are

$$\widehat{\beta}_0 = \bar{x} - \widehat{\beta}_1 \bar{t}$$

for the intercept, and

$$\widehat{\beta}_1 = \frac{\sum_{t=1}^{n}(x_t - \bar{x})(t - \bar{t})}{\sum_{t=1}^{n}(t - \bar{t})^2}$$

for the slope, where $\bar{x} = n^{-1}\sum_{t=1}^{n} x_t$ and $\bar{t} = n^{-1}\sum_{t=1}^{n} t = (n+1)/2$. Details are provided in the next section. The residuals,

$$\widehat{w}_t = x_t - \widehat{\beta}_0 - \widehat{\beta}_1 t, \tag{1.39}$$

form the ***detrended series*** and should relatively free of any increasing trend. It should be noted that periods of constantly increasing and decreasing activity

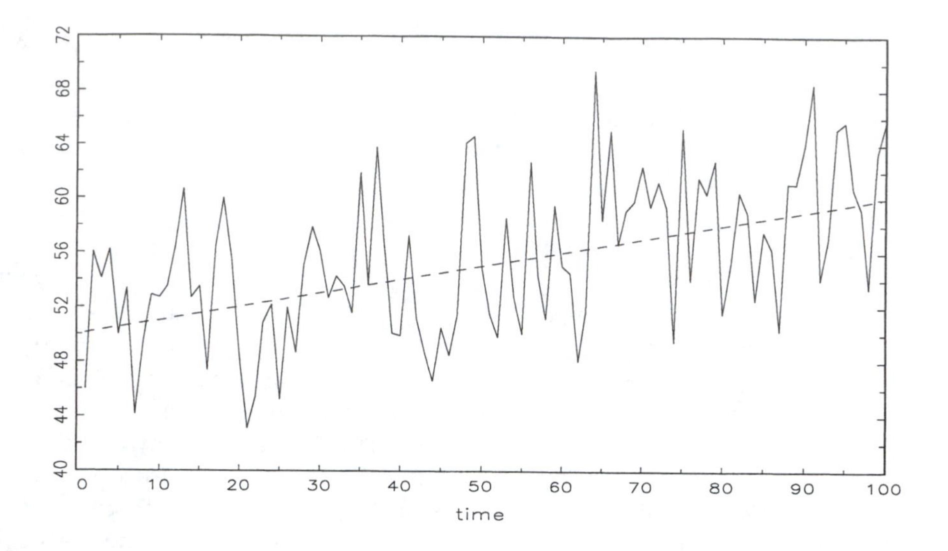


**Figure 1.14:** Simulated data, $x_t$, for $t = 1, ..., 100$, from the model (1.38) with $\beta_0 = 50$, $\beta_1 = 0.1$, and where the $w_t$ are generated as independent Gaussian variates with mean 0 and $\sigma_w = 5$. The straight line $50 + 0.1t$ is shown as a dashed line.

together may still be present. In particular, long regular periods will not be eliminated by detrending.

**Example 1.22 Detrending Global Temperature**

The original global temperature data are shown in Figure 1.2, and we might compare the general appearance of the temperature data in Figure 1.2 to the simulated data in Figure 1.14.

The top graph of Figure 1.15 shows the detrended series using the estimated intercept $\widehat{\beta}_0 = -.395$ and slope $\widehat{\beta}_1 = .006$. This implies, from the model (1.38), that the temperature increases .006 degrees Centigrade per year or .6 degrees per 100 years. The standard error of this slope estimate is .04 degrees per 100 years, and this is one item quoted as evidence of global warming. Apart from this consideration, the autocorrelation function of the original series, shown in Figure 1.16, exhibits slow decay indicative of nonstationary behavior, and most of the early points exceed the 95% limits specified using (1.33). The ACF of the detrended series, shown in Figure 1.16, improves the behavior slightly, but does not completely eliminate the nonstationary behavior. A long cycle occurs in

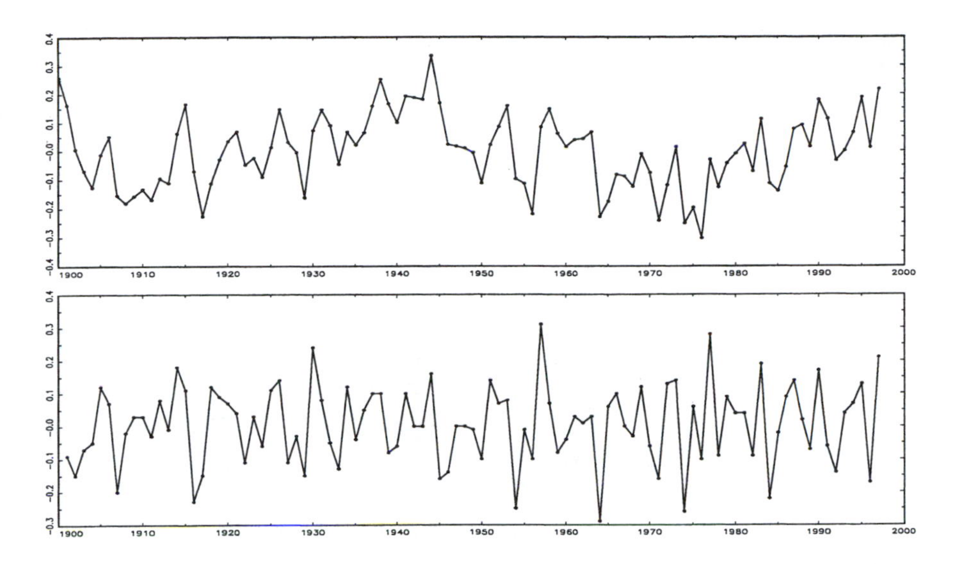


**Figure 1.15:** Detrended (top) and differenced (bottom) global temperature series. The original data are shown in Figure 1.2.

the middle of the series that is probably the cause of the remaining slow decay in the ACF.

An alternative to detrending that is often used is ***differencing***, which applies successive operations of the form

$$\nabla x_t = x_t - x_{t-1} \tag{1.40}$$

to achieve a stationary series. The first difference eliminates a linear trend, whereas a second difference, that is, the difference of (1.40), can eliminate a quadratic trend so that a single long cycle, not eliminated by the detrending procedure will be attennuated by differencing. In order to define higher differences, we need a variation in notation that we use, for the first time here, and often in our discussion of ARIMA models in Chapter 2. Suppose we define the ***backshift operator***

$$Bx_t = x_{t-1} \tag{1.41}$$

and extend it to powers $B^2x_t = B(Bx_t) = Bx_{t-1} = x_{t-2}$, so $B^kx_t = x_{t-k}$. Then, we may rewrite (1.40) as

$$\nabla x_t = (1 - B)x_t. \tag{1.42}$$

Higher order differences are defined as

$$\nabla^d x_t = (1 - B)^d x_t, \tag{1.43}$$

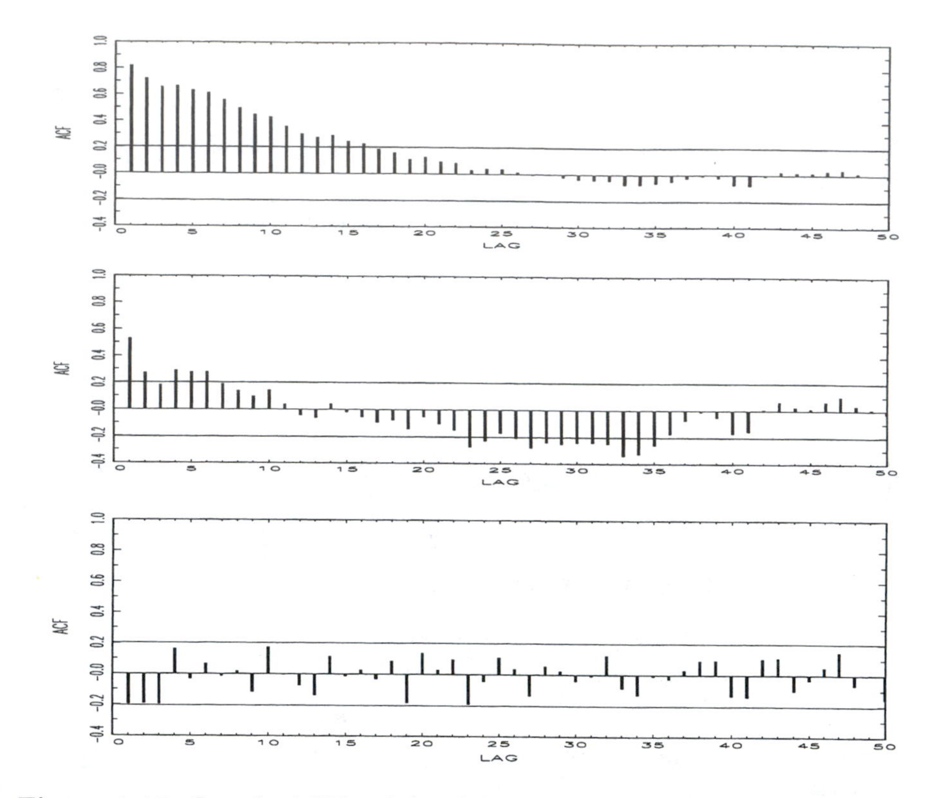


**Figure 1.16:** Sample ACF's of the global temperature (top), and of the detrended (middle) and the differenced (bottom) series.

where we may expand the operator $(1-B)^d$ algebraically to evaluate for higher integer values of $d$. For example, the second difference becomes

$$\begin{aligned} \nabla^2 x_t &= (1-B)^2 x_t \\ &= (1-2B+B^2)x_t \\ &= x_t - 2x_{t-1} + x_{t-2} \end{aligned}$$

by the linearity of the operator. To check, just take the difference of the first difference $\nabla x_t = x_t - x_{t-1}$.

The first difference (1.40) is an example of a ***linear filter*** applied to eliminate a trend. Other filters, formed by averaging values near $x_t$, can produce adjusted series that eliminate other kinds of unwanted fluctuations, as in Chapter 3. The differencing technique is an important component of the ARIMA model of Box and Jenkins (1970) (see also Box et al, 1994), to be discussed in Chapter 2.

**Example 1.23 Differencing Global Temperature**

The first difference of the global temperature series, also shown in Figure 1.15 does not contain the long middle cycle we observe in the detrended series. The ACF of this series is also shown in Figure 1.16, the behavior of this series seems more stationary; only a few values exceed the limits and no obvious regions exist where the function decays slowly. This characteristic would appear to make it superior to detrending, but we will see in Chapter 3 that it is possible that important kinds of oscillations are restricted by differencing.

An alternative to differencing is a less-severe operation that still assumes stationarity of the underlying time series. This alternative, called ***fractional differencing***, extends the notion of the difference operator (1.43) to fractional powers $-.5 < d < .5$, which still define stationary processes. The resulting ***long memory*** time series, introduced by Granger and Joyeux (1980) and by Hosking (1981), is often used as a model for environmental time series arising in hydrology. The application of the fractional difference operator proceeds by expanding

$$(1-B)^d = \sum_{j=0}^{\infty} \pi_j B^j \tag{1.44}$$

in a Taylor's series, leading to a set of recursions for the coefficients of the form $\pi_0 = 1$ and

$$\pi_{j+1} = \frac{(j-d)\pi_j}{(j+1)} \tag{1.45}$$

for $j = 0, 1, \cdots$. The fractional difference of the series $x_t$ can then be written as

$$\nabla^d x_t = \sum_{j=0}^{\infty} \pi_j x_{t-j} \tag{1.46}$$

for $j = 0, 1, \ldots$. We may cut the sum off at $j = t-1$ and use the resulting sum as a reasonable approximation using only observed data, for $t$ large enough.

Often, obvious aberrations are present that can contribute nonstationary as well as nonlinear behavior in observed time series. In such cases, ***transformations*** may be useful to equalize the variability over the length of a single series. A particularly useful transformation is

$$y_t = \ln x_t, \tag{1.47}$$

which tends to suppress larger fluctuations that occur over portions of the series where the underlying values are larger. Other possibilities are ***power transformations*** in the Box-Cox family of the form

$$y_t = \begin{cases} (x_t^\lambda - 1)/\lambda, & \lambda \neq 0 \\ \ln x_t, & \lambda = 0. \end{cases} \tag{1.48}$$

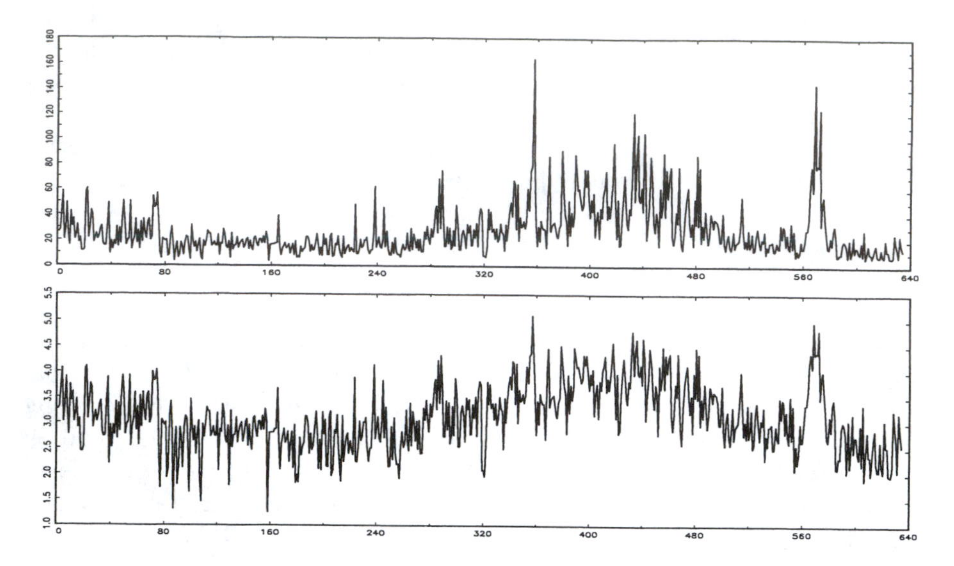


**Figure 1.17:** Glacial varve thicknesses (top) from Massachusetts for $n = 634$ years compared with log transformed thicknesses (bottom).

Methods for choosing the power $\lambda$ are available (see Johnson and Wichern, 1992, Section 4.7) but we do not pursue them here. Often, transformations are also used to improve the approximation to normality or to improve linearity in predicting the value of one series from another.

### Example 1.24 Paleoclimatic Glacial Varves

Melting glaciers deposit yearly layers of sand and silt during the spring melting seasons, which can be reconstructed yearly over a period ranging from the time deglaciation began in New England (about 12,600 years ago) to the time it ended (about 6,000 years ago). Such sedimentary deposits, called ***varves***, can be used as proxies for paleoclimatic parameters, such as temperature, because, in a warm year, more sand and silt are deposited from the receding glacier. Figure 1.17 shows the thicknesses of the yearly varves collected from one location in Massachusetts for 634 years, beginning 11,834 years ago. For further information, see Shumway and Verosub (1992). Because the variation in thicknesses increases in proportion to the amount deposited, a logarithmic transformation could improve the nonstationarity observable in the variance as a function of time. Figure 1.17 shows the original and transformed varves, and it is clear that this improvement has occurred. We may also plot the histogram of the original and transformed data, as in Problem 1.23, to argue that the approximation to normality is improved. The ordinary first differences (1.42) are also computed in Problem 1.23, and we note that the first differences have an autocorrelation function with a peak at lag $h = 1$. Later, in Chapter 2, we will show that perhaps the varve series has long memory and will propose computing the fractionally differenced series (1.46).

As a final preliminary data processing technique, we mention the use of ***scatterplot matrices*** for the purpose of visualizing the relations between series at different lags. In the definition of the ACF, we are essentially interested in relations between $x_t$ and $x_{t-h}$; the autocorrelation function tells us whether a substantial linear relation exists between the series and its own lagged values. The ACF gives a profile of the linear correlation at all possible lags and shows which values of $h$ lead to the best predictability. The restriction of this idea to linear predictability, however, may mask a possible nonlinear relation between current values, $x_t$, and past values, $x_{t-h}$. To check for nonlinear relations of this form, it is convenient to display a lagged scatterplot matrix, as in Figure 1.18, that displays values of $x_t$ on the vertical axis plotted against $x_{t-h}$ on the horizontal axis for the SOI $x_t$. Similarly, we might want to look at values of one series $y_t$ plotted against another series at various lags, $x_{t-h}$, to look for possible nonlinear relations between the two series. Because, for example, we might wish to predict the Recruitment series, say, $y_t$, from current or past values of the SOI series, $x_{t-h}$, for $h = 0, 1, 2, ...$ it would be worthwhile to examine the scatterplot matrix. Figure 1.19 shows the lagged scatterplot of the Recruitment series $y_t$ on the vertical axis plotted against the SOI index $x_{t-h}$ on the horizontal axis.

**Example 1.25 Scatterplot Matrices, SOI, and Recruitment Series**

Consider the possibility of looking for nonlinear functional relations at lags in the SOI series, $x_{t-h}$, for $h = 0, 1, 2, ...$, and the Recruitment series, $y_t$. Noting first the top panel in Figure 1.18, we see strong positive and linear relations at lags $h = 1, 2, 11, 12$, that is, between $x_t$ and $x_{t-1}, x_{t-2}, x_{t-11}, x_{t-12}$, and a negative linear relation at lags $h = 6, 7$. These results match up well with peaks noticed in the ACF in Figure 1.13. Figure 1.19 shows linearity in relating the Recruitment series $y_t$ to the SOI index at $x_{t-5}, x_{t-6}, x_{t-7}, x_{t-8}$, indicating the SOI series tends to lead the Recruitment series and the coefficients are negative, implying that increases in the SOI lead to decreases in the Recruitment, and vice-versa. Some possible nonlinear behavior shows as the relation tends to flatten out at both extremes, indicating a logistic type transformation may be useful.

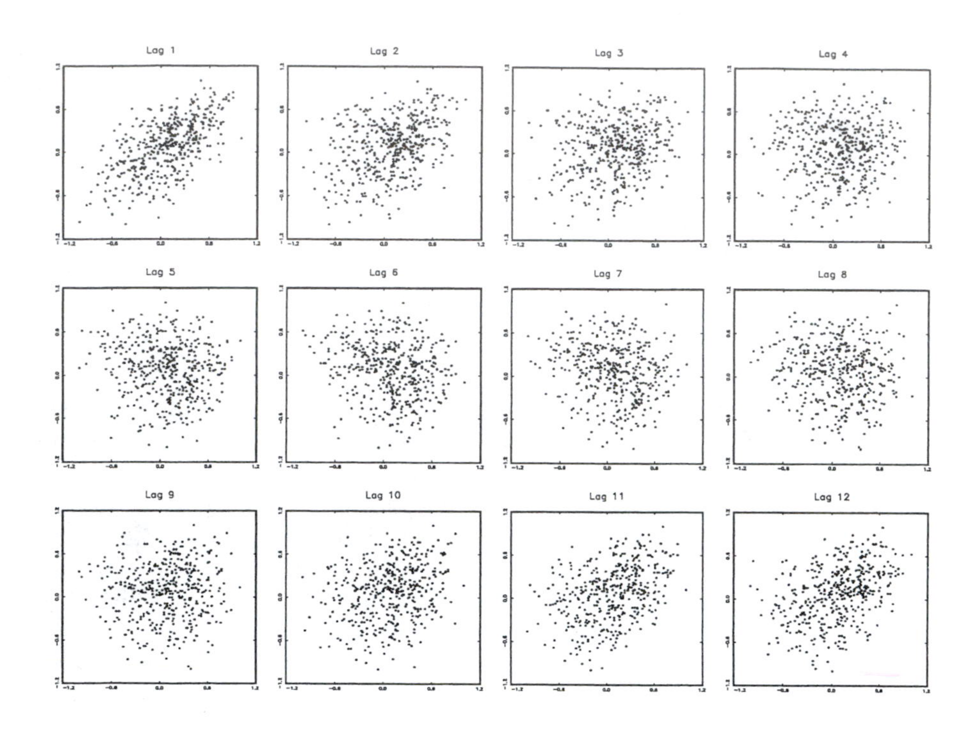


**Figure 1.18:** Scatterplot matrix relating current SOI values to past SOI values at lags $h = 1, 2, ..., 12$.

# 1.8 Classical Regression and Smoothing in the Time Series Context

We begin our discussion of linear regression in the time series context by assuming some output or ***dependent*** time series, say, $x_t, t = 1, \dots, n$, that is being influenced by a collection of possible input or ***independent*** series, say, $z_{t1}, z_{t2}, \dots, z_{tq}$, where we first regard the inputs as fixed and known. This assumption, necessary for applying conventional linear regression, will be relaxed later on. We express this relation through the ***linear regression model***

$$x_t = \beta_1 z_{t1} + \beta_2 z_{t2} + \cdots + \beta_q z_{tq} + w_t, \tag{1.49}$$

where $\beta_1, \beta_2, \dots, \beta_q$ are unknown fixed regression coefficients and $w_t$ is a random error or noise, ordinarily assumed to be white with mean zero and variance $\sigma_w^2$. Again, we will relax this assumption later. A more general setting within which to embed mean square estimation and linear regression is given in Chap-

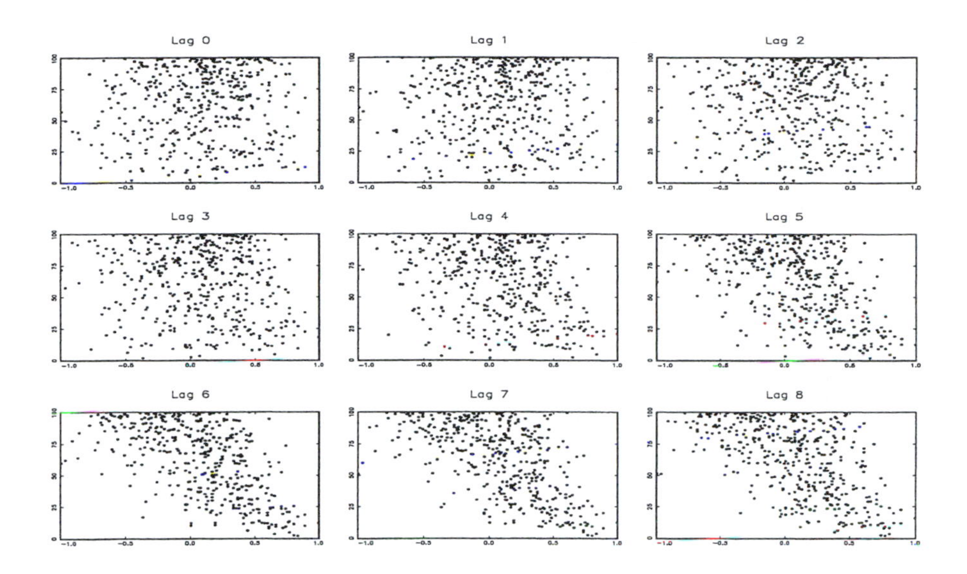


**Figure 1.19:** Scatterplot matrix of the Recruitment series $y_t$ on the vertical axis plotted against the SOI index $x_{t-h}$ on the horizontal axis at lags $h = 0, 1, ..., 8$.

ter 2, Section T2.15, where we introduce Hilbert spaces and the Projection Theorem.

**Example 1.26 Detrending**

We have assumed implicitly that the model

$$x_t = \beta_1 + \beta_2 t + w_t$$

is reasonable in our discussion of detrending in Example 1.22. This is in the form of the regression model (1.49) when we make the identification $q = 2$, $z_{t1} = 1, z_{t2} = t$. The problem in detrending is to find the coefficients and detrend by constructing the estimated residual series $\widehat{w}_t$. We obtained the estimated coefficients $\widehat{\beta}_1 = -.395$, $\widehat{\beta}_2 = .006$ yielding an estimated increase of .6 degrees centigrade per 100 years. We discuss the precise way in which the solution is accomplished below.

The linear model described by (1.49) above can be conveniently written in a more general notation by defining the column vectors $\boldsymbol{z}_t = (z_{t1}, z_{t2}, \ldots, z_{tq})'$ and $\boldsymbol{\beta} = (\beta_1, \beta_2, \ldots, \beta_q)'$, where $'$ denotes transpose, so (1.49) can be written in the alternate form

$$x_t = \boldsymbol{\beta}' \boldsymbol{z}_t + w_t. \tag{1.50}$$

It is natural to consider estimating the unknown coefficient vector $\boldsymbol{\beta}$ by minimizing the residual sum of squares

$$RSS = \sum_{t=1}^{n} (x_t - \boldsymbol{\beta}' \boldsymbol{z}_t)^2, \tag{1.51}$$

with respect to $\beta_1, \beta_2, \ldots, \beta_q$. Minimizing $RSS$ yields the ***ordinary least squares estimator***. This minimization can be accomplished by differentiating (1.51) with respect to the vector $\boldsymbol{\beta}$ or by using the properties of projections. In the notation above, this procedure gives the ***normal equations***

$$\left( \sum_{t=1}^{n} \boldsymbol{z}_t \boldsymbol{z}_t' \right) \hat{\boldsymbol{\beta}} = \sum_{t=1}^{n} \boldsymbol{z}_t x_t. \tag{1.52}$$

A further simplification of notation results from defining the matrix $Z = (\boldsymbol{z}_1, \boldsymbol{z}_2, \ldots, \boldsymbol{z}_n)'$ as the $n \times q$ matrix composed of the $n$ samples of the input variables and the observed $n \times 1$ vector $\boldsymbol{x} = (x_1, x_2, \ldots, x_n)'$. This identification yields

$$(Z'Z)\, \hat{\boldsymbol{\beta}} = Z' \boldsymbol{x} \tag{1.53}$$

and the solution

$$\widehat{\boldsymbol{\beta}} = (Z'Z)^{-1} Z' \boldsymbol{x} \tag{1.54}$$

when the matrix $Z'Z$ is of rank $q$. The minimized residual sum of squares (1.51) has the equivalent matrix forms

$$\begin{aligned} RSS &= (\boldsymbol{x} - Z\widehat{\boldsymbol{\beta}})'(\boldsymbol{x} - Z\widehat{\boldsymbol{\beta}}) \\ &= \boldsymbol{x}'\boldsymbol{x} - \widehat{\boldsymbol{\beta}}' Z' \boldsymbol{x} \\ &= \boldsymbol{x}'\boldsymbol{x} - \boldsymbol{x}' Z (Z'Z)^{-1} Z' \boldsymbol{x}, \end{aligned} \tag{1.55}$$

to give some useful versions for later reference. The ordinary least squares estimators are unbiased, i.e., $E(\widehat{\boldsymbol{\beta}}) = \boldsymbol{\beta}$, and have the smallest variance within the class of linear unbiased estimators.

If the errors $w_t$ are normally distributed (Gaussian), $\widehat{\boldsymbol{\beta}}$ is also the maximum likelihood estimator for $\boldsymbol{\beta}$ and is normally distributed with

$$\begin{aligned} \operatorname{cov}(\widehat{\boldsymbol{\beta}}) &= \sigma_w^2 \left( \sum_{t=1}^{n} \boldsymbol{z}_t \boldsymbol{z}_t' \right)^{-1} \\ &= \sigma_w^2 (Z'Z)^{-1} \\ &= \sigma_w^2 C, \end{aligned} \tag{1.56}$$

where

$$C = (Z'Z)^{-1} \tag{1.57}$$

is a convenient notation for later equations. An unbiased estimator for the variance $\sigma_w^2$ is

$$s_w^2 = \frac{RSS}{n - q}, \tag{1.58}$$

**Table 1.3** Analysis of Variance for Regression

| Source | df | Sum of Squares | Mean Square |
|---|---|---|---|
| $z_{t,q_1+1}, \ldots, z_{t,q}$ | $q - q_1$ | $SS_{reg} = RSS_1 - RSS$ | $MS_{reg} = SS_{reg}/(q - q_1)$ |
| Error | $n - q$ | $RSS$ | $s_w^2 = RSS/(n - q)$ |
| Total | $n - q_1$ | $RSS_1$ | |

contrasted with the maximum likelihood estimator $\widehat{\sigma}_w^2 = RSS/n$, which has the divisor $n$. Under the normal assumption, $s_w^2$ is distributed proportionally to a ***chi-squared*** random variable with $n - q$ degrees of freedom, denoted by $\chi^2_{n-q}$, and independently of $\widehat{\beta}$. It follows that

$$t_{n-q} = \frac{(\widehat{\beta}_i - \beta_i)}{s_w\sqrt{c_{ii}}} \tag{1.59}$$

has the ***t-distribution*** with $n - q$ degrees of freedom; $c_{ii}$ denotes the $i^{th}$ diagonal element of $C$, as defined in (1.57).

Various competing models are of interest to isolate or select the best subset of independent variables. Suppose a proposed model specifies that only a subset $q_1 < q$ independent variables, say, $\boldsymbol{z}_{1t} = (z_{t1}, z_{t2}, \ldots, z_{tq_1})'$ is influencing the dependent variable $x_t$, so the model

$$x_t = \boldsymbol{\beta}_1' \boldsymbol{z}_{1t} + w_t \tag{1.60}$$

becomes the null hypothesis, where $\boldsymbol{\beta}_1 = (\beta_1, \beta_2, \ldots, \beta_{q_1})'$ is a subset of coefficients of the original $q$ variables. We can test the reduced model (1.60) against the full model (1.50) by comparing the residual sums of squares under the two models using the ***F-statistic***

$$F_{q-q_1,n-q} = \frac{RSS_1 - RSS}{RSS} \frac{n-q}{q-q_1}, \tag{1.61}$$

which has the central $F$-distribution with $q - q_1$ and $n - q$ degrees of freedom when (1.60) is the correct model. The statistic, which follows from applying the likelihood ratio criterion, has the improvement per number of parameters added in the numerator compared with the error sum of squares under the full model in the denominator. The information involved in the test procedure is often summarized in an ***Analysis of Variance (ANOVA)*** table as given in Table 1.3 for this particular case. The difference in the numerator is often called the ***regression sum of squares***

In terms of Table 1.3, it is conventional to write the $F$-statistic (1.61) as the ratio of the two mean squares, obtaining

$$F_{q-q_1,n-q} = \frac{MS_{reg}}{s_w^2}. \tag{1.62}$$

A special case of interest is $q_1 = 1$ and $z_{1t} = 1$, so the model in (1.60) becomes

$$x_t = \beta_1 + w_t,$$

and we may measure the ***proportion of variation*** accounted for by the other variables using

$$R_{xz}^2 = \frac{RSS_0 - RSS}{RSS_0}, \tag{1.63}$$

where the residual sum of squares under the reduced model

$$RSS_0 = \sum_{t=1}^{n}(x_t - \bar{x})^2, \tag{1.64}$$

in this case, is just the sum of squared deviations from the mean $\bar{x}$. The measure $R_{xz}^2$ is also the ***squared multiple correlation*** between $x_t$ and the variables $z_{t2}, z_{t3}, \ldots, z_{tq}$.

The techniques discussed in the previous paragraph can be used to test various models against one another using the $F$ test given in (1.61), (1.62), and the ANOVA Table. These tests have been used in the past in a stepwise manner, where variables are added or deleted when the values from the $F$-test either exceed or fail to exceed some predetermined levels. The procedure, called ***stepwise multiple regression***, is useful in arriving at a set of useful variables. An alternative is to focus on a procedure for ***model selection*** that does not proceed sequentially, but simply evaluates each model on its own merits. Suppose we consider a regression model with $k$ coefficients and denote the ***maximum likelihood estimator*** for the variance as

$$\widehat{\sigma}_k^2 = \frac{RSS_k}{n}, \tag{1.65}$$

where $RSS_k$ denotes the residual sum of squares under the model with $k$ regresssion coefficients. Then, Akaike (1969, 1973, 1974) suggested measuring the goodness of fit for this particular model by

$$\text{AIC} = \ln\, \widehat{\sigma}_k^2 + \frac{2k}{n}. \tag{1.66}$$

The value of $k$ yielding the minimum AIC specifies the best model. The idea is roughly that minimizing $\widehat{\sigma}_k^2$ would be a reasonable objective, except that it decreases monotonically as $k$ increases. Therefore, we ought penalize the error variance by a term proportional to the number of parameters. The choice for the penalty term given by (1.66) is not the only one and a considerable literature is available advocating different penalty terms. A corrected form, suggested by Sugiura (1978), and expanded by Hurvich and Tsai (1989), can be based on small-sample distributional results for the linear regression model(details are provided in Problem 1.27). The corrected form is defined as

$$\text{AICc} = \ln\, \widehat{\sigma}_k^2 + \frac{n+k}{n-k-2}. \tag{1.67}$$

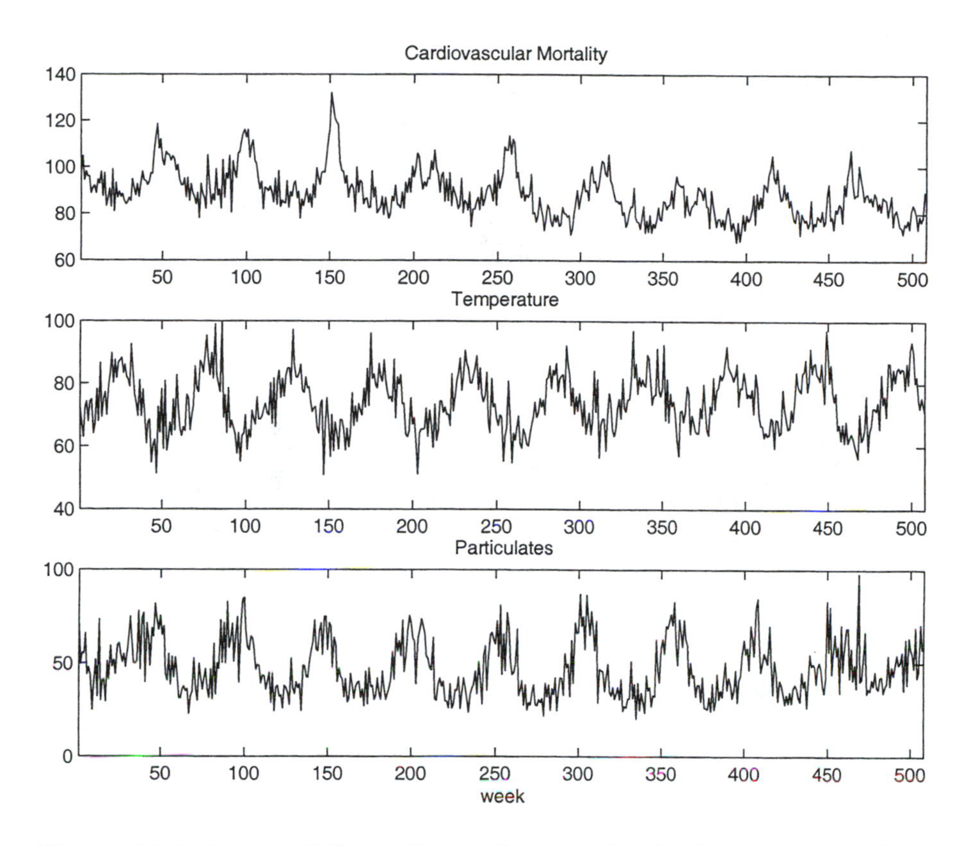


**Figure 1.20:** Average daily cardiovascular mortality (top), temperature (middle) and particulate pollution (bottom) in Los Angeles County. There are 508 six-day smoothed averages obtained by filtering daily values over the 10 year period 1970-1979.

We may also derive a correction term based on Bayesian arguments, as in Schwarz (1978), which leads to

$$\text{SIC} = \ln\ \widehat{\sigma}_k^2 + \frac{k \log n}{n}. \tag{1.68}$$

(See also Rissanen, 1978, for an approach yielding the same statistic based on a minimum description length argument.) Various simulation studies have tended to verify that SIC does well at getting the correct order in large samples whereas AICc tends to be superior in smaller samples where the relative number of parameters is large (see McQuarrie and Tsai, 1998 for detailed comparisons). In fitting regression models, two measures that have been used in the past are ***adjusted R-squared***, which is essentially $s_w^2$, and ***Mallows*** $C_p$, Mallows (1973), which we do not consider in this context.

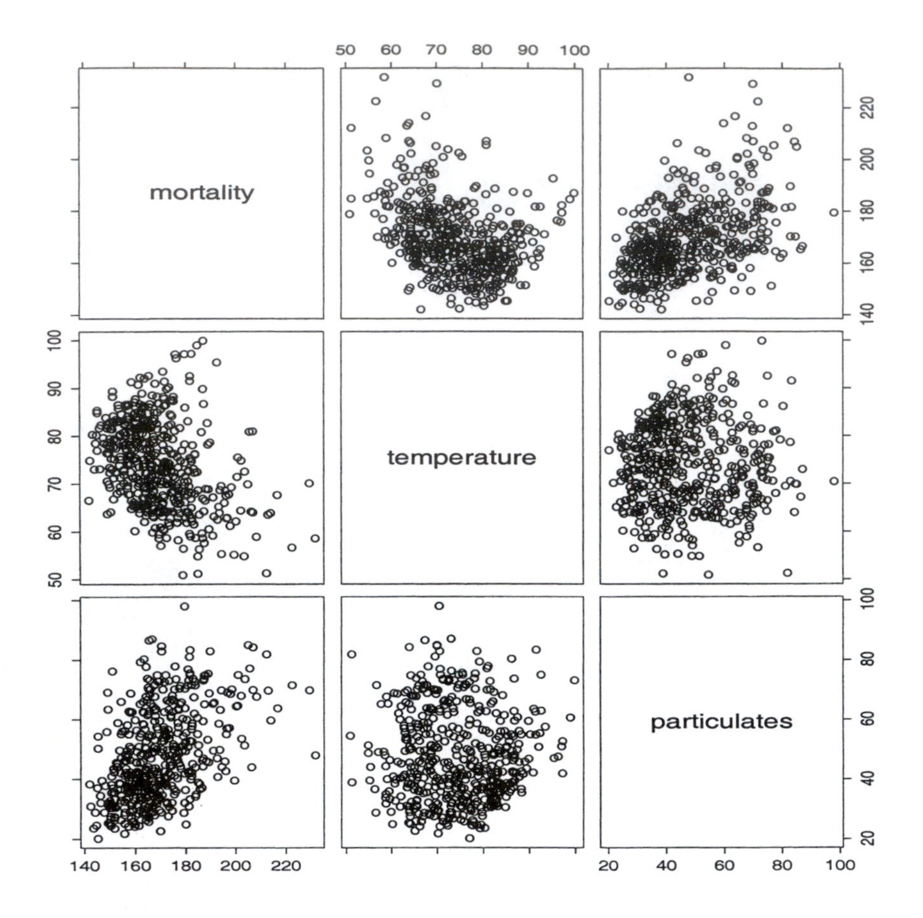


**Figure 1.21:** Scatterplot matrix showing plausible relations between mortality, temperature, and pollution.

### Example 1.27 Pollution, Temperature and Mortality

The data shown in Figure 1.20 are extracted series from a study by Shumway et al (1988) of the possible effects of temperature and pollution on daily mortality in Los Angeles County. Note the strong seasonal components in all of the series, corresponding to winter-summer variations and the downward trend in the cardiovascular mortality over the 10-year period.

A scatterplot matrix, shown in Figure 1.21, indicates a possible linear relation between mortality and the pollutant particulates and a possible relation to temperature. Note the curvilinear shape of the temperature mortality curve, indicating that higher temperatures as well as lower temperatures are associated with increases in cardiovascular mortality.

**Table 1.4** Summary Statistics for Mortality Models

| Model | RSS(1.51) | $s_w^2$(1.58) | $R^2$(1.63) | AICc(1.67) |
|---|---|---|---|---|
| (1.69) | 40,020 | 79.09 | .21 | 5.38 |
| (1.70) | 31,413 | 62.20 | .38 | 5.14 |
| (1.71) | 27,985 | 55.52 | .45 | 5.03 |
| (1.72) | 20,509 | 40.77 | .60 | 4.72 |

Based on the scatterplot matrix, we entertain, tentatively four models where $M_t$ denotes cardiovascular mortality, $T_t$ denotes temperature and $P_t$ denotes the particulate levels. They are

$$M_t = \beta_0 + \beta_1 t + w_t \tag{1.69}$$
$$M_t = \beta_0 + \beta_1 t + \beta_2(T_t - T_\cdot) + w_t \tag{1.70}$$
$$M_t = \beta_0 + \beta_1 t + \beta_2(T_t - T_\cdot) + \beta_3(T_t - T_\cdot)^2 + w_t \tag{1.71}$$
$$M_t = \beta_0 + \beta_1 t + \beta_2(T_t - T_\cdot) + \beta_3(T_t - T_\cdot)^2 + \beta_4 P_t + w_t \tag{1.72}$$

where we adjust temperature for its mean, $T_\cdot = 74.6$, to avoid scaling problems. It is clear that (1.69) is a ***trend*** only model, (1.70) is ***linear temperature***, (1.71) is ***curvilinear temperature*** and (1.72) is ***curvilinear temperature and pollution***. We summarize some the statistics given for this particular case in Table 1.4. The values of $R^2$ were computed by noting that $RSS_0 = 50,687$ using (1.64).

We note that each model does substantially better than the one before it and that the model including both temperature, temperature squared and particulates does the best, accounting for some 60% of the variability and with the best value for AICc. Note that one can compare any two models using the residual sums of squares and (1.61). Hence, a model with only trend could be compared to the full model using $q = 5, q_1 = 2, n = 508$, so

$$\begin{aligned} F_{3,503} &= \frac{(40,020 - 20,509)}{20,509} \frac{503}{3} \\ &= 160, \end{aligned}$$

which exceeds $F_{3,\infty}(.001) = 5.42$. We obtain the best prediction model,

$$\begin{aligned} \widehat{M}_t = \; & 81.59 - .027_{(.002)} t - .473_{(.032)}(T_t - 74.6) \\ & + .023_{(.003)}(T_t - 74.6)^2 \\ & + .255_{(.019)} P_t, \end{aligned}$$

for mortality, where the standard errors, computed from (1.56)-(1.58), are given in parentheses. As expected, a negative trend is present in time as well as a negative coefficient for adjusted temperature. The quadratic effect of temperature can clearly be seen in the scatterplots of Figure 1.21. Pollution weights positively and can be interpreted as the incremental contribution to daily deaths per unit of particulate pollution. It would still be essential to check the residuals $\widehat{w}_t = M_t - \widehat{M}_t$ for autocorrelation, but we defer this question to the section on correlated least squares, in which the incorporation of time correlation changes the estimated standard errors.

## Smoothing Time Series

In Section 1.3, we introduced the concept of smoothing a time series, and in Example 1.8, we discussed using a moving average to smooth a time series. This method is useful in discovering certain traits in a time series, such as long-term trend and seasonal components. In particular, if $x_t$ represents the observations,

$$y_t = \sum_{j=-k}^{k} a_j x_{t-j}, \tag{1.73}$$

where $a_j = a_{-j} \geq 0$ and $\sum_{j=-k}^{k} a_j = 1$ is a symmetric moving average. In Figure 1.7, a moving average smoother, $y_t$, is not as choppy as the data $x_t$, and can reveal some information about the nature of the data. For example, the top of Figure 1.22 shows mortality (taken from the data set discussed in Example 1.27), a five-point moving average ($k = 2$) that helps bring out the seasonal component and a 53-point moving average ($k = 26$) that helps bring out the trend in total mortality. In both cases, the weights $a_{-k}, ..., a_0, ..., a_k$ are all the same, and equal to $1/(2k + 1)$.

Many other ways are available for smoothing times series data based on methods from ***scatterplot smoothers***. The general setup for a time plot is

$$x_t = y_t + w_t, \tag{1.74}$$

where $y_t$ is some smooth function, say, $y_t = f(t)$, of time. Some obvious choices for $y_t$ in (1.74) are ***polynomial regression***

$$y_t = \beta_0 + \beta_1 t + \cdots + \beta_p t^p \tag{1.75}$$

or ***periodic regression***

$$\begin{aligned} y_t &= \alpha_0 + \alpha_1 \cos(2\pi\omega_1 t) + \beta_1 \sin(2\pi\omega_1 t) \\ &\quad + \cdots + \alpha_p \cos(2\pi\omega_p t) + \beta_p \sin(2\pi\omega_p t), \end{aligned} \tag{1.76}$$

where $\omega_1, ..., \omega_p$ are distinct, specified frequencies. In addition, one might consider combining (1.75) and (1.76). Of course, these smoothers can be applied using classical linear regression.

Modern regression techniques are used to fit general smoothers to the pairs of points $(t, x_t)$. Many of these techniques can easily be applied to time series data using the S-plus statistical package; see Venables and Ripley (1994, Chapter 10) for details on applying these methods. For example, the moving average fits shown in Figure 1.22 were done using the S-plus `filter` function.

One approach to smoothing a time plot uses the function `supsmu` in S-plus. It is based on $k$-nearest neighbors linear regression, wherein one uses the $k/2$ values bigger than the value of $x_t$, and the $k/2$ values smaller than the value of $x_t$, to predict $x_t$ using linear regression. For example, the middle of Figure 1.22 shows total mortality, and the nearest neighbor method using `supsmu` based on $k = 6$ to highlight the seasonal component of the data, and one based on the maximum allowable value of $k$ to examine the trend component. In general, `supsmu` uses a variable window for smoothing (see Friedman, 1984), but it can be used for correlated data by fixing the smoothing window, as was done here.

The bottom plot in Figure 1.22 shows ***kernel smoothing***, where $y_t$ in (1.74) is found as follows:

$$y_t = \sum_{i=1}^{n} w_t(i) x_t, \tag{1.77}$$

where

$$w_t(i) = K\left(\frac{t-i}{b}\right) \Big/ \sum_{j=1}^{n} K\left(\frac{t-j}{b}\right). \tag{1.78}$$

This method is called the Naradaya–Watson density estimator (Watson, 1966). In (1.78), $K(\cdot)$ is a kernel function; typically, the normal kernel, $K(z) = \frac{1}{\sqrt{2\pi}} \exp(-z^2/2)$, is used. To implement this in S-plus, one uses the `ksmooth` function. The wider the ***bandwidth***, $b$, the smoother the result. In Figure 1.22, the values of $b$ for this example were $b = 4$ for the seasonal component, and $b = 100$ for the trend component.

One extension of polynomial regression is to first divide time $t = 1, ..., n$ into $k$ intervals, $t \in [t_0 = 1, t_1]$, $t \in [t_1 + 1, t_2]$ , . . . , $t \in [t_{k-1} + 1, t_k = n]$. The values $t_0, t_1, ..., t_k$ are called *knots*. Then, in each interval, one fits a regression of the form (1.75); typically, $p = 3$, and this is called ***cubic splines***. In S-plus, one can use the function `bs` for B-splines, or `ns` for natural splines, an extension of B-splines, to fit cubic splines to the time plot.

A related method is ***smoothing splines***, which minimizes a compromise between the fit and the degree of smoothness given by

$$\sum_{t=1}^{n} [x_t - f(t)]^2 + \lambda \int \left(f''(t)\right)^2 dt, \tag{1.79}$$

where $y_t = f(t)$ is a cubic spline with a knot at each $t$. The degree of smoothness is controlled by $\lambda > 0$. The top of Figure 1.23 shows smoothing splines on total mortality using $\lambda = 5 \times 10^{-8}$ for the seasonal component, and $\lambda = 0.1$ for

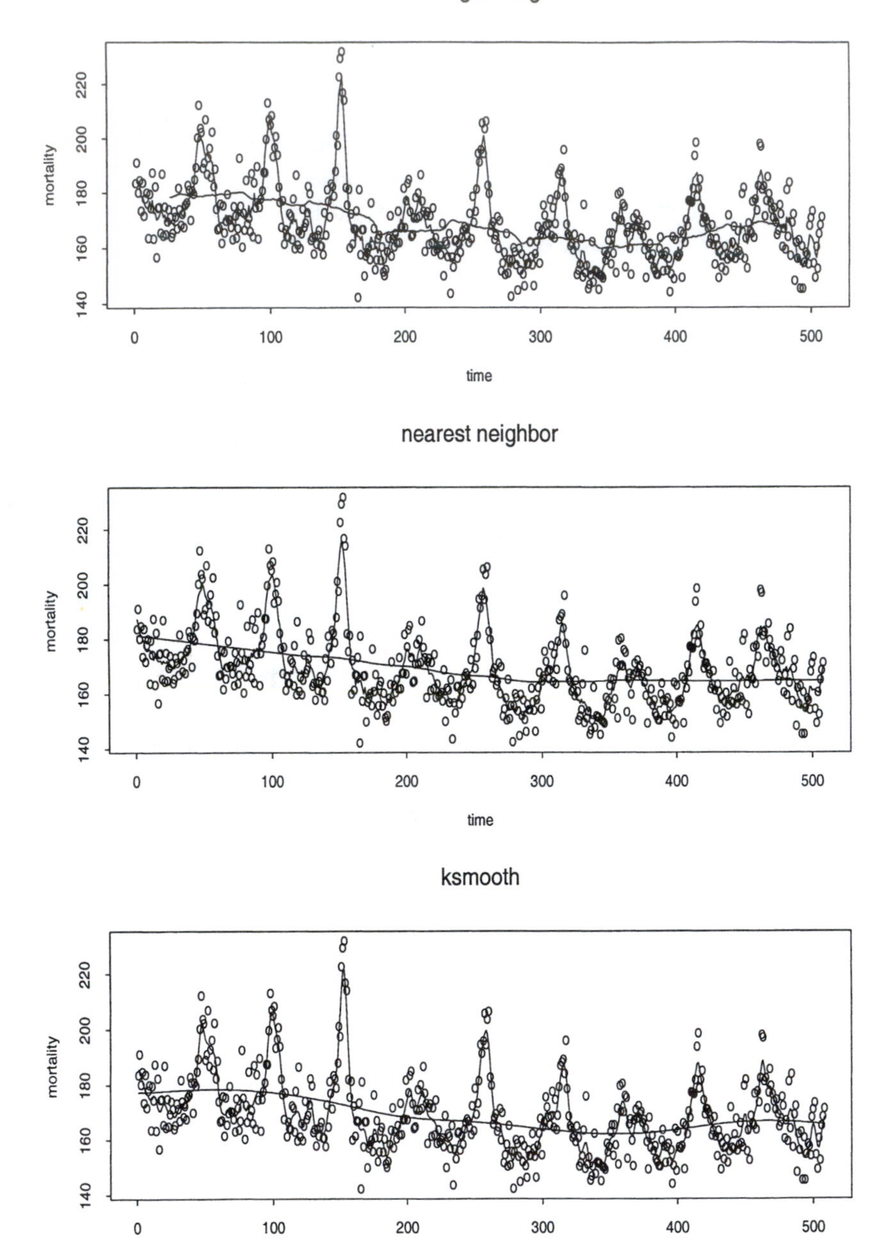


**Figure 1.22:** Smoothers of the mortality time plot using moving averages, nearest neighbor, and kernel smoothing techniques.

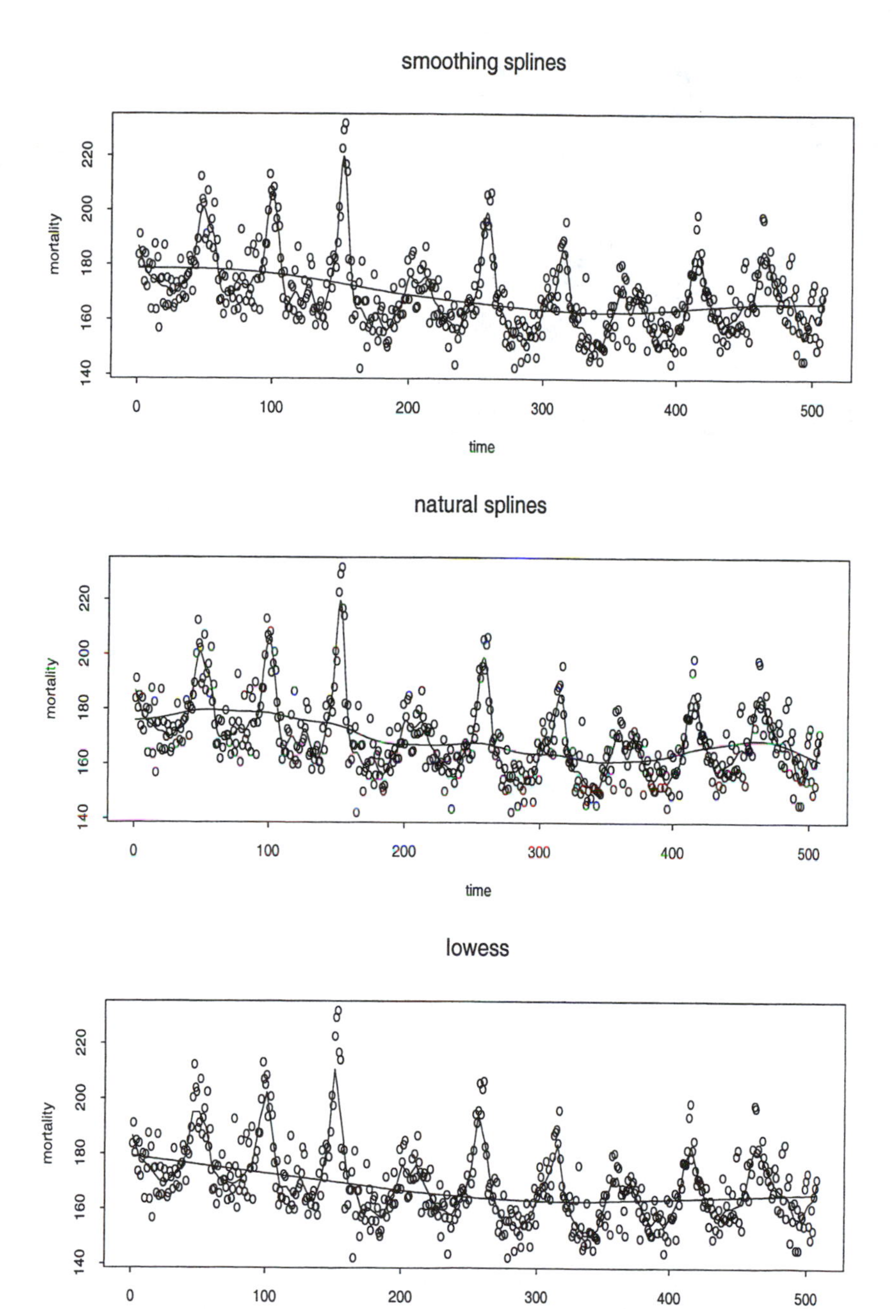


**Figure 1.23:** Smoothers of the mortality time plot using smoothing splines, natural splines, and locally weighted regression.

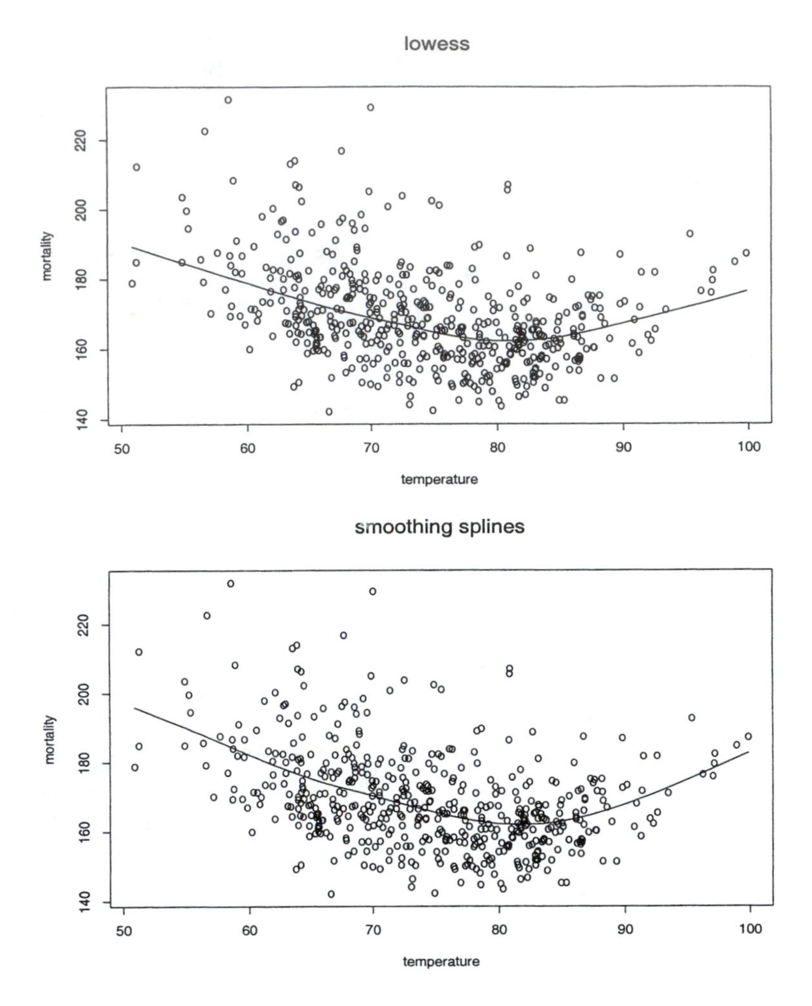


**Figure 1.24:** Smoothers of mortality as a function of temperature using lowess and smoothing splines.

the trend. This was done using the `smooth.spline` function in S-plus. The middle of Figure 1.23 shows a similar result using natural splines.

The bottom of Figure 1.23 shows smoothing of total mortality using `lowess` (see Cleveland, 1979). This method of smoothing is rather complex, but the basic idea is close to nearest neighbor regression. First, a certain proportion of nearest neighbors (in value, not in time) to $x_t$ are included in a weighting scheme; values closer to $x_t$ get more weight. Then, a robust weighted regression is used to predict $x_t$ and obtain the smoothed estimate, $y_t$. The larger the fraction of nearest neighbors included, the smoother the $y_t$ will be. In Figure 1.23, the smoother uses about two-thirds of the data to obtain an estimate of the trend component, and the seasonal component uses 2% of the 508 observations.

In addition to smoothing time plots, smoothing techniques can be applied to smoothing a time series as a function of another time series. In this case, we smooth the scatterplot of two contemporaneously measured time series, one series as the function of the other. As an example, Figure 1.24 shows scatter plots of total mortality, $M_t$, and temperature, $T_t$, along with $M_t$ is smoothed as a function of $T_t$ using lowess and using smoothing splines. In both cases, mortality increases at extreme temperatures, but in an asymmetric way; mortality is higher at colder temperatures than at hotter temperatures.

As a final word of caution, the methods mentioned above do not particularly take into account the fact that the data are serially correlated, and most of the techniques mentioned have been designed for independent observations. That is, for example, the smoothers shown in Figure 1.24 are calculated under the false assumption that the pairs $(M_t, T_t)$, for $t = 1, ..., 508$, are iid pairs of observations. In addition, the degree of smoothness used in the previous examples were chosen arbitrarily to bring out what might be considered obvious features in the data set.

## 1.9 Vector-Valued and Multidimensional Series

We frequently encounter situations in which the relations between a number of jointly measured time series are of interest. For example, the previous section involved measuring two series, the SOI and the number of new fish (Recruitment), and then considering searching for various possible associations between the two series.

Hence, it will be useful to consider the notion of a ***vector time series*** $\boldsymbol{x}_t = (x_{t1}, x_{t2}, \ldots, x_{tp})'$, which contains as its components $p$ univariate time series. We denote the $p \times 1$ column vector of the observed series as $\boldsymbol{x}_t$. The row vector $\boldsymbol{x}_t'$ is its transpose. For the stationary case, the $p \times 1$ *mean vector*

$$\boldsymbol{\mu} = E(\boldsymbol{x}_t) \tag{1.80}$$

of the form $\boldsymbol{\mu} = (\mu_{t1}, \mu_{t2}, \ldots, \mu_{tp})'$ and the $p \times p$ *autocovariance matrix*

$$\Gamma(h) = E[(\boldsymbol{x}_{t+h} - \boldsymbol{\mu})(\boldsymbol{x}_t - \boldsymbol{\mu})'] \tag{1.81}$$

can be defined, where the elements of the matrix $\Gamma(h)$ are the cross-covariance functions

$$\gamma_{ij}(h) = E[(x_{t+h,i} - \mu_i)(x_{tj} - \mu_j)] \tag{1.82}$$

for $i, j = 1, \ldots, p$. Because $\gamma_{ij}(h) = \gamma_{ji}(-h)$, it follows that

$$\Gamma(-h) = \Gamma'(h). \tag{1.83}$$

Now, the ***sample autocovariance matrix*** of the vector series $\boldsymbol{x}_t$ is the $p \times p$ matrix of sample cross-covariances, defined as

$$\widehat{\Gamma}(h) = n^{-1} \sum_{t=1}^{n-h} (\boldsymbol{x}_{t+h} - \bar{\boldsymbol{x}})(\boldsymbol{x}_t - \bar{\boldsymbol{x}})', \tag{1.84}$$

where

$$\bar{\boldsymbol{x}} = n^{-1} \sum_{t=1}^{n} \boldsymbol{x}_t \tag{1.85}$$

denotes the $p \times 1$ ***sample mean vector***. The symmetry property of the theoretical autocovariance (1.83) extends to the sample autocovariance (1.84), which is defined for negative values by taking

$$\widehat{\Gamma}(-h) = \widehat{\Gamma}(h)'. \tag{1.86}$$

In many applied problems, an observed series may be indexed by more than time alone. For example, the position in space of an experimental unit might be described by two coordinates, say, $s_1$ and $s_2$. We may proceed in these cases by defining a ***multidimensional process*** $x_{\boldsymbol{s}}$ as a function of the $r \times 1$ vector $\boldsymbol{s} = (s_1, s_2, \ldots, s_r)'$ where $s_i$ denotes the coordinate of the $i^{th}$ index.

**Example 1.28 Soil Surface Temperatures**

As an example, the two-dimensional ($r = 2$) temperature series $x_{s_1,s_2}$ in Figure 1.25 is indexed by a row number $s_1$ and a column number $s_2$ which represent positions on a $64 \times 36$ spatial grid set out on an agricultural field. The value of the temperature measured at row $s_1$ and column $s_2$, is denoted by $x_{\boldsymbol{s}} = x_{s1,s2}$. We can note from the two-dimensional plot that a distinct change occurs in the character of the two-dimensional surface character starting at about row 40, where the oscillations along the row axis become fairly stable and periodic. For example, averaging over the 36 columns, we may compute an average value for each $s_1$ as in Figure 1.26. It is clear that the noise present in the first part of the two-dimensional series is nicely averaged out and we see a clear and consistent temperature signal.

The ***autocovariance function*** of a stationary multidimensional process, $x_{\boldsymbol{s}}$, can be defined as a function of the multidimensional lag vector, say, $\boldsymbol{h} = (h_1, h_2, \ldots, h_r)'$, as

$$\gamma(\boldsymbol{h}) = E[(x_{\boldsymbol{s}+\boldsymbol{h}} - \mu)(x_{\boldsymbol{s}} - \mu)], \tag{1.87}$$

where

$$\mu = E(x_{\boldsymbol{s}}) \tag{1.88}$$

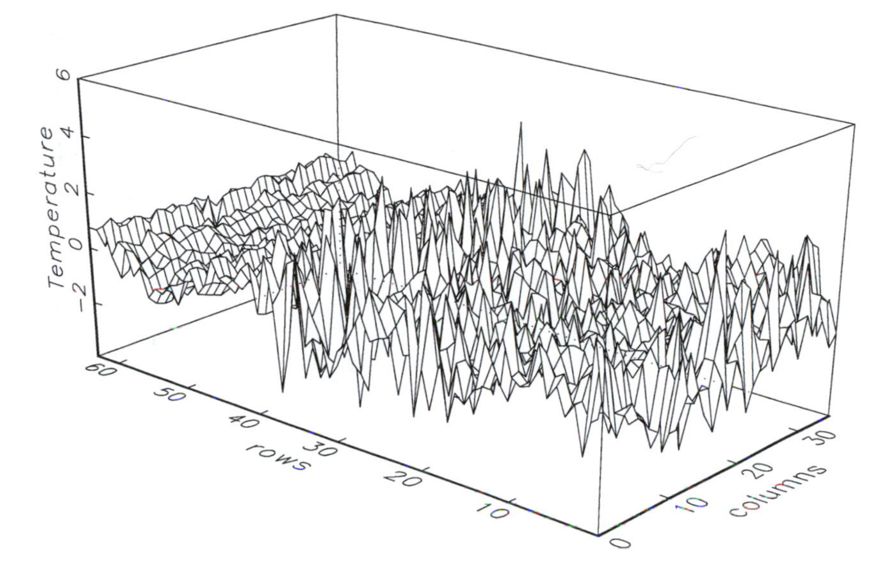


**Figure 1.25:** Two-dimensional time series of temperature measurements taken on a rectangular field ($64 \times 36$ with 17-foot spacing). Data are from Bazza et al (1988).

does not depend on the spatial coordinate $\boldsymbol{s}$. For the two dimensional temperature process, (1.87) becomes

$$\gamma(h_1, h_2) = E[(x_{s_1+h_1, s_2+h_2} - \mu)(x_{s_1,s_2} - \mu)], \tag{1.89}$$

which is a function of lag, both in the row ($h_1$) and column ($h_2$) directions.

The ***multidimensional sample autocovariance function*** is defined as

$$\widehat{\gamma}(\boldsymbol{h}) = (S_1 S_2 \cdots S_r)^{-1} \sum_{s_1} \sum_{s_2} \cdots \sum_{s_r} (x_{\boldsymbol{s}+\boldsymbol{h}} - \bar{x})(x_{\boldsymbol{s}} - \bar{x}), \tag{1.90}$$

where $\boldsymbol{s} = (s_1, s_2, \dots, s_r)'$ and the range of summation for each argument is $1 \le s_i \le S_i - h_i, i = 1, \dots, r$. The mean is computed over the r-dimensional array, that is,

$$\bar{x} = (S_1 S_2 \cdots S_r)^{-1} \sum_{s_1} \sum_{s_2} \cdots \sum_{s_r} x_{s_1, s_2, \cdots, s_r}, \tag{1.91}$$

where the arguments $s_i$ are summed over $1 \le s_i \le S_i$. The multidimensional sample autocorrelation function follows, as usual, by taking the scaled ratio

$$\widehat{\rho}(\boldsymbol{h}) = \frac{\widehat{\gamma}(\boldsymbol{h})}{\widehat{\gamma}(\boldsymbol{0})}. \tag{1.92}$$

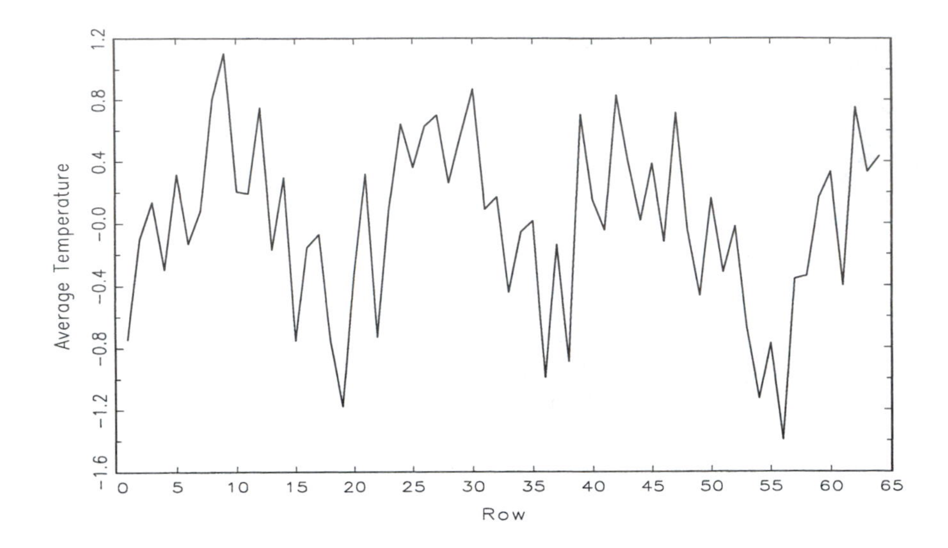


**Figure 1.26:** Row averages of the two-dimensional soil temperature profile. $\bar{x}_{s_1} = \sum_{s_2} x_{s_1,s_2}/36$.

**Example 1.29 Sample ACF of the Soil Temperature Series**

The autocorrelation function of the two-dimensional temperature process can be written in the form

$$\widehat{\rho}(h_1, h_2) = \frac{\widehat{\gamma}(h_1, h_2)}{\widehat{\gamma}(0, 0)},$$

where

$$\widehat{\gamma}(h_1, h_2) = (S_1 S_2)^{-1} \sum_{s_1} \sum_{s_2} (x_{s_1+h_1, s_2+h_2} - \bar{x})(x_{s_1,s_2} - \bar{x})$$

Figure 1.27 shows the autocorrelation function for the temperature data and we note the systematic periodic variation that appears along the rows. The autocovariance over columns seems to be strongest for $h_1 = 0$, implying columns may form replicates of some underlying process that has a periodicity over the rows. This idea can be investigated by examining the mean series over columns as shown in Figure 1.26.

The sampling requirements for multidimensional processes are rather severe because values must be available over some uniform grid in order to compute the ACF. In some areas of application, such as in soil science, we may prefer to sample a limited number of rows or *transects* and hope these are essentially

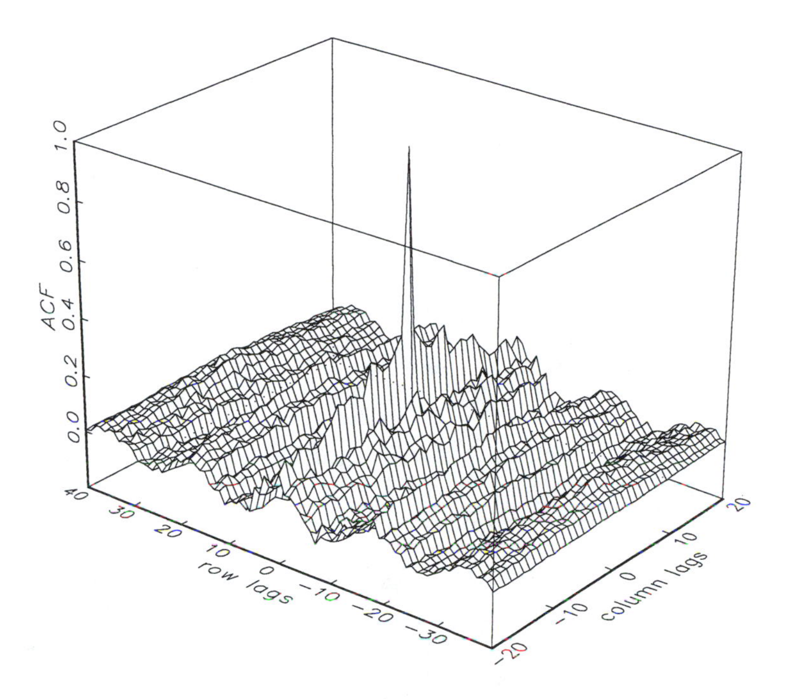


**Figure 1.27:** Two-dimensional autocorrelation function for the soil temperature data.

replicates of the basic underlying phenomenon of interest. One-dimensional methods can then be applied. When observations are irregular in time space, modifications to the estimators need to be made. Systematic approaches to the problems introduced by irregularly spaced observations have been developed by Journel and Huijbregts (1978) or Cressie (1993). We shall not pursue such methods in detail here, but it is worth noting that the introduction of the ***variogram***

$$2V_x(\boldsymbol{h}) = \text{var}\{x_{\boldsymbol{s}+\boldsymbol{h}} - x_{\boldsymbol{s}}\} \tag{1.93}$$

and its sample estimator

$$2\widehat{V}_x(\boldsymbol{h}) = \frac{1}{N(\boldsymbol{h})} \sum_{\boldsymbol{s}} (x_{\boldsymbol{s}+\boldsymbol{h}} - x_{\boldsymbol{s}})^2 \tag{1.94}$$

play key roles, where $N(\boldsymbol{h})$ denotes both the number of points located within $\boldsymbol{h}$ and the sum runs over the points in the neighborhood. Clearly, substantial indexing difficulties will develop from estimators of the kind, and often it will be difficult to find non-negative definite estimators for the covariance function. Problem 1.30 investigates the relation between the variogram and the autocovariance function in the stationary case.

## T1.10 Convergence Modes

The study of the optimality properties of various estimators (such as the sample autocorrelation function) depends, in part, on being able to assess the large-sample behavior of these estimators. We summarize briefly here the kinds of convergence useful in this setting, namely, ***mean square convergence***, ***convergence in probability***, and ***convergence in distribution***.

We consider first a particular class of random variables that plays an important role in the study of ***second-order time series***, namely, the class of random variables belonging to the space $L^2$, satisfying $E|x|^2 < \infty$. In proving certain properties of the class $L^2$ we will often use the ***Cauchy–Schwarz inequality***

$$|E(xy)|^2 \leq E(|x|^2)E(|y|^2), \tag{1.95}$$

the ***Minkowski inequality***

$$E^{1/2}(|x+y|^2) \leq E^{1/2}(|x|^2) + E^{1/2}(|y|^2) \tag{1.96}$$

and the ***Tchebycheff inequality***

$$P\{|x| \geq a\} \leq \frac{E(|x|^2)}{a^2} \tag{1.97}$$

for $a > 0$.

We then define ***mean square convergence*** of a sequence of $L^2$ random variables $x_n, n = 1, 2, \ldots$ to a random variable $x$, denoted by

$$x_n \stackrel{ms}{\to} x, \tag{1.98}$$

if and only if

$$E|x_n - x|^2 \to 0 \tag{1.99}$$

as $n \to \infty$. We summarize some of the properties of mean square convergence as follows. If $x_n \stackrel{ms}{\to} x, y_n \stackrel{ms}{\to} y$, then

(i) $E(x_n) \to E(x)$;

(ii) $E(|x_n|^2) \to E(|x|^2)$;

(iii) $E(x_n y_n) \to E(xy)$.

To prove (i), by the Tchebycheff inequality,

$$|E(x_n y) - E(xy)| \quad = \quad |E[(x_n - x)y]|$$

$$\leq \quad E^{1/2}|x_n - x|^2 E^{1/2}|y|^2,$$

which converges to zero by the mean square convergence of $x_n$. Specializing to $y = 1$, we obtain (i). To prove (ii), we may write $x_n = x_n - x + x$ and $x = x - x_n + x_n$ and apply the Minkowski inequality, so

$$E^{1/2}|x_n|^2 \leq E^{1/2}|x_n - x|^2 + E^{1/2}|x|^2$$

and

$$E^{1/2}|x|^2 \leq E^{1/2}|x - x_n|^2 + E^{1/2}|x_n|^2$$

or

$$|E^{1/2}|x_n|^2 - E^{1/2}|x|^2| \leq E^{1/2}|x_n - x|^2,$$

which converges to zero. To prove (iii),

$$\begin{aligned} |E(x_n y_n) - E(xy)| &= |E[x_n(y_n - y) + E[(x_n - x)y| \\ &\leq |E[x_n(y_n - y)| + |E[(x_n - x)y]| \\ &\leq E^{1/2}|x_n|^2 E^{1/2}|y_n - y|^2 + E^{1/2}|x_n - x|^2 E^{1/2}|y|^2 \end{aligned}$$

using the Minkowski and Cauchy–Schwarz inequalities in the last two steps and noting $E(x_n^2) \to E(x^2)$ by property (ii).

We also note the $L^2$ completeness theorem known as the ***Riesz–Fisher Theorem*** .

**Theorem 1.1:** *Let $x_n$ be in $L^2$. Then, there exists an $x$ in $L^2$ such that $x_n \stackrel{ms}{\to} x$ if and only if*

$$E|x_m - x_n|^2 \to 0 \tag{1.100}$$

*for $m, n \to \infty$.*

Often the condition of Theorem 1.1 is easier to verify to establish that a mean square limit $x$ exists without knowing what it is. For ordinary sequences, Theorem 1.1 is just the Cauchy condition.

#### Example 1.30 Mean Square Convergence of the Sample Mean

Consider the white noise sequence $w_t$ and the *signal plus noise* series

$$x_t = \mu + w_t.$$

Then, because

$$E|\bar{x} - \mu|^2 = \frac{\sigma_w^2}{n}$$

converges to zero as $n \to \infty$, $\bar{x} \stackrel{ms}{\to} \mu$.

As a more important example of the use of the Riesz–Fisher Theorem 1.1 and the properties (i), (ii), and (iii) of mean square convergent series given before it, a ***time-invariant linear filter*** is defined as a convolution of the form

$$y_t = \sum_{j=-\infty}^{\infty} a_j x_{t-j} \tag{1.101}$$

for each $t = 0, \pm 1, \pm 2, \ldots$, where $x_t$ is a weakly stationary input series and $a_j, j = 0, \pm 1, \pm 2, \ldots$ are constants satisfying

$$\sum_{j=-\infty}^{\infty} |a_j| < \infty. \tag{1.102}$$

The output series $y_t$ defines a ***filtering*** or ***smoothing*** of the input series that changes the character of the time series in a predictable way. We need to know the conditions under which the outputs $y_t$ in (1.101) and the linear process (1.26) exist. We discuss the case here in which $x_t$ is assumed to be in $L^2$, i.e., $E(x_t^2) < K < \infty$.

Considering the sequence

$$y_t^n = \sum_{j=-n}^{n} a_j x_{t-j}, \tag{1.103}$$

$n = 1, 2, \ldots$, we need to show first that $y_t^n$ has a mean square limit. By Theorem 1.1, it is enough to show that

$$E|y_t^m - y_t^n|^2 \to 0$$

as $m, n \to \infty$. For $m > n$,

$$\begin{aligned} E^{1/2}|\sum_{j=-m}^{m} a_j x_{t-j} - \sum_{j=-n}^{n} a_j x_{t-j}|^2 \quad &\le \quad E^{1/2}|\sum_{j=n+1}^{m} a_j x_{t-j}|^2 \\ &\quad + E^{1/2}|\sum_{j=-(n+1)}^{-m} a_j x_{t-j}|^2, \end{aligned}$$

using the Minkowski inequality. Then, the first term on the right-hand side of the inequality becomes

$$\begin{aligned} E^{1/2} \sum_{j,k=n+1}^{m} |a_j x_{t-j} a_k x_{t-k}| \quad &\le \quad \left( \sum_{j,k=n+1}^{m} |a_j||a_k| E\left(|x_{t-j}||x_{t-k}|\right) \right)^{1/2} \\ &\le \quad \left( \sum_{j,k=n+1}^{m} |a_j||a_k| E^{1/2}|x_{t-j}|^2 E^{1/2}|x_{t-k}|^2 \right)^{1/2} \\ &= \quad K^{1/2} \sum_{j=n+1}^{m} |a_j|, \end{aligned}$$

using the Cauchy–Schwarz inequality. The same argument works on the second term of the right-hand side of the inequality, and (1.102) guarantees the bound converges to zero.

Now, having established that the filter output exists as a mean square limit $y_t$, we can get its mean and autocovariance function using properties (i) and (iii). For example, because $y_t^n \to y_t$, $E(y_t^n) \to E(y_t)$, i.e.

$$E(y_t^n) = \sum_{j=-n}^{n} a_j \mu_x$$

converges to

$$E(y_t) = \mu_x \sum_{j=-\infty}^{\infty} a_j. \tag{1.104}$$

Similarly, by (iii),

$$E[(y_{t+h}^n - Ey_{t+h}^n)(y_t^n - Ey_t^n)] \to E[(y_{t+h} - Ey_{t+h})(y_t - Ey_t)].$$

In this case,

$$\begin{aligned} E[(y_{t+h}^n - Ey_{t+h}^n)(y_t^n - Ey_t^n)] &= E \sum_{j,k=-n}^{n} a_k(x_{t+h-k} - \mu_x)a_j(x_{t-j} - \mu_x) \\ &= \sum_{j,k=-n}^{n} a_k \gamma_x(j+h-k)a_j, \end{aligned}$$

showing that

$$\gamma_y(h) = \sum_{j=-\infty}^{\infty} \sum_{k=-\infty}^{\infty} a_j \gamma_x(j+h-k)a_k. \tag{1.105}$$

A second important kind of convergence is ***convergence in probability***. The sequence $x_n, n = 1, 2, \dots$ converges in probability to a random variable $x$, denoted by

$$x_n \stackrel{p}{\to} x, \tag{1.106}$$

if and only if

$$P\{|x_n - x| > \epsilon\} \to 0 \tag{1.107}$$

for all $\epsilon > 0$, as $n \to \infty$. An immediate consequence of the Tchebycheff inequality (1.97) is that

$$P\{|x_n - x| \geq \epsilon\} \leq \frac{E(|x_n - x|^2)}{\epsilon^2},$$

so convergence in mean square implies convergence in probability, i.e.,

$$x_n \stackrel{ms}{\to} x \ \Rightarrow \ x_n \stackrel{p}{\to} x. \tag{1.108}$$

This result implies, for example, that the filter (1.101) exists as a limit in probability because it converges in mean square. We mention, at this point, the useful ***Weak Law of Large Numbers*** which states that, for an independent identically distributed sequence $x_n$ of random variables with mean $\mu$, we have

$$\bar{x} \xrightarrow{p} \mu \tag{1.109}$$

as $n \to \infty$, where $\bar{x} = n^{-1} \sum_{t=1}^{n} x_t$ is the usual sample mean.

We also will make use of the term ***order in probability*** and sometimes write $x_n - x = o_p(a_n)$. This result has is useful in that we can specify more carefully the rate at which convergence occurs. Generally, we say that

$$x_n = o_p(a_n) \tag{1.110}$$

if and only if

$$\frac{x_n}{a_n} \xrightarrow{p} 0. \tag{1.111}$$

Under this convention, the notation for $x_n \xrightarrow{p} x$ becomes $|x_n - x| = o_p(1)$. Finally, we use, on occasion, the notion of ***boundedness in probability***, written $x_n = O_p(a_n)$ when, for every $\epsilon > 0$, there exists a $\delta(\epsilon) > 0$ such that

$$P\{|\frac{x_n}{a_n}| > \delta(\epsilon)\} \leq \epsilon \tag{1.112}$$

for all $n$. The definitions can be compared with their nonrandom counterparts, namely, for a fixed sequence $x_n = o(1)$ if $x_n \to 0$ and $x_n = O(1)$ if $x_n, n = 1, 2, \ldots$ is bounded. Some handy properties of $o_p(\cdot)$ and $O_p(\cdot)$ are as follows.

(i) If $x_n = o_p(a_n), y_n = o_p(b_n)$, then $x_n y_n = o_p(a_n b_n)$ and $x_n + y_n = o_p(\max(a_n, b_n))$.

(ii) If $x_n = o_p(a_n), y_n = O_p(b_n)$, then $x_n y_n = o_p(a_n b_n)$.

(iii) Statement (i) is true if $O_p(\cdot)$ replaces $o_p(\cdot)$.

**Example 1.31 Convergence and Order in Probability for the Sample Mean**

For the sample mean, by the Tchebycheff inequality,

$$\begin{aligned} P\{|\bar{x} - \mu| > \epsilon\} &\leq \frac{E[(\bar{x} - \mu)^2]}{\epsilon^2} \\ &= \frac{\sigma_w^2}{n\epsilon^2} \to 0, \end{aligned}$$

as $n \to \infty$. It follows that $\bar{x} \xrightarrow{p} \mu$ and

$$|\bar{x} - \mu| = o_p(1).$$

To find the rate, it follows that that, for $\delta(\epsilon) > 0$,

$$\begin{aligned} P\left\{\frac{|\bar{x}-\mu|}{n^{-1/2}} > \delta(\epsilon)\right\} &\leq \frac{n\sigma_w^2}{n\delta^2(\epsilon)} \\ &= \frac{\sigma_w^2}{\delta^2(\epsilon)} \end{aligned}$$

by Tchebycheff's inequality, so taking $\epsilon = \sigma_w^2/\delta^2(\epsilon)$ shows that $\delta(\epsilon) = \sigma_w/\sqrt{\epsilon}$ does the job and

$$|\bar{x}-\mu| = O_p(n^{-1/2}).$$

For $r \times 1$ random vectors $\boldsymbol{x}_n$, convergence in probability, written $\boldsymbol{x}_n \to \boldsymbol{x}$ or $\boldsymbol{x}_n - \boldsymbol{x} = o_p(1)$ is defined as element-by-element convergence in probability, or equivalently, as convergence in terms of the Euclidian distance

$$||\boldsymbol{x}_n - \boldsymbol{x}|| \xrightarrow{p} 0, \tag{1.113}$$

where $||\boldsymbol{a}|| = \sum_j a_j^2$ for any vector $\boldsymbol{a}$. In this context, we note the result that if $\boldsymbol{x}_n \xrightarrow{p} \boldsymbol{x}$ and $g(\boldsymbol{x}_n)$ is a continuous mapping,

$$g(\boldsymbol{x}_n) \xrightarrow{p} g(\boldsymbol{x}). \tag{1.114}$$

**Example 1.32 Convergence in Probability of the Sample Variance**

Suppose we have a sequence $x_n$ of independent, identically distributed random variables with mean $\mu$ and variance $\sigma^2$. Consider the sample variance

$$\begin{aligned} s^2 &= n^{-1}\sum_{t=1}^{n}(x_t-\bar{x})^2 \\ &= n^{-1}\sum_{t=1}^{n}x_t^2 - \bar{x}^2. \end{aligned}$$

Now, because $Ex_t^2 = \sigma^2 + \mu^2$, we have by the Weak Law of Large Numbers that

$$n^{-1}\sum_{t=1}^{n}x_t^2 \xrightarrow{p} \sigma^2 + \mu^2$$

and that $\bar{x} \xrightarrow{p} \mu$, so, by (1.114), $\bar{x}^2 \xrightarrow{p} \mu^2$. The sample variance is the sum of two terms, so, by Property (i)

$$n^{-1}\sum_{t=1}^{n}x_t^2 - \bar{x}^2 - [(\sigma^2+\mu^2)-\mu^2] = o_p(1),$$

and we have the result that $s^2 \xrightarrow{p} \sigma^2$.

Furthermore, if $\boldsymbol{x}_n - \boldsymbol{a} = O_p(\delta_n)$ with $\delta_n \to 0$ and $g(\cdot)$ is a function with continuous first derivatives continuous in a neighborhood of $\boldsymbol{a} = (a_1, a_2, \dots, a_k)'$, we have the ***Taylor series expansion in probability***

$$g(\boldsymbol{x}_n) = g(\boldsymbol{a}) + \left.\frac{\partial g(\boldsymbol{x})}{\partial \boldsymbol{x}}\right|_{\boldsymbol{x}=\boldsymbol{a}}' (\boldsymbol{x}_n - \boldsymbol{a}) + o_p(\delta_n), \tag{1.115}$$

where

$$\left.\frac{\partial g(\boldsymbol{x})}{\partial \boldsymbol{x}}\right|_{\boldsymbol{x}=\boldsymbol{a}} = \left( \left.\frac{\partial g(\boldsymbol{x})}{\partial x_1}\right|_{\boldsymbol{x}=\boldsymbol{a}}, \dots, \left.\frac{\partial g(\boldsymbol{x})}{\partial x_k}\right|_{\boldsymbol{x}=\boldsymbol{a}} \right)'$$

denotes the vector of partial derivatives with respect to $x_1, x_2, \dots, x_k$, evaluated at $\boldsymbol{a}$.

#### Example 1.33 Expansion for the Logarithm of the Sample Mean

Consider $g(\bar{x}) = \log \bar{x}$, which has a derivative at $\mu, \mu > 0$. Then, because $|\bar{x} - \mu| = O_p(n^{-1/2})$ from Example 1.30, the conditions for the Taylor expansion in probability, (1.115), are satisfied and we have

$$\log \bar{x} = \log \mu + \mu^{-1}(\bar{x} - \mu) + o_p(n^{-1/2}).$$

The large sample distributions of sample mean and sample autocorrelation functions defined earlier can be developed using the notion of convergence in distribution. A sequence of $r \times 1$ random vectors $\boldsymbol{x}_n, n = 1, 2, \dots$ is said to converge in distribution, written

$$\boldsymbol{x}_n \xrightarrow{d} \boldsymbol{x} \tag{1.116}$$

if

$$F_n(\boldsymbol{x}) \to F(\boldsymbol{x}) \tag{1.117}$$

at the continuity points of distribution function $F(\cdot)$. If $\boldsymbol{x}_n \xrightarrow{d} \boldsymbol{x}$, the distribution of $\boldsymbol{x}_n$ can be approximated by the distribution of $\boldsymbol{x}$ in large samples.

#### Example 1.34 Convergence in Distribution

Consider a sequence $x_n, n = 1, 2, \dots$ of iid normal random variables with mean zero and variance $1/n$. Now, using the normal cdf (1.7), we have $F_n(x) = \Phi(\sqrt{n}x)$, so

$$F_n(x) \to \begin{cases} 0 & x < 0, \\ 1/2, & x = 0 \\ 1, & x > 0 \end{cases}$$

and we may take

$$F(x) = \begin{cases} 0, & x < 0 \\ 1, & x \geq 0, \end{cases}$$

because the point where the two functions differ is not a continuity point of $F(x)$.

The distribution function relates uniquely to the ***characteristic function*** through the Fourier transform, defined as a function with vector argument $\boldsymbol{\lambda} = (\lambda_1, \lambda_2, \ldots, \lambda_r)'$, say

$$\begin{aligned} \phi(\boldsymbol{\lambda}) &= E(\exp\{i\boldsymbol{\lambda}'\boldsymbol{x}\}) \\ &= \int \exp\{i\boldsymbol{\lambda}'\boldsymbol{x}\}\, dF(\boldsymbol{x}). \end{aligned} \tag{1.118}$$

Hence, for a sequence $\boldsymbol{x}_n, n = 1, 2, \ldots$, we may characterize convergence in distribution of $F_n(\cdot)$ in terms of convergence of the sequence of characteristic functions $\phi_n(\cdot)$, i.e.,

$$\phi_n(\boldsymbol{\lambda}) \to \phi(\boldsymbol{\lambda}) \;\Leftrightarrow\; F_n(\boldsymbol{x}) \xrightarrow{d} F(\boldsymbol{x}), \tag{1.119}$$

where $\Leftrightarrow$ means that the implication goes both directions. In this connection, the ***Cramér-Wold device*** says that for every $\boldsymbol{c} = (c_1, c_2, \ldots, c_p)'$

$$\boldsymbol{c}'\boldsymbol{x}_n \xrightarrow{d} \boldsymbol{c}'\boldsymbol{x} \;\Leftrightarrow \boldsymbol{x}_n \xrightarrow{d} \boldsymbol{x}. \tag{1.120}$$

Also, convergence in probability implies convergence in distribution, namely,

$$\boldsymbol{x}_n \xrightarrow{p} \boldsymbol{x} \;\Rightarrow\; \boldsymbol{x}_n \xrightarrow{d} \boldsymbol{x}, \tag{1.121}$$

but that the converse is only true when $\boldsymbol{x}_n \xrightarrow{d} \boldsymbol{c}$, where $\boldsymbol{c}$ is a constant vector. If $\boldsymbol{x}_n \xrightarrow{d} \boldsymbol{x}$ and $\boldsymbol{y}_n \xrightarrow{d} \boldsymbol{c}$ are two sequences of random vectors and $\boldsymbol{c}$ is a constant vector,

$$\boldsymbol{x}_n + \boldsymbol{y}_n \xrightarrow{d} \boldsymbol{x} + \boldsymbol{c} \tag{1.122}$$

and

$$\boldsymbol{y}_n'\boldsymbol{x}_n \xrightarrow{d} \boldsymbol{c}'\boldsymbol{x}. \tag{1.123}$$

For a continuous mapping $h(\boldsymbol{x})$,

$$\boldsymbol{x}_n \xrightarrow{d} \boldsymbol{x} \;\Rightarrow\; h(\boldsymbol{x}_n) \xrightarrow{d} h(\boldsymbol{x}). \tag{1.124}$$

A number of results in time series depend on making a series of approximations to prove convergence in distribution. For example, we have that if $\boldsymbol{x}_n \xrightarrow{d} \boldsymbol{x}$ can be *approximated* by the sequence $\boldsymbol{y}_n$ in the sense that

$$\boldsymbol{y}_n - \boldsymbol{x}_n = o_p(1), \tag{1.125}$$

then we have that $\boldsymbol{y}_n \xrightarrow{d} \boldsymbol{x}$, so the approximating sequence $\boldsymbol{y}_n$ has the same limiting distribution as $\boldsymbol{x}$. We present the following ***Basic Approximation Theorem (BAT)*** that will be used later to derive asymptotic distributions for the sample mean and ACF.

**Theorem 1.2:** *Let $\boldsymbol{x}_n$, $n = 1, 2, \ldots$ and $\boldsymbol{y}_{mn}$, $m = 1, 2, \ldots$ be random $r \times 1$ vectors such that*

(i) $\boldsymbol{y}_{mn} \stackrel{d}{\to} \boldsymbol{y}_m$ *as* $n \to \infty$ *for each* $m$;

(ii) $\boldsymbol{y}_m \stackrel{d}{\to} \boldsymbol{y}$ *as* $m \to \infty$;

(iii) $\lim_{m\to\infty} \limsup_{n\to\infty} P\{|\boldsymbol{x}_n - \boldsymbol{y}_{mn}| > \epsilon\} = 0$ *for every* $\epsilon > 0$.

*Then,* $\boldsymbol{x}_n \stackrel{d}{\to} \boldsymbol{y}$.

As a practical matter, condition (iii) is implied by the Tchebycheff inequality if

$$E\{|x_n - y_{mn}|^2\} \to 0$$

as $m, n \to \infty$, and this latter condition is often much easier to establish.

The theorem allows approximation of the underlying sequence in two steps, through the intermediary sequence $\boldsymbol{y}_{mn}$, depending on two arguments. In the time series case, $n$ is generally the sample length and $m$ is generally the number of terms in an approximation to the linear process of the form (1.103).

The proof of the theorem is a simple exercise in using the characteristic functions and appealing to (1.119). We need to show

$$|\phi_{\boldsymbol{x}_n} - \phi_{\boldsymbol{y}}| \to 0,$$

where $\phi_{\boldsymbol{y}} = \phi_{\boldsymbol{y}}(\cdot)$ denotes the characteristic function of the random vector $\boldsymbol{y}$. First,

$$|\phi_{\boldsymbol{x}_n} - \phi_{\boldsymbol{y}}| \le |\phi_{\boldsymbol{x}_n} - \phi_{\boldsymbol{y}_{mn}}| + |\phi_{\boldsymbol{y}_{mn}} - \phi_{\boldsymbol{y}_m}| + |\phi_{\boldsymbol{y}_m} - \phi_{\boldsymbol{y}}|.$$

By the condition (ii) and (1.119), the last term converges to zero, and by condition (i) and (1.119), the second term converges to zero and we only need consider the first term

$$\begin{aligned}
|\phi_{\boldsymbol{x}_n} - \phi_{y_{mn}}| &= |E(e^{i\boldsymbol{\lambda}'\boldsymbol{x}_n} - e^{i\boldsymbol{\lambda}'\boldsymbol{y}_{mn}})| \\
&\le E|e^{i\boldsymbol{\lambda}'\boldsymbol{x}_n}(1 - e^{i\boldsymbol{\lambda}'(\boldsymbol{y}_{mn} - \boldsymbol{x}_n)})| \\
&= E|1 - e^{i\boldsymbol{\lambda}'(\boldsymbol{y}_{mn} - \boldsymbol{x}_n)}| \\
&= E\Big\{|1 - e^{i\boldsymbol{\lambda}'(\boldsymbol{y}_{mn} - \boldsymbol{x}_n)}| I_{\{|\boldsymbol{y}_{mn} - \boldsymbol{x}_n| < \delta\}}\Big\} \\
&\quad + E\Big\{|1 - e^{i\boldsymbol{\lambda}'(\boldsymbol{y}_{mn} - \boldsymbol{x}_n)}| I_{\{|\boldsymbol{y}_{mn} - \boldsymbol{x}_n| \ge \delta\}}\Big\},
\end{aligned}$$

where $\delta > 0$ and $I_A$ denotes the indicator function of the set $A$, i.e., $I_A = 1$ if $x$ is in $A$ and is zero otherwise. For the first term,

$$\begin{aligned}
|1 - e^{i\boldsymbol{\lambda}'(\boldsymbol{y}_{mn} - \boldsymbol{x}_n)}| &\le \sqrt{2\{1 - \cos[\boldsymbol{\lambda}'(\boldsymbol{y}_{mn} - \boldsymbol{x}_n)\}} \\
&\le |\boldsymbol{\lambda}'(\boldsymbol{y}_{mn} - \boldsymbol{x}_n)|
\end{aligned}$$

$$< \quad \epsilon$$

if $|\boldsymbol{y}_{mn} - \boldsymbol{x}_n| < \epsilon$ and the first term goes to zero. For the second term, note that

$$|1 - e^{i\boldsymbol{\lambda}'(\boldsymbol{y}_{mn} - \boldsymbol{x}_n)}| \leq 2$$

and we have

$$E\left\{|1 - e^{i\boldsymbol{\lambda}'(\boldsymbol{y}_{mn} - \boldsymbol{x}_n)}| I_{|\boldsymbol{y}_{mn} - \boldsymbol{x}_n| \geq \delta}\right\} \leq 2P\{|\boldsymbol{y}_{mn} - \boldsymbol{x}_n| \geq \delta\},$$

which converges to zero by property (iii).

# T1.11 Central Limit Theorems

We will generally be concerned with the large-sample properties of estimators that turn out to be normally distributed as $n \to \infty$. A sequence of random variables $x_n$ is said to be ***asymptotically normal with mean*** $\mu_n$ ***and variance*** $\sigma_n^2$ if, for $n$ sufficiently large

$$\sigma_n^{-1}(x_n - \mu_n) \xrightarrow{d} z,$$

where $z$ has the standard normal distribution. We shall abbreviate this as

$$x_n \sim AN(\mu_n, \sigma_n^2), \tag{1.126}$$

where $\sim$ will denote ***is distributed as***. We state the important ***Central Limit Theorem***, as follows.

**Theorem 1.3:** *Let $x_n$ be independent and identically distributed with mean $\mu$ and variance $\sigma^2$. Then, if $\bar{x} = n^{-1}(x_1 + x_2 + \ldots + x_n)$ denotes the sample mean, we have that*

$$\bar{x} \sim AN(\mu, \sigma^2/n), \tag{1.127}$$

*equivalently stated as*

$$n^{1/2}(\bar{x} - \mu) \xrightarrow{d} y \sim N(0, \sigma^2). \tag{1.128}$$

For a proof of this theorem using the characteristic function, see Brockwell and Davis (1991).

Often, we will be concerned with $r \times 1$ vectors $\boldsymbol{x}_n$, and we will define asymptotic normality for this case as

$$\boldsymbol{x}_n \sim AN(\boldsymbol{\mu}_n, \Sigma_n) \tag{1.129}$$

if

$$\boldsymbol{c}'\boldsymbol{x}_n \sim AN(\boldsymbol{c}'\boldsymbol{\mu}_n, \boldsymbol{c}'\Sigma_n\boldsymbol{c}) \tag{1.130}$$

for all $\boldsymbol{c}$ and $\Sigma_n$ is positive definite. The definition is motivated by the Cramér-Wold device considered earlier. Now, we will use the result in what follows that, if $\boldsymbol{x}_n \sim AN(\boldsymbol{\mu}, c_n^2\Sigma)$, where $\Sigma$ is symmetric with $c_n \to 0$ and $\boldsymbol{g}(\boldsymbol{x})$ is a $k \times 1$ continuously differentiable vector function of $\boldsymbol{x}$,

$$\boldsymbol{g}(\boldsymbol{x}_n) \sim AN(\boldsymbol{g}(\boldsymbol{\mu}), c_n^2 D\Sigma D'), \tag{1.131}$$

where $D$ is the $k \times r$ matrix with elements

$$d_{ij} = \left.\frac{\partial g_i(\boldsymbol{x})}{\partial x_j}\right|_{\boldsymbol{\mu}}.$$

In order to begin to consider what happens for dependent data in the limiting case, it is necessary to define, first of all, a particular kind of dependence known as ***M-dependence.*** We say that a time series $x_t$ is ***M-dependent*** if the set of values $x_s, s \leq t$ is independent of the set of values $x_s, s \geq t + M + 1$, so time points separated by more than $M$ units are independent. A central limit theorem for such dependent processes, used in conjunction with the Basic Approximation Theorem, will allow us to develop large-sample distributional results for the sample mean $\bar{x}$ and the sample ACF $\widehat{\rho}_x(h)$ in the stationary case.

In the arguments that follow, we often make use of the formula for the variance of $\bar{x}$ in the stationary case, namely,

$$\text{var}\ \bar{x} = n^{-1} \sum_{u=-(n-1)}^{(n-1)} \left(1 - \frac{|u|}{n}\right)\gamma(u). \tag{1.132}$$

To prove the above formula, letting $u = s - t$ and $v = t$ in

$$\begin{aligned}
n^2 E[(\bar{x} - \mu)^2] &= \sum_{s=1}^{n}\sum_{t=1}^{n} E[(x_s - \mu)(x_t - \mu)] \\
&= \sum_{s=1}^{n}\sum_{t=1}^{n} \gamma(s-t) \\
&= \sum_{u=-(n-1)}^{-1} \sum_{v=-(u-1)}^{n} \gamma(u) + \sum_{u=0}^{n-1}\sum_{v=1}^{n-u} \gamma(u) \\
&= \sum_{u=-(n-1)}^{-1} (n+u)\gamma(u) + \sum_{u=0}^{n-1} (n-u)\gamma(u) \\
&= \sum_{u=-(n-1)}^{(n-1)} (n - |u|)\gamma(u)
\end{aligned}$$

gives the required result. We shall also use the fact that, for

$$\sum_{u=-\infty}^{\infty} |\gamma(u)| < \infty,$$

we would have, by dominated convergence[2],

$$n \text{ var } \bar{x} \to \sum_{u=-\infty}^{\infty} \gamma(u), \tag{1.133}$$

because $|(1 - |u|/n)\gamma(u)| \leq |\gamma(u)|$ and $(1 - |u|/n)\gamma(u) \to \gamma(u)$. We may now state the ***M-Dependent Central Limit Theorem*** as follows.

**Theorem 1.4:** *If $x_t$ is a strictly stationary M-dependent sequence of random variables with mean zero and autocovariance function $\gamma(\cdot)$ and if*

$$V_M = \sum_{u=-M}^{M} \gamma(u), \tag{1.134}$$

*where $V_M \neq 0$,*

$$\bar{x} \sim AN(0, V_M/n). \tag{1.135}$$

To prove the theorem, using the Basic Approximation Theorem, we may construct a sequence of variables $y_{mn}$ approximating

$$n^{1/2}\bar{x} = n^{-1/2} \sum_{t=1}^{n} x_t$$

in the dependent case and then simply verify conditions (i), (ii), and (iii)of Theorem 1.2. For $n > 2m$, we may first consider the approximation

$$\begin{aligned} y_{mn} &= n^{-1/2}[(x_1 + \cdots + x_{m-M}) + (x_{m+1} + \cdots + x_{2m-M}) \\ &\quad + (x_{2m+1} + \cdots + x_{3m-M}) + \cdots + (x_{(r-1)m+1} + \cdots + x_{rm-M})] \\ &= n^{-1/2}(z_1 + z_2 + \cdots + z_r), \end{aligned}$$

where $r = [n/m]$, with $[n/m]$ denoting the greatest integer less than or equal to $n/m$. This approximation contains only part of $n^{1/2}\bar{x}$, but the random variables $z_1, z_2, \ldots, z_r$ are independent because they are separated by more than $M$ time points, e.g., $m - (m - M - 1) = M + 1$ points separate $z_1$ and $z_2$. Because of strict stationarity, $z_1, z_2, \ldots, z_r$ are identically distributed with zero means and variances

$$S_{m-M} = \sum_{|u| \leq M} (m - M - |u|)\gamma(u)$$

[2]Dominated convergence technically relates to convergent sequences (with respect to a sigma-additive measure $\mu$) of measurable functions $f_n \to f$ bounded by an integrable function $g$, $\int g \, d\mu < \infty$. For such a sequence,

$$\int f_n \, d\mu \to \int f \, d\mu.$$

For the case in point, take $f_n(u) = (1 - |u|/n)\gamma(u)$ for $|u| < n$ and as zero for $|u| \geq n$. Take $\mu(u) = 1, u = \pm 1, \pm 2, \ldots$ to be counting measure.

by a computation similar to that producing (1.132). We first verify condition (i) of the Basic Approximation Theorem.

(i): Applying the Central Limit Theorem to the sum $y_{mn}$ gives

$$\begin{aligned} y_{mn} &= n^{-1/2}\sum_{i=1}^{r} z_i \\ &= (n/r)^{-1/2} r^{-1/2}\sum_{i=1}^{r} z_i. \end{aligned}$$

Because $(n/r)^{-1/2} \to m^{-1/2}$ and

$$r^{-1/2}\sum_{i=1}^{r} z_i \xrightarrow{d} N(0, S_{m-M}),$$

it follows from (1.123) that

$$y_{mn} \xrightarrow{d} y_n \sim N(0, S_{m-M}/m).$$

as $n \to \infty$, for a fixed $m$.

Next, verify (ii) as below.

(ii): First, the variance of $y_m$, $S_{m-M}/m \to V_M$, using dominated convergence. Hence, the characteristic function of $y_m$, say,

$$\begin{aligned} \phi_n(\lambda) &= \exp\left\{-\frac{1}{2}\lambda^2\, \frac{S_{m-M}}{m}\right\} \\ &\to \exp\left\{-\frac{1}{2}\lambda^2\, V_M\right\}, \end{aligned}$$

which is the characteristic function of a random variable $y \sim N(0, V_M)$ and the result follows because of (1.119).

(iii): To verify the last condition of the BAT theorem,

$$\begin{aligned} n^{1/2}\bar{x} - y_{mn} &= n^{-1/2}[(x_{m-M+1} + \cdots + x_m) + (x_{2m-M+1} + \cdots + x_{2m}) \\ &\quad +(x_{(r-1)m-M+1} + \cdots + x_{(r-1)m}) + \cdots \\ &\quad +(x_{rm-M+1} + \cdots + x_n)] \\ &= n^{-1/2}(w_1 + w_2 + \cdots + w_r), \end{aligned}$$

so the error is expressed as a scaled sum of iid variables with variance $S_M$ for the first $r-1$ variables and

$$\text{var}(w_r) = \sum_{|u|\le M}\Big(n - [n/m]m + M - |u|\Big)\gamma(u)$$

$$\leq \sum_{|u| \leq M} (m + M - |u|)\gamma(u).$$

Hence,

$$\text{var}\,[n^{1/2}\bar{x} - y_{mn}] = n^{-1}[(r-1)S_M + \text{var}\,w_r],$$

which converges to $m^{-1}S_M$ as $n \to \infty$. Because $m^{-1}S_M \to 0$ as $m \to \infty$, the condition of (iii) holds by the Tchebycheff inequality.

## T1.12 The Mean and Autocorrelation Functions

The background material in the previous two sections can be used to develop the asymptotic properties of the sample mean and ACF used to evaluate statistical significance. In particular, we are interested in verifying Property 1.1.

We begin with the distribution of the sample mean $\bar{x}$, noting that (1.133) suggests a form for the limiting variance. In all of the asymptotics, we will use the assumption that $x_t$ is a linear process, as defined in (1.26) and (1.27). It is worth mentioning, at this point, that the linear process includes the ARIMA models considered in Chapter 2 as special cases.

Before proceeding further, we should note that the exact sampling distribution of $\bar{x}$ is available if the distribution of the underlying vector $\boldsymbol{x} = (x_1, x_2, \ldots, x_n)'$ is multivariate normal. Then, $\bar{x}$ is just a linear combination of jointly normal variables that will have the normal distribution

$$\bar{x} \sim N\left(\mu_x,\, n^{-1} \sum_{|u|<n} \left(1 - \frac{|u|}{n}\right)\gamma(u)\right), \tag{1.136}$$

by (1.132). In the case where $x_t$ are not jointly normally distributed, we have the following theorem.

**Theorem 1.5:** *If $x_t$ is a stationary linear process of the form (1.26) and $\sum_j \psi_j \neq 0$, then*

$$\bar{x} \sim AN(\mu_x, n^{-1}V), \tag{1.137}$$

*where*

$$V = \sum_{h=-\infty}^{\infty} \gamma(h) = \sigma_w^2 \left(\sum_{j=-\infty}^{\infty} \psi_j\right)^2 \tag{1.138}$$

*and $\gamma(\cdot)$ is the autocovariance function of $x_t$.*

To prove the above, we can again use the Basic Approximation Theorem 1.2 by first defining the ***2m-dependent*** linear process with finite limits

$$x_t^m = \sum_{j=-m}^{m} \psi_j w_{t-j}$$

as an approximation to $x_t$ to use in the approximating mean

$$\bar{x}_m = n^{-1} \sum_{t=1}^{n} x_t^m.$$

Then, take

$$y_{mn} = n^{1/2}(\bar{x}_m - \mu_x)$$

as an approximation to $x_n = n^{1/2}(\bar{x} - \mu_x)$.

(i): Apply Theorem 1.4 to note that

$$y_{mn} \xrightarrow{d} y_m \sim N(0, V_m),$$

as $n \to \infty$, where

$$\begin{aligned} V_m &= \sum_{h=-m}^{m} \gamma(h) \\ &= \sigma_w^2 \Big( \sum_{j=-n}^{n} \psi_j \Big)^2. \end{aligned}$$

To verify the above, we note that for the general linear process with infinite limits, (1.28) implies that

$$\begin{aligned} \sum_{h=-\infty}^{\infty} \gamma(h) &= \sigma_w^2 \sum_{h=-\infty}^{\infty} \sum_{j=-\infty}^{\infty} \psi_{j+h}\psi_j \\ &= \sigma_w^2 \sum_{j=-\infty}^{\infty} \psi_j \sum_{h=-\infty}^{\infty} \psi_{j+h} \\ &= \sigma_w^2 \Big( \sum_{j=-\infty}^{\infty} \psi_j \Big)^2, \end{aligned}$$

so taking the special case $\psi_j = 0, |j| > m$, we obtain $V_m$.

(ii): Because $V_m \to V$ in (1.138) as $m \to \infty$, we may use the same characteristic function argument as under (ii) in the proof of Theorem 1.4 to note that

$$y_m \xrightarrow{d} y \sim N(0, V),$$

where $V$ is given by (1.138).

(iii): Now,

$$n^{1/2}(\bar{x} - \mu_x) - y_{mn} = n^{-1/2} \sum_{t=1}^{n} (x_t - x_t^m)$$

$$= n^{-1/2} \sum_{t=1}^{n} e_t^m,$$

where the error process $e_t^m$ is

$$e_t^m = \sum_{|j|>m} \psi_j w_{t-j}.$$

If we denote the autocovariance function of the process $e_t^m$ by $\gamma_e(\cdot)$, it follows from (1.133) that

$$\begin{aligned} \text{var}\,[n^{1/2}(\bar{x} - \mu_x) - y_{mn}] &\to \sum_{u=-\infty}^{\infty} \gamma_e(u) \\ &= \sigma_w^2 \Big( \sum_{|j|>n} \psi_j \Big)^2, \end{aligned}$$

as $n \to \infty$. The right side of the last expression converges to zero as $m \to \infty$, establishing the required result.

In order to develop the sampling distribution of the sample autocovariance function, $\widehat{\gamma}(h)$, and the sample autocorrelation function, $\widehat{\rho}_x(h)$, we need to develop some idea as to the mean and variance of $\widehat{\gamma}(h)$ under some reasonable assumptions. These computations for $\widehat{\gamma}(h)$ are messy, and we consider a comparable quantity

$$\tilde{\gamma}(h) = n^{-1} \sum_{t=1}^{n} (x_{t+h} - \mu_x)(x_t - \mu_x) \tag{1.139}$$

as an approximation. By Problem 1.36,

$$n^{1/2}[\tilde{\gamma}(h) - \widehat{\gamma}(h)] = o_p(1),$$

so that limiting distributional results proved for $n^{1/2}\tilde{\gamma}(h)$ will hold for $n^{1/2}\widehat{\gamma}(h)$ by (1.125).

We begin by proving formulas for the variance and for the limiting variance of $\tilde{\gamma}(h)$ under the assumptions that $x_t$ is a linear process of the form (1.26), satisfying (1.27) with the white noise variates $w_t$ having variance $\sigma_w^2$ as before, but also required to have fourth moments satisfying

$$E(w_t^4) = \eta\sigma_w^4 < \infty, \tag{1.140}$$

where $\eta$ is some constant. We seek results comparable with (1.132) and (1.133) for $\tilde{\gamma}(h)$. Using, (1.139), $E[\tilde{\gamma}(h)] = \gamma(h)$. Under the above assumptions, we show now that, for $p, q = 0, 1, 2, \ldots$,

$$\text{cov}\,[\tilde{\gamma}(p), \tilde{\gamma}(q)] = n^{-1} \sum_{u=-(n-1)}^{(n-1)} \left(1 - \frac{|u|}{n}\right) V_u, \tag{1.141}$$

where

$$V_u = \gamma(u)\gamma(u-p+q) + \gamma(u+q)\gamma(u-p) + (\eta - 3)\sigma_w^4 \sum_i \psi_{i+u+q}\psi_{i+u}\psi_{i+p}\psi_i. \tag{1.142}$$

The absolute summability of the $\psi_j$ can then be shown to imply the absolute summability of the $V_u$.[3] Thus, the dominated convergence theorem implies

$$\begin{aligned} n \text{ cov}\,[\tilde{\gamma}(p), \tilde{\gamma}(q)] &\to \sum_{u=-\infty}^{\infty} V_u \\ &= (\eta - 3)\sigma_w^4 \gamma(p)\gamma(q) \\ &\quad + \sum_{u=-\infty}^{\infty} \Big[\gamma(u)\gamma(u-p+q) \\ &\quad + \gamma(u+q)\gamma(u-p)\Big]. \end{aligned} \tag{1.143}$$

To verify (1.141) is somewhat tedious, so we only go partially through the calculations, leaving the repetitive details to the reader. First, rewrite (1.26) as

$$x_t = \mu + \sum_{i=-\infty}^{\infty} \psi_{t-i} w_i,$$

so that

$$E[\tilde{\gamma}(p)\tilde{\gamma}(q)] = n^{-2} \sum_{s,t} \sum_{i,j,k,\ell} \psi_{s+p-i}\psi_{s-j}\psi_{t+q-k}\, \psi_{t-\ell} E(w_i w_j w_k w_\ell).$$

Then, evaluate, using the easily verified properties of the $w_t$ series

$$E(w_i w_j w_k w_\ell) = \begin{cases} \eta\sigma_w^4 & \text{if } i = j = k = \ell \\ \sigma_w^4 & \text{if } i = j \neq k = \ell \\ 0 & \text{if } i \neq j, i \neq k \text{ and } i \neq \ell. \end{cases}$$

To apply the rules, we break the sum over the subscripts $i, j, k, \ell$ into four terms, namely,

$$\begin{aligned} \sum_{i,j,k,\ell} &= \sum_{i=j=k=\ell} + \sum_{i=j\neq k=\ell} + \sum_{i=k\neq j=\ell} + \sum_{i=\ell\neq j=k} \\ &= S_1 + S_2 + S_3 + S_4. \end{aligned}$$

Now,

$$S_1 = \eta\sigma_w^4 \sum_i \psi_{s+p-i}\psi_{s-i}\psi_{t+q-i}\psi_{t-i}$$

[3]Note: $\sum_{j=-\infty}^{\infty} |a_j| < \infty$ and $\sum_{j=-\infty}^{\infty} |b_j| < \infty$ implies $\sum_{j=-\infty}^{\infty} |a_j b_j| < \infty$.

$$= \eta\sigma_w^4 \sum_i \psi_{i+s-t+p}\psi_{i+s-t}\psi_{i+q}\psi_i,$$

where we have let $i' = t - i$ to get the final form. For the second term,

$$\begin{aligned} S_2 &= \sum_{i=j\neq k=\ell} \psi_{s+p-i}\psi_{s-j}\psi_{t+q-k}\psi_{t-\ell}E(w_i w_j w_k w_\ell) \\ &= \sum_{i\neq k} \psi_{s+p-i}\psi_{s-i}\psi_{t+q-k}\psi_{t-k}E(w_i^2)E(w_k^2). \end{aligned}$$

Then, using the fact that

$$\sum_{i\neq k} = \sum_{i,k} - \sum_{i=k},$$

we have

$$\begin{aligned} S_2 &= \sigma_w^4 \sum_{i,k} \psi_{s+p-i}\psi_{s-i}\psi_{t+q-k}\psi_{t-k} - \sigma_w^4 \sum_i \psi_{s+p-i}\psi_{s-i}\psi_{t+q-i}\psi_{t-i} \\ &= \sigma_w^2\gamma(p)\gamma(q) - \sigma_w^4 \sum_i \psi_{i+s-t+p}\psi_{i+s-t}\psi_{i+q}\psi_i, \end{aligned}$$

letting $i' = s - i, k' = t - k$ in the first term and $i' = s - i$ in the second term. Repeating the argument for $S_3$ and $S_4$ and substituting into the covariance expression yields

$$\begin{aligned} E[\tilde{\gamma}(p)\tilde{\gamma}(q)] &= n^{-2} \sum_{s,t} \Big[ \gamma(p)\gamma(q) + \gamma(s-t)\gamma(s-t-p+q) \\ &\quad + \gamma(s-t)\gamma(s-t-q) \\ &\quad + (\eta - 3)\sigma_w^4 \sum_i \psi_{i+s-t+p}\psi_{i+s-t}\psi_{i+q}\psi_i \Big]. \end{aligned}$$

Then, letting $u = s - t$ and subtracting $E[\tilde{\gamma}(p)]E[\tilde{\gamma}(q)] = \gamma(p)\gamma(q)$ from the summation leads to the result (1.142). Summing (1.142) over $u$ and applying dominated convergence leads to (1.143).

The above results for the variances and covariances of the approximating statistics $\tilde{\gamma}(\cdot)$ enable proving the following central limit theorem for the autocovariance functions $\widehat{\gamma}(\cdot)$.

**Theorem 1.6:** *If $x_t$ is a stationary linear process of the form (1.26) satisfying the fourth moment condition (1.140), then*

$$\begin{pmatrix} \widehat{\gamma}(0) \\ \widehat{\gamma}(1) \\ \vdots \\ \widehat{\gamma}(K) \end{pmatrix} \sim AN \left[ \begin{pmatrix} \gamma(0) \\ \gamma(1) \\ \vdots \\ \gamma(K) \end{pmatrix}, n^{-1}V \right],$$

*where $V$ is the matrix with elements given by (1.143), namely,*

$$v_{pq} = (\eta - 3)\sigma_w^4 \gamma(p)\gamma(q) + \sum_{u=-\infty}^{\infty} \Big[ \gamma(u)\gamma(u-p+q) + \gamma(u+q)\gamma(u-p) \Big]. \tag{1.144}$$

It suffices to show the result for the approximate autocovariance (1.139) for $\tilde{\gamma}(\cdot)$ by the remark given below it (see also Problem 1.36). First, define the strictly stationary $(2m+K)$-dependent $(K+1)\times 1$ vector

$$\boldsymbol{y}_t^m = \begin{pmatrix} (x_t^m - \mu)^2 \\ (x_{t+1}^m - \mu)(x_t^m - \mu) \\ \vdots \\ (x_{t+K}^m - \mu)(x_t^m - \mu) \end{pmatrix},$$

where

$$x_t^m = \mu + \sum_{j=-m}^{m} \psi_j w_{t-j}$$

is the usual approximation. The sample mean of the above vector is

$$\bar{\boldsymbol{y}}_{mn} = n^{-1} \sum_{t=1}^{n} \boldsymbol{y}_t^m = \begin{pmatrix} \tilde{\gamma}^{mn}(0) \\ \tilde{\gamma}^{mn}(1) \\ \vdots \\ \tilde{\gamma}^{mn}(K) \end{pmatrix},$$

where

$$\tilde{\gamma}^{mn}(h) = n^{-1} \sum_{t=1}^{n} (x_{t+h}^m - \mu)(x_t^m - \mu)$$

denotes the sample autocovariance of the approximating series. Also,

$$E\boldsymbol{y}_t^m = \begin{pmatrix} \gamma^m(0) \\ \gamma^m(1) \\ \vdots \\ \gamma^m(K) \end{pmatrix},$$

where $\gamma^m(h)$ is the theoretical covariance function of the series $x_t^m$. Then, consider the vector

$$\boldsymbol{y}_{mn} = n^{1/2}[\bar{\boldsymbol{y}}_{mn} - E(\bar{\boldsymbol{y}}_{mn})]$$

as an approximation to

$$n^{1/2} \left[ \begin{pmatrix} \tilde{\gamma}(0) \\ \tilde{\gamma}(1) \\ \vdots \\ \tilde{\gamma}(K) \end{pmatrix} - \begin{pmatrix} \gamma(0) \\ \gamma(1) \\ \vdots \\ \gamma(K) \end{pmatrix} \right],$$

where $E(\bar{\boldsymbol{y}}_{mn})$ is the same as $E(\boldsymbol{y}_t^m)$ given above. The elements of the vector approximation are clearly $n^{1/2}(\tilde{\gamma}^{mn}(h) - \gamma^m(h))$. To apply the Basic Approximation Theorem 1.2, verify (i), (ii), and (iii) as below.

(i): First, apply the central limit theorem to the $(2m+K)-$dependent series $\boldsymbol{c}'\boldsymbol{y}_{mn}$ using the Cramér-Wold device (1.120). We obtain

$$\boldsymbol{c}'y_{mn} = n^{1/2}\boldsymbol{c}'[\bar{\boldsymbol{y}}_{mn} - E(\bar{\boldsymbol{y}}_{mn})] \xrightarrow{d} y_m \sim N(0, \boldsymbol{c}'V_m\boldsymbol{c}),$$

as $n \to \infty$, where $V_m$ is a matrix containing the finite analogs of the elements $v_{pq}$ defined in (1.144).

(ii) Note that, since $V_m \to V$ as $m \to \infty$, it follows that

$$y_m \xrightarrow{d} y \sim N(0, \boldsymbol{c}'V\boldsymbol{c}),$$

so, by the Cramér-Wold device, the limiting multivariate normal variable is $N(0, V)$.

(iii): To show condition (iii) of the Basic Approximation Theorem, note that element-by-element probabilities of the form

$$P\{|n^{1/2}\boldsymbol{x}_n - \boldsymbol{y}_{mn}| > \epsilon\}$$

can be bounded by

$$n\left[\text{var } \tilde{\gamma}^{mn}(h) + \text{var } \tilde{\gamma}^m(h) - 2 \text{ cov } [\tilde{\gamma}^{mn}(h), \tilde{\gamma}^m(h)]\right]/\epsilon^2,$$

using the Tchebycheff inequality. The preceding expression approaches

$$(v_{hh} + v_{hh} - 2v_{hh})/\epsilon^2 = 0,$$

as $m, n \to \infty$.

To obtain a result comparable to Theorem 1.6 for the autocorrelation function ACF, we note the following theorem.

**Theorem 1.7:** *If $x_t$ is a stationary linear process of the form (1.26) satisfying the fourth moment condition (1.140), then*

$$\begin{pmatrix} \widehat{\rho}(1) \\ \vdots \\ \widehat{\rho}(K) \end{pmatrix} \sim AN\left[\begin{pmatrix} \rho(1) \\ \vdots \\ \rho(K) \end{pmatrix}, n^{-1}W\right],$$

*where $W$ is the matrix with elements given by*

$$w_{pq} \quad = \quad \sum_{u=-\infty}^{\infty}\Big[\rho(u+p)\rho(u+q) + \rho(u-p)\rho(u+q) + 2\rho(p)\rho(q)\rho^2(u)$$

$$- 2\rho(p)\rho(u)\rho(u+q) - 2\rho(q)\rho(u)\rho(u+p)\Big]$$

$$= \sum_{u=1}^{\infty}[\rho(u+p)+\rho(u-p)-2\rho(p)\rho(u)]$$
$$\times\ [\rho(u+q)+\rho(u-q)-2\rho(q)\rho(u)], \tag{1.145}$$

*where the last form is more convenient.*

To prove the theorem, use the result (1.131) for the limiting distribution of a general function of the form

$$\boldsymbol{g}(x_0, x_1, \ldots, x_K) = (x_1/x_0, x_2/x_0, \ldots, x_K/x_0)',$$

where $g_i(x_0, x_1, \ldots, x_K) = x_i/x_0$ denotes the ith element of the vector $\boldsymbol{g}(\cdot)$. If $x_h = \widehat{\gamma}(h)$ are the sample covariance functions,

$$\boldsymbol{g}\left(\widehat{\gamma}(0), \widehat{\gamma}(1), \ldots, \widehat{\gamma}(K)\right) = (\widehat{\rho}(1), \ldots, \widehat{\rho}(K))'$$

is asymptotically normal with mean vector $(\rho(1), \ldots, \rho(K))'$ and covariance matrix

$$n^{-1}W = n^{-1}DVD',$$

where $V$ is defined by (1.144) and $D$ is the $(K+1)\times K$ matrix of partial derivatives

$$D = \frac{1}{x_0^2}\begin{pmatrix} -x_1 & x_0 & 0 & \ldots & 0 \\ -x_2 & 0 & x_0 & \ldots & 0 \\ \vdots & \vdots & \vdots & \ddots & \vdots \\ -x_K & 0 & 0 & \ldots & x_0, \end{pmatrix}$$

Substituting $\gamma(h)$ for $x_h$, we note that $D$ can be written as the patterned matrix

$$D = \frac{1}{\gamma(0)}\left(-\rho \quad I_K\right),$$

where $\rho = (\rho(1), \rho(2), \ldots, \rho(K))'$ is the $K \times 1$ matrix of autocorrelations and $I_K$ is the $K \times K$ identity matrix. Then, it follows from writing the matrix $V$ in the partitioned form

$$V = \begin{pmatrix} v_{00} & \boldsymbol{v}_1' \\ \boldsymbol{v}_1 & V_{22} \end{pmatrix}$$

that

$$W = \gamma^{-2}(0)\left[v_{00}\rho\rho' - \rho\boldsymbol{v}_1' - \boldsymbol{v}_1\rho' + V_{22}\right],$$

where $\boldsymbol{v}_1 = (v_{10}, v_{20}, \ldots, v_K0)'$ and $V_{22} = \{v_{pq}, p, q = 1, \ldots, K\}$. Hence,

$$w_{pq} = \gamma^{-2}(0)\left[v_{pq} - \rho(p)v_{0q} - \rho(q)v_{p0} + \rho(p)\rho(q)v_{00}\right]$$

$$= \sum_{u=-\infty}^{\infty}\Big[\rho(u)\rho(u-p+q) + \rho(u-p)\rho(u+q) + 2\rho(p)\rho(q)\rho^2(u)$$

$$- \rho(p)\rho(u)\rho(u+q) - 2\rho(q)\rho(u)\rho(u-p)\Big].$$

Interchanging the summations, we get the $w_{pq}$ specified in the statement of the theorem.

Specializing the theorem to the case of interest in this chapter, we note that, for white noise, $w_{ij} = 1, i = j$ and is zero otherwise. In this case, the $\rho^n(h)$ are uncorrelated and jointly normal with

$$\widehat{\rho}(h) \sim AN(0, n^{-1}). \tag{1.146}$$

This justifies the use of (1.33) and the discussion below it as a method for testing whether a series is white noise.

For the cross-correlation, it has been noted that the same kind of approximation holds and we quote the following theorem for the bivariate case, which can be proved using similar arguments (see Brockwell and Davis, 1991, p. 410).

**Theorem 1.8:** *If*

$$x_t = \sum_{j=-\infty}^{\infty} \alpha_j w_{t-j,1}$$

*and*

$$y_t = \sum_{j=-\infty}^{\infty} \beta_j w_{t-j,2}$$

*are two linear processes with absolutely summable coefficients and the two white noise sequences are independent of each other with variances $\sigma_1^2$ and $\sigma_2^2$, then for $h \geq 0$,*

$$\widehat{\rho}_{xy}(h) \sim AN\Big(\rho_{xy}(h), n^{-1}\sum_j \rho_x(j)\rho_y(j)\Big) \tag{1.147}$$

*and the joint distribution of $(\widehat{\rho}_{xy}(h), \widehat{\rho}_{xy}(k))'$ is asymptotically normal with mean vector zero and*

$$\text{cov}\ (\widehat{\rho}_{xy}(h), \widehat{\rho}_{xy}(k)) = n^{-1}\sum_j \rho_x(j)\rho_y(j+k-h). \tag{1.148}$$

Again, specializing to the case of interest in this chapter, as long as at least one of the two series is white noise, we obtain

$$\widehat{\rho}_{xy}(h) \sim AN\big(0, n^{-1}\big), \tag{1.149}$$

which justifies Property 1.2.

# Problems

*Section 1.3*

**1.1** Consider a signal plus noise model of the general form $x_t = s_t + w_t$, where $w_t$ is Gaussian white noise with $\sigma_w^2 = 1$. Simulate and plot $n = 200$ observations from each of the following two models (*Save the data generated here for use in Problem 1.21* ):

(a) $x_t = s_t + w_t$, for $t = 1, ..., 200$, where

$$s_t = \begin{cases} 0, & t = 1, ..., 100 \\ 10 \exp\{-\frac{(t-100)}{20}\} \cos(2\pi t/4), & t = 101, ..., 200. \end{cases}$$

(b) $x_t = s_t + w_t$, for $t = 1, ..., 200$, where

$$s_t = \begin{cases} 0, & t = 1, ..., 100 \\ 10 \exp\{-\frac{(t-100)}{200}\} \cos(2\pi t/4), & t = 101, ..., 200. \end{cases}$$

(c) Compare the general appearance of the series (a) and (b) with the earthquake series and the explosion series shown in Figure 1.6. In addition, plot (or sketch) and compare the signal modulators (a) $\exp\{-t/20\}$ and (b) $\exp\{-t/200\}$, for $t = 1, 2, ..., 100$.

**1.2** As in the previous problem, we consider a signal plus noise model whose signal is generated by an autoregression given by $y_t = -.90 y_{t-2} + w_t$, which is similar to (1.2). Simulate and plot $n = 200$ observations from each of the following two models (*Save the data generated here for use in Problem 1.21*):

(a)

$$x_t = \begin{cases} w_t, & t = 1, ..., 100 \\ 10 \exp\{-\frac{(t-100)}{20}\} y_t, & t = 101, ..., 200. \end{cases}$$

(b)

$$x_t = \begin{cases} w_t, & t = 1, ..., 100 \\ 10 \exp\{-\frac{(t-100)}{200}\} y_t, & t = 101, ..., 200. \end{cases}$$

(c) Compare the general appearance of the series (a) and (b) with the earthquake series and the explosion series shown in Figure 1.6.

*Section 1.4*

**1.3** Show that the autocovariance function

$$\gamma(s, t) = E[(x_s - \mu_s)(x_t - \mu_t)] = E(x_s x_t) - \mu_s \mu_t,$$

where $E[x_t] = \mu_t$.

**1.4** For the two series, $x_t$, in Problem 1.1 (a) and (b):

(a) compute and sketch the mean functions $\mu_x(t)$; for $t = 1, ..., 200$.

(b) calculate the autocovariance functions, $\gamma_x(s,t)$, for $s, t = 1, ..., 200$.

**1.5** Consider the time series

$$x_t = \beta_1 + \beta_2 t + w_t,$$

where $\beta_1$ and $\beta_2$ are known constants and $w_t$ is a white noise process with variance $\sigma^2$.

(a) Determine whether $x_t$ is stationary. If $x_t$ is not stationary, exhibit a transformation that produces a stationary process.

(b) Show that the mean of the moving average

$$y_t = \frac{1}{2q+1} \sum_{j=-q}^{q} x_{t-j}$$

is $\beta_1 + \beta_2 t$, and give a simplified expression for the autocovariance function.

**1.6** A real-valued function $f(t)$, defined on the integers, is non-negative definite if and only if

$$\sum_{s=1}^{n} \sum_{t=1}^{n} a_s f(s-t) a_t \geq 0$$

for all positive integers $n$ and for all vectors $\boldsymbol{a} = (a_1, a_2, \ldots, a_n)'$. For the matrix $F = \{f(s-t), s, t = 1, 2, \ldots, n\}$, this implies that $\boldsymbol{a}' F \boldsymbol{a} \geq 0$ for all vectors $\boldsymbol{a}$.

(a) Prove that $\gamma(h)$, the autocovariance function of a stationary process, is a non-negative definite function.

(b) Verify that the sample autocovariance $\widehat{\gamma}(h)$ is a non-negative definite function.

*Section 1.5*

**1.7** For a moving average process of the form

$$x_t = w_{t-1} + 2w_t + w_{t+1},$$

where $w_t$ are independent with zero means and variance $\sigma_w^2$, determine the autocovariance and autocorrelation functions as a function of lag $h = s - t$ and plot.

**1.8** (***Random Walk Model***). Let $w_t = 1, 2, \ldots$ be zero-mean independent random variables with variance $\sigma_w^2$. Define the process

$$x_t = \sum_{k=1}^{t} w_k$$

(a) Find the mean, and show that the autocovariance function of this process is

$$\gamma(s,t) = \sigma_w^2 \min(s,t),$$

where $\min(s,t)$ denotes the minimum of $s$ and $t$.

(b) Show that the series is nonstationary.

(c) Suggest a transformation to make the series stationary, and prove that the transformed series is stationary.

**1.9** A time series with a periodic component can be constructed from

$$x_t = u_1 \sin(2\pi\nu_0 t) + u_2 \cos(2\pi\nu_0 t),$$

where $u_1$ and $u_2$ are independent random variables with zero means and $E(u_1^2) = E(u_2^2) = \sigma^2$. The constant $\nu_0$ determines the period or time it takes the process to make one complete cycle. Show that this series is weakly stationary with autocovariance function

$$\gamma(h) = \sigma^2 \cos(2\pi\nu_0 h).$$

**1.10** Consider a process consisting of a linear trend with an additive noise term consisting of independent random variables $w_t$ with zero means and variances $\sigma_w^2$, that is,

$$x_t = \beta_0 + \beta_1 t + w_t,$$

where $\beta_0, \beta_1$ are fixed constants.

(a) Prove $x_t$ is nonstationary.

(b) Prove that the first difference series $\nabla x_t = x_t - x_{t-1}$ is stationary by finding its mean and autocovariance function.

**1.11** Suppose we would like to predict a single stationary series $x_t$ with zero mean and autocorrelation function $\gamma(h)$ at some time in the future, say, $t + \ell, \ell > 0$.

(a) If we predict using only $x_t$ and some scale multiplier $A$, show that the mean-square prediction error

$$MSE(A) = E[(x_{t+\ell} - Ax_t)^2]$$

is minimized by the value

$$A = \rho(\ell).$$

(b) Show that the minimum mean-square prediction error is

$$MSE(A) = \gamma(0)[1 - \rho^2(\ell)].$$

(c) Show that if $x_{t+\ell} = Ax_t$, $\rho(\ell) = 1$ if $A > 0$ and $\rho(\ell) = -1$ if $A < 0$.

**1.12** Consider the linear process defined in (1.26).

(a) Verify that the autocovariance function of the process is given by (1.28). Use the result to verify your answer to Problem 1.7.
(b) Show that $x_t$ exists as a limit in mean square if (1.27) holds.

**1.13** For two weakly stationary series $x_t$ and $y_t$, verify (1.25).

**1.14** Consider the two series

$$x_t = w_t$$

$$y_t = w_t - \theta w_{t-1} + u_t,$$

where $w_t$ and $u_t$ are independent white noise series with variances $\sigma_w^2$ and $\sigma_u^2$, respectively, and $\theta$ is an unspecified constant.

(a) Express the ACF $\rho_y(h), h = 0, \pm 1, \pm 2, \ldots$ of the series $y_t$ as a function of $\sigma_w^2, \sigma_u^2$, and $\theta$.
(b) Determine the CCF $\rho_{xy}(h)$ relating $x_t$ and $y_t$.
(c) Show that $x_t$ and $y_t$ are jointly stationary.

**1.15** Let $x_t$ be a stationary *normal process* with mean $\mu_x$ and autocovariance function $\gamma(h)$. Define the nonlinear time series

$$y_t = \exp\{x_t\}.$$

(a) Express the mean value function $E(y_t)$ in terms of $\mu_x$ and $\gamma(0)$. The moment generating function of a normal random variable $x$ with mean $\mu$ and variance $\sigma^2$ is

$$M_x(\lambda) = E[\exp\{\lambda x\}] = \exp\left\{\mu\lambda + \frac{1}{2}\sigma^2\lambda^2\right\}.$$

(b) Determine the autocovariance function of $y_t$. The sum of the two normal random variables $x_{t+h} + x_t$ is still a normal random variable.

**1.16** Let $w_t, t = 0, \pm 1, \pm 2, \ldots$ be a normal white noise process, and consider the series

$$x_t = w_t w_{t-1}.$$

Determine the mean and autocovariance function of $x_t$, and state whether it is stationary.

**1.17** Consider the series

$$x_t = \sin(2\pi u t),$$

$t = 1, 2, \ldots$, where $u$ has a uniform probability distribution on the interval $(0, 1)$.

(a) Prove $x_t$ is weakly stationary.

(b) Prove $x_t$ is not strictly stationary. [Hint: consider the joint bivariate cdf (1.16) at the points $t = 1, s = 2$ with $h = 1$, and find values of $c_t, c_s$ where strict stationarity does not hold.]

**1.18** Suppose we have the linear process $x_t$ generated by

$$x_t = w_t - \theta w_{t-1},$$

$t = 0, 1, 2, \ldots$, where $\{w_t\}$ is independent and identically distributed with characteristic function $\phi_w(\cdot)$, and $\theta$ is a fixed constant.

(a) Express the joint characteristic function of $x_1, x_2, \ldots, x_n$, say,

$$\phi_{x_1, x_2, \ldots, x_n}(\lambda_1, \lambda_2, \ldots, \lambda_n),$$

in terms of $\phi_w(\cdot)$.

(b) Deduce from (a) that $x_t$ is strictly stationary.

**1.19** Suppose that $x_t$ is a linear process of the form (1.26) satisfying the absolute summability condition (1.27). Prove

$$\sum_{h=-\infty}^{\infty} |\gamma(h)| < \infty.$$

*Section 1.6*

**1.20** Let $x_t$ be a weakly stationary process with mean $\mu$ and autocovariance function $\gamma(h), h = 0, \pm 1, \pm 2, \ldots$ Consider estimating the mean by

$$\bar{x} = n^{-1} \sum_{t=1}^{n} x_t,$$

the sample mean of the data points over time.

(a) Prove the estimator is unbiased, that is,

$$E(\bar{x}) = \mu.$$

(b) Show that the variance of the sample mean can be written as

$$E[(\bar{x}-\mu)^2] = n^{-1}\gamma(0) + 2n^{-1}\sum_{k=1}^{n}\left(1-\frac{k}{n}\right)\gamma(k).$$

(c) Show that the variance in (b) reduces to $\sigma^2/n$ when $x_t$ are independent zero mean variables with variance $\sigma^2$.

**1.21** Although the models in Problems 1.1 and 1.2 are not stationary (Why?), the sample ACF can be informative. For the data that you generated in those problems, calculate and plot the sample ACF, and then comment.

**1.22** Simulate series of lengths $n = 10, 100, 1000$ of the simple three-point moving average series in Example 1.16.

(a) Compare the ACF's and their confidence intervals for $n = 10, 100$ and 1000, with the theoretical values listed in (1.11).

(b) Plot the scatter diagrams for $n = 100$ relating $x_t$ to

$$x_{t-1}, x_{t-2}, \ldots, x_{t-9},$$

and explain the results.

*Section 1.7*

**1.23** The glacial varve record plotted in Figure 1.17 exhibits some nonstationarity that can be improved by transforming to logarithms and some additional nonstationarity that can be corrected by differencing the logarithms.

(a) Verify that the untransformed glacial varves has intervals over which $\hat{\gamma}(0)$ changes by computing the zero-lag autocovariance over two different intervals. Argue that the transformation $y_t = \ln x_t$ stabilizes the variance over the series. Plot the histograms of $x_t$ and $y_t$ to see whether the approximation to normality is improved by transforming the data.

(b) Show that the series $y_t$ still exhibits nonstationary behavior by examining $\hat{\rho}_y(h)$. Compute the first difference $u_t = y_t - y_{t-1}$ of the log transformed varve records, and examine the autocorrelation function $\hat{\rho}_u(h)$ for evidence of nonstationarity. Can you think of a practical interpretation for $u_t$? Do any time intervals, on the order of 100 years in this data, where one can observe behavior comparable to that observed in the global temperature records in Figure 1.2?

(c) Plot the autocorrelation of the series $u_t$, and argue that a first difference produces a reasonably stationary series.

(d) Compute the ACF of the differenced transformed series, and argue that a generalization of the model given by Example 1.19 might be reasonable. Assume

$$u_t = \mu_u + w_t - \theta w_{t-1}$$

is stationary when the inputs $w_t$ are assumed independent with mean 0 and variance $\sigma_w^2$. Show that

$$\gamma_u(h) = \begin{cases} \sigma_w^2(1+\theta^2) & \text{if } h = 0 \\ -\theta\ \sigma_w^2 & \text{if } h = \pm 1 \\ 0 & \text{if } |h| \geq 1. \end{cases}$$

Using the sample ACF and the printed autocovariance $\widehat{\gamma}_u(0)$, derive estimators for $\theta$ and $\sigma^2$. This is an application of the method of moments from classical statistics, where estimators of the parameters are derived by equating sample moments to theoretical moments.

**1.24** Consider the two time series representing average wholesale U.S. gas and oil prices over 180 months, beginning in July, 1973 and ending in December, 1987. Analyze the data using some of the techniques in this chapter with the idea that we should be looking at how changes in oil prices influence changes in gas prices. For further reading, see Liu(1991). In particular,

(a) Plot the raw data, and look at the autocorrelation functions to argue that the untransformed data series are nonstationary.

(b) It is often argued in economics that price changes are important, in particular, the percentage change in prices from one month to the next. On this basis, argue that a transformation of the form $y_t = \ln x_t - \ln x_{t-1}$ might be applied to the data, where $x_t$ is the oil or gas price series.

(c) Use lagged multiple scatterplots and the autocorrelation and cross-correlation functions of the transformed oil and gas price series to investigate the properties of these series. Is it possible to guess whether gas prices are raised more quickly in response to increasing oil prices than they are decreased when oil prices are decreased? Use the cross-correlation function over the first 100 months compared with the cross-correlation function over the last 80 months. Do you think that it might be possible to predict log percentage changes in gas prices from log percentage changes in oil prices? Plot the two series on the same scale.

*Section 1.8*

**1.25** For the Johnson & Johnson data, say $y_t$, for $t = 1, ..., 84$, shown in Figure 1.1, let $x_t = \ln(y_t)$.

(a) Fit the regression model

$$x_t = \beta t + \alpha_1 Q_1(t) + \alpha_2 Q_2(t) + \alpha_3 Q_3(t) + \alpha_4 Q_4(t) + w_t$$

where $Q_i(t) = 1$ if time $t$ corresponds to quarter $i = 1, 2, 3, 4$, and zero otherwise. The $Q_i(t)$'s are called indicator variables. We will assume for now that $w_t$ is a Gaussian white noise sequence. What is the interpretation of the parameters $\beta$, $\alpha_1$, $\alpha_2$, $\alpha_3$, and $\alpha_4$?

(b) What happens if you include an intercept term in the model in (a)?

(c) Compare the data, $x_t$, to the fitted values,

$$\widehat{x}_t = \widehat{\beta} t + \widehat{\alpha}_1 Q_1(t) + \widehat{\alpha}_2 Q_2(t) + \widehat{\alpha}_3 Q_3(t) + \widehat{\alpha}_4 Q_4(t).$$

Does it appear that the model fits the data well?

(d) Examine the residuals, $x_t - \widehat{x}_t$, assessing the Gaussian assumption and use the ACF to assess the white noise assumption of the model in (a). State your conclusions.

**1.26** For the data plotted in Figure 1.4, let $S_t$ denote the SOI index series, and let $R_t$ denote the Recruitment series.

(a) Reexamine the scatterplot matrix of $R_t$ versus $S_{t-h}$ shown in Figure 1.19 and the CCF of the two series shown in Figure 1.13, and fit the regression

$$\begin{aligned} R_t &= \alpha + \beta_0 S_t + \beta_1 S_{t-1} + \beta_2 S_{t-2} + \beta_3 S_{t-3} + \beta_4 S_{t-4} \\ &\quad + \beta_5 S_{t-5} + \beta_6 S_{t-6} + \beta_7 S_{t-7} + \beta_8 S_{t-8} + w_t. \end{aligned}$$

Compare the magnitudes and signs of the coefficients $\beta_0, ..., \beta_8$ with the scatterplots in Figure 1.19 and with the CCF in Figure 1.13.

(b) Use some of the smoothing techniques described in Section 1.8 to discover whether a trend exists in the Recruitment series, $R_t$, and to explore the periodic behavior of the data.

(c) In Example 1.25, some nonlinear behavior exists between the current value of Recruitment and past values of the SOI index. Use the smoothing techniques described in Section 1.8 to explore this possibility, concentrating on the scatterplot of $R_t$ versus $S_{t-6}$.

**1.27** ***Kullback-Leibler Information.*** Given the random vector $\boldsymbol{y}$, we define the information for discriminating between two densities in the same family, indexed by a parameter $\boldsymbol{\theta}$, say $f(\boldsymbol{y};\boldsymbol{\theta}_1)$ and $f(\boldsymbol{y};\boldsymbol{\theta}_2)$, as

$$I(\boldsymbol{\theta}_1;\boldsymbol{\theta}_2) = \frac{1}{n} E_1 \ln \frac{f(\boldsymbol{y};\boldsymbol{\theta}_1)}{f(\boldsymbol{y};\boldsymbol{\theta}_2)}, \tag{1.150}$$

where $E_1$ denotes expectation with respect to the density determined by $\boldsymbol{\theta}_1$. For the regression model, the parameters are $\boldsymbol{\theta} = (\boldsymbol{\beta}', \sigma^2)'$. Show that we obtain

$$I(\boldsymbol{\theta}_1;\boldsymbol{\theta}_2) = \frac{1}{2}\left(\frac{\sigma_1^2}{\sigma_2^2} - \ln\frac{\sigma_1^2}{\sigma_2^2} - 1\right) + \frac{1}{2}\frac{(\boldsymbol{\beta}_1 - \boldsymbol{\beta}_2)'Z'Z(\boldsymbol{\beta}_1 - \boldsymbol{\beta}_2)}{n\sigma_2^2} \tag{1.151}$$

in that case.

**1.28** ***Model Selection.*** Both selection criteria (1.66) and (1.67) are derived from information theoretic arguments, based on the well known ***Kullback-Leibler discrimination information*** numbers (see Kullback and Leibler, 1951, Kullback, 1978). We give an argument due to Hurvich and Tsai (1989). We think of the measure (1.151) as measuring the discrepancy between the two densities, characterized by the parameter values $\boldsymbol{\theta}_1' = (\boldsymbol{\beta}_1', \sigma_1^2)'$ and $\boldsymbol{\theta}_2' = (\boldsymbol{\beta}_2', \sigma_2^2)'$. Now, if the true value of the parameter vector is $\boldsymbol{\theta}_1$, we argue that the best model would be one that minimizes the discrepancy between the theoretical value and the sample, say $I(\boldsymbol{\theta}_1;\widehat{\boldsymbol{\theta}})$. Because $\boldsymbol{\theta}_1$ will not be known, Hurvich and Tsai (1989) considered finding an unbiased estimator for $E_1[I(\boldsymbol{\beta}_1, \sigma_1^2; \hat{\boldsymbol{\beta}}, \hat{\sigma}^2)]$, where

$$I(\boldsymbol{\beta}_1, \sigma_1^2; \hat{\boldsymbol{\beta}}, \hat{\sigma}^2) = \frac{1}{2}\left(\frac{\sigma_1^2}{\hat{\sigma}^2} - \ln\frac{\sigma_1^2}{\hat{\sigma}^2} - 1\right) + \frac{1}{2}\frac{(\boldsymbol{\beta}_1 - \hat{\boldsymbol{\beta}})'Z'Z(\boldsymbol{\beta}_1 - \hat{\boldsymbol{\beta}})}{n\hat{\sigma}^2}$$

and $\boldsymbol{\beta}$ is a $k \times 1$ regression vector. Show that

$$E_1[I(\boldsymbol{\beta}_1, \sigma_1^2; \hat{\boldsymbol{\beta}}, \hat{\sigma}^2)] = \frac{1}{2}\left(-\ln\sigma_1^2 + E_1 \ln\widehat{\sigma}^2 + \frac{n+k}{n-k-2}\right), \tag{1.152}$$

using the distributional properties of the regression coefficients and error variance. An unbiased estimator for $E_1 \log\widehat{\sigma}^2$ is $\log\widehat{\sigma}^2$. Hence, we have shown that the expectation of the above discrimination information is as claimed. As models with differing dimensions $k$ are considered, only the second two terms in (1.152) will vary and we only need unbiased estimators for those two terms. This gives the form of AICc quoted in (1.67) in the chapter. You will need the two distributional results

$$\frac{n\widehat{\sigma}^2}{\sigma_1^2} \sim \chi_{n-k}^2$$

and

$$\frac{(\widehat{\boldsymbol{\beta}} - \boldsymbol{\beta}_1)'Z'Z(\widehat{\boldsymbol{\beta}} - \boldsymbol{\beta}_1)}{\sigma_1^2} \sim \chi_k^2$$

The two quantities are distributed independently as chi-squared distributions with the indicated degrees of freedom. If $x \sim \chi^2_n$, $E(1/x) = 1/(n-2)$.

*Section 1.9*

**1.29** Consider a collection of time series $x_{1t}, x_{2t}, \ldots, x_{Nt}$ that are observing some common signal $\mu_t$ observed in noise processes $e_{1t}, e_{2t}, \ldots, e_{Nt}$, with a model for the jth observed series given by

$$x_{jt} = \mu_t + e_{jt}.$$

Suppose the noise series have zero means and are uncorrelated for different $j$. The common autocovariance functions of all series are given by $\gamma_e(s,t)$. Define the sample mean

$$\bar{x}_t = \frac{1}{N}\sum_{j=1}^{N} x_{jt}.$$

(a) Show that $E[\bar{x}_t] = \mu_t$.

(b) Show that $E[(\bar{x}_t - \mu)^2)] = N^{-1}\gamma(t,t)$.

(c) How can we use the results in estimating the common signal?

**1.30** A concept used in ***geostatistics***, see Journel and Huijbregts (1978) or Cressie (1993), is that of the ***variogram***, defined for a spatial process $x_{\boldsymbol{s}}$, $\boldsymbol{s} = (s_1, s_2)$, for $s_1, s_2 = 0, \pm 1, \pm 2, \ldots$, as

$$V_x(\boldsymbol{h}) = \frac{1}{2}E[(x_{\boldsymbol{s}+\boldsymbol{h}} - x_{\boldsymbol{s}})^2],$$

where $\boldsymbol{h} = (h_1, h_2)$, for $h_1, h_2 = 0, \pm 1, \pm 2, \ldots$ Show that, for a stationary process, the variogram and autocovariance functions can be related through

$$V_x(\boldsymbol{h}) = \gamma(\boldsymbol{0}) - \gamma(\boldsymbol{h}),$$

where $\gamma(\boldsymbol{h})$ is the usual lag $\boldsymbol{h}$ covariance function and $\boldsymbol{0} = (0,0)$. Note the easy extension to any spatial dimension.

*Section T1.10*

**1.31** Let $x_n, n = 1, 2, \ldots$ be a sequence of $L^2$ random variables, and suppose that

$$E(x_n^2) = O(a_n^2).$$

Prove that $x_n = O_p(a_n)$.

**1.32** If the sequence of $L^2$ random variables $x_n$ is such that $E(x_n) \to \mu$ and

$$E[(x_n - Ex_n)^2] \to 0,$$

$x_n \xrightarrow{p} \mu$.

**1.33** Show that, if $x_n \xrightarrow{d} x, y_n \xrightarrow{d} y$, with $x_n$ and $y_n$ independent, then $x_n + y_n \xrightarrow{d} x + y$, with $x$ and $y$ independent.

*Section T1.12*

**1.34** Suppose

$$x_t = \beta_0 + \beta_1 t,$$

where $\beta_0$ and $\beta_1$ are constants. Prove as $n \to \infty$,

$$\widehat{\rho}_x(h) \to 1$$

for fixed $h$, where $\widehat{\rho}_x(h)$ is the ACF (1.32).

**1.35** Suppose $x_t$ is a weakly stationary time series with mean zero and with absolutely summable autocovariance function, $\gamma(h)$, such that

$$\sum_{h=-\infty}^{\infty} \gamma(h) = 0.$$

Prove that $\sqrt{n}\,\bar{x} \xrightarrow{p} 0$, where $\bar{x}$ is the sample mean (1.30).

**1.36** Let $x_t$ be a linear process of the form (1.26), satisfying (1.27). If we define

$$\tilde{\gamma}(h) = n^{-1} \sum_{t=1}^{n} (x_{t+h} - \mu_x)(x_t - \mu_x),$$

show that

$$n^{1/2}\big(\tilde{\gamma}(h) - \widehat{\gamma}(h)\big) = o_p(1).$$

Hint: The Markov Inequality

$$P\{|x| \ge \epsilon\} < \frac{E|x|}{\epsilon}$$

can be helpful for the cross-product terms.

**1.37** For a linear process of the form

$$x_t = \sum_{j=0}^{\infty} \phi_1^j w_{t-j},$$

with $|\phi_1| < 1$, show that

$$\sqrt{n}\frac{(\widehat{\rho}_x(1) - \rho_x(1))}{\sqrt{1 - \rho_x^2(1)}} \xrightarrow{d} N(0,1),$$

and construct a 95% confidence interval for $\phi_1$ when $\widehat{\rho}_x(1) = .64$.

# CHAPTER 2

# Time Series Regression and ARIMA Models

## 2.1 Introduction

In Chapter 1, we introduced autocorrelation and cross-correlation functions (ACF's and CCF's) as tools for clarifying relations that may occur within and between time series at various lags. In addition, we have explained how to build linear models based on classical regression theory for exploiting the associations indicated by large values of the ACF or CCF. The time domain methods of this chapter, contrasted with the frequency domain methods introduced in later chapters, are appropriate when we are dealing with possibly nonstationary, shorter time series; these series are the rule rather than the exception in applications arising in economics and the social sciences. In addition, the emphasis in these fields is usually on forecasting future values, which is easily treated as a regression problem. This chapter develops a number of regression techniques for time series that are all related to classical ordinary and weighted or correlated least squares.

Classical regression is often insufficient for explaining all of the interesting dynamics of a time series. For example, the ACF of the residuals of the simple linear regression fit to the global temperature data (see Example 1.22 of Chapter 1) reveals additional structure in the data that the regression did not capture. Instead, the introduction of correlation as a phenomenon that may be generated through lagged linear relations leads to proposing the ***autoregressive (AR)*** and ***autoregressive moving average (ARMA)*** models. Adding nonstationary models to the mix leads to the ***autoregressive integrated moving average (ARIMA)*** model popularized in the landmark work by Box and Jenkins (1970). The ***Box–Jenkins method*** for identifying a plausible ARIMA model is given in this chapter along with techniques for ***parameter estimation*** and ***forecasting*** for these models. In the later sections, we present ***long memory ARMA***, ***threshold autoregressive models***, ***regression with ARMA errors***, and an extension of the Box–Jenkins method for predicting a single output from a collection of possible input series is considered where the inputs themselves may follow ARIMA models, commonly referred to as ***transfer function models***. Finally, we present ***ARCH models*** and the analysis of volatility.

## 2.2 Autoregressive Moving Average Models

The classical regression model in Section 1.8 of Chapter 1 was developed for the static case, namely, we only allow the dependent variable to be influenced by current values of the independent variables. In the time series case, it is desirable to allow the dependent variable to be influenced by the past values of the independent variables and possibly by its own past values. If the present can be plausibly modeled in terms of only the past values of the independent inputs, we have the enticing prospect that forecasting will be possible.

### Introduction to Autoregressive Models

***Autoregressive models*** are created with the idea that the present value of the series, $x_t$, can be explained as a function of $p$ past values, $x_{t-1}, x_{t-2}, \ldots, x_{t-p}$, where $p$ determines the number of steps into the past needed to forecast the current value. As a typical case, recall Example 1.9 in which data were generated using the model

$$x_t = x_{t-1} - .90x_{t-2} + w_t,$$

where $w_t$ is white Gaussian noise with $\sigma_w^2 = 1$. We have now assumed the current value is a particular *linear* function of past values. The regularity that persists in Figure 1.8 gives an indication that forecasting for such a model might be a distinct possibility, say, through some version such as

$$x_{t+1}^t = x_t - .90x_{t-1},$$

where the quantity on the left-hand side denotes the forecast at the next period $t+1$ based on current and past observed values $x_1, x_2, ..., x_t$. We will make this notion more precise in our discussion of forecasting (Section 2.5).

The extent to which it might be possible to forecast a real data series from its own past values can be assessed by looking at the autocorrelation function and the lagged scatterplot matrices discussed in Chapter 1. For example, the lagged scatterplot matrix for the Southern Oscillation Index (SOI), shown in Figure 1.18, gives a distinct indication that lags 1 and 2, for example, are linearly associated with the present value. The ACF shown in Figure 1.13 shows relatively large positive values at lags 1, 2, 12, 24, and 36 and large negative values at 18, 30, and 42. We note also the possible relation between the SOI and Recruitment series indicated in the scatterplot matrix shown in Figure 1.19. We will indicate in later sections on transfer function and vector AR modeling how to handle the dependence on values taken by other series.

The preceding discussion motivates the definition of an ***autoregressive model of order p***, abbreviated as ***AR(p)***, of the form

$$x_t = \phi_1 x_{t-1} + \phi_2 x_{t-2} + \ldots + \phi_p x_{t-p} + w_t, \tag{2.1}$$

where $\phi_1, \phi_2, \ldots, \phi_p$ are constants and $w_t$ is a white noise series with mean zero and variance $\sigma_w^2$. We assume for simplicity in notation that the mean of $x_t$ is zero. If the mean, $\mu$, of $x_t$ is not zero, we can replace $x_t$ by $x_t - \mu$ in (2.1), or write

$$x_t = \alpha + \phi_1 x_{t-1} + \phi_2 x_{t-2} + \ldots + \phi_p x_{t-p} + w_t, \tag{2.2}$$

where $\alpha = \mu(1 - \phi_1 - \cdots - \phi_p)$. We note several different ways (2.1) can be written that will be used in the sequel. First, define $\boldsymbol{\phi} = (\phi_1, \phi_2, \ldots, \phi_p)'$ and $\boldsymbol{x}_{t-1} = (x_{t-1}, x_{t-2}, \ldots, x_{t-p})'$ so that

$$x_t = \boldsymbol{\phi}' \boldsymbol{x}_{t-1} + w_t \tag{2.3}$$

and the AR($p$) model becomes the regression model of Section 1.8. Some technical difficulties, however, develop from applying that model because $\boldsymbol{x}_{t-1}$ has random components, whereas $\boldsymbol{z}_t$ was assumed to be fixed. A second useful form follows by using the backshift operator (1.41) to write the AR($p$) model, (2.1), as

$$(1 - \phi_1 B - \phi_2 B^2 - \ldots - \phi_p B^p) x_t = w_t, \tag{2.4}$$

or even more concisely as

$$\phi(B) x_t = w_t, \tag{2.5}$$

where the ***autoregressive operator***

$$\phi(B) = 1 - \phi_1 B - \phi_2 B^2 - \ldots - \phi_p B^p \tag{2.6}$$

is an operator whose properties are important in solving (2.5) for $x_t$.

We initiate the investigation of AR models by considering the first-order model, AR(1), given by $x_t = \phi x_{t-1} + w_t$. Iterating backwards $k$ times, we get

$$\begin{aligned} x_t &= \phi x_{t-1} + w_t = \phi(\phi x_{t-2} + w_{t-1}) + w_t \\ &= \phi^2 x_{t-2} + \phi w_{t-1} + w_t \\ &\vdots \\ &= \phi^k x_{t-k} + \sum_{j=0}^{k-1} \phi^j w_{t-j}. \end{aligned}$$

This method suggests that, by continuing to iterate backwards, and provided that $|\phi| < 1$ and the variance of $x_t$ is bounded, we can represent an AR(1) model by

$$x_t = \sum_{j=0}^{\infty} \phi^j w_{t-j}, \tag{2.7}$$

in the mean square sense (see Section T1.10). This conclusion follows from the fact that

$$\lim_{k\to\infty} E\left(x_t - \sum_{j=0}^{k-1}\phi^j w_{t-j}\right)^2 = \lim_{k\to\infty}\phi^{2k}E\left(x_{t-k}^2\right) = 0.$$

Alternately, we could simply have defined an AR(1) model to be the stationary process given in equation (2.7), because, with $|\phi| < 1$,

$$\begin{aligned} x_t &= \sum_{j=0}^{\infty}\phi^j w_{t-j} = (\sum_{j=1}^{\infty}\phi^j w_{t-j}) + w_t \\ &= \phi(\sum_{j=0}^{\infty}\phi^j w_{t-1-j}) + w_t = \phi x_{t-1} + w_t. \end{aligned} \tag{2.8}$$

The AR(1) process defined by (2.7) is stationary with mean

$$E(x_t) = \sum_{j=0}^{\infty}\phi^j E(w_{t-j}) = 0,$$

and autocovariance function,

$$\begin{aligned} \gamma(h) &= \text{cov}(x_{t+h}, x_t) = E\left[\left(\sum_{j=0}^{\infty}\phi^j w_{t+h-j}\right)\left(\sum_{k=0}^{\infty}\phi^j w_{t-k}\right)\right] \\ &= \sigma_w^2\sum_{j=0}^{\infty}\phi^j\phi^{j+h} = \sigma_w^2\phi^h\sum_{j=0}^{\infty}\phi^{2j} = \frac{\sigma_w^2\phi^h}{1-\phi^2}, \quad h \geq 0. \end{aligned} \tag{2.9}$$

Recall that $\gamma(h) = \gamma(-h)$, so we will only exhibit the autocovariance function for $h \geq 0$. From (2.9), the ACF of an AR(1) is

$$\rho(h) = \frac{\gamma(h)}{\gamma(0)} = \phi^h, \quad h \geq 0, \tag{2.10}$$

and $\rho(h)$ satisfies the recursion

$$\rho(h) = \phi\rho(h-1), \quad h \geq 1. \tag{2.11}$$

Well will discuss the ACF of a general AR($p$) model in Section 2.4.

**Example 2.1 The Sample Path of an AR(1) Process**

Figure 2.1 shows a time plot of two AR(1) processes, one with $\phi = 0.9$ and one with $\phi = -0.9$; in both cases, $\sigma_w^2 = 1$. In the first case, $\rho(h) = .9^h$, for $h \geq 0$, so the observations close together in time are positively correlated with each other. This result means that the observations at

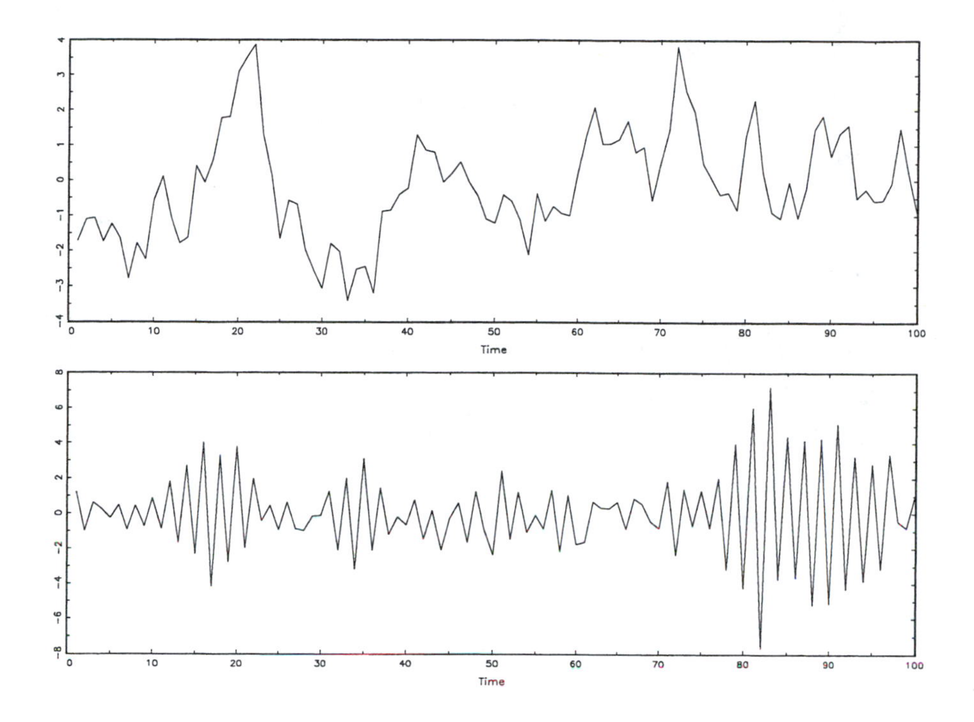


**Figure 2.1:** Simulated AR(1) models: $\phi = 0.9$ (top); $\phi = -0.9$ (bottom).

contiguous time points will tend be close in value to each other; this fact shows up in top of Figure 2.1 as a very smooth sample path for $x_t$. Now, contrast this to the case in which $\phi = -0.9$, so that $\rho(h) = (-.9)^h$, for $h \geq 0$. This result means that observations at contiguous time points are negatively correlated but observations two time points apart are positively correlated. This fact shows up in the bottom of Figure 2.1, where if an observation, $x_t$, is positive [negative], the next observation, $x_{t+1}$, is typically negative [positive], and the next observation, $x_{t+2}$ is typically positive [negative]. Thus, in this case, the sample path is very choppy.

### Example 2.2 Explosive AR Models and Causality

In Chapter 1, Problem 1.8, it was discovered that the random walk $x_t = x_{t-1} + w_t$ is not stationary. We might wonder whether there is a stationary AR(1) process with $|\phi| > 1$. Such processes are called explosive because the values of the time series quickly become large in magnitude. Clearly, $\sum_{j=0}^{k-1} \phi^j w_{t-j}$ will not converge in mean square as $k \to \infty$, so the intuition used to get (2.7) will not work directly. We can, however, modify that argument to obtain a stationary model as follows. Write $x_{t+1} = \phi x_t + w_{t+1}$, in which case,

$$\begin{aligned} x_t &= \phi^{-1} x_{t+1} - \phi^{-1} w_{t+1} = \phi^{-1}\left(\phi^{-1} x_{t+2} - \phi^{-1} w_{t+2}\right) - \phi^{-1} w_{t+1} \\ &\vdots \\ &= \phi^{-k} x_{t+k} - \sum_{j=1}^{k-1} \phi^{-j} w_{t+j}, \end{aligned} \tag{2.12}$$

by iterating forward $k$ steps. Because $|\phi^{-1}| < 1$, this result suggests the stationary future dependent AR(1) model

$$x_t = -\sum_{j=1}^{\infty} \phi^{-j} w_{t+j}.$$

The reader can verify that this is stationary and of the AR(1) form $x_t = \phi x_{t-1} + w_t$. Unfortunately, this model is useless because it requires us to know the future to be able to predict the future. When a process does not depend on the future, such as the AR(1) when $|\phi| < 1$, we will say the process is ***causal.*** In the explosive case of this example, the process is stationary, but it is also future dependent, and not causal.

The technique of iterating backwards to get an idea of the stationary solution of AR models works well when $p = 1$, but not for larger orders. A general technique is that of matching coefficients. Consider the AR(1) model in operator form

$$\phi(B) x_t = w_t, \tag{2.13}$$

where $\phi(B) = 1 - \phi B$, and $|\phi| < 1$. Also, write the model in equation (2.7) using operator form as

$$x_t = \sum_{j=0}^{\infty} \psi_j w_{t-j} = \psi(B) w_t, \tag{2.14}$$

where $\psi(B) = \sum_{j=0}^{\infty} \psi_j B^j$ and $\psi_j = \phi^j$. Suppose we did not know that $\psi_j = \phi^j$. We could substitute $\phi(B)x_t$ from (2.13) for $w_t$ in (2.14) to obtain

$$x_t = \psi(B) w_t = \psi(B)\phi(B) x_t. \tag{2.15}$$

Equating coefficients on the left- and right-hand sides of (2.15), we get

$$1 = (1 + \psi_1 B + \psi_2 B^2 + \cdots + \psi_j B^j + \cdots)(1 - \phi B). \tag{2.16}$$

Reorganizing the coefficients in (2.16),

$$1 = 1 + (\psi_1 - \phi)B + (\psi_2 - \psi_1\phi)B^2 + \cdots + (\psi_j - \psi_{j-1}\phi)B^j + \cdots,$$

we see that for each $j = 1, 2, ...$, the coefficient of $B^j$ on the right, must be zero (because it is zero on the left). The coefficient of $B$ on the right is $(\psi_1 - \phi)$, and equating this to zero, $\psi_1 - \phi = 0$, leads to $\psi_1 = \phi$. Continuing, the coefficient of $B^2$ is $(\psi_2 - \psi_1\phi)$, so $\psi_2 = \phi^2$. In general, $\psi_j - \psi_{j-1}\phi = 0$, which leads to the general solution $\psi_j = \phi^j$.

This example makes it clear that $\psi(B)$ is also the inverse of the operator $\phi(B)$. In operator form, we took the following steps starting with the AR(1) model, $\phi(B)x_t = w_t$, where $\phi(B) = (1 - \phi B)$.

(i) Multiply each side by the inverse operator (assuming it exists)

$$\phi^{-1}(B)\phi(B)x_t = \phi^{-1}(B)w_t.$$

(ii) Write the result as $x_t = \psi(B)w_t$, where we defined $\psi(B) = \phi^{-1}(B)$.

(iii) Solve for $\phi^{-1}(B)$ by matching the coefficients in $\psi(B)\phi(B) = 1$.

The solution, of course, was $\phi^{-1}(B) = 1 + \phi B + \phi^2 B^2 + \cdots + \phi^j B^j + \cdots$. Notice the operators behave like polynomials. That is, consider the polynomial $\phi(z) = 1 - \phi z$, where $z$ is a complex number and $|\phi| < 1$. Then,

$$\phi^{-1}(z) = \frac{1}{(1 - \phi z)} = 1 + \phi z + \phi^2 z^2 + \cdots + \phi^j z^j + \cdots, \quad |z| \leq 1.$$

These results will be generalized in our discussion of ARMA models. We will find the polynomials corresponding to the operators useful in exploring the general properties of ARMA models.

### Introduction to Moving Average Models

As an alternative to the autoregressive representation in which the $x_t$ on the left-hand side of the equation are assumed to be combined linearly, the ***moving average model of order q***, abbreviated as ***MA(q)***, assumes the white noise $w_t$ on the right-hand side of the defining equation are combined linearly to form the observed data. In such cases, we write

$$x_t = w_t + \theta_1 w_{t-1} + \theta_2 w_{t-2} + \ldots + \theta_q w_{t-q} \tag{2.17}$$

where there are $q$ lags in the moving average and $\theta_1, \theta_2, \ldots, \theta_q$ are parameters that determine the overall pattern of the process. The system is the same as the infinite moving average defined as the linear process (2.14), where $\psi_0 = 1$, $\psi_j = \theta_j, j = 1, \ldots, q$, and $\psi_j = 0$ for other values. We may also write the MA($q$) process in the equivalent form

$$x_t = \theta(B)w_t, \tag{2.18}$$

where the ***moving average operator***

$$\theta(B) = 1 + \theta_1 B + \theta_2 B^2 + \ldots + \theta_q B^q \tag{2.19}$$

defines a linear combination of values in the shift operator $B^k w_t = w_{t-k}$ as before.

Unlike the autoregressive process, the moving average process is stationary for any values of the parameters $\theta_1, ..., \theta_q$; details of this result are provided in Section 2.4.

**Example 2.3 Autocorrelation and Sample Path of an MA(1) Process**

Consider the MA(1) model $x_t = w_t + \theta w_{t-1}$. Then,

$$\gamma(h) = \begin{cases} (1+\theta^2)\sigma_w^2, & h = 0 \\ \theta\sigma_w^2, & h = 1 \\ 0, & h > 1, \end{cases}$$

and the autocorrelation function is

$$\rho(h) = \begin{cases} \frac{\theta}{(1+\theta^2)}, & h = 1 \\ 0, & h > 1. \end{cases}$$

The ACF of a general MA($q$) model will be presented in Section 2.4.

Note $|\rho(1)| \leq 1/2$ for all values of $\theta$ (Problem 2.1). The time series is "one-dependent;" that is, $x_t$ is correlated with $x_{t-1}$, but not with $x_{t-2}, x_{t-3}, \ldots$ . Contrast this with the case of the AR(1) model in which the correlation between $x_t$ and $x_{t-k}$ is never zero. When $\theta = 0.5$, for example, $x_t$ and $x_{t-1}$ are positively correlated, and $\rho(1) = 0.4$. When $\theta = -0.5$, $x_t$ and $x_{t-1}$ are negatively correlated, $\rho(1) = -0.4$. Figure 2.2 shows a time plot of these two processes with $\sigma_w^2 = 1$. The series in Figure 2.2, where $\theta = 0.5$, is smoother than the series in Figure 2.2, where $\theta = -0.5$.

**Example 2.4 Non-uniqueness of MA Models and Invertibility**

From Example 2.3, for an MA(1) model, $\rho(h)$ is the same for $\theta$ and $\frac{1}{\theta}$; try 5 and $\frac{1}{5}$, for example. In addition, the pair $\sigma_w^2 = 1$ and $\theta = 5$ yield the same autocovariance function as the pair $\sigma_w^2 = 25$ and $\theta = 1/5$, namely,

$$\gamma(h) = \begin{cases} 26, & h = 0 \\ 5, & h = 1 \\ 0, & h > 1. \end{cases}$$

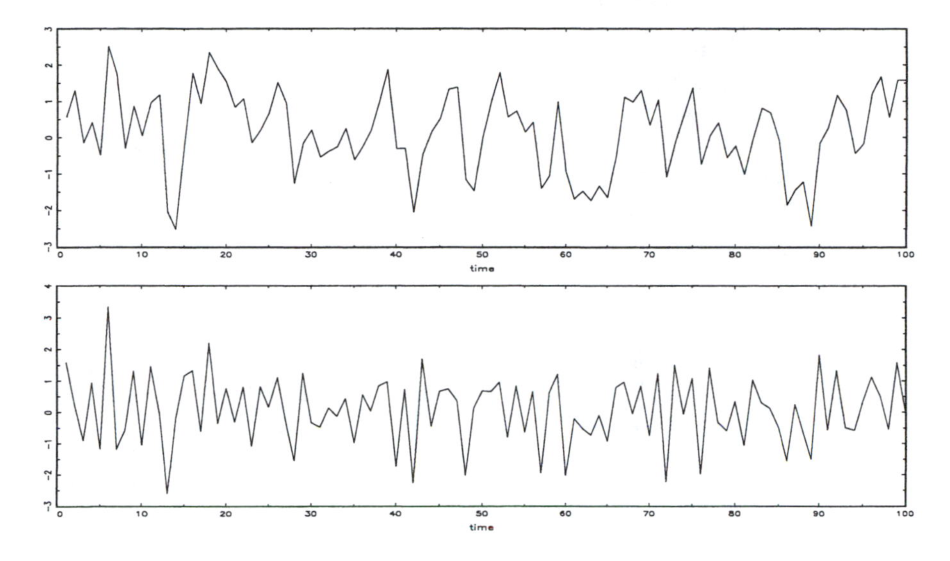


**Figure 2.2:** Simulated MA(1) models: $\theta = 0.5$ (top); $\theta = -0.5$ (bottom).

Thus, the MA(1) processes

$$x_t = w_t + \frac{1}{5}w_{t-1}, \quad w_t \sim \text{iid } \text{N}(0, 25)$$

and

$$x_t = v_t + 5v_{t-1}, \quad v_t \sim \text{iid } \text{N}(0, 1)$$

are the same. We can only observe the time series $x_t$ and not the noise, $w_t$ or $v_t$, so we cannot distinguish between the models. Hence, we will have to choose only one of them. For convenience, by mimicking the criterion of causality for AR models, we will choose the model with an infinite AR representation. Such a process is called an ***invertible*** process.

To discover which model is the invertible model, we can reverse the roles of $x_t$ and $w_t$ (because we are mimicking the AR case) and write the MA(1) model as $w_t = -\theta w_{t-1} + x_t$. Following the steps that led to (2.40), if $|\theta| < 1$, then $w_t = \sum_{j=0}^{\infty}(-\theta)^j x_{t-j}$, which is the desired infinite AR representation of the model. Hence, given a choice, we will choose the model with $\sigma_w^2 = 25$ and $\theta = 1/5$ because it is invertible.

As in the AR case, the polynomials, $\theta(z)$, corresponding to the moving average operators, $\theta(B)$, will be useful in exploring general properties of MA processes. For example, following the steps of equations (2.13)-(2.16), we can write the MA(1) model as $x_t = \theta(B)w_t$, where $\theta(B) = 1 + \theta B$. If $|\theta| < 1$, then we can write the model as $\pi(B)x_t = w_t$, where $\pi(B) = \theta^{-1}(B)$. Let $\theta(z) = 1 + \theta z$, for $|z| \leq 1$, then $\pi(z) = \theta^{-1}(z) = 1/(1+\theta z) = \sum_{j=0}^{\infty}(-\theta)^j z^j$, and we determine that $\pi(B) = \sum_{j=0}^{\infty}(-\theta)^j B^j$.

AUTOREGRESSIVE MOVING AVERAGE MODELS

We now proceed with the general development of autoregressive, moving average, and mixed ***autoregressive moving average (ARMA)*** models for stationary time series. A time series $x_t$, for $t = 0, \pm1, \pm2, ...$, is said to be ARMA$(p,q)$ if $x_t$ is stationary and

$$x_t = \phi_1 x_{t-1} + \cdots + \phi_p x_{t-p} + w_t + \theta_1 w_{t-1} + \cdots + \theta_q w_{t-q}, \tag{2.20}$$

with $\phi_p \neq 0$, $\theta_q \neq 0$, and $\sigma_w^2 > 0$. The parameters $p$ and $q$ are called the autoregressive and the moving average orders, respectively. As before, if $x_t$ has a nonzero mean $\mu$, we set $\alpha = \mu(1 - \phi_1 - \cdots - \phi_p)$ and write the model as

$$x_t = \alpha + \phi_1 x_{t-1} + \cdots \phi_p x_{t-p} + w_t + \theta_1 w_{t-1} + \cdots \theta_q w_{t-q}. \tag{2.21}$$

As previously noted, when $q = 0$, the model is called an autoregressive model of order $p$, AR$(p)$, and when $p = 0$, the model is called a moving average model of order $q$, MA$(q)$. To aid in the investigation of ARMA models, it will be useful to write them using the AR operator, (2.6), and the MA operator, (2.19). In particular, the ARMA$(p,q)$ model in (2.20) can then can be written in concise form as

$$\phi(B)x_t = \theta(B)w_t. \tag{2.22}$$

Before we discuss the conditions under which (2.20) is causal and invertible, we point out a potential problem with the ARMA model.

**Example 2.5 Parameter Redundancy**

Consider a white noise process $x_t = w_t$. Equivalently, we can write this as $0.5x_{t-1} = 0.5w_{t-1}$ by shifting back one unit of time and multiplying by 0.5. Now, subtract the two representations to obtain

$$x_t - 0.5x_{t-1} = w_t - 0.5w_{t-1},$$

or

$$x_t = 0.5x_{t-1} - 0.5w_{t-1} + w_t,$$

which looks like an ARMA(1,1) model. Of course, $x_t$ is still white noise; nothing has changed in this regard, but we have hidden the fact that $x_t$ is white noise because of the ***parameter redundancy*** or overparameterization. Write the parameter redundant model in operator form:

$$(1 - 0.5B)x_t = (1 - 0.5B)w_t.$$

Apply the operator $(1 - 0.5B)^{-1}$ to both sides to obtain

$$x_t = (1 - 0.5B)^{-1}(1 - 0.5B)x_t = (1 - 0.5B)^{-1}(1 - 0.5B)w_t = w_t,$$

which is the original model. We can easily detect the problem of over-parameterization with the use of polynomials by writing the AR polynomial $\phi(z) = (1 - 0.5z)$, the MA polynomial $\theta(z) = (1 - 0.5z)$, and noting that both polynomials have a ***common factor***, namely $(1 - 0.5z)$. This common factor immediately identifies the parameter redundancy. Discarding the common factor in each leaves $\phi(z) = 1$ and $\theta(z) = 1$, and we deduce that the model is actually white noise. The consideration of parameter redundancy will be crucial when we discuss estimation for general ARMA models. As this example points out, we might fit an ARMA(1,1) model to white noise data and find that the parameter estimates are significant. If we were unaware of parameter redundancy, we might claim the data are correlated when in fact they are not (Problem 2.19).

Examples 2.2, 2.4, and 2.5 point to a number of problems with the general definition of ARMA$(p, q)$ models, as given by (2.20), or, equivalently, by (2.22). To summarize, we have seen the following problems:

(i) parameter redundant models,

(ii) stationary AR models that depend on the future, and

(iii) MA models that are not unique.

To overcome these problems, we will require some additional restrictions on the model parameters. First, we define the ***AR and MA polynomials*** as

$$\phi(z) = 1 - \phi_1 z - \cdots - \phi_p z^p, \quad \phi_p \neq 0, \tag{2.23}$$

and

$$\theta(z) = 1 + \theta_1 z + \cdots + \theta_q z^q, \quad \theta_q \neq 0, \tag{2.24}$$

respectively, where $z$ is a complex number.

To address the first problem, we will henceforth refer to an ARMA$(p, q)$ model to mean that it is in its simplest form. That is, in addition to the original definition given in equation (2.20), ***we will also require that $\phi(z)$ and $\theta(z)$ have no common factors***. So, the process, $x_t = 0.5x_{t-1} - 0.5w_{t-1} + w_t$, discussed in Example 2.5 is not referred to as an ARMA(1,1) process because, in its reduced form, $x_t$ is white noise.

To address the problem of future-dependent models, we formally introduce the concept of ***causality***. An ARMA$(p, q)$ model, $\phi(B)x_t = \theta(B)w_t$, is said to be causal, if the time series $x_t$, $t = 0, \pm 1, \pm 2, ...$, can be written as a one-sided linear process:

$$x_t = \sum_{j=0}^{\infty} \psi_j w_{t-j} = \psi(B)w_t, \tag{2.25}$$

where $\psi(B) = \sum_{j=0}^{\infty} \psi_j B^j$, and $\sum_{j=0}^{\infty} |\psi_j| < \infty$; we set $\psi_0 = 1$.

In Example 2.2, the AR(1) process, $x_t = \phi x_{t-1} + w_t$, is causal only when $|\phi| < 1$. Equivalently, the process is causal only when the root of $\phi(z) = 1 - \phi z$ is bigger than one in absolute value. That is, the root, say, $z_0$, of $\phi(z)$ is $z_0 = 1/\phi$ [because $\phi(z_0) = 0$] and $|z_0| > 1$ because $|\phi| < 1$. In general, we have the following property.

***Property P2.1: Causality of an ARMA(p, q) Process***
*An ARMA(p,q) model is causal only when the roots of $\phi(z)$ lie outside the unit circle; that is, $\phi(z) = 0$ only when $|z| > 1$. The coefficients of the linear process given in (2.25) can be determined by solving*

$$\psi(z) = \sum_{j=0}^{\infty} \psi_j z^j = \frac{\theta(z)}{\phi(z)}, \quad |z| \le 1.$$

Finally, to address the problem of uniqueness discussed in Example 2.4, we choose the model that allows an infinite autoregressive representation. In particular, an ARMA$(p, q)$ model, $\phi(B)x_t = \theta(B)w_t$, is said to be ***invertible***, if the time series $x_t$, $t = 0, \pm 1, \pm 2, \ldots$, can be written as

$$\pi(B)x_t = \sum_{j=0}^{\infty} \pi_j x_{t-j} = w_t, \tag{2.26}$$

where $\pi(B) = \sum_{j=0}^{\infty} \pi_j B^j$, and $\sum_{j=0}^{\infty} |\pi_j| < \infty$; we set $\pi_0 = 1$. Analogous to Property P2.1, we have the following property.

***Property P2.2: Invertibility of an ARMA(p, q) Process***
*An ARMA(p,q) model is invertible only when the roots of $\theta(z)$ lie outside the unit circle. The coefficients $\pi_j$ of $\pi(B)$ given in (2.26) can be determined by solving*

$$\pi(z) = \sum_{j=0}^{\infty} \pi_j z^j = \frac{\phi(z)}{\theta(z)}, \quad |z| \le 1.$$

The proof of Property P2.1 is given in Section T2.16 (the proof of Property P2.2 is similar and, hence, is not provided). The following examples illustrate these concepts.

**Example 2.6 Parameter Redundancy, Causality, and Invertiblity**

Consider the process

$$x_t = 0.4x_{t-1} + 0.45x_{t-2} + w_{t-1} + 0.25w_{t-2} + w_t,$$

or, in operator form,

$$(1 - 0.4B - 0.45B^2)x_t = (1 + B + 0.25B^2)w_t.$$

At first, $x_t$ appears to be an ARMA(2,2) process. But, the associated polynomials $\phi(z) = 1 - 0.4z - 0.45z^2 = (1+0.5z)(1-0.9z)$, and, $\theta(z) = (1+z+0.25z^2) = (1+0.5z)^2$, have a common factor that can be cancelled. After cancellation, the polynomials become $\phi(z) = (1-0.9z)$ and $\theta(z) = (1+0.5z)$, so the model is an ARMA(1,1) model, $(1-0.9B)x_t = (1+0.5B)w_t$, or

$$x_t = 0.9x_{t-1} + 0.5w_{t-1} + w_t. \tag{2.27}$$

The model is causal because $\phi(z) = (1-0.9z) = 0$ when $z = 10/9$, which is outside the unit circle. The model is also invertible because the root of $\theta(z) = (1+0.5z)$ is $z = -2$, which is outside the unit circle.

To write the model as a linear process, we can obtain the $\psi$-weights using Property P2.1:

$$\begin{aligned}\psi(z) &= \frac{\theta(z)}{\phi(z)} = \frac{(1+0.5z)}{(1-0.9z)} \\ &= (1+0.5z)(1+0.9z+0.9^2z^2+0.9^3z^3+\cdots) \quad |z| \le 1.\end{aligned}$$

The coefficient of $z^j$ in $\psi(z)$ is $\psi_j = (0.5+0.9)0.9^{j-1}$, for $j \ge 1$, so (2.27) can be written as

$$x_t = w_t + 1.4\sum_{j=1}^{\infty} 0.9^{j-1} w_{t-j}.$$

Similarly, to find the invertible representation using Property P2.2:

$$\pi(z) = \frac{\phi(z)}{\theta(z)} = (1-0.9z)(1-0.5z+0.5^2z^2-0.5^3z^3+\cdots) \quad |z| \le 1.$$

In this case, the $\pi$-weights are given by $\pi_j = (-1)^j(0.9+0.5)0.5^{j-1}$, for $j \ge 1$, and hence, we can also write (2.27) as

$$x_t = 1.4\sum_{j=1}^{\infty}(-0.5)^{j-1}x_{t-j} + w_t.$$

### Example 2.7 Causal Conditions for an AR(2) Process

For an AR(1) model, $(1-\phi B)x_t = w_t$, to be causal, the root of $\phi(z) = 1-\phi z$ must lie outside of the unit circle. In this case, the root is $z = 1/\phi$, so that it is easy to go from the causal requirement on the root, that is, $|1/\phi| > 1$, to a requirement on the parameter, that is, $|\phi| < 1$. It is not so easy to establish this relationship for higher order models.

For example, the AR(2) model, $(1-\phi_1 B-\phi_2 B^2)x_t = w_t$, is causal when the two roots of $\phi(z) = 1-\phi_1 z-\phi_2 z^2$ lie outside of the unit circle. Using the quadratic formula, this requirement can be written as

$$\left|\frac{\phi_1 \pm \sqrt{\phi_1^2+4\phi_2}}{-2\phi_2}\right| > 1.$$

The roots of $\phi(z)$ may be real and distinct, real and equal, or a complex conjugate pair. If we denote those roots by $z_1$ and $z_2$, we can write $\phi(z) = (1-z_1^{-1}z)(1-z_2^{-1}z)$; note that $\phi(z_1) = \phi(z_2) = 0$. The model can be written in operator form as $(1-z_1^{-1}B)(1-z_2^{-1}B)x_t = w_t$. From this representation, it follows that $\phi_1 = (z_1^{-1}+z_2^{-1})$ and $\phi_2 = -(z_1 z_2)^{-1}$. This relationship can be used to establish the following equivalent condition for causality:

$$\phi_1+\phi_2 < 1, \quad \phi_2-\phi_1 < 1, \quad \text{and} \quad |\phi_2| < 1. \tag{2.28}$$

This causality condition specifies a triangular region in the parameter space. We leave the details of the equivalence to the reader (Problem 2.4).

## 2.3 Homogeneous Difference Equations

The study of the behavior of ARMA processes is greatly enhanced by the use of homogeneous difference equations. This topic is also useful in the study of time domain models and stochastic processes in general. We will give a brief and heuristic account of the topic along with some examples of the usefulness of the theory. For details, the reader is referred to Mickens (1987).

Suppose we have a sequence of numbers $u_0, u_1, u_2, \ldots$ such that

$$u_n - \alpha u_{n-1} = 0, \quad \alpha \neq 0, \quad n = 1,2,\ldots \tag{2.29}$$

For example, recall (2.11) in which we showed that the ACF of an AR(1) process is a sequence, $\rho(h)$, satisfying $\rho(h) = \phi\rho(h-1)$, for $h = 1,2,\ldots$ Equation (2.29) represents a ***homogeneous difference equation of order 1***. To solve the equation, we write:

$$\begin{aligned}
u_1 &= \alpha u_0 \\
u_2 &= \alpha u_1 = \alpha^2 u_0 \\
&\vdots \\
u_n &= \alpha u_{n-1} = \alpha^n u_0.
\end{aligned}$$

Given an initial condition $u_0 = c$, we may solve (2.29), namely, $u_n = \alpha^n c$.

In operator notation, (2.29) can be written as $(1 - \alpha B)u_n = 0$. The polynomial associated with (2.29) is $\alpha(z) = 1 - \alpha z$, and the root, say, $z_0$, of this polynomial is $z_0 = 1/\alpha$; that is $\alpha(z_0) = 0$. We know the solution to (2.29), with initial condition $u_0 = c$, is

$$u_n = \alpha^n c = \left(z_0^{-1}\right)^n c.$$

That is, the solution to the difference equation (2.29) depends only on the initial condition and the inverse of the root to the associated polynomial $\alpha(z)$.

Now suppose that the sequence satisfies

$$u_n - \alpha_1 u_{n-1} - \alpha_2 u_{n-2} = 0, \quad \alpha_2 \neq 0, \quad n = 2, 3, \ldots \tag{2.30}$$

This equation is a ***homogeneous difference equation of order 2***. The corresponding polynomial is

$$\alpha(z) = 1 - \alpha_1 z - \alpha_2 z^2,$$

which has two roots, say, $z_1$ and $z_2$; that is, $\alpha(z_1) = \alpha(z_2) = 0$. We will consider two cases. First suppose $z_1 \neq z_2$. Then the general solution to (2.30) is

$$u_n = c_1 z_1^{-n} + c_2 z_2^{-n}, \tag{2.31}$$

where $c_1$ and $c_2$ depend on the initial conditions. This claim can be verified by direct substitution of (2.31) into (2.30):

$$\begin{aligned}
c_1 z_1^{-n} + c_2 z_2^{-n} & - \alpha_1 \left(c_1 z_1^{-(n-1)} + c_2 z_2^{-(n-1)}\right) - \alpha_2 \left(c_1 z_1^{-(n-2)} + c_2 z_2^{-(n-2)}\right) \\
&= c_1 z_1^{-n} \left(1 - \alpha_1 z_1 - \alpha_2 z_1^2\right) + c_2 z_2^{-n} \left(1 - \alpha_1 z_2 - \alpha_2 z_2^2\right) \\
&= c_1 z_1^{-n} \alpha(z_1) + c_2 z_2^{-n} \alpha(z_2) \\
&= 0.
\end{aligned}$$

Given two initial conditions $u_0$ and $u_1$, we may solve for $c_1$ and $c_2$:

$$\begin{aligned}
u_0 &= c_1 + c_2 \\
u_1 &= c_1 z_1^{-1} + c_2 z_2^{-1},
\end{aligned}$$

where $z_1$ and $z_2$ can be solved for in terms of $\alpha_1$ and $\alpha_2$ using the quadratic formula, for example.

When the roots are equal, $z_1 = z_2$ $(= z_0)$, the general solution to (2.30) is

$$u_n = z_0^{-n}(c_1 + c_2 n). \tag{2.32}$$

This claim can also be verified by direct substitution of (2.32) into (2.30):

$$\begin{aligned}
z_0^{-n}(c_1 + c_2 n) & - \alpha_1 \left(z_0^{-(n-1)}[c_1 + c_2(n-1)]\right) - \alpha_2 \left(z_0^{-(n-2)}[c_1 + c_2(n-2)]\right) \\
&= z_0^{-n}(c_1 + c_2 n)\left(1 - \alpha_1 z_0 - \alpha_2 z_0^2\right) + c_2 z_0^{-n+1}\left(\alpha_1 + 2\alpha_2 z_0\right) \\
&= c_2 z_0^{-n+1}\left(\alpha_1 + 2\alpha_2 z_0\right).
\end{aligned}$$

To show that $(\alpha_1 + 2\alpha_2 z_0) = 0$, write $1 - \alpha_1 z - \alpha_2 z^2 = (1 - z_0^{-1} z)^2$, and take derivatives with respect to $z$ on both sides of the equation to obtain $(\alpha_1 + 2\alpha_2 z) = 2z_0^{-1}(1 - z_0^{-1} z)$. Thus, $(\alpha_1 + 2\alpha_2 z_0) = 2z_0^{-1}(1 - z_0^{-1} z_0) = 0$, as was to be shown. Finally, given two initial conditions, $u_0$ and $u_1$, we can solve for $c_1$ and $c_2$:

$$\begin{aligned} u_0 &= c_1 \\ u_1 &= (c_1 + c_2) z_0^{-1}. \end{aligned}$$

To summarize these results, in the case of distinct roots, the solution to the homogeneous difference equation of degree two was

$$\begin{aligned} u_n = & \; z_1^{-n} \times (\text{a polynomial in } n \text{ of degree } m_1 - 1) \\ & + z_2^{-n} \times (\text{a polynomial in } n \text{ of degree } m_2 - 1), \end{aligned}$$

where $m_1$ is the multiplicity of the root $z_1$ and $m_2$ is the multiplicity of the root $z_2$. In this example, of course, $m_1 = m_2 = 1$, and we called the polynomials of degree zero $c_1$ and $c_2$, respectively. In the case of the repeated root, the solution was

$$u_n = z_0^{-n} \times (\text{a polynomial in } n \text{ of degree } m_0 - 1),$$

where $m_0$ is the multiplicity of the root $z_0$; that is, $m_0 = 2$. In this case, we wrote the polynomial of degree one as $c_1 + c_2 n$. In both cases, we solved for $c_1$ and $c_2$ given two initial conditions, $u_0$ and $u_1$.

**Example 2.8 The ACF of an AR(2) Process**

Suppose $x_t = \phi_1 x_{t-1} + \phi_2 x_{t-2} + w_t$ is a causal AR(2) process. Multiply each side of the model by $x_{t-h}$ for $h > 0$, and take expectation: $E(x_t x_{t-h}) = \phi_1 E(x_{t-1} x_{t-h}) + \phi_2 E(x_{t-2} x_{t-h}) + E(w_t x_{t-h})$. The result is

$$\gamma(h) = \phi_1 \gamma(h-1) + \phi_2 \gamma(h-2), \quad h = 1, 2, \ldots . \tag{2.33}$$

For $h > 0$, $E(w_t x_{t-h}) = 0$ because, for a causal model, $x_{t-h}$ is a linear function of $\{w_{t-h}, w_{t-h-1}, \ldots\}$, which is uncorrelated with $w_t$. Divide (2.33) through by $\gamma(0)$ to obtain the difference equation for the ACF of the process:

$$\rho(h) - \phi_1 \rho(h-1) - \phi_2 \rho(h-2) = 0, \quad h = 1, 2, \ldots . \tag{2.34}$$

The initial conditions are $\rho(0) = 1$ and $\rho(-1) = \phi_1/(1 - \phi_2)$, which is obtained by evaluating (2.34) for $h = 1$ and noting that $\rho(1) = \rho(-1)$.

Using the results for the homogeneous difference equation of order two, let $z_1$ and $z_2$ be the roots of the associated polynomial, $\phi(z) = 1 - \phi_1 z - \phi_2 z^2$. Because the model is causal, we know the roots are outside the unit circle: $|z_1| > 1$ and $|z_2| > 1$. Now, consider the solution for three cases:

(i) When $z_1$ and $z_2$ are real and distinct, then

$$\rho(h) = c_1 z_1^{-h} + c_2 z_2^{-h},$$

so $\rho(h) \to 0$ exponentially fast as $h \to \infty$.

(ii) When $z_1 = z_2 (= z_0)$ are real and equal, then

$$\rho(h) = z_0^{-h}(c_1 + c_2 h),$$

so $\rho(h) \to 0$ exponentially fast $h \to \infty$.

(iii) When $z_1 = \bar{z}_2$ are a complex conjugate pair, then $c_2 = \bar{c}_1$ [because $\rho(h)$ is real], and

$$\rho(h) = c_1 z_1^{-h} + \bar{c}_1 \bar{z}_1^{-h}.$$

Write $c_1$ and $z_1$ in polar coordinates, for example, $z_1 = |z_1|e^{i\theta}$, where $\theta$ is the angle whose tangent is the ratio of the imaginary part and the real part of $z_1$ [sometimes called $\arg(z_1)$; the range of $\theta$ is $[-\pi, \pi]$]. Then, using the fact that $e^{i\alpha} + e^{-i\alpha} = 2\cos(\alpha)$, the solution has the form

$$\rho(h) = a|z_1|^{-h} \cos(h\theta + b),$$

where $a$ and $b$ are determined by the initial conditions. Again, $\rho(h)$ dampens to zero exponentially fast as $h \to \infty$, but it does so in a sinusoidal fashion. The implication of this result is shown in the next example.

### Example 2.9 The Sample Path of an AR(2) With Complex Roots

Figure 2.3 shows $n = 144$ observations from the AR(2) model

$$x_t = 1.5x_{t-1} - .75x_{t-2} + w_t,$$

with $\sigma_w^2 = 1$, and with complex roots chosen so the process exhibits pseudo-cyclic behavior at the rate of one cycle every 12 time points. The autoregressive polynomial for this model is $\phi(z) = 1 - 1.5z + .75z^2$. The roots of $\phi(z)$ are $1 \pm i/\sqrt{3}$, and $\theta = \tan^{-1}(1/\sqrt{3}) = 2\pi/12$ radians per unit time. To convert the angle to cycles per unit time, divide by $2\pi$ to get $1/12$ cycles per unit time. The ACF for this model is shown in Section 2.4, Figure 2.4.

We now exhibit the solution for the general ***homogeneous difference equation of order p***:

$$u_n - \alpha_1 u_{n-1} - \cdots - \alpha_p u_{n-p} = 0, \quad \alpha_p \neq 0, \quad n = p, p+1, \ldots . \tag{2.35}$$

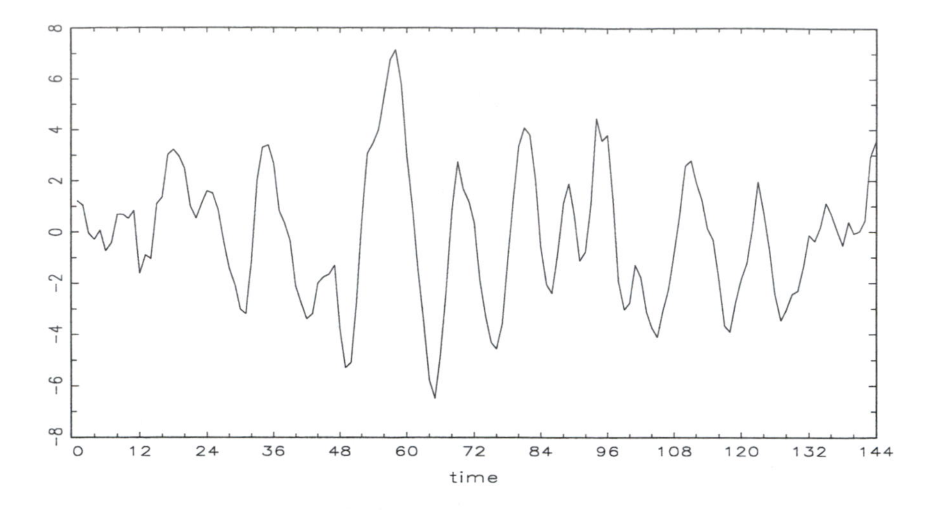


**Figure 2.3:** Simulated AR(2) model, $n = 144$ with $\phi_1 = 1.5$ and $\phi_2 = -0.75$.

The associated polynomial is

$$\alpha(z) = 1 - \alpha_1 z - \cdots - \alpha_p z^p.$$

Suppose $\alpha(z)$ has $r$ distinct roots, $z_1$ with multiplicity $m_1$, $z_2$ with multiplicity $m_2$, ..., and $z_r$ with multiplicity $m_r$, such that $m_1 + m_2 + \cdots m_r = p$. The general solution to the difference equation (2.35) is

$$u_n = z_1^{-n} P_1(n) + z_2^{-n} P_2(n) + \cdots + z_r^{-n} P_r(n), \tag{2.36}$$

where $P_j(n)$, for $j = 1, 2, ..., r$, is a polynomial in $n$, of degree $m_j - 1$. Given $p$ initial conditions $u_0, ..., u_{p-1}$, we can solve for the $P_j(n)$ explicitly.

### Example 2.10 Determining the $\psi$-weights for a Causal ARMA$(p, q)$

For a causal ARMA$(p, q)$ model, $\phi(B)x_t = \theta(B)w_t$, where the zeros of $\phi(z)$ are outside the unit circle, recall that we may write

$$x_t = \sum_{j=0}^{\infty} \psi_j w_{t-j},$$

where the $\psi$-weights are determined using Property P2.1.

For the pure MA$(q)$ model, $\psi_0 = 1$, $\psi_j = \theta_j$, for $j = 1, ..., q$, and $\psi_j = 0$, otherwise. For the general case of ARMA$(p, q)$ models, the task of solving for the $\psi$-weights is much more complicated, as was demonstrated in Example 2.6. The use of the theory of homogeneous difference equations can help here. To solve for the $\psi$-weights in general, we must match the coefficients in $\psi(z)\phi(z) = \theta(z)$:

$$(\psi_0 + \psi_1 z + \psi_2 z^2 + \cdots)(1 - \phi_1 z - \phi_2 z^2 + \cdots) = (1 + \theta_1 z + \theta_2 z^2 + \cdots).$$

The first few values are

$$\begin{aligned} \psi_0 &= 1 \\ \psi_1 - \phi_1\psi_0 &= \theta_1 \\ \psi_2 - \phi_1\psi_1 - \phi_2\psi_0 &= \theta_2 \\ \psi_3 - \phi_1\psi_2 - \phi_2\psi_1 - \phi_3\psi_0 &= \theta_3 \\ &\vdots \end{aligned}$$

where we would take $\phi_j = 0$ for $j > p$, and $\theta_j = 0$ for $j > q$. The $\psi$-weights satisfy the homogeneous difference equation given by

$$\psi_j - \sum_{k=1}^{p} \phi_k \psi_{j-k} = 0, \quad j \geq \max(p, q+1), \tag{2.37}$$

with initial conditions

$$\psi_j - \sum_{k=1}^{j} \phi_k \psi_{j-k} = \theta_j, \quad 0 \leq j \leq \max(p, q+1). \tag{2.38}$$

The general solution depends on the roots of the AR polynomial $\phi(z) = 1 - \phi_1 z - \cdots - \phi_p z^p$, as seen from (2.37). The specific solution will, of course, depend on the initial conditions.

Consider the ARMA process given in (2.27), $x_t = 0.9x_{t-1} + 0.5w_{t-1} + w_t$. Because $\max(p, q+1) = 2$, using (2.38), we have $\psi_0 = 1$ and $\psi_1 = 0.9 + 0.5 = 1.4$. By (2.37), for $j = 2, 3, \ldots$, the $\psi$-weights satisfy $\psi_j - 0.9\psi_{j-1} = 0$. The general solution is $\psi_j = c\,0.9^j$. To find the specific solution, use the initial condition $\psi_1 = 1.4$, so $1.4 = 0.9c$ or $c = 1.4/0.9$. Finally, $\psi_j = 1.4(0.9)^{j-1}$, for $j \geq 1$, as we saw in Example 2.6.

## 2.4 Autocorrelation and Partial Autocorrelation Functions

We begin by exhibiting the ACF of an MA($q$) process, $x_t = \theta(B)w_t$, where $\theta(B) = 1 + \theta_1 B + \cdots + \theta_q B^q$. Because $x_t$ is a finite linear combination of white noise terms, the process is stationary with mean

$$E(x_t) = \sum_{j=0}^{q} \theta_j E(w_{t-j}) = 0,$$

where we have written $\theta_0 = 1$, and with autocovariance function

$$\begin{aligned}\gamma(h) = \text{cov}\,(x_{t+h}, x_t) &= E\left[\left(\sum_{j=0}^{q} \theta_j w_{t+h-j}\right)\left(\sum_{k=0}^{q} \theta_j w_{t-k}\right)\right] \\ &= \begin{cases} \sigma_w^2 \sum_{j=0}^{q-h} \theta_j \theta_{j+h}, & 0 \le h \le q \\ 0, & h > q. \end{cases} \end{aligned} \tag{2.39}$$

Recall that $\gamma(h) = \gamma(-h)$, so we will only display the values for $h \ge 0$. The cutting off of $\gamma(h)$ after $q$ lags is the signature of the MA($q$) model. Dividing (2.39) by $\gamma(0)$ yields the ***ACF of an MA(q)***:

$$\rho(h) = \begin{cases} \frac{\sum_{j=0}^{q-h} \theta_j \theta_{j+h}}{1+\theta_1^2+\cdots+\theta_q^2}, & 1 \le h \le q \\ 0, & h > q. \end{cases} \tag{2.40}$$

For a causal ARMA($p, q$) model, $\phi(B)x_t = \theta(B)w_t$, where the zeros of $\phi(z)$ are outside the unit circle, write

$$x_t = \sum_{j=0}^{\infty} \psi_j w_{t-j}.$$

It follows immediately that $E(x_t) = 0$. Also, the autocovariance function of $x_t$ can be written as:

$$\gamma(h) = \text{cov}(x_{t+h}, x_t) = \sigma_w^2 \sum_{j=0}^{\infty} \psi_j \psi_{j+h}, \quad h \ge 0. \tag{2.41}$$

We could then use (2.37) and (2.38) to solve for the $\psi$-weights. In turn, we could solve for $\gamma(h)$, and the ACF $\rho(h) = \gamma(h)/\gamma(0)$. As in Example 2.8, it is also possible to obtain a homogeneous difference equation directly in terms of $\gamma(h)$. First, we write

$$\begin{aligned}\gamma(h) &= \text{cov}(x_{t+h}, x_t) = E\left[\left(\sum_{j=1}^{p} \phi_j x_{t+h-j} + \sum_{j=0}^{q} \theta_j w_{t+h-j}\right) x_t\right] \\ &= \sum_{j=1}^{p} \phi_j \gamma(h-j) + \sigma_w^2 \sum_{j=h}^{q} \theta_j \psi_{j-h}, \quad h \ge 0, \end{aligned} \tag{2.42}$$

where we have used the fact that for $h \ge 0$,

$$E(x_{t+h} w_t) = E\left[\left(\sum_{j=0}^{\infty} \psi_j w_{t+h-j}\right) w_t\right] = \psi_h \sigma_w^2.$$

From (2.42), we can write a general homogeneous equation:

$$\gamma(h) - \phi_1\gamma(h-1) - \cdots - \phi_p\gamma(h-p) = 0, \quad h \geq \max(p, q+1), \tag{2.43}$$

with initial conditions

$$\gamma(h) - \sum_{j=1}^{p} \phi_j\gamma(h-j) = \sigma_w^2 \sum_{j=h}^{q} \theta_j\psi_{j-h}, \quad 0 \leq h < \max(p, q+1). \tag{2.44}$$

Dividing (2.43) and (2.44) through by $\gamma(0)$ will allow us to solve for the ACF, $\rho(h) = \gamma(h)/\gamma(0)$.

**Example 2.11 The ACF of an ARMA(1,1)**

Consider the causal ARMA(1,1) process $x_t = \phi x_{t-1} + \theta w_{t-1} + w_t$, where $|\phi| < 1$. Based on (2.43), the autocovariance function satisfies

$$\gamma(h) - \phi\gamma(h-1) = 0, \quad h = 2, 3, ...,$$

so the general solution is $\gamma(h) = c\phi^h$, for $h = 1, 2, \ldots$ . To solve for $c$, we use (2.44):

$$\begin{aligned} \gamma(0) &= \phi\gamma(1) + \sigma_w^2[1 + \theta\phi + \theta^2] \\ \gamma(1) &= \phi\gamma(0) + \sigma_w^2\theta. \end{aligned}$$

Solving for $\gamma(0)$ and $\gamma(1)$, we obtain:

$$\begin{aligned} \gamma(0) &= \sigma_w^2 \frac{1 + 2\theta\phi + \theta^2}{1 - \phi^2} \\ \gamma(1) &= \sigma_w^2 \frac{(1 + \theta\phi)(\phi + \theta)}{1 - \phi^2}. \end{aligned}$$

Because $\gamma(1) = c\phi$, we have $c = \gamma(1)/\phi$, so the general solution is

$$\gamma(h) = \sigma_w^2 \frac{(1 + \theta\phi)(\phi + \theta)}{1 - \phi^2} \phi^{h-1}.$$

Finally, dividing through by $\gamma(0)$ yields the ACF

$$\rho(h) = \frac{(1 + \theta\phi)(\phi + \theta)}{1 + 2\theta\phi + \theta^2} \phi^{h-1}, \quad h \geq 1. \tag{2.45}$$

**Example 2.12 The ACF of an AR($p$)**

For a causal AR($p$), it follows immediately from (2.43) that

$$\rho(h) - \phi_1\rho(h-1) - \cdots - \phi_p\rho(h-p) = 0, \quad h \geq p. \tag{2.46}$$

Let $z_1, ..., z_r$ denote the roots of $\phi(z)$, each with multiplicity $m_1, ..., m_r$, respectively, where $m_1 + \cdots + m_r = p$. Then, from (2.37), the general solution is

$$\rho(h) = z_1^{-h} P_1(h) + z_2^{-h} P_2(h) + \cdots + z_r^{-h} P_r(h), \quad h \geq p, \tag{2.47}$$

where $P_j(h)$ is a polynomial in $h$ of degree $m_j - 1$.

Recall that for a causal model, all of the roots are outside the unit circle, $|z_i| > 1$, for $i = 1, ..., r$. If all the roots are real, then $\rho(h)$ dampens exponentially fast to zero as $h \to \infty$. If some of the roots are complex, then they will be in conjugate pairs and $\rho(h)$ will dampen, in a sinusoidal fashion, exponentially fast to zero as $h \to \infty$. In the case of complex roots, the time series will appear to be cyclic in nature. This, of course, is also true for ARMA models in which the AR part has complex roots.

## The Partial Autocorrelation Function (PACF)

We have seen in (2.40) that, for MA($q$) models, the ACF will be zero for lags greater than $q$. Moreover, because $\theta_q \neq 0$, the ACF will not be zero at lag $q$. Thus, the ACF provides a considerable amount of information about the order of the dependence when the process is a moving average process. If the process, however, is ARMA or AR, the ACF alone tells us little about the orders of dependence. Hence, it is worthwhile pursuing a function that will behave like the ACF for AR models, namely, the ***partial autocorrelation function (PACF)***.

To motivate the idea, consider a causal AR(1) model, $x_t = \phi x_{t-1} + w_t$. Then,

$$\begin{aligned}\gamma(2) = \text{cov}(x_t, x_{t-2}) &= \text{cov}(\phi x_{t-1} + w_t, x_{t-2}) \\ &= \text{cov}(\phi^2 x_{t-2} + \phi w_{t-1} + w_t, x_{t-2}) = \phi^2 \gamma(0).\end{aligned}$$

This result follows from causality because $x_{t-2}$ involves $\{w_{t-2}, w_{t-3}, ...\}$, which are all uncorrelated with $w_t$ and $w_{t-1}$. The correlation between $x_t$ and $x_{t-2}$ is not zero, as it would be for an MA(1), because $x_t$ is dependent on $x_{t-2}$ through $x_{t-1}$. Suppose we break this chain of dependence by removing (*partial out*) $x_{t-1}$. That is, we consider the correlation between $x_t - \phi x_{t-1}$ and $x_{t-2} - \phi x_{t-1}$, because it is the correlation between $x_t$ and $x_{t-2}$ with the linear dependence of each on $x_{t-1}$ removed. In this way, we have broken the dependence chain between $x_t$ and $x_{t-2}$. In fact,

$$\text{cov}(x_t - \phi x_{t-1}, x_{t-2} - \phi x_{t-1}) = \text{cov}(w_t, x_{t-2} - \phi x_{t-1}) = 0.$$

To formally define the PACF for mean-zero stationary time series, let $x_h^{h-1}$ denote the best linear predictor of $x_h$ based on $\{x_1, x_2, ..., x_{h-1}\}$. We will discuss prediction in detail in the next section, but for now, we note $x_h^{h-1}$ has the form:

$$x_h^{h-1} = \beta_1 x_{h-1} + \beta_2 x_{h-2} + \cdots + \beta_{h-1} x_1, \tag{2.48}$$

where the $\beta$'s are chosen to minimize the mean square linear prediction error, $E(x_h - x_h^{h-1})^2$. In addition, let $x_0^{h-1}$ denote the minimum mean square linear predictor of $x_0$ based on $\{x_1, x_2, ..., x_{h-1}\}$. As will be seen in the next section, $x_0^{h-1}$ can be written as

$$x_0^{h-1} = \beta_1 x_1 + \beta_2 x_2 + \cdots + \beta_{h-1} x_{h-1}. \tag{2.49}$$

Equation (2.48) can be thought of as the linear regression of $x_h$ on the past, $x_{h-1}, ..., x_1$, and (2.49) can be thought of as the linear regression of $x_0$ on the future, $x_1, ..., x_{h-1}$. The coefficients, $\beta_1, ..., \beta_{h-1}$ are the same in (2.48) and (2.49), which means that, for stationary processes, linear prediction backward in time is equivalent to linear prediction forward in time. We will discuss this result further in the next section.

Formally, for a stationary time series, $x_t$, we define the ***partial autocorrelation function (PACF)***, $\phi_{hh}$, $h = 1, 2, ...$, by

$$\phi_{11} = \text{corr}(x_1, x_0) = \rho(1) \tag{2.50}$$

and

$$\phi_{hh} = \text{corr}(x_h - x_h^{h-1}, x_0 - x_0^{h-1}), \quad h \geq 2. \tag{2.51}$$

Both $(x_h - x_h^{h-1})$ and $(x_0 - x_0^{h-1})$ are uncorrelated with $\{x_1, x_2, ..., x_{h-1}\}$. By stationarity, the PACF, $\phi_{hh}$, is the correlation between $x_t$ and $x_{t-h}$ with the linear effect of $\{x_{t-1}, ..., x_{t-(h-1)}\}$, on each, removed. If the process $x_t$ is Gaussian, then $\phi_{hh} = \text{corr}(x_t, x_{t-h} | \, x_{t-1}, ..., x_{t-(h-1)})$. That is, $\phi_{hh}$ is the correlation coefficient between $x_t$ and $x_{t-h}$ in the bivariate distribution of $(x_t, x_{t-h})$ conditional on $\{x_{t-1}, ..., x_{t-(h-1)}\}$.

### Example 2.13 The PACF of a Causal AR(1)

Consider the PACF of the AR(1) process given by $x_t = \phi x_{t-1} + w_t$, with $|\phi| < 1$ . By definition, $\phi_{11} = \rho(1) = \phi$. To calculate $\phi_{22}$, consider the prediction of $x_2$ based on a linear function of $x_1$, say, $x_2^1 = \alpha x_1$. We choose $\alpha$ to minimize

$$E(x_2 - \alpha x_1)^2 = \gamma(0) - 2\alpha\gamma(1) + \alpha^2\gamma(0).$$

Taking derivatives and setting the result equal to zero, we have $\alpha = \gamma(1)/\gamma(0) = \rho(1) = \phi$. Thus, $x_2^1 = \phi x_1$. Next, consider the prediction of $x_0$ based on a linear function of $x_1$: $x_0^1 = \alpha x_1$. We choose $\alpha$ to minimize

$$E(x_0 - \alpha x_1)^2 = \gamma(0) - 2\alpha\gamma(1) + \alpha^2\gamma(0).$$

Analogously, we have $x_0^1 = \phi x_1$, which agrees with the claim that prediction forward in time is equivalent to prediction backward in time. Hence, $\phi_{22} = \text{corr}(x_2 - \phi x_1, x_0 - \phi x_1)$. But, note

$$\text{cov}(x_2 - \phi x_1, x_0 - \phi x_1) = \gamma(2) - 2\phi\gamma(1) + \phi^2\gamma(0) = 0$$

since $\gamma(h) = \gamma(0)\phi^h$. Thus, $\phi_{22} = 0$. In the next example, we will see that in this case $\phi_{hh} = 0$, for all $h > 1$.

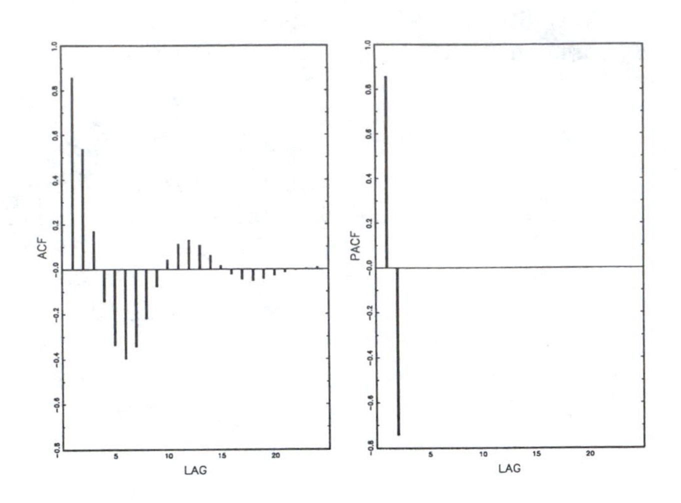


**Figure 2.4:** The ACF and PACF, to lag 24, of an AR(2) model, with $\phi_1 = 1.5$ and $\phi_2 = -0.75$.

### Example 2.14 The PACF of a Causal AR(p)

Let $x_t = \sum_{j=1}^{p} \phi_j x_{t-j} + w_t$, where the roots of $\phi(z)$ are outside the unit circle. When $h > p$, then

$$x_h^{h-1} = \sum_{j=1}^{p} \phi_j x_{h-j}.$$

We have not proven this obvious result yet, but we will prove it in the next section. Thus, when $h > p$,

$$\begin{aligned} \phi_{hh} &= \text{corr}(x_h - x_h^{h-1}, x_0 - x_0^{h-1}) \\ &= \text{corr}(w_h, x_0 - x_0^{h-1}) = 0, \end{aligned}$$

since, by causality, $x_0 - x_0^{h-1}$ depends only on $\{w_{h-1}, w_{h-2}, ...\}$; recall equation (2.49). When $h \le p$, $\phi_{pp}$ is not zero, and $\phi_{11}, ..., \phi_{p-1,p-1}$ are not necessarily zero. Figure 2.4 shows the ACF and the PACF of the AR(2) model presented in Example 2.9.

### Example 2.15 The PACF of an invertible MA(q)

For an invertible MA(q), we can write $x_t = \sum_{j=1}^{\infty} \pi_j x_{t-j} + w_t$. Moreover, no finite representation exists. From this result, it should be apparent that the PACF will never cut off, as in the case of an AR(p).

**Table 2.1** Behavior of the ACF and PACF for Causal and Invertible ARMA Models

| | AR($p$) | MA($q$) | ARMA($p,q$) |
|---|---|---|---|
| ACF | Tails off | Cuts off after lag $q$ | Tails off |
| PACF | Cuts off after lag $p$ | Tails off | Tails off |

For an MA(1), $x_t = w_t + \theta w_{t-1}$, with $|\theta| < 1$, calculations similar to Example 2.13 will yield $\phi_{22} = (-\theta)^2/(1+\theta^2+\theta^4)$. For the MA(1) in general, we can show that

$$\phi_{hh} = \frac{(-\theta)^h(1-\theta^2)}{1-\theta^{2(h+1)}}, \quad h \geq 1.$$

In the next section, we will discuss methods of calculating the PACF. The PACF for MA models behaves much like the ACF for AR models. Also, the PACF for AR models behaves much like the ACF for MA models. Because an invertible ARMA model has an infinite AR representation, the PACF will not cut off. We may summarize these results in Table 2.1.

**Example 2.16 Preliminary Analysis of the Recruitment Series**

We consider the problem of modeling the Recruitment series (number of new fish) shown in Figure 1.4. There are 453 months of observed recruitment ranging over the years 1950-1987. The ACF and the PACF given in Figure 2.5 are consistent with the behavior of an AR(2). The ACF has cycles corresponding roughly to a 12-month period, and the PACF has large values for $h = 1, 2$ and then is essentially zero for higher order lags. Based on Table 2.1, these results suggest that a second-order ($p = 2$) autoregressive model might provide a good fit. Although we will discuss estimation in detail in Section 2.6, we ran a regression (see Section 1.8) using the data triplets $\{(x_3, x_2, x_1), (x_4, x_3, x_2), ..., (x_{453}, x_{452}, x_{451})\}$ to fit a model of the form

$$x_t = \phi_0 + \phi_1 x_{t-1} + \phi_2 x_{t-2} + w_t$$

for $t = 3, 4, \ldots, 453$. The values of the estimates were $\widehat{\phi}_0 = 6.74(1.11)$, $\widehat{\phi}_1 = 1.35(.04), \widehat{\phi}_2 = -.46(.04)$, and $\widehat{\sigma}_w^2 = 90.31$, where the estimated standard errors are in parentheses.

## 2.5 Forecasting

In ***forecasting***, the goal is to predict future values of a time series, $x_{n+m}$, $m = 1, 2, ...$, based on the data collected to the present, $\boldsymbol{x} = \{x_n, x_{n-1}, ..., x_1\}$. Throughout this section, we will assume $x_t$ is stationary and the model parameters are known. The problem of forecasting when the model parameters are unknown will be discussed in the next section; also, see Problem 2.25. The ***minimum mean square error predictor*** of $x_{n+m}$ is $x^n_{n+m} = E(x_{n+m}|x_n, x_{n-1}, ..., x_1)$ because the conditional expectation minimizes the mean square error

$$E\{x_{n+m} - g(\boldsymbol{x})\}^2, \tag{2.52}$$

where $g(\boldsymbol{x})$ is a (measurable) function of the observations $\boldsymbol{x}$. This result follows by iterating the expectation, $E\{x_{n+m} - g(\boldsymbol{x})\}^2 = E[E\{[x_{n+m} - g(\boldsymbol{x})]^2 \mid \boldsymbol{x}\}]$, and then observing that the inner expectation is minimized when $x^n_{n+m} = E(x_{n+m} \mid \boldsymbol{x})$; see Problem 2.13.

First, we will restrict attention to predictors that are linear functions of the data, that is, predictors of the form

$$x^n_{n+m} = \alpha_0 + \sum_{k=1}^{n} \alpha_k x_k, \tag{2.53}$$

where $\alpha_0, \alpha_1, ..., \alpha_n$ are real numbers. Linear predictors of the form (2.53) that minimize the mean square prediction error (2.52) are called ***best linear***

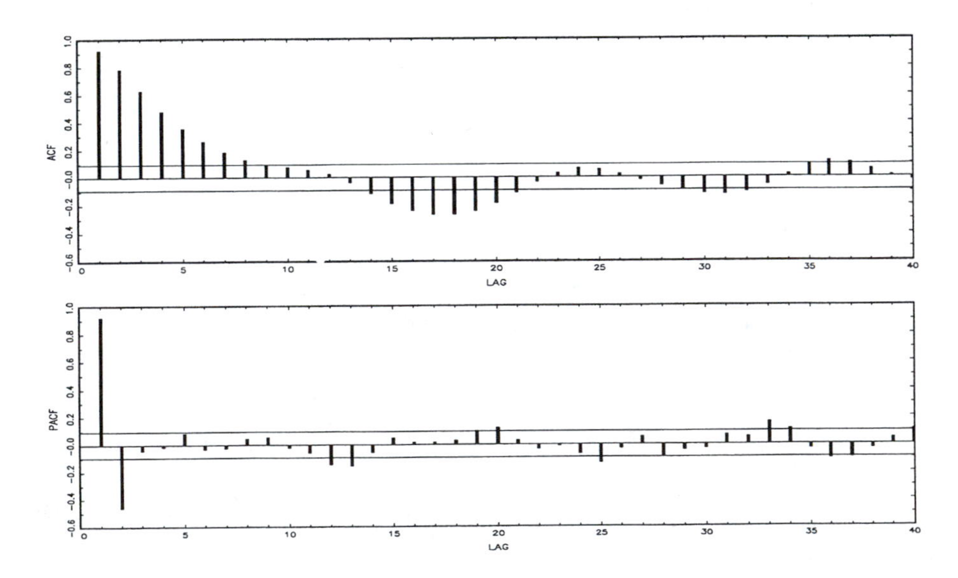


**Figure 2.5:** ACF and PACF of the Recruitment series.

***predictors***. As we shall see, linear prediction depends only on the second-order moments of the process, which are easy to estimate from the data. Much of the material in this section is enhanced by the theoretical material presented in Section T2.15. For example, Theorem 2.3 states that if the process is Gaussian, minimum mean square error predictors and best linear predictors are the same. The following property, which is based on the projection theorem, Theorem 2.1 of Section T2.15, is a key result.

***Property P2.3: Best Linear Prediction for Stationary Processes***
*Given data* $x_1, ..., x_n$, *the best linear predictor,* $x_{n+m}^n = \alpha_0 + \sum_{k=1}^n \alpha_k x_k$, *of* $x_{n+m}$, *for* $m \geq 1$, *is found by solving*

$$\begin{aligned} &E\left[x_{n+m} - x_{n+m}^n\right] = 0; \\ &E\left[\left(x_{n+m} - x_{n+m}^n\right) x_k\right] = 0, \quad k = 1, ..., n. \end{aligned} \tag{2.54}$$

The equations specified in (2.54) are called the ***prediction equations***, and they are used to solve for the coefficients $\{\alpha_0, \alpha_1, ..., \alpha_n\}$. If $E(x_t) = \mu$, the first equation of (2.54) is $E(x_{n+m}^n) = E(x_{n+m}) = \mu$, which implies $\alpha_0 = \mu(1 - \sum_{k=1}^n \alpha_k)$. Hence, the form of the BLP is $x_{n+m}^n = \mu + \sum_{k=1}^n \alpha_k (x_k - \mu)$. Thus, until we discuss estimation, there is no loss of generality in considering the case that $\mu = 0$, in which case, $\alpha_0 = 0$.

Consider, first, ***one-step-ahead prediction***. That is, given $\{x_1, ..., x_n\}$, we wish to forecast the value of the time series at the next time point, $x_{n+1}$. The BLP of $x_{n+1}$ is

$$x_{n+1}^n = \phi_{n1} x_n + \phi_{n2} x_{n-1} + \cdots + \phi_{nn} x_1, \tag{2.55}$$

where, for purposes that will become clear shortly, we have written $\alpha_k$ in (2.54), as $\phi_{n,n+1-k}$ in (2.55), for $k = 1, ..., n$. Using Property P2.3, the coefficients $\{\phi_{n1}, \phi_{n2}, ..., \phi_{nn}\}$ satisfy

$$E\left[\left(x_{n+1} - \sum_{j=1}^n \phi_{nj} x_{n+1-j}\right) x_{n+1-k}\right] = 0, \quad k = 1, ..., n,$$

or

$$\sum_{j=1}^n \phi_{nj} \gamma(k - j) = \gamma(k), \quad k = 1, ..., n. \tag{2.56}$$

The prediction equations (2.56) can be written in matrix notation as

$$\Gamma_n \boldsymbol{\phi}_n = \boldsymbol{\gamma}_n, \tag{2.57}$$

where $\Gamma_n = \{\gamma(k - j)\}_{j,k=1}^n$ is an $n \times n$ matrix, $\boldsymbol{\phi}_n = (\phi_{n1}, ..., \phi_{nn})'$ is an $n \times 1$ vector, and $\boldsymbol{\gamma}_n = (\gamma(1), ..., \gamma(n))'$ is an $n \times 1$ vector.

The matrix $\Gamma_n$ is nonnegative definite. If $\Gamma_n$ is singular, there are many solutions to (2.57), but, by the projection theorem (Section T2.15), $x_{n+1}^n$ is unique. If $\Gamma_n$ is nonsingular, the elements of $\boldsymbol{\phi}_n$ are unique, and are given by

$$\boldsymbol{\phi}_n = \Gamma_n^{-1}\boldsymbol{\gamma}_n. \tag{2.58}$$

For ARMA models, the fact that $\sigma_w^2 > 0$ and $\gamma(h) \to 0$ as $h \to \infty$ is enough to ensure that $\Gamma_n$ is positive definite (Problem 2.10). It is sometimes convenient to write the one-step-ahead forecast in vector notation

$$x_{n+1}^n = \boldsymbol{\phi}_n'\boldsymbol{x}, \tag{2.59}$$

where $\boldsymbol{x} = (x_n, x_{n-1}, ..., x_1)'$.

The ***mean square one-step-ahead prediction error*** is

$$P_{n+1}^n = E(x_{n+1} - x_{n+1}^n)^2 = \gamma(0) - \boldsymbol{\gamma}_n'\Gamma_n^{-1}\boldsymbol{\gamma}_n. \tag{2.60}$$

To verify (2.60) using (2.58) and (2.59),

$$\begin{aligned}
E(x_{n+1} - x_{n+1}^n)^2 &= E(x_{n+1} - \boldsymbol{\phi}_n'\boldsymbol{x})^2 = E(x_{n+1} - \boldsymbol{\gamma}_n'\Gamma_n^{-1}\boldsymbol{x})^2 \\
&= E(x_{n+1}^2 - 2\boldsymbol{\gamma}_n'\Gamma_n^{-1}\boldsymbol{x}x_{n+1} + \boldsymbol{\gamma}_n'\Gamma_n^{-1}\boldsymbol{x}\boldsymbol{x}'\Gamma_n^{-1}\boldsymbol{\gamma}_n) \\
&= \gamma(0) - 2\boldsymbol{\gamma}_n'\Gamma_n^{-1}\boldsymbol{\gamma}_n + \boldsymbol{\gamma}_n'\Gamma_n^{-1}\Gamma_n\Gamma_n^{-1}\boldsymbol{\gamma}_n \\
&= \gamma(0) - \boldsymbol{\gamma}_n'\Gamma_n^{-1}\boldsymbol{\gamma}_n.
\end{aligned}$$

### Example 2.17 Prediction for an AR(2)

Suppose we have a causal AR(2) process $x_t = \phi_1 x_{t-1} + \phi_2 x_{t-2} + w_t$, and one observation $x_1$. Then, using equation (2.58), the one-step-ahead prediction of $x_2$ based on $x_1$ is

$$x_2^1 = \phi_{11}x_1 = \frac{\gamma(1)}{\gamma(0)}x_1 = \rho(1)x_1.$$

Now, suppose we want the one-step-ahead prediction of $x_3$ based on two observations $x_1$ and $x_2$. We could use (2.58) again and solve

$$x_3^2 = \phi_{21}x_2 + \phi_{22}x_1 = (\gamma(1), \gamma(2))\begin{pmatrix}\gamma(0) & \gamma(1)\\ \gamma(1) & \gamma(0)\end{pmatrix}^{-1}\begin{pmatrix}x_2\\ x_1\end{pmatrix},$$

but, it should be apparent from the model that $x_3^2 = \phi_1 x_2 + \phi_2 x_1$. Because $\phi_1 x_2 + \phi_2 x_1$ satisfies the prediction equations (2.54),

$$E\{[x_3 - (\phi_1 x_2 + \phi_2 x_1)]x_1\} = E(w_3 x_1) = 0,$$

$$E\{[x_3 - (\phi_1 x_2 + \phi_2 x_1)]x_2\} = E(w_3 x_2) = 0,$$

it follows that, indeed, $x_3^2 = \phi_1 x_2 + \phi_2 x_1$, and by the uniqueness of the coefficients in this case, that $\phi_{21} = \phi_1$ and $\phi_{22} = \phi_2$. Continuing in this way, it is easy to verify that, for $n \geq 2$,

$$x_{n+1}^n = \phi_1 x_n + \phi_2 x_{n-1}.$$

That is, $\phi_{n1} = \phi_1, \phi_{n2} = \phi_2$, and $\phi_{nj} = 0$, for $j = 3, 4, ..., n$.

From Example 2.16, it should be clear (Problem 2.47) that, if the time series is a causal AR($p$) process, then, for $n \geq p$,

$$x_{n+1}^n = \phi_1 x_n + \phi_2 x_{n-1} + \cdots + \phi_p x_{n-p+1}. \tag{2.61}$$

For ARMA models in general, the prediction equations will not be as simple as the pure AR case. In addition, for $n$ large, the use of (2.58) is prohibitive because it requires the inversion of a large matrix. There are, however, iterative solutions that do not require any matrix inversion. In particular, we mention the recursive solution due to Levinson (1947) and Durbin (1960).

***Property P2.4: The Durbin–Levinson Algorithm***
*Equations (2.58) and (2.60) can be solved iteratively as follows:*

$$\phi_{00} = 0, \quad P_1^0 = \gamma(0). \tag{2.62}$$

*For $n \geq 1$,*

$$\phi_{nn} = \frac{\rho(n) - \sum_{k=1}^{n-1} \phi_{n-1,k}\ \rho(n-k)}{1 - \sum_{k=1}^{n-1} \phi_{n-1,k}\ \rho(k)}, \quad P_{n+1}^n = P_n^{n-1}(1 - \phi_{nn}^2), \tag{2.63}$$

*where, for $n \geq 2$,*

$$\phi_{nk} = \phi_{n-1,k} - \phi_{nn}\phi_{n-1,n-k}, \quad k = 1, 2, ..., n-1. \tag{2.64}$$

The proof of Property P2.4 is left as an exercise; see Problem 2.11.

**Example 2.18 Using the Durbin–Levinson Algorithm**

To use the algorithm, start with $\phi_{00} = 0$, $P_1^0 = \gamma(0)$. Then, for $n = 1$,

$$\phi_{11} = \rho(1) \quad \text{and} \quad P_2^1 = \gamma(0)[1 - \phi_{11}^2].$$

For $n = 2$,

$$\begin{aligned}
\phi_{22} &= \frac{\rho(2) - \phi_{11}\ \rho(1)}{1 - \phi_{11}\ \rho(1)} = \frac{\rho(2) - \rho(1)^2}{1 - \rho(1)^2} \\
\phi_{21} &= \phi_{11} - \phi_{22}\phi_{11} = \rho(1)[1 - \phi_{22}] \\
P_3^2 &= \gamma(0)[1 - \phi_{11}^2][1 - \phi_{22}^2].
\end{aligned}$$

For $n = 3$,

$$\phi_{33} = \frac{\rho(3) - \phi_{21}\ \rho(2) - \phi_{22}\ \rho(1)}{1 - \phi_{21}\ \rho(1) - \phi_{22}\ \rho(2)},$$

and so on.

An important consequence of the Durbin–Levinson algorithm is (see Problem 2.11) as follows.

***Property P2.5: Iterative Solution for the PACF***
*The PACF of a stationary process $x_t$, can be obtained iteratively via (2.63) as $\phi_{nn}$, for $n = 1, 2, \ldots$ .*

**Example 2.19 The PACF of an AR(2)**

From Example 2.14 we know that for an AR(2), $\phi_{hh} = 0$ for $h > 2$, but we will use the results of Example 2.17 and Property P2.5 to calculate the first three values of the PACF. Recall (Example 2.8) that for an AR(2), $\rho(1) = \phi_1/(1 - \phi_2)$, and in general $\rho(h) - \phi_1\rho(h-1) - \phi_2\rho(h-2) = 0$, for $h \geq 2$. Then,

$$\begin{aligned}
\phi_{11} &= \rho(1) = \frac{\phi_1}{1 - \phi_2} \\
\phi_{22} &= \frac{\rho(2) - \rho(1)^2}{1 - \rho(1)^2} = \frac{\left[\phi_1\left(\frac{\phi_1}{1-\phi_2}\right) + \phi_2\right] - \left(\frac{\phi_1}{1-\phi_2}\right)^2}{1 - \left(\frac{\phi_1}{1-\phi_2}\right)^2} = \phi_2 \\
\phi_{21} &= \phi_1 \\
\phi_{33} &= \frac{\rho(3) - \phi_1\rho(2) - \phi_2\rho(1)}{1 - \phi_1\rho(1) - \phi_2\rho(2)} = 0.
\end{aligned}$$

So far, we have concentrated on one-step-ahead prediction, but Property P2.3 allows us to calculate the BLP of $x_{n+m}$ for any $m \geq 1$. Given data, $\{x_1, \ldots, x_n\}$, the ***m-step-ahead predictor*** is

$$x_{n+m}^n = \phi_{n1}^{(m)} x_n + \phi_{n2}^{(m)} x_{n-1} + \cdots + \phi_{nn}^{(m)} x_1, \tag{2.65}$$

where $\{\phi_{n1}^{(m)}, \phi_{n2}^{(m)}, \ldots, \phi_{nn}^{(m)}\}$ satisfy the prediction equations,

$$\sum_{j=1}^{n} \phi_{nj}^{(m)} E(x_{n+1-j}x_{n+1-k}) = E(x_{n+m}x_{n+1-k}), \quad k = 1, \ldots, n,$$

or

$$\sum_{j=1}^{n} \phi_{nj}^{(m)}\ \gamma(k - j) = \gamma(m + k - 1), \quad k = 1, \ldots, n. \tag{2.66}$$

The prediction equations can again be written in matrix notation as

$$\Gamma_n \boldsymbol{\phi}_n^{(m)} = \boldsymbol{\gamma}_n^{(m)}, \tag{2.67}$$

where $\boldsymbol{\gamma}_n^{(m)} = (\gamma(m), \gamma(m+1), ..., \gamma(m+n-1))'$, and $\boldsymbol{\phi}_n^{(m)} = (\phi_{n1}^{(m)}, ..., \phi_{nn}^{(m)})'$ are $n \times 1$ vectors.

The ***mean square m-step-ahead prediction error*** is

$$P_{n+m}^n = E\left(x_{n+m} - x_{n+m}^n\right)^2 = \gamma(0) - \boldsymbol{\gamma}_n^{(m)'} \Gamma_n^{-1} \boldsymbol{\gamma}_n^{(m)}. \tag{2.68}$$

Another useful algorithm for calculating forecasts was given by Brockwell and Davis (1991, Chapter 5). This algorithm follows directly from applying the projection theorem (Section T2.15) to the ***innovations***, $x_t - x_t^{t-1}$, for $t = 1, ..., n$, using the fact that the innovations $x_t - x_t^{t-1}$ and $x_s - x_s^{s-1}$ are uncorrelated for $s \neq t$ (see Problem 2.48). We present the case in which $x_t$ is a mean-zero stationary time series.

***Property P2.6: The Innovations Algorithm***

*The one-step-ahead predictors, $x_{t+1}^t$, and their mean-squared errors, $P_{t+1}^t$, can be calculated iteratively as*

$$x_1^0 = 0, \quad P_1^0 = \gamma(0)$$

$$x_{t+1}^t = \sum_{j=1}^{t} \theta_{tj}(x_{t+1-j} - x_{t+1-j}^{t-j}), \quad t = 1, 2, ... \tag{2.69}$$

$$P_{t+1}^t = \gamma(0) - \sum_{j=0}^{t-1} \theta_{t,t-j}^2 P_{j+1}^j \quad t = 1, 2, ..., \tag{2.70}$$

*where, for $j = 0, 1, ..., t-1$,*

$$\theta_{t,t-j} = \left(\gamma(t-j) - \sum_{k=0}^{j-1} \theta_{k,j-k}\theta_{t,t-k}P_{k+1}^k\right)\left(P_{j+1}^j\right)^{-1}. \tag{2.71}$$

Given data $x_1, ..., x_n$, the innovations algorithm can be calculated successively for $t = 1$, then $t = 2$ and so on, in which case the calculation of $x_{n+1}^n$ and $P_{n+1}^n$ is made at the final step $t = n$. The $m$-step-ahead predictor and its mean-square error based on the innovations algorithm (Problem 2.48) are given by

$$x_{n+m}^n = \sum_{j=m}^{n+m-1} \theta_{n+m-1,j}(x_{n+m-j} - x_{n+m-j}^{n+m-j-1}), \tag{2.72}$$

$$P_{n+m}^n = \gamma(0) - \sum_{j=m}^{n+m-1} \theta_{n+m-1,j}^2 P_{n+m-j}^n, \tag{2.73}$$

where the $\theta_{n+m-1,j}$ are obtained by continued iteration of (2.71).

**Example 2.20 Prediction for an MA(1)**

The innovations algorithm lends itself well to prediction for moving average processes. Consider an MA(1) model, $x_t = w_t + \theta w_{t-1}$. Recall that $\gamma(0) = (1+\theta^2)\sigma_w^2$, $\gamma(1) = \theta\sigma_w^2$, and $\gamma(h) = 0$ for $h > 1$. Then, using Property P2.6, we have

$$\begin{aligned} \theta_{n1} &= \theta\sigma_w^2/P_n^{n-1} \\ \theta_{nj} &= 0, \quad j = 2, ..., n \\ P_1^0 &= (1+\theta^2)\sigma_w^2 \\ P_{n+1}^n &= (1+\theta^2 - \theta\theta_{n1})\sigma_w^2. \end{aligned}$$

Finally, from (2.69), the one-step-ahead predictor is

$$x_{n+1}^n = \theta\left(x_n - x_n^{n-1}\right)\sigma_w^2/P_n^{n-1}.$$

FORECASTING ARMA PROCESSES

The general prediction equations (2.54) provide little insight into forecasting for ARMA models in general. There are a number of different ways to express these forecasts, and each aids in understanding the special structure of ARMA prediction. Throughout, we assume $x_t$ is a causal and invertible ARMA$(p,q)$ process, $\phi(B)x_t = \theta(B)w_t$. First, we consider two types of forecasts. We write $x_{n+m}^n$ to mean the minimum mean square error predictor of $x_{n+m}$ based on the data $\{x_n, ..., x_1\}$, that is,

$$x_{n+m}^n = E(x_{n+m} \mid x_n, ..., x_1).$$

For ARMA models, it is easier to calculate the predictor of $x_{n+m}$, assuming we have the complete history of the process $\{x_n, x_{n-1}, ...\}$. We will denote the predictor of $x_{n+m}$ ***based on the infinite past*** as

$$\widetilde{x}_{n+m} = E(x_{n+m} \mid x_n, x_{n-1}, ...).$$

The idea here is that, for large samples, $\widetilde{x}_{n+m}$ will provide a good approximation to $x_{n+m}^n$.

Now, write $x_{n+m}$ in its causal and invertible forms:

$$x_{n+m} = \sum_{j=0}^{\infty} \psi_j w_{n+m-j}, \quad \psi_0 = 1 \tag{2.74}$$

$$w_{n+m} = \sum_{j=0}^{\infty} \pi_j x_{n+m-j}, \quad \pi_0 = 1. \tag{2.75}$$

Then, taking conditional expectations in (2.74), we have

$$\widetilde{x}_{n+m} = \sum_{j=0}^{\infty} \psi_j \widetilde{w}_{n+m-j} = \sum_{j=m}^{\infty} \psi_j w_{n+m-j}, \tag{2.76}$$

because, by (2.75),

$$\widetilde{w}_t \equiv E(w_t | x_n, x_{n-1}, ...) = \begin{cases} 0, & t > n \\ w_t, & t \leq n. \end{cases}$$

Similarly, taking conditional expectations in (2.75), we have

$$0 = \widetilde{x}_{n+m} + \sum_{j=1}^{\infty} \pi_j \widetilde{x}_{n+m-j},$$

or

$$\widetilde{x}_{n+m} = - \sum_{j=1}^{m-1} \pi_j \widetilde{x}_{n+m-j} - \sum_{j=m}^{\infty} \pi_j x_{n+m-j}, \tag{2.77}$$

using the fact $E(x_t \mid x_n, x_{n-1}, ...) = x_t$, for $t \leq n$. Prediction is accomplished recursively using (2.77), starting with the one-step-ahead predictor, $m = 1$, and then continuing for $m = 2, 3, ....$ Using (2.76), we can write

$$x_{n+m} - \widetilde{x}_{n+m} = \sum_{j=0}^{m-1} \psi_j w_{n+m-j},$$

so the ***mean square prediction error*** can be written as

$$P_{n+m}^n = E(x_{n+m} - \widetilde{x}_{n+m})^2 = \sigma_w^2 \sum_{j=0}^{m-1} \psi_j^2. \tag{2.78}$$

Also, we note, for a fixed sample size, $n$, the prediction errors are correlated. That is, for $k \geq 1$,

$$E\{(x_{n+m} - \widetilde{x}_{n+m})(x_{n+m+k} - \widetilde{x}_{n+m+k})\} = \sigma_w^2 \sum_{j=0}^{m-1} \psi_j \psi_{j+k}. \tag{2.79}$$

When $n$ is small, the general prediction equations (2.54) can be used easily. When $n$ is large, we would use (2.77) by truncating, because only the data $x_1, x_2, ..., x_n$ are available. In this case, we can truncate (2.77) by setting $\sum_{j=n+m}^{\infty} \pi_j x_{n+m-j} = 0$. The ***truncated predictor*** is then written as

$$\widetilde{x}_{n+m}^n = - \sum_{j=1}^{m-1} \pi_j \widetilde{x}_{n+m-j}^n - \sum_{j=m}^{n+m-1} \pi_j x_{n+m-j}, \tag{2.80}$$

which is also calculated recursively, $m = 1, 2, ....$ The mean square prediction error, in this case, is approximated using (2.78).

For AR($p$) models, and when $n > p$, equation (2.61) yields the exact predictor, $x_{n+m}^n$, of $x_{n+m}$, and there is no need for approximations. That is, for $n > p$, $\widetilde{x}_{n+m}^n = \widetilde{x}_{n+m} = x_{n+m}^n$. Also, in this case, the one-step-ahead prediction error is $E(x_{n+1} - x_{n+1}^n)^2 = \sigma_w^2$. For general ARMA($p, q$) models, the truncated predictors (Problem 2.15) for $m = 1, 2, ...$, are

$$\widetilde{x}_{n+m}^n = \phi_1 \widetilde{x}_{n+m-1}^n + \cdots + \phi_p \widetilde{x}_{n+m-p}^n + \theta_1 \widetilde{w}_{n+m}^n + \cdots + \theta_q \widetilde{w}_{n+m-q+1}^n, \quad (2.81)$$

where $\widetilde{x}_t^n = x_t$ for $1 \leq t \leq n$ and $\widetilde{x}_t^n = 0$ for $t \leq 0$. The truncated prediction errors are given by: $\widetilde{w}_t^n = 0$ for $t \leq 0$ or $t > n$, and $\widetilde{w}_t^n = \phi(B)\widetilde{x}_t^n - \theta_1 \widetilde{w}_{t-1}^n - \cdots - \theta_q \widetilde{w}_{t-q}^n$ for $1 \leq t \leq n$.

**Example 2.21 Forecasting an ARMA(1,1) Series**

Given data $x_1, ..., x_n$, for forecasting purposes, write the model as

$$x_{n+1} = \phi x_n + w_{n+1} + \theta w_n.$$

Then, based on (2.81), the one-step-ahead truncated forecast is

$$\widetilde{x}_{n+1}^n = \phi x_n + 0 + \theta \widetilde{w}_n^n.$$

For $m \geq 2$, we have

$$\widetilde{x}_{n+m}^n = \phi \widetilde{x}_{n+m-1}^n,$$

which can be calculated recursively, $m = 2, 3, ...$ .

To calculate $\widetilde{w}_n^n$, which is needed to initialize the successive forecasts, the model can be written as $w_t = x_t - \phi x_{t-1} - \theta w_{t-1}$ for $t = 1, ...n$. For truncated forecasting, put $\widetilde{w}_0^n = 0$ and then iterate the errors forward in time (we set $x_0 = 0$)

$$\widetilde{w}_t^n = x_t - \phi x_{t-1} - \theta \widetilde{w}_{t-1}^n, \quad t = 1, ..., n.$$

The approximate forecast variance is computed from (2.78) using the $\psi$-weights determined as in Example 2.10. In particular, the $\psi$-weights satisfy $\psi_j = (\phi + \theta)\phi^{j-1}$, for $j \geq 1$. This result gives

$$\begin{aligned} P_{n+m}^n &= \sigma_w^2 \left[ 1 + (\phi + \theta)^2 \sum_{j=1}^{m-1} \phi_1^{2(j-1)} \right] \\ &= \sigma_w^2 \left[ 1 + \frac{(\phi + \theta_1)^2 (1 - \phi^{2(m-1)})}{(1 - \phi^2)} \right]. \end{aligned}$$

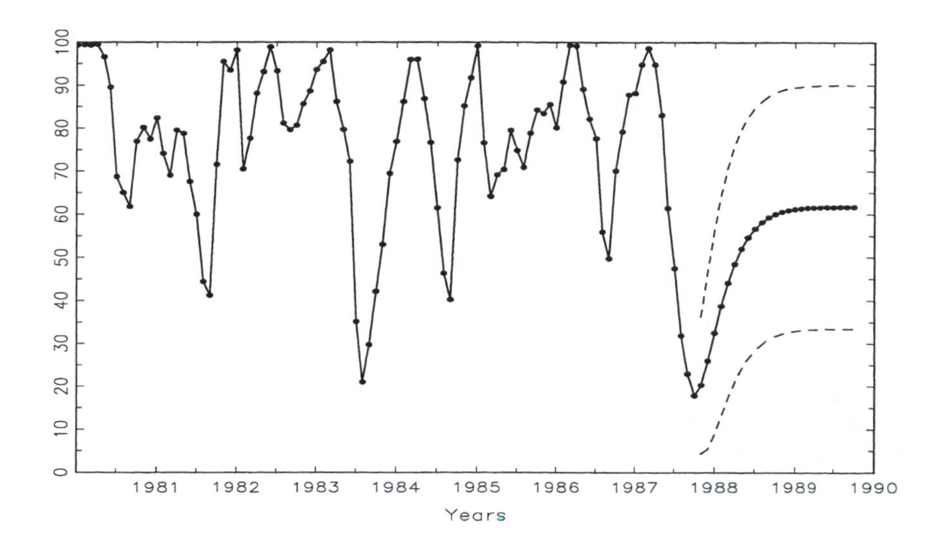


**Figure 2.6:** Twenty-four month forecasts for the Recruitment series. The actual data shown are from January, 1980 to September, 1987, and then forecasts plus and minus one standard error are displayed.

To assess the precision of the forecasts, ***prediction intervals*** are typically calculated along with the forecasts. In general, $(1-\alpha)$ prediction intervals are of the form

$$x_{n+m}^{n} \pm c_{\frac{\alpha}{2}} \sqrt{P_{n+m}^{n}}, \tag{2.82}$$

where $c_{\alpha/2}$ is chosen to get the desired degree of confidence. For example, if the process is Gaussian, then choosing $c_{\alpha/2} = 2$ will yield an approximate 95% prediction interval for $x_{n+m}$. From Tchebycheff's inequality (1.97), we know that using $c_{\alpha/2} = 2$ will provide, at least, a 75% prediction interval, and setting $c_{\alpha/2} = 3$ will provide, at least, an 89% prediction interval. If we are interested in establishing prediction intervals over more than one time period, then $c_{\alpha/2}$ should be adjusted appropriately, for example, by using Bonferroni's inequality [see (3.68) in Chapter 3 or Johnson and Wichern, 1992, Chapter 5].

**Example 2.22 Forecasting the Recruitment Series.**

Using the parameter estimates as the actual parameter values, Figure 2.6 shows the result of forecasting the Recruitment series given in Example 2.16 over a 24-month horizon, $m = 1, 2, ..., 24$. The actual forecasts are calculated as

$$x_{n+m}^{n} = 6.74 + 1.35 x_{n+m-1}^{n} - 0.46 x_{n+m-2}^{n}$$

for $n = 453$ and $m = 1, 2, ..., 12$. Recall that $x_t^s = x_t$ when $t \leq s$. The forecasts errors $P_{n+m}^n$ are calculated using (2.110). Recall that $\widehat{\sigma}_w^2 = 90.31$, and using (2.37) from Example 2.10, we have $\psi_j = 1.35\psi_{j-1} - 0.46\psi_{j-2}$ for $j \geq 2$, where $\psi_0 = 1$ and $\psi_1 = 1.35$. Thus, for $n = 453$,

$$\begin{aligned} P_{n+1}^n &= 90.31, \\ P_{n+2}^n &= 90.31(1 + 1.35^2), \\ P_{n+3}^n &= 90.31(1 + 1.35^2 + [1.35^2 - .46]^2), \end{aligned}$$

and so on.

Note how the forecast levels off quickly and the prediction intervals are wide, even though in this case the forecast limits are only based on one standard error; that is, $x_{n+m}^n \pm \sqrt{P_{n+m}^n}$.

We complete this section with a brief discussion of ***backcasting***. In backcasting, we want to predict $x_{1-m}$, $m = 1, 2, ...$, based on the data $\{x_1, ..., x_n\}$. Write the backcast as

$$x_{1-m}^n = \sum_{j=1}^n \alpha_j x_j. \tag{2.83}$$

Analogous to (2.66), the prediction equations (assuming $\mu = 0$) are

$$\sum_{j=1}^n \alpha_j E(x_j x_k) = E(x_{1-m} x_k), \quad k = 1, ..., n, \tag{2.84}$$

or

$$\sum_{j=1}^n \alpha_j \gamma(k - j) = \gamma(m + k - 1), \quad k = 1, ..., n. \tag{2.85}$$

These equations are precisely the prediction equations for forward prediction. That is, $\alpha_j \equiv \phi_{nj}^{(m)}$, for $j = 1, ...n$, where the $\phi_{nj}^{(m)}$ are given by (2.67). Finally, the backcasts are given by

$$x_{1-m}^n = \phi_{n1}^{(m)} x_1 + \cdots + \phi_{nn}^{(m)} x_n, \quad m = 1, 2, .... \tag{2.86}$$

**Example 2.23 Backcasting an ARMA(1,1)**

Consider a causal and invertible ARMA(1,1) process, $x_t = \phi x_{t-1} + \theta w_{t-1} + w_t$; we will call this the forward model. We have just seen that prediction backward in time is the same as prediction forward in time for stationary models. Thus, the process can equivalently be generated by the backward model $x_t = \phi x_{t+1} + \theta v_{t+1} + v_t$, where $\{v_t\}$ is a white noise process with variance $\sigma_w^2$ (using spectral densities, Chapter 3, there is a simple proof that the two representations are equivalent).

We may write $x_t = \sum_{j=0}^{\infty} \psi_j v_{t+j}$, where $\psi_0 = 1$; this means that $x_t$ is uncorrelated with $\{v_{t-1}, v_{t-2}, ...\}$, in analogy to the forward model.

Given data $\{x_1, ...., x_n\}$, truncate $v_n^n = E(v_n \mid x_1, ...., x_n)$ to zero. That is, put $\widetilde{v}_n^n = 0$, as an initial approximation, and then generate the errors backward

$$\widetilde{v}_t^n = x_t - \phi x_{t+1} + \theta \widetilde{v}_{t+1}^n, \quad t = (n-1), (n-2), ..., 1.$$

Then,

$$\widetilde{x}_0^n = \phi x_1 + \theta \widetilde{v}_1^n + \widetilde{v}_0^n = \phi x_1 + \theta \widetilde{v}_1^n,$$

because $\widetilde{v}_t^n = 0$ for $t \leq 0$. Continuing, the general truncated backcasts are given by

$$\widetilde{x}_{1-m}^n = \phi \widetilde{x}_{2-m}^n, \quad m = 2, 3, ... .$$

## 2.6 Estimation

Throughout this section, we assume we have $n$ observations, $x_1, ..., x_n$, from a causal and invertible ARMA$(p,q)$ process in which the order parameters, $p$ and $q$, are known. Our goal is to estimate the parameters, $\phi_1, ..., \phi_p, \theta_1, ..., \theta_q$, and $\sigma_w^2$. We will discuss the problem of determining $p$ and $q$ later.

We begin with ***method of moments*** estimators. The idea behind these estimators is that of equating population moments to sample moments and then solving for the parameters in terms of the sample moments. We immediately see that, if $E(x_t) = \mu$, then the method of moments estimator of $\mu$ is the sample average, $\bar{x}$. Thus, while discussing method of moments, we will assume $\mu = 0$. Although the method of moments can produce good estimators, they can sometimes lead to suboptimal estimators. We first consider the case in which the method leads to optimal (efficient) estimators, that is, AR$(p)$ models.

When the process is AR$(p)$,

$$x_t = \phi_1 x_{t-1} + \cdots + \phi_p x_{t-p} + w_t,$$

the first $p+1$ equations of (2.43) and (2.44) are called the ***Yule–Walker equations***:

$$\begin{aligned} \gamma(0) &= \phi_1 \gamma(1) + \cdots + \phi_p \gamma(p) + \sigma_w^2 \\ \gamma(h) &= \phi_1 \gamma(h-1) + \cdots + \phi_p \gamma(h-p), \quad h = 1, 2, ..., p. \end{aligned} \tag{2.87}$$

In matrix notation, the Yule–Walker equations are

$$\Gamma_p \boldsymbol{\phi} = \boldsymbol{\gamma}_p, \quad \sigma_w^2 = \gamma(0) - \boldsymbol{\phi}' \boldsymbol{\gamma}_p, \tag{2.88}$$

where $\Gamma_p = \{\gamma(k-j)\}_{j,k=1}^p$ is a $p \times p$ matrix, $\boldsymbol{\phi} = (\phi_1, ..., \phi_p)'$ is a $p \times 1$ vector, and $\boldsymbol{\gamma}_p = (\gamma(1), ..., \gamma(p))'$ is a $p \times 1$ vector. Using the method of moments, we replace $\gamma(h)$ in (2.88) by $\widehat{\gamma}(h)$ (see equation 1.31) and solve

$$\widehat{\boldsymbol{\phi}} = \widehat{\Gamma}_p^{-1}\widehat{\boldsymbol{\gamma}}_p, \quad \widehat{\sigma}_w^2 = \widehat{\gamma}(0) - \widehat{\boldsymbol{\gamma}}_p'\widehat{\Gamma}_p^{-1}\widehat{\boldsymbol{\gamma}}_p. \tag{2.89}$$

These estimators are typically called the ***Yule–Walker estimators***. For calculation purposes, it is sometimes more convenient to work with the sample ACF. By factoring $\widehat{\gamma}(0)$ in (2.89), we can write the Yule–Walker estimates as

$$\widehat{\boldsymbol{\phi}} = \widehat{\boldsymbol{R}}_p^{-1}\widehat{\boldsymbol{\rho}}_p, \quad \widehat{\sigma}_w^2 = \widehat{\gamma}(0)\left[1 - \widehat{\boldsymbol{\rho}}_p'\widehat{\boldsymbol{R}}_p^{-1}\widehat{\boldsymbol{\rho}}_p\right], \tag{2.90}$$

where $\widehat{R}_p = \{\widehat{\rho}(k-j)\}_{j,k=1}^p$ is a $p \times p$ matrix and $\widehat{\boldsymbol{\rho}}_p = (\widehat{\rho}(1), ..., \widehat{\rho}(p))'$ is a $p \times 1$ vector.

For AR($p$) models, if the sample size is large, the Yule–Walker estimators are approximately normally distributed, and $\widehat{\sigma}_w^2$ is close to the true value of $\sigma_w^2$. We state these results in Property P2.7. For details, see Section T2.17.

***Property P2.7: Large Sample Results for Yule–Walker Estimators***
*The asymptotic ($n \to \infty$) behavior of the Yule–Walker estimators in the case of causal AR(p) processes is as follows:*

$$\sqrt{n}\left(\widehat{\boldsymbol{\phi}} - \boldsymbol{\phi}\right) \xrightarrow{d} \mathrm{N}\left(\mathbf{0}, \sigma_w^2\boldsymbol{\Gamma}_p^{-1}\right), \qquad \widehat{\sigma}_w^2 \xrightarrow{p} \sigma_w^2. \tag{2.91}$$

The Durbin–Levinson algorithm, (2.62)-(2.64), can be used to calculate $\widehat{\boldsymbol{\phi}}$ without inverting $\widehat{R}_p$, by replacing $\gamma(h)$ by $\widehat{\gamma}(h)$ in the algorithm. In running the algorithm, we will iteratively calculate the $h \times 1$ vector, $\widehat{\boldsymbol{\phi}}_h = (\widehat{\phi}_{h1}, ..., \widehat{\phi}_{hh})'$, for $h = 1, 2, ....$ Thus, in addition to obtaining the desired forecasts, the Durbin-Levinson algorithm yields $\widehat{\phi}_{hh}$, the sample PACF. Using (2.91), we can show the following property.

***Property P2.8: Large Sample Distribution of the PACF***
*For a causal AR(p) process, asymptotically ($n \to \infty$),*

$$\sqrt{n}\,\widehat{\phi}_{hh} \xrightarrow{d} \mathrm{N}(0,1), \quad \text{for} \quad h > p. \tag{2.92}$$

**Example 2.24 Yule–Walker Estimation for an AR(2) Process**

The data shown in Figure 2.3 were $n = 144$ simulated observations from the AR(2) model $x_t = 1.5x_{t-1} - .75x_{t-2} + w_t$, where $w_t \sim$ iid N(0,1). For this data, $\widehat{\gamma}(0) = 8.434$, $\widehat{\rho}(1) = .834$, and $\widehat{\rho}(2) = .476$. Thus,

$$\widehat{\boldsymbol{\phi}} = \begin{pmatrix} \widehat{\phi}_1 \\ \widehat{\phi}_2 \end{pmatrix} = \begin{bmatrix} 1 & .834 \\ .834 & 1 \end{bmatrix}^{-1} \begin{pmatrix} .834 \\ .476 \end{pmatrix} = \begin{pmatrix} 1.439 \\ -.725 \end{pmatrix}$$

and

$$\widehat{\sigma}_w^2 = 8.434 \left[1 - (.834, .476) \begin{pmatrix} 1.439 \\ -.725 \end{pmatrix}\right] = 1.215.$$

By Property P2.7, the asymptotic variance–covariance matrix of $\widehat{\boldsymbol{\phi}}$,

$$\frac{1}{144}\frac{1.215}{8.434}\begin{bmatrix} 1 & .834 \\ .834 & 1 \end{bmatrix}^{-1} = \begin{bmatrix} .057^2 & -.003 \\ -.003 & .057^2 \end{bmatrix},$$

can be used to get confidence regions for, or make inferences about $\widehat{\boldsymbol{\phi}}$ and its components. For example, an approximate 95% confidence interval for $\phi_2$ is $-0.725 \pm 2(.057)$, or $(-0.839, -0.611)$, which contains the true value of $\phi_2 = -0.75$.

For this data, the first three sample partial autocorrelations were $\widehat{\phi}_{11} = \widehat{\rho}(1) = .834$, $\widehat{\phi}_{22} = \widehat{\phi}_2 = -.725$, and $\widehat{\phi}_{33} = -.075$. According to Property P2.8, the asymptotic standard error of $\widehat{\phi}_{33}$ is $1/\sqrt{144} = .083$, and the observed value, $-.075$, is less than one standard deviation from $\phi_{33} = 0$.

In the case of AR($p$) models, the Yule–Walker estimators given in (2.90) are optimal in the sense that the asymptotic distribution, (2.91), is the best asymptotic normal distribution. This is because, given initial conditions, AR($p$) models are linear models, and the Yule–Walker estimators are essentially least squares estimators. If we use method of moments for MA or ARMA models, we will not get optimal estimators because such processes are nonlinear in the parameters.

**Example 2.25 Yule–Walker Estimation for an MA(1) Process**

Consider the time series $x_t = w_t + \theta w_{t-1}$, where $|\theta| < 1$. The model can then be written as

$$x_t = \sum_{j=1}^{\infty} (-\theta)^j x_{t-j} + w_t,$$

which is nonlinear in $\theta$. The Yule–Walker equations are $\gamma(0) = \sigma_w^2(1+\theta^2)$, and $\gamma(1) = \sigma_w^2\theta$, so the estimate of $\theta$ is found by solving:

$$\widehat{\rho}(1) = \frac{\widehat{\theta}}{1 + \widehat{\theta}^2},$$

where $\widehat{\rho}(1)$ is the sample ACF at lag-one. Two solutions exist, so we would pick the invertible one. If $|\widehat{\rho}(1)| \le \frac{1}{2}$, then the solutions are real, otherwise, a real solution does not exist. Even though $|\rho(1)| < \frac{1}{2}$ for an invertible MA(1), it may happen that $|\widehat{\rho}(1)| \ge \frac{1}{2}$ because it is an estimator. When $|\widehat{\rho}(1)| < \frac{1}{2}$, the invertible estimate is

$$\widehat{\theta} = \frac{1 - \sqrt{1 - 4\widehat{\rho}(1)^2}}{2\widehat{\rho}(1)}.$$

Using the results of (1.100) and Theorem 1.7, we have that

$$\widehat{\theta} \sim \text{AN}\left(\theta, \ \frac{1+\theta^2+4\theta^4+\theta^6+\theta^8}{n(1-\theta^2)^2}\right).$$

The maximum likelihood estimator (which we discuss next) of $\theta$, in this case, has an asymptotic variance of $(1-\theta^2)/n$. When $\theta = 0.5$, for example, the ratio of the asymptotic variance of the Yule–Walker estimator to the maximum likelihood estimator of $\theta$ is about 3.5. That is, for large samples, the variance of the method of moments estimator is about 3.5 times larger than the variance of the MLE of $\theta$ when $\theta = 0.5$.

### Maximum Likelihood and Least Squares Estimation

To fix ideas, we first focus on the AR(1) case. Let $(x_t - \mu) = \phi(x_{t-1} - \mu) + w_t$, where $|\phi| < 1$ and $w_t \sim \text{N}(0, \sigma_w^2)$. Given data $x_1, x_2, ..., x_n$, we seek the likelihood

$$L(\mu, \phi, \sigma_w) = f_{\mu,\phi,\sigma_w}(x_1, x_2, ..., x_n).$$

In the case of an AR(1), we may write the likelihood as

$$L(\mu, \phi, \sigma_w) = f(x_1) f(x_2 \mid x_1) \cdots f(x_n \mid x_{n-1}),$$

where we have dropped the parameter subscripts on the densities $f(\cdot)$ to ease the notation. Because $x_t \mid x_{t-1} \sim \text{N}\left(\mu + \phi(x_{t-1} - \mu), \sigma_w^2\right)$, we have

$$f(x_t \mid x_{t-1}) = f_w[(x_t - \mu) - \phi(x_{t-1} - \mu)],$$

where $f_w(\cdot)$ is the density of $w_t$, that is, the normal density with mean zero and variance $\sigma_w^2$. We may then write the likelihood as

$$L(\mu, \phi, \sigma_w) = f(x_1) \prod_{t=2}^{n} f_w\left[(x_t - \mu) - \phi(x_{t-1} - \mu)\right].$$

To find $f(x_1)$, we can use the causal representation of an AR(1), $(x_t - \mu) = \sum_{j=0}^{\infty} \phi^j w_{t-j}$, to see that $x_1$ is normal, with mean $\mu$ and variance $\sigma_w^2/(1-\phi^2)$. Finally, for an AR(1), the likelihood of the data is

$$L(\mu, \phi, \sigma_w) = (2\pi\sigma_w^2)^{-n/2}(1-\phi^2)^{1/2} \exp\left[-\frac{S(\mu, \phi)}{2\sigma_w^2}\right], \tag{2.93}$$

where

$$S(\mu, \phi) = (1-\phi^2)(x_1 - \mu)^2 + \sum_{t=2}^{n}\left[(x_t - \mu) - \phi(x_{t-1} - \mu)\right]^2. \tag{2.94}$$

Typically, $S(\mu, \phi)$ is called the ***unconditional sum of squares***. We could have also considered the estimation of $\mu$ and $\phi$, using ***unconditional least***

***squares***, that is, estimation by minimizing the unconditional sum of squares, $S(\mu, \phi)$. Using (2.93), the maximum likelihood estimate of $\sigma_w^2$ is

$$\widehat{\sigma}_w^2 = n^{-1} S(\widehat{\mu}, \widehat{\phi}), \tag{2.95}$$

where $\widehat{\mu}$ and $\widehat{\phi}$ are the MLEs of $\mu$ and $\phi$, respectively. If we replace $n$ in (2.95) by $n-2$, and $\widehat{\mu}$ and $\widehat{\phi}$ by the unconditional least squares estimators, we would obtain the unconditional least squares estimate of $\sigma_w^2$.

If, in (2.93), we take logs, replace $\sigma_w^2$ by its MLE, and ignore constants, $\widehat{\mu}$ and $\widehat{\phi}$ are the values that minimize the criterion function

$$l(\mu, \phi) = \ln \left[ n^{-1} S(\mu, \phi) \right] - n^{-1} \ln(1 - \phi^2). \tag{2.96}$$

That is, $l(\mu, \phi) \propto -2 \ln L(\mu, \phi, \widehat{\sigma}_w)$. Because (2.94) and (2.96) are complicated functions of the parameters, the minimization of $l(\mu, \phi)$ or $S(\mu, \phi)$ is accomplished numerically. In the case of AR models, we have the advantage that, conditional on initial values, they are linear models. That is, we can drop the term in the likelihood that causes the nonlinearity. Conditioning on $x_1$, the ***conditional likelihood***becomes

$$\begin{aligned} L(\mu, \phi, \sigma_w | x_1) &= \prod_{t=2}^{n} f_w \left[ (x_t - \mu) - \phi(x_{t-1} - \mu) \right] \\ &= (2\pi\sigma_w^2)^{-(n-1)/2} \exp\left[ -\frac{S_c(\mu, \phi)}{2\sigma_w^2} \right], \end{aligned} \tag{2.97}$$

where the ***conditional sum of squares*** is

$$S_c(\mu, \phi) = \sum_{t=2}^{n} \left[ (x_t - \mu) - \phi(x_{t-1} - \mu) \right]^2. \tag{2.98}$$

The conditional MLE of $\sigma_w^2$ is

$$\widehat{\sigma}_w^2 = S_c(\widehat{\mu}, \widehat{\phi})/(n-1), \tag{2.99}$$

and $\widehat{\mu}$ and $\widehat{\phi}$ are the values that minimize the conditional sum of squares, $S_c(\mu, \phi)$. Letting $\alpha = \mu(1 - \phi)$, the conditional sum of squares can be written as

$$S_c(\mu, \phi) = \sum_{t=2}^{n} \left[ x_t - (\alpha + \phi x_{t-1}) \right]^2. \tag{2.100}$$

The problem is now the linear regression problem stated in Section 1.8. Following the results from least squares estimation, we have $\widehat{\alpha} = \bar{x}_2 - \widehat{\phi}\bar{x}_1$, where $\bar{x}_1 = (n-1)^{-1} \sum_{t=1}^{n-1} x_t$, $\bar{x}_2 = (n-1)^{-1} \sum_{t=2}^{n} x_t$, and the conditional estimates are then

$$\widehat{\mu} = \frac{\bar{x}_2 - \widehat{\phi}\bar{x}_1}{1 - \widehat{\phi}} \tag{2.101}$$

$$\widehat{\phi} = \frac{\sum_{t=2}^{n}(x_t - \bar{x}_2)(x_{t-1} - \bar{x}_1)}{\sum_{t=2}^{n}(x_{t-1} - \bar{x}_1)^2}. \tag{2.102}$$

From (2.101) and (2.102), we see that $\widehat{\mu} \approx \bar{x}$ and $\widehat{\phi} \approx \widehat{\rho}(1)$. That is, the Yule–Walker estimators and the conditional least squares estimators are approximately the same. The only difference is the inclusion or exclusion of terms involving the end points, $x_1$ and $x_n$. We can also adjust the estimate of $\sigma_w^2$ in (2.99) to be equivalent to the least squares estimator, that is, divide $S_c(\widehat{\mu}, \widehat{\phi})$ by $(n-3)$ instead of $(n-1)$ in (2.99).

For general AR($p$) models, maximum likelihood estimation, unconditional least squares, and conditional least squares follow analogously to the AR(1) example. For general ARMA models, it is difficult to write the likelihood as an explicit function of the parameters. Instead, it is advantageous to write the likelihood in terms of the ***innovations***, or one-step-ahead prediction errors, $x_t - x_t^{t-1}$. This will also be useful in Chapter 4 when we study state-space models.

Suppose $x_t$ is a causal ARMA($p, q$) process with $w_t \sim \mathrm{N}(0, \sigma_w^2)$. Let $\boldsymbol{\beta} = (\mu, \phi_1, ..., \phi_p, \theta_1, ..., \theta_q)'$ be the $(p+q+1) \times 1$ vector of the model parameters. The likelihood can be written as

$$L(\boldsymbol{\beta}, \sigma_w^2) = \prod_{t=1}^{n} f(x_t \mid x_{t-1}, \dots, x_1).$$

The conditional distribution of $x_t$ given $x_{t-1}, ..., x_1$ is Gaussian with mean $x_t^{t-1}$ and variance $P_t^{t-1}$. In addition, for ARMA models, we may write $P_t^{t-1} = \sigma_w^2 r_t^{t-1}$ where $r_t^{t-1}$ does not depend on $\sigma_w^2$ (this can readily be seen from Proposition P2.4 by noting $P_1^0 = \gamma(0) = \sigma_w^2 \sum_{j=0}^{\infty} \psi_j^2$).

The likelihood of the data can now be written as

$$L(\boldsymbol{\beta}, \sigma_w^2) = (2\pi\sigma_w^2)^{-n/2}(r_1^0 r_2^1 \cdots r_n^{n-1})^{-1/2} \exp\left[-\frac{S(\boldsymbol{\beta})}{2\sigma_w^2}\right], \tag{2.103}$$

where

$$S(\boldsymbol{\beta}) = \sum_{t=1}^{n} \left[\frac{(x_t - x_t^{t-1})^2}{r_t^{t-1}}\right]. \tag{2.104}$$

Both $x_t^{t-1}$ and $r_t^{t-1}$ are functions of $\boldsymbol{\beta}$, and given values for $\boldsymbol{\beta}$ and $\sigma_w^2$, the likelihood may be evaluated using the techniques of Section 2.5. Maximum likelihood estimation would now proceed by maximizing (2.103) with respect to $\boldsymbol{\beta}$ and $\sigma_w^2$. As in the AR(1) example, we have

$$\widehat{\sigma}_w^2 = n^{-1} S(\widehat{\boldsymbol{\beta}}),$$

where $\widehat{\boldsymbol{\beta}}$ is the value of $\boldsymbol{\beta}$ that minimizes the criterion function

$$l(\boldsymbol{\beta}) = \ln\left[n^{-1} S(\boldsymbol{\beta})\right] + n^{-1} \sum_{t=1}^{n} \ln r_t^{t-1}. \tag{2.105}$$

Unconditional least squares would be performed by minimizing (2.104) with respect to $\boldsymbol{\beta}$. Conditional least squares estimation would involve minimizing (2.104) with respect to $\boldsymbol{\beta}$ but where, to ease the computational burden, the predictions and their errors are obtained by conditioning on initial values of the data. In general, numerical optimization routines are used to obtain the actual estimates and their standard errors.

### Example 2.26 The Newton–Raphson and Scoring Algorithms

Two common numerical optimization routines for accomplishing maximum likelihood estimation are Newton–Raphson and scoring. We will give a brief account of the mathematical ideas here. The actual implementation of these algorithms is much more complicated than our discussion might imply. For details, the reader is referred to any of the *Numerical Recipes* books, for example, Press et al (1993).

Let $l(\boldsymbol{\beta})$ be a criterion function of $k$ parameters $\boldsymbol{\beta} = (\beta_1, ..., \beta_k)$, that we wish to minimize with respect to $\boldsymbol{\beta}$. For example, consider the likelihood function given by (2.96) or by (2.105). Suppose $l(\widehat{\boldsymbol{\beta}})$ is the extremum that we are interested in finding, and $\widehat{\boldsymbol{\beta}}$ is found by solving $\partial l(\boldsymbol{\beta})/\partial\beta_j = 0$, for $j = 1, ..., k$. Let $l^{(1)}(\boldsymbol{\beta})$ denote the $k \times 1$ vector of partials

$$l^{(1)}(\boldsymbol{\beta}) = \left(\frac{\partial l(\boldsymbol{\beta})}{\partial\beta_1}, ..., \frac{\partial l(\boldsymbol{\beta})}{\partial\beta_k}\right)'.$$

Note, $l^{(1)}(\widehat{\boldsymbol{\beta}}) = \mathbf{0}$, the $k \times 1$ zero vector. Let $l^{(2)}(\boldsymbol{\beta})$ denote the $k \times k$ matrix of second order partials

$$l^{(2)}(\boldsymbol{\beta}) = \left\{-\frac{\partial l^2(\boldsymbol{\beta})}{\partial\beta_i\partial\beta_j}\right\}_{i,j=1}^{k},$$

and assume $l^{(2)}(\boldsymbol{\beta})$ is nonsingular. Let $\boldsymbol{\beta}_0$ be an initial estimator of $\boldsymbol{\beta}$. Then, using a Taylor expansion, we have the following approximation:

$$\mathbf{0} = l^{(1)}(\widehat{\boldsymbol{\beta}}) \approx l^{(1)}(\boldsymbol{\beta}_0) - l^{(2)}(\boldsymbol{\beta}_0)\left[\widehat{\boldsymbol{\beta}} - \boldsymbol{\beta}_0\right].$$

Setting the right-hand-side equal to zero and solving for $\widehat{\boldsymbol{\beta}}$, we get

$$\widehat{\boldsymbol{\beta}}_{(1)} = \boldsymbol{\beta}_0 + \left[l^{(2)}(\boldsymbol{\beta}_0)\right]^{-1} l^{(1)}(\boldsymbol{\beta}_0).$$

The Newton–Raphson algorithm proceeds by iterating this result, replacing $\boldsymbol{\beta}_0$ by $\widehat{\boldsymbol{\beta}}_{(1)}$ to get $\widehat{\boldsymbol{\beta}}_{(2)}$, and so on, until convergence. Under a set of appropriate conditions, the sequence of estimators, $\widehat{\boldsymbol{\beta}}_{(1)}, \widehat{\boldsymbol{\beta}}_{(2)}, \ldots$, will converge to $\widehat{\boldsymbol{\beta}}$.

For maximum likelihood estimation, the criterion function used is $l(\boldsymbol{\beta}) = -\ln L(\boldsymbol{\beta})$; any constants can be ignored. In scoring, we replace $l^{(2)}(\boldsymbol{\beta})$ by $E[l^{(2)}(\boldsymbol{\beta})]$, the ***information*** matrix. Under appropriate conditions, the inverse of the information matrix is the asymptotic variance-covariance matrix of the estimator $\widehat{\boldsymbol{\beta}}$. In the numerical procedure, this matrix is often approximated by the inverse of $l^{(2)}(\widehat{\boldsymbol{\beta}})$, where $\widehat{\boldsymbol{\beta}}$ is the value of the estimate at the time of convergence. In pseudo maximum likelihood estimation, we use numerical techniques to approximate the derivatives.

We now discuss least squares for ARMA$(p,q)$ models via ***Gauss–Newton***. For general and complete details of the Gauss–Newton procedure, the reader is referred to Fuller (1995). Let $x_t$ be a causal and invertible Gaussian ARMA$(p,q)$ process. Write $\boldsymbol{\beta} = (\phi_1, ..., \phi_p, \theta_1, ..., \theta_q)'$, and for the ease of discussion, we will put $\mu = 0$. We write the model in terms of the errors

$$w_t(\boldsymbol{\beta}) = x_t - \sum_{j=1}^{p} \phi_j x_{t-j} - \sum_{k=1}^{q} \theta_k w_{t-k}(\boldsymbol{\beta}), \tag{2.106}$$

emphasizing the dependence of the errors on the parameters.

For conditional least squares, we approximate the residual sum of squares by conditioning on $x_1, ..., x_p$ $(p > 0)$ and $w_p = w_{p-1} = w_{-2} = \cdots = w_{1-q} = 0$ $(q > 0)$, in which case we may evaluate (2.106) for $t = p+1, p+2, ..., n$. Using this conditioning argument, the conditional sum of squares is

$$S_c(\boldsymbol{\beta}) = \sum_{t=p+1}^{n} w_t^2(\boldsymbol{\beta}).$$

Minimizing $S_c(\boldsymbol{\beta})$ with respect to $\boldsymbol{\beta}$ yields the conditional least squares estimates. If $q = 0$, the problem is linear regression, and no numerical technique is needed to minimize $S_c(\phi_1, ..., \phi_p)$. If $q > 0$, the problem becomes nonlinear regression and we will have to rely on numerical optimization.

When $n$ is large, conditioning on a few initial values will have little influence on the final parameter estimates. In the case of small to moderate sample sizes, one may wish to rely on unconditional least squares. The unconditional least squares problem is to choose $\boldsymbol{\beta}$ to minimize the unconditional sum of squares, which we have generically denoted by $S(\boldsymbol{\beta})$ in this section. The unconditional sum of squares can be written in various ways, and one useful form in the case of ARMA$(p,q)$ models is derived in Box et al (1994, Appendix A7.3). They showed (see Problem 2.18) the unconditional sum of squares can be written as

$$S(\boldsymbol{\beta}) = \sum_{t=-\infty}^{n} \widehat{w}_t^2(\boldsymbol{\beta}),$$

where $\widehat{w}_t(\boldsymbol{\beta}) = E(w_t \mid x_1, ..., x_n)$. When $t \leq 0$, the $\widehat{w}_t(\boldsymbol{\beta})$ are obtained by backcasting. As a practical matter, we approximate $S(\boldsymbol{\beta})$ by starting the sum at

$t = -M+1$, where $M$ is chosen large enough to guarantee $\sum_{t=-\infty}^{-M} \widehat{w}_t^2(\boldsymbol{\beta}) \approx 0$. In the case of unconditional least squares estimation, a numerical optimization technique is needed even when $q = 0$.

To employ Gauss–Newton, let $\widehat{\boldsymbol{\beta}}_0 = (\phi_1^{(0)}, ..., \phi_p^{(0)}, \theta_1^{(0)}, ..., \theta_q^{(0)})'$ be an initial estimate of $\boldsymbol{\beta}$. For example, we could obtain $\widehat{\boldsymbol{\beta}}_0$ by method of moments. The first-order Taylor expansion of $w_t(\boldsymbol{\beta})$ is

$$w_t(\boldsymbol{\beta}) \approx w_t(\widehat{\boldsymbol{\beta}}_0) - \left(\boldsymbol{\beta} - \widehat{\boldsymbol{\beta}}_0\right)' \boldsymbol{z}_t(\widehat{\boldsymbol{\beta}}_0), \tag{2.107}$$

where

$$\boldsymbol{z}_t(\widehat{\boldsymbol{\beta}}_0) = \left(-\frac{\partial w_t(\widehat{\boldsymbol{\beta}}_0)}{\partial \beta_1}, ..., -\frac{\partial w_t(\widehat{\boldsymbol{\beta}}_0)}{\partial \beta_{p+q}}\right)', \quad t = 1, ..., n.$$

The linear approximation of $S_c(\boldsymbol{\beta})$ is

$$Q(\boldsymbol{\beta}) = \sum_{t=p+1}^{n} \left[ w_t(\widehat{\boldsymbol{\beta}}_0) - \left(\boldsymbol{\beta} - \widehat{\boldsymbol{\beta}}_0\right)' \boldsymbol{z}_t(\widehat{\boldsymbol{\beta}}_0) \right]^2 \tag{2.108}$$

and this is the quantity that we will minimize. For approximate unconditional least squares, we would start the sum in (2.108) at $t = -M+1$, for a large value of $M$, and work with the backcasted values.

Using the results of ordinary least squares (Section 1.8), we know

$$(\widehat{\boldsymbol{\beta} - \boldsymbol{\beta}_0}) = \left(n^{-1} \sum_{t=p+1}^{n} \boldsymbol{z}_t(\widehat{\boldsymbol{\beta}}_0) \boldsymbol{z}_t'(\widehat{\boldsymbol{\beta}}_0)\right)^{-1} \left(n^{-1} \sum_{t=p+1}^{n} \boldsymbol{z}_t(\widehat{\boldsymbol{\beta}}_0) w_t(\widehat{\boldsymbol{\beta}}_0)\right) \tag{2.109}$$

minimizes $Q(\boldsymbol{\beta})$. From (2.109), we write the ***one-step Gauss–Newton estimate*** as

$$\widehat{\boldsymbol{\beta}}_{(1)} = \widehat{\boldsymbol{\beta}}_0 + \Delta(\widehat{\boldsymbol{\beta}}_0), \tag{2.110}$$

where $\Delta(\boldsymbol{\beta}_0)$ denotes the right-hand-side of (2.109). Gauss–Newton estimation is accomplished by replacing $\widehat{\boldsymbol{\beta}}_0$ by $\widehat{\boldsymbol{\beta}}_{(1)}$ in (2.110). This process is repeated by calculating, at iteration $j = 2, 3, \ldots,$

$$\widehat{\boldsymbol{\beta}}_{(j)} = \widehat{\boldsymbol{\beta}}_{(j-1)} + \Delta(\widehat{\boldsymbol{\beta}}_{(j-1)})$$

until convergence.

### Example 2.27 Gauss–Newton for an MA(1)

Consider an invertible MA(1) process, $x_t = w_t + \theta w_{t-1}$. Write the truncated errors as

$$w_t(\theta) = x_t - \theta w_{t-1}(\theta), \quad t = 1, ..., n, \tag{2.111}$$

where we condition on $w_0(\theta) = 0$. Taking derivatives,

$$-\frac{\partial w_t(\theta)}{\partial \theta} = w_{t-1}(\theta) + \theta \frac{\partial w_{t-1}(\theta)}{\partial \theta}, \quad t = 1, ..., n, \tag{2.112}$$

where $\partial w_0(\theta)/\partial\theta = 0$. We can also write (2.112), using the notation of (2.107), as

$$z_t(\theta) = w_{t-1} - \theta z_{t-1}(\theta), \quad t = 1, ..., n, \tag{2.113}$$

where $z_0(\theta) = 0$.

Let $\widehat{\theta}_0$ be an initial estimate of $\theta$, for example, the estimate given in Example 2.25. Then, the Gauss–Newton procedure for conditional least squares is given by

$$\widehat{\theta}_{j+1} = \widehat{\theta}_j + \frac{\sum_{t=1}^n z_t(\widehat{\theta}_j) w_t(\widehat{\theta}_j)}{\sum_{t=1}^n z_t^2(\widehat{\theta}_j)}, \quad j = 0, 1, 2, ..., \tag{2.114}$$

where the values in (2.114) are calculated recursively using (2.111) and (2.113). The calculations are stopped when $|\widehat{\theta}_{j+1} - \widehat{\theta}_j|$, or $|Q(\widehat{\theta}_{j+1}) - Q(\widehat{\theta}_j)|$, are smaller than some preset amount.

**Example 2.28 Fitting the Glacial Varve Series**

Consider the series of glacial varve thicknesses from Massachusetts for $n = 634$ years, as analyzed in Figure 1.17 and in Problem 1.25, where it was argued that a first-order moving average model might fit the logarithmically transformed and differenced varve series, say,

$$\nabla[\ln(x_t)] = \ln(x_t) - \ln(x_{t-1}) = \ln\left(\frac{x_t}{x_{t-1}}\right),$$

which can be interpreted as being proportional to the percentage change in the thickness.

The sample ACF and PACF, shown in Figure 2.7, confirm the tendency of $\nabla[\ln(x_t)]$ to behave as a first-order moving average process as the ACF has only a significant peak at lag one and the PACF decreases exponentially. Using Table 2.1, this sample behavior fits that of the MA(1) very well.

Nine iterations of the Gauss–Newton procedure, (2.114), starting with $\widehat{\theta}_0 = -0.1$ yielded the values

$$-0.442, -0.624, -0.717, -0.750, -0.763, -0.768, -0.771, -0.772, -0.772$$

for $\widehat{\theta}_{(1)}, ..., \widehat{\theta}_{(9)}$, and a final estimated error variance $\widehat{\sigma}_w^2 = 0.236$ as in (1.58). Using the final value of $\widehat{\theta} = -0.772$ and the vectors $z_t$ of partial derivatives in (2.113) leads to a standard error of 0.025 and a $t$-value of 30.45 using (1.59) with 632 degrees of freedom (one is lost in differencing).

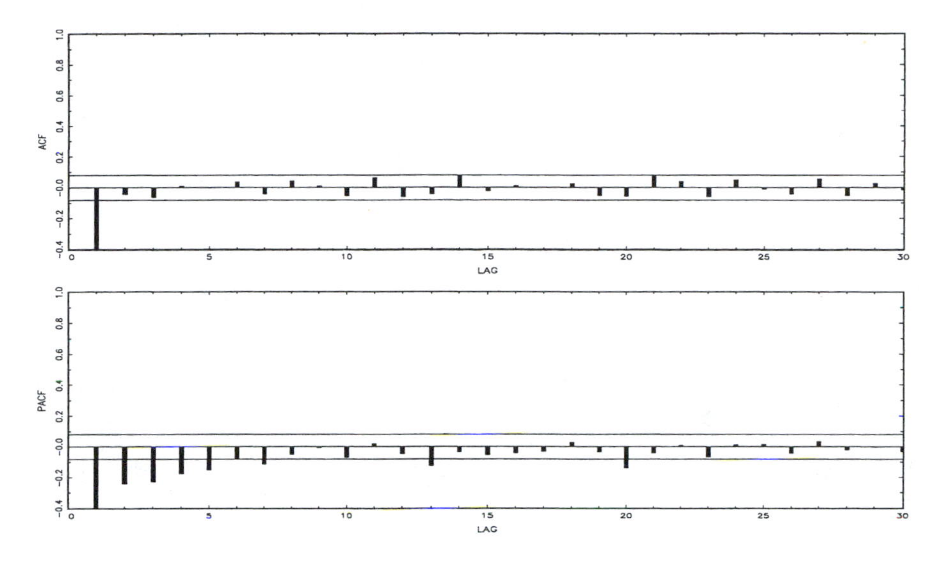


**Figure 2.7:** ACF and PACF of transformed glacial varves.

In the general case of causal and invertible ARMA$(p,q)$ models, maximum likelihood estimation and conditional and unconditional least squares estimation (and Yule–Walker estimation in the case of AR models) all lead to optimal estimators. The proof of this general result can be found in a number of texts on theoretical time series analysis (for example, Brockwell and Davis, 1991, or Hannan, 1970, to mention a few). We will denote the ARMA coefficient parameters by $\boldsymbol{\beta} = (\phi_1, ..., \phi_p, \theta_1, ..., \theta_q)'$.

***Property P2.9: Large Sample Distribution of the Estimators***
*The maximum likelihood, unconditional least squares, and conditional least squares estimators, each initialized by the method of moments estimator, all provide optimal estimators of $\boldsymbol{\beta}$, in the sense that the asymptotic distribution of the of the estimator, $\widehat{\boldsymbol{\beta}}$, say, is the best asymptotic normal distribution. In particular, as $n \to \infty$,*

$$\sqrt{n}\left(\widehat{\boldsymbol{\beta}} - \boldsymbol{\beta}\right) \xrightarrow{d} \mathrm{N}\left(\mathbf{0}, \sigma_w^2\, \boldsymbol{\Gamma}_{p,q}^{-1}\right). \tag{2.115}$$

In (2.115), the variance–covariance matrix of the estimator $\widehat{\boldsymbol{\beta}}$ is the inverse of the ***information*** matrix. In this case, the $(p+q) \times (p+q)$ matrix $\Gamma_{p,q}$, has the form

$$\Gamma_{p,q} = \begin{pmatrix} \Gamma_{\phi\phi} & \Gamma_{\phi\theta} \\ \Gamma_{\theta\phi} & \Gamma_{\theta\theta} \end{pmatrix}. \tag{2.116}$$

The $p \times p$ matrix $\Gamma_{\phi\phi}$ is given by (2.88), that is, the $ij$-th element of $\Gamma_{\phi\phi}$, for $i, j = 1, ..., p$, is $\gamma_x(i-j)$ from an AR($p$) process, $\phi(B)x_t = w_t$. Similarly, $\Gamma_{\theta\theta}$ is a $q \times q$ matrix with the $ij$-th element, for $i, j = 1, ..., q$, equal to $\gamma_y(i-j)$ from an AR($q$) process, $\theta(B)y_t = w_t$. The $p \times q$ matrix $\Gamma_{\phi\theta} = \{\gamma_{xy}(i-j)\}$, for $i = 1, ..., p$; $j = 1, ..., q$; that is, the $ij$-th element is the cross-covariance between the two AR processes given by $\phi(B)x_t = w_t$ and $\theta(B)y_t = w_t$. Finally, $\Gamma_{\theta\phi} = \Gamma'_{\phi\theta}$ is $q \times p$. Further discussion of Property P2.9, including a proof for the case of least squares estimators for AR($p$) processes, can be found in Section T2.17.

**Example 2.29 Some Specific Asymptotic Distributions**

The following are some specific cases of Property P2.9.

**AR(1):** $\gamma_x(0) = \sigma_w^2/(1-\phi^2)$, so $\sigma_w^2 \Gamma_{1,0}^{-1} = (1-\phi^2)$. Thus,

$$\widehat{\phi} \sim \text{AN}\left[\phi, n^{-1}(1-\phi^2)\right]. \tag{2.117}$$

**AR(2):** The reader can verify that

$$\gamma_x(0) = \left(\frac{1-\phi_2}{1+\phi_2}\right) \frac{\sigma_w^2}{(1-\phi_2)^2 - \phi_1^2}$$

and $\gamma_x(1) = \phi_1\gamma_x(0) + \phi_2\gamma_x(1)$. From these facts, we can compute $\Gamma_{2,0}^{-1}$. In particular, we have

$$\begin{pmatrix} \widehat{\phi}_1 \\ \widehat{\phi}_2 \end{pmatrix} \sim \text{AN}\left[\begin{pmatrix} \phi_1 \\ \phi_2 \end{pmatrix}, \; n^{-1}\begin{pmatrix} 1-\phi_2^2 & -\phi_1(1+\phi_2) \\ \text{sym} & 1-\phi_2^2 \end{pmatrix}\right]. \tag{2.118}$$

**MA(1):** In this case, write $\theta(B)y_t = w_t$, or $y_t + \theta y_{t-1} = w_t$. Then, analogous to the AR(1) case, $\gamma_y(0) = \sigma_w^2/(1-\theta^2)$, so $\sigma_w^2\Gamma_{0,1}^{-1} = (1-\theta^2)$. Thus,

$$\widehat{\theta} \sim \text{AN}\left[\theta, n^{-1}(1-\theta^2)\right]. \tag{2.119}$$

**MA(2):** Write $y_t + \theta_1 y_{t-1} + \theta_2 y_{t-2} = w_t$, so , analogous to the AR(2) case, we have

$$\begin{pmatrix} \widehat{\theta}_1 \\ \widehat{\theta}_2 \end{pmatrix} \sim \text{AN}\left[\begin{pmatrix} \theta_1 \\ \theta_2 \end{pmatrix}, \; n^{-1}\begin{pmatrix} 1-\theta_2^2 & \theta_1(1+\theta_2) \\ \text{sym} & 1-\theta_2^2 \end{pmatrix}\right]. \tag{2.120}$$

**ARMA(1,1):** To calculate $\Gamma_{\phi\theta}$, we must find $\gamma_{xy}(0)$, where $x_t - \phi x_{t-1} = w_t$ and $y_t + \theta y_{t-1} = w_t$. We have

$$\begin{aligned} \gamma_{xy}(0) &= \text{cov}(x_t, y_t) = \text{cov}(\phi x_{t-1} + w_t, -\theta y_{t-1} + w_t) \\ &= -\phi\theta\gamma_{xy}(0) + \sigma_w^2. \end{aligned}$$

Solving, we find, $\gamma_{xy}(0) = \sigma_w^2/(1+\phi\theta)$. Thus,

$$\begin{pmatrix} \widehat{\phi} \\ \widehat{\theta} \end{pmatrix} \sim \mathrm{AN}\left[\begin{pmatrix} \phi \\ \theta \end{pmatrix}, \; n^{-1}\begin{bmatrix} (1-\phi^2)^{-1} & (1+\phi\theta)^{-1} \\ \text{sym} & (1-\theta^2)^{-1} \end{bmatrix}^{-1}\right]. \tag{2.121}$$

We leave it to the reader to complete the task of computing the asymptotic variance–covariance matrix in (2.121).

The reader might wonder, for example, why the asymptotic distributions of $\widehat{\phi}$ from an AR(1) [equation (2.117)] and $\widehat{\theta}$ from an MA(1) [equation (2.119)] are of the same form. It is possible to explain this unexpected result heurisitically using the intuition of linear regression. That is, for the normal regression model presented in Section 1.8 with no intercept term, $x_t = \beta z_t + w_t$, we know $\widehat{\beta}$ is normally distributed with mean $\beta$, and from (1.56),

$$\mathrm{var}\left\{\sqrt{n}\left(\widehat{\beta}-\beta\right)\right\} = n\sigma_w^2\left(\sum_{t=1}^{n} z_t^2\right)^{-1} = \sigma_w^2\left(n^{-1}\sum_{t=1}^{n} z_t^2\right)^{-1}.$$

For the causal AR(1) model given by $x_t = \phi x_{t-1} + w_t$, the intuition of regression tells us to expect that, for $n$ large,

$$\sqrt{n}\left(\widehat{\phi}-\phi\right)$$

is approximately normal with mean zero and with variance given by

$$\sigma_w^2\left(n^{-1}\sum_{t=2}^{n} x_{t-1}^2\right)^{-1}.$$

Now, $n^{-1}\sum_{t=2}^{n} x_{t-1}^2$ is the sample variance (recall that the mean of $x_t$ is zero) of the $x_t$, so as $n$ becomes large we would expect it to approach $\mathrm{var}(x_t) = \gamma(0) = \sigma_w^2/(1-\phi^2)$. Thus, the large sample variance of $\sqrt{n}\left(\widehat{\phi}-\phi\right)$ is

$$\sigma_w^2\gamma_x(0)^{-1} = \sigma_w^2\left(\frac{\sigma_w^2}{1-\phi^2}\right)^{-1} = (1-\phi^2);$$

that is, (2.117) holds.

In the case of an MA(1), we may use the discussion of Example 2.27 to write an approximate regression model for the MA(1). That is, consider the approximation (2.113) as the regression model

$$z_t(\widehat{\theta}) = -\theta z_{t-1}(\widehat{\theta}) + w_{t-1},$$

where now, $z_{t-1}(\widehat{\theta})$ as defined in Example 2.27, plays the role of the regressor. Continuing with the analogy, we would expect the asymptotic distribution of $\sqrt{n}\left(\widehat{\theta}-\theta\right)$ to be normal, with mean zero, and approximate variance

$$\sigma_w^2 \left( n^{-1} \sum_{t=2}^{n} z_{t-1}^2(\widehat{\theta}) \right)^{-1}.$$

As in the AR(1) case, $n^{-1}\sum_{t=2}^{n} z_{t-1}^2(\widehat{\theta})$ is the sample variance of the $z_t(\widehat{\theta})$ so, for large $n$, this should be $\mathrm{var}\{z_t(\theta)\} = \gamma_z(0)$, say. But note, as seen from (2.113), $z_t(\theta)$ is approximately an AR(1) process with parameter $-\theta$. Thus,

$$\sigma_w^2 \gamma_z(0)^{-1} = \sigma_w^2 \left( \frac{\sigma_w^2}{1-(-\theta)^2} \right)^{-1} = (1-\theta^2),$$

which agrees with (2.119). Finally, the asymptotic distributions of the AR parameters estimates and the MA parameter estimates are of the same form because in the MA case, the "regressors" are the differential processes $z_t(\theta)$ that have AR structure, and it is this structure that determines the asymptotic variance of the estimators.

In Example 2.28, the estimated standard error of $\widehat{\theta}$ was 0.025. In the example, this value was calculated as the square root of

$$s_w^2 \left( n^{-1} \sum_{t=2}^{n} z_{t-1}^2(\widehat{\theta}) \right)^{-1},$$

where $n = 633$, $s_w^2 = 0.236$, and $\widehat{\theta} = -0.772$. Using (2.119), we could have also calculated this value as the square root of $(1-0.772^2)/633$, which is also 0.025.

The asymptotic behavior of the parameter estimators gives us an additional insight into the problem of fitting ARMA models to data. For example, suppose a time series follows an AR(1) process and we decide to fit an AR(2) to the data. Does any problem occur in doing this? More generally, why not simply fit large-order AR models to make sure that we capture the dynamics of the process? After all, if the process is truly an AR(1), the other autoregressive parameters will not be significant. The answer is that if we ***overfit***, we will lose efficiency. For example, if we fit an AR(1) to an AR(1) process, for large $n$, $\mathrm{var}(\widehat{\phi}_1) \approx n^{-1}(1-\phi_1^2)$. But if we fit an AR(2) to the AR(1) process, for large $n$, $\mathrm{var}(\widehat{\phi}_1) \approx n^{-1}(1-\phi_2^2) = n^{-1}$ because $\phi_2 = 0$. Thus, the variance of $\phi_1$ has been inflated, making the estimator less precise. We do want to mention that overfitting can be used as a diagnostic tool. For example, if we fit an AR(2) model to the data and are satisfied with that model, then adding one more parameter and fitting an AR(3) should lead to approximately the same model as in the AR(2) fit. We will discuss model diagnostics in more detail in Section 2.8.

If $n$ is small, or if the parameters are close to the boundaries, the asymptotic approximations can be quite poor. The ***bootstrap*** can be helpful in this case; for a broad treatment of the bootstrap, see Efron and Tibshirani (1994). We discuss the case of an AR(1) here and leave the general discussion for Chapter 4. For now, we give a simple example of the bootstrap for an AR(1) process.

**Example 2.30 Bootstrapping an AR(1)**

We consider an AR(1) model with a regression coefficient near the boundary of causality and an error process that is symmetric but not normal. Specifically, consider the stationary and causal model

$$x_t = \mu + \phi(x_{t-1} - \mu) + w_t, \tag{2.122}$$

where $\mu = 50$, $\phi = .95$, and $w_t$ are iid double exponential with location zero, and scale parameter $\beta = 2$. The density of $w_t$ is given by

$$f_{w_t}(w) = \frac{1}{2\beta} \exp\{-|w|/\beta\} \quad -\infty < w < \infty.$$

In this example, $E(w_t) = 0$ and $\text{var}(w_t) = 2\beta^2 = 8$. Figure 2.8 shows $n = 100$ simulated observations from this process. This particular realization is interesting; the data look like they were generated from a nonstationary process with three different mean levels. In fact, the data were generated from a well-behaved, albeit nonnormal, stationary and causal model, and we might not be inclined to fit an AR(1) model to this data. To show the advantages of the bootstrap, we will act as if we do not know the actual error distribution and we will proceed as if it was normal; of course, this means that the normal estimate of $\phi$ will not be the actual MLE because the data are not normal.

Using the data shown in Figure 2.8, we obtained the Yule–Walker estimates $\widehat{\mu} = 40.048$, $\widehat{\phi} = .959$, and $s_w^2 = 15.302$, where $s_w^2$ is the estimate of $\text{var}(w_t)$. Based on Property P2.9, we would say that $\widehat{\phi}$ is approximately normal with mean $\phi$ (which we supposedly do not know) and variance $(1-\phi^2)/100$, which we would approximate by $(1 - .959^2)/100 = 0.028^2$.

To assess the finite sample distribution of $\widehat{\phi}$ when $n = 100$, we simulated 1000 realizations of this AR(1) process and estimated the parameters via Yule–Walker. The finite sampling density of the Yule–Walker estimate of $\phi$, based on the 1000 repeated simulations, is shown in Figure 2.9. Clearly the sampling distribution is not close to normality for this sample size. The mean of the distribution shown in Figure 2.9 is 0.907, and the variance of the distribution is $0.052^2$; these values are considerably

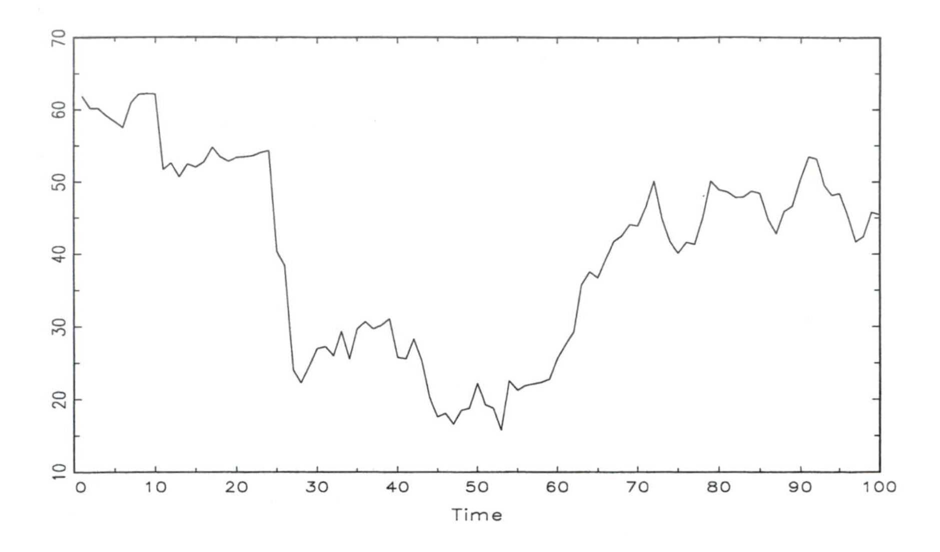


**Figure 2.8:** One hundred observations generated from the AR(1) model in Example 2.30.

different than the asymptotic values. Some of the quantiles of the finite sample distribution are .805 (5%), .837 (10%), 0.879 (25%), 0.919 (50%), .945 (75%), .961 (90%), and 0.971 (95%).

Before discussing the bootstrap, we first investigate the sample innovation process, $x_t - x_t^{t-1}$, with corresponding variances $P_t^{t-1}$. For the AR(1) model in this example, $x_t - x_t^{t-1} = x_t - [\mu + \phi(x_{t-1} - \mu)]$, for $t = 2, ..., 100$; from this, it follows that $P_t^{t-1} = \sigma_w^2$ for $t = 2, ..., 100$. When $t = 1$, we have $x_1 - x_1^0 = x_1 - \mu$, and $P_1^0 = \sigma_w^2/(1 - \phi^2)$. The innovations have zero mean but different variances; in order that all of the innovations have the same variance, $\sigma_w^2$, we will write them as

$$\begin{aligned} \epsilon_1 &= (x_1 - \mu)\sqrt{(1 - \phi^2)} \\ \epsilon_t &= (x_t - \mu) - \phi(x_{t-1} - \mu), \quad \text{for} \quad t = 2, ..., 100. \end{aligned} \tag{2.123}$$

From these equations, we can write the model in terms of the innovations $\epsilon_t$ as

$$\begin{aligned} x_1 &= \mu + \epsilon_1/\sqrt{(1 - \phi^2)} \\ x_t &= \mu + \phi(x_{t-1} - \mu) + \epsilon_t \quad \text{for} \quad t = 2, ..., 100. \end{aligned} \tag{2.124}$$

Next, replace the parameters with their estimates in (2.123), that is, $n = 100$, $\widehat{\mu} = 40.048$, and $\widehat{\phi} = .959$, and denote the resulting sample

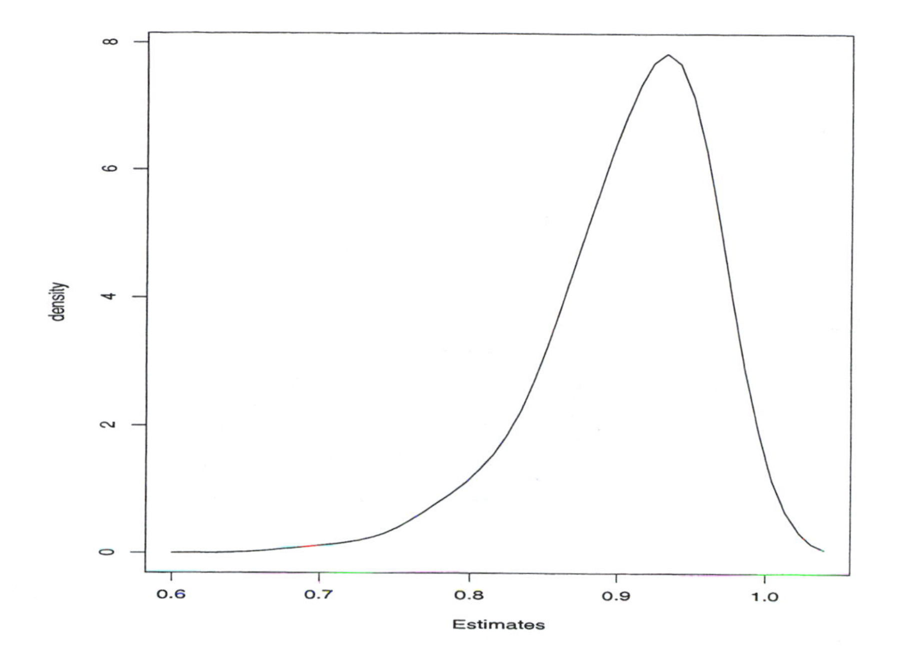


**Figure 2.9:** Finite sample density of the Yule–Walker estimate of $\phi$ in Example 2.30.

innovations as $\{\widehat{\epsilon}_1, ..., \widehat{\epsilon}_{100}\}$. To obtain one bootstrap sample, first randomly sample, with replacement, $n = 100$ values from the set of sample innovations; call the sampled values $\{\epsilon_1^*, ..., \epsilon_{100}^*\}$. Now, generate a bootstrapped data set sequentially by setting

$$\begin{aligned} x_1^* &= 40.048 + \epsilon_1^* / \sqrt{(1 - .959^2)} \\ x_t^* &= 40.048 + .959(x_{t-1}^* - 40.048) + \epsilon_t^*, \quad t = 2, ..., n. \end{aligned} \tag{2.125}$$

Next, estimate the parameters as if the data were $x_t^*$. Call these estimates $\widehat{\mu}(1)$, $\widehat{\phi}(1)$, and $s_w^2(1)$. Repeat this process a large number, $B$, of times, generating a collection of bootstrapped parameter estimates, $\{\widehat{\mu}(b), \widehat{\phi}(b), s_w^2(b), b = 1, ..., B\}$. We can then approximate the finite sample distribution of an estimator from the bootstrapped parameter values. For example, we can approximate the distribution of $\widehat{\phi} - \phi$ by the empirical distribution of $\widehat{\phi}(b) - \widehat{\phi}$, for $b = 1, ..., B$.

Figure 2.10 shows the bootstrap histogram of 200 bootstrapped estimates of $\phi$ using the data shown in Figure 2.8. In particular, the mean of the distribution of $\widehat{\phi}(b)$ is 0.918 with a variance of $.046^2$. Some quantiles of this distribution are .832 (5%), .848 (10%), .897 (25%), .928 (50%), .954

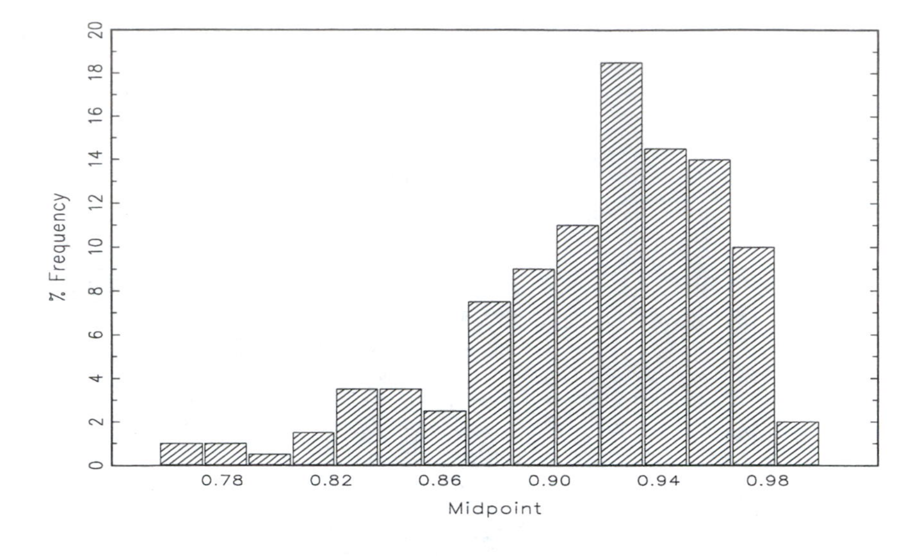


**Figure 2.10:** Bootstrap histogram of $\widehat{\phi}$ based on 200 bootstraps.

(75%), .968 (90%), and .975 (95%). Clearly, the bootstrap distribution of $\widehat{\phi}$ is closer to the distribution of $\widehat{\phi}$ shown in Figure 2.9, than to the asymptotic (normal) approximation.

## 2.7 Integrated Models for Nonstationary Data

In Chapter 1, we saw that if $y_t$ is a random walk, $y_t = y_{t-1} + w_t$; then by differencing $y_t$, we find that $\nabla y_t = w_t$ is stationary. In many situations, time series can be thought of as being composed of two components, a nonstationary trend component and a zero-mean stationary component. For example, we might observe

$$y_t = \mu_t + x_t, \tag{2.126}$$

where $\mu_t = \beta_0 + \beta_1 t$ and $x_t$ is stationary. Differencing such a process will lead to a stationary process:

$$\nabla y_t = y_t - y_{t-1} = \beta_1 + x_t - x_{t-1} = \beta_1 + \nabla x_t.$$

Note, $\nabla x_t$ is stationary, and in general, a (finite) linear combination of stationary processes is stationary. Another model that leads to first differencing is the case in which $\mu_t$ in (2.126) is stochastic and slowly varying according to a random walk. That is, in (2.126)

$$\mu_t = \mu_{t-1} + v_t$$

where $v_t$ is stationary. In this case,

$$\nabla y_t = v_t + \nabla x_t,$$

is stationary. If $\mu_t$ in (2.126) is a $k$-th order polynomial, $\mu_t = \sum_{j=0}^{k} \beta_j t^j$, then (Problem 2.26) the differenced series $\nabla^k y_t$ is stationary. Stochastic trend models can also lead to higher order differencing. For example, suppose in (2.126)

$$\mu_t = \mu_{t-1} + v_t \quad \text{and} \quad v_t = v_{t-1} + e_t,$$

where $e_t$ is stationary. Then, $\nabla y_t = v_t + \nabla x_t$ is not stationary, but $\nabla^2 y_t = e_t + \nabla^2 x_t$ is stationary.

The ***integrated*** ARMA model, ARIMA$(p, d, q)$, is a broadening of the class of ARMA models to include differencing. A process, $x_t$ is said to be ***ARIMA(p, d, q)*** if $\nabla^d x_t = (1 - B)^d x_t$ is ARMA$(p, q)$. In general, we will write the model as

$$\phi(B)(1 - B)^d x_t = \theta(B) w_t. \tag{2.127}$$

If $E(\nabla^d x_t) = \mu$, then we can write the model as $\phi(B)(1-B)^d x_t = \alpha + \theta(B) w_t$, where $\alpha = \mu(1 - \phi_1 - \cdots - \phi_p)$.

**Example 2.31 IMA(1,1) and Exponentially Weighted Moving Averages**

The ARIMA(0,1,1), or IMA(1,1) model is of interest because many economic time series can be successfully modeled this way. In addition, the model leads to a frequently used, and abused, forecasting method called exponentially weighted moving averages (EWMA). We will write the model as

$$x_t = x_{t-1} + w_t - \theta w_{t-1}; \tag{2.128}$$

this model formulation is easier to work with here, and it leads to the standard representation for EWMA. When $|\theta| < 1$, the model has an invertible representation,

$$x_t = \sum_{j=1}^{\infty} (1 - \theta) \theta^{j-1} x_{t-j} + w_t. \tag{2.129}$$

Verification of (2.129) is left to the reader (Problem 2.27). From (2.129), we have that the one-step-ahead prediction, using the notation of Section

2.5, is

$$\begin{aligned}\tilde{x}_{n+1} &= \sum_{j=1}^{\infty}(1-\theta)\theta^{j-1}x_{n+1-j} \\ &= (1-\theta)x_n + \theta\sum_{j=1}^{\infty}(1-\theta)\theta^{j-1}x_{n-j} \\ &= (1-\theta)x_n + \theta\tilde{x}_n. \end{aligned} \tag{2.130}$$

Based on (2.130), the truncated forecasts are obtained by setting $\tilde{x}_1^0 = 0$, and then updating as follows:

$$\tilde{x}_{n+1}^n = (1-\theta)x_n + \theta\tilde{x}_n^{n-1}, \quad n \geq 1. \tag{2.131}$$

From (2.131), we see that the new forecast is a linear combination of the old forecast and the new observation. In EWMA, the parameter $\alpha$ is called the ***smoothing constant*** and is restricted to be between zero and one. Larger values of $\theta$ lead to smoother forecasts. This method of forecasting is popular because it is easy to use; we need only retain the previous forecast value and the current observation to forecast the next time period. Unfortunately, as previously suggested, the method is often abused because some forecasters do not verify that the observations follow an IMA(1,1) process, and often arbitrarily pick values of $\theta$.

Finally, the model for the glacial varve series in Example 2.28 is an IMA(1,1) on the logarithms of the data. Recall that the fitted model there was $\ln x_t = \ln x_{t-1} + w_t - 0.772 w_{t-1}$ and $\text{var}(w_t) = 0.236$.

## 2.8 Building ARIMA Models

There are a few basic steps to fitting ARIMA models to time series data. These steps involve ***plotting the data***, ***possibly transforming the data***, ***identifying the dependence orders of the model***, ***parameter estimation***, and ***diagnostics***. First, as with any data analysis, we should plot the data, $x_t$ versus $t$, and inspect the graph for any anomalies. If, for example, the variability in the data grows with time, it will be necessary to transform the data to stabilize the variance. In such cases, the Box–Cox class of power transformations, equation (1.48), could be employed. Also, the particular application might suggest an appropriate transformation. For example, suppose a process evolves as a fairly small and stable percent change, such as an investment. For example, we might have

$$x_t = (1 + p_t)x_{t-1},$$

where $x_t$ is the value of the investment at time $t$ and $p_t$ is the percentage change from period $t-1$ to $t$, which may be negative. Taking logs and differencing, we have

$$\nabla[\ln(x_t)] = \ln(x_t) - \ln(x_{t-1}) = \ln(1 + p_t).$$

If the percent change $p_t$ stays relatively small in magnitude, then $\ln(1+p_t) \approx p_t$ and, thus,

$$\nabla[\ln(x_t)] \approx p_t,$$

will be a relatively stable process. Frequently, $\nabla[\ln(x_t)]$ is called the ***return*** or ***growth rate***. This general idea was used in Example 2.28, and we will use it again in Example 2.32.

After suitably transforming the data, the next step is to identify preliminary values of the autoregressive order, $p$, the order of differencing, $d$, and the moving average order, $q$. We have already addressed, in part, the problem of selecting $d$. A time plot of the data will typically suggest whether any differencing is needed. If differencing is called for, then difference the data once, $d = 1$, and inspect the time plot of $\nabla x_t$. If additional differencing is necessary, then try differencing again and inspect a time plot of $\nabla^2 x_t$. Be careful not to overdifference because this may introduce dependence where none exists. For example, $x_t = w_t$ is serially uncorrelated, but $\nabla x_t = w_t - w_{t-1}$ is MA(1). In addition to time plots, the sample ACF can help in indicating whether differencing is needed. Since the polynomial $\phi(z)(1-z)^d$ has a unit root, the sample ACF, $\widehat{\rho}(h)$, will not decay to zero fast as $h$ increases. Thus, a slow decay in $\widehat{\rho}(h)$ is an indication that differencing may be needed.

When preliminary values of $d$ have been settled, the next step is to look at the sample ACF and PACF of $\nabla^d x_t$ for whatever values of $d$ have been chosen. Using Table 2.1 as a guide, preliminary values of $p$ and $q$ are chosen. Recall that, if $p = 0$ and $q > 0$, the ACF cuts off after lag $q$, and the PACF tails off. If $q = 0$ and $p > 0$, the PACF cuts off after lag $p$, and the ACF tails off. If $p > 0$ and $q > 0$, both the ACF and PACF will tail off. Because we are dealing with estimates, it will not always be clear whether the sample ACF or PACF is tailing off or cutting off. Also, two models that are seemingly different can actually be very similar. With this in mind, we should not worry about being so precise at this stage of the model fitting. At this stage, a few preliminary values of $p$, $d$, and $q$ should be at hand, and we can start estimating the parameters.

**Example 2.32 Analysis of GNP Data**

In this example, we consider the analysis of quarterly U.S. GNP from 1947(1) to 1991(1), $n = 177$. The series was obtained from the Citibase database and is seasonally adjusted. Figure 2.11 shows a plot of the data, say, $y_t$. Because strong trend hides any other effect, it is not clear from Figure 2.11 that the variance is increasing with time. The sample ACF of the data is shown in Figure 2.12. Figure 2.13 shows the first difference of the data, $\nabla y_t$, and now, with the trend removed, clearly,

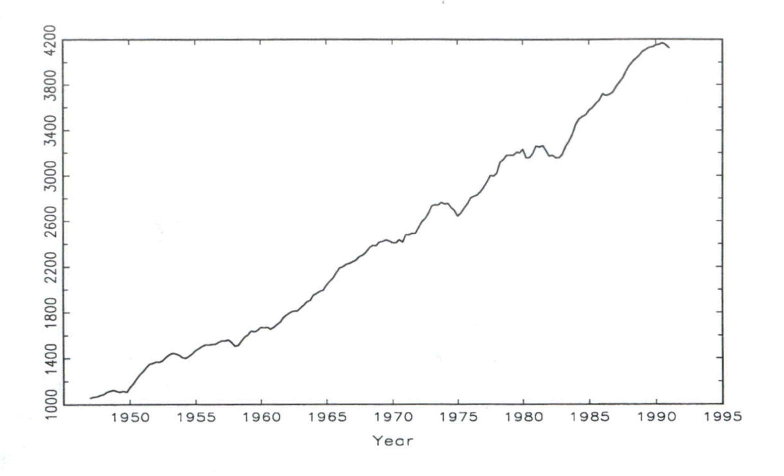


**Figure 2.11:** Quarterly U.S. GNP from 1947(1) to 1991(1).

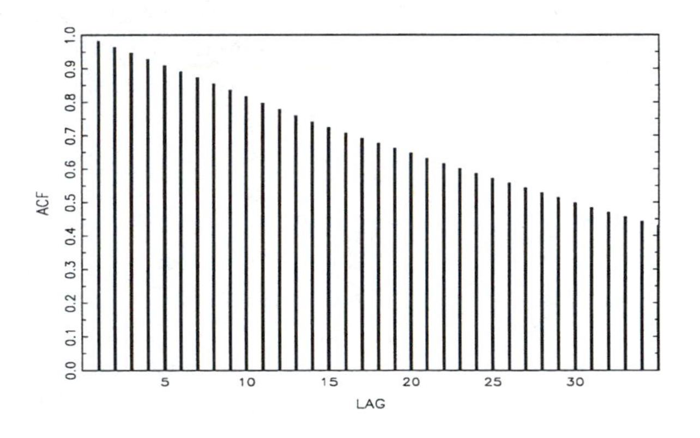


**Figure 2.12:** Sample ACF of GNP data.

the variability increases with time. Hence, we will first log the data, and then remove the trend by differencing, say, $x_t = \nabla \ln(y_t)$. The growth rate, $x_t$, is plotted in Figure 2.14, and, appears to be a stable process.

The sample ACF and PACF of the quarterly growth rate are plotted in Figure 2.15. Inspecting the sample ACF and PACF, we might feel that the ACF is cutting off at lag 2 and the PACF is tailing off. This would suggest the GNP growth rate follows an MA(2) process, or log GNP follows an ARIMA(0,1,2) model. Rather than focus on one model, we will also suggest that it appears that the ACF is tailing off and the PACF

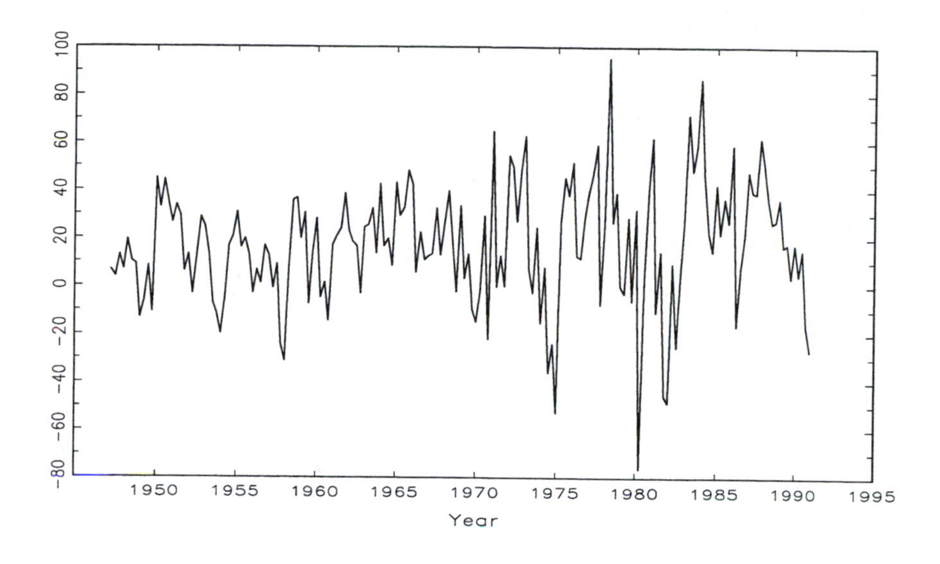


**Figure 2.13:** First difference of the U.S. GNP data.

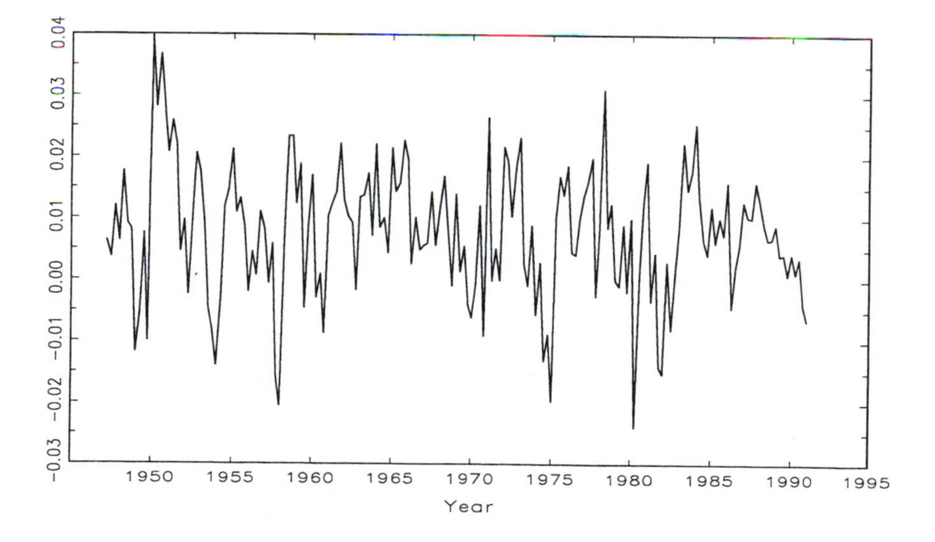


**Figure 2.14:** U.S. GNP quarterly growth rate.

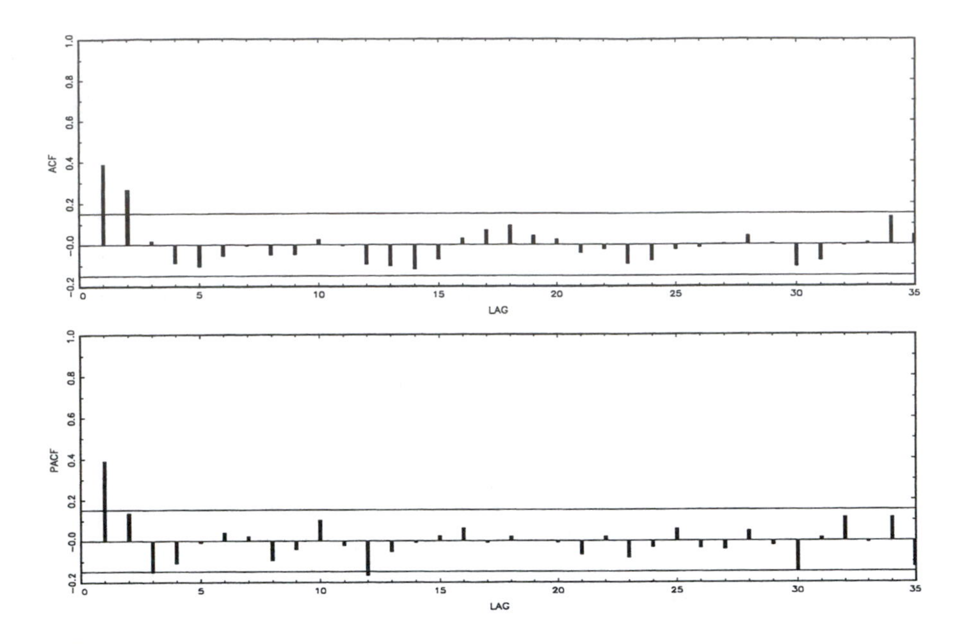


**Figure 2.15:** Sample ACF and PACF of GNP quarterly growth rate.

is cutting off at lag 3. This suggests an AR(3) model for the growth rate, or ARIMA(3,1,0) for log GNP. As a preliminary analysis, we will fit both models.

Using unconditional least squares to fit the MA(2) model for the growth rate, $x_t$, the estimated model is

$$x_t = .008_{(.001)} + .313_{(.073)}\widehat{w}_{t-1} + .274_{(.074)}\widehat{w}_{t-2} + \widehat{w}_t, \tag{2.132}$$

where $\widehat{\sigma}_w = .0014$ is based on 173 degrees of freedom. The values in parentheses are the corresponding estimated standard errors. All of the regression coefficients are significant, including the constant. We make a special note of this because typically, as a default, computer packages do not fit a constant in a differenced model. In this example, not including a constant leads to the wrong conclusions about the nature of the model. We leave it to the reader to investigate what happens when the constant is not included.

The estimated AR(3) model is

$$\begin{aligned} x_t &= .005_{(.001)} + .350_{(.076)}x_{t-1} + .181_{(.079)}x_{t-2} \\ &- .145_{(.076)}x_{t-3} + \widehat{w}_t, \end{aligned} \tag{2.133}$$

where $\widehat{\sigma}_w = .0014$ on 172 degrees of freedom. We will discuss diagnostics next, but assuming both of these models fit well, how are we to reconcile the apparent differences of the estimated models (2.132) and (2.133)? In fact, the fitted models are practically the same. To show this, consider an MA(2) model of the form in (2.132) without a constant term; that is,

$$x_t = .31w_{t-1} + .27w_{t-2} + w_t,$$

and write it in its invertible form, $w_t = \sum_{j=0}^{\infty} \pi_j x_{t-j}$. Then, using the techniques of Section 2.3, $\pi_0 = 1, \pi_1 = -.31, \pi_2 = -.18, \pi_3 = .14, \pi_4 = 0, \pi_5 = -.04, \pi_6 = .01, \pi_7 = .01, \pi_8 = -.01, \pi_9 = 0, \pi_{10} = 0$, and so forth. Thus,

$$x_t \approx .31x_{t-1} + .18x_{t-2} - .14x_{t-3} + w_t,$$

which is very similar to the AR(3) model in (2.133).

The next step in model fitting is diagnostics. This investigation includes the analysis of the residuals as well as model comparisons. Again, the first step involves a time plot of the ***innovations*** (or residuals), $x_t - \widehat{x}_t^{t-1}$, or of the ***standardized innovations***

$$e_t = \left(x_t - \widehat{x}_t^{t-1}\right) \Big/ \sqrt{\widehat{P}_t^{t-1}}, \tag{2.134}$$

where $\widehat{x}_t^{t-1}$ is the one-step-ahead prediction of $x_t$ based on the fitted model and $\widehat{P}_t^{t-1}$ is the estimated one-step-ahead error variance. If the model fits well, the standardized residuals should behave as an iid sequence with mean zero and variance one. The time plot should be inspected for any obvious departures from this assumption. Unless the time series is Gaussian, it is not enough that the residuals are uncorrelated. For example, the ***bilinear model*** given by

$$\epsilon_t = \alpha w_{t-1}\epsilon_{t-2} + w_t,$$

where $\alpha^2\sigma_w^2 < 1$, is a stationary process. For this process, however,

$$\text{corr}(\epsilon_s, \epsilon_t) = 0, \quad s \neq t,$$

but the process $\epsilon_t^2$ has the autocorrelation structure of an ARMA(2,1). Details can be found in Granger and Andersen (1978), Gabr and Subba-Rao (1981), or Subba-Rao (1981). Another example of this property is ***ARCH models***, which we discuss in Section 2.14. If, after a model fit, the residuals have some dependence structure, our model has not done a thorough job of describing the dynamics of the process. Thus, it pays to assess the normality of the residuals.

Investigation of marginal normality can be accomplished visually by looking at a histogram of the residuals. In addition to this, a ***Q-Q plot*** can help in identifying departures from normality. Consider the ordered residuals, say, $e_{(1)} \leq e_{(2)} \leq \cdots \leq e_{(n)}$. Empirically, the proportion of residuals less than or equal to $e_{(j)}$, is $j/n$. Using a continuity correction, that proportion is approximated by $(j - \frac{1}{2})/n$. If the residuals are normal, then $e_{(j)}$ should be approximately the same as the $(j-\frac{1}{2})/n$ quantile of a standard normal, say, $q_{(j)}$. That is, if $z \sim \text{N}(0,1)$, then $\text{pr}[z \leq q_{(j)}] = (j - \frac{1}{2})/n$. For example, for $n = 10$ and $j = 1$, $(j - \frac{1}{2})/n = .05$, and $q_{(1)} = -1.645$, because $\text{pr}[z \leq -1.645] = .05$. A Q-Q plot is a graph of $(q_{(j)}, e_{(j)})$, for $j = 1, ..., n$. If the residuals are normal, then the pairs will be approximately linearly related. Tests of the strength of the linearity can be performed via the correlation among the $(q_{(j)}, e_{(j)})$ pairs. See Johnson and Wichern (1992, Chapter 4) for details of this test as well as additional tests for multivariate normality.

There are several tests of randomness, for example the runs test, that could be applied to the residuals. We could also inspect the sample autocorrelations of the residuals, say, $\widehat{\rho}_e(h)$, for any patterns or large values. Recall that, for a white noise sequence, the sample ACF are approximately independently and normally distributed with zero means and variances $1/n$. Hence, a good check on the correlation structure of the residuals is to plot $\widehat{\rho}_e(h)$ versus $h$ along with the error bounds of $\pm 2/\sqrt{n}$. The residuals from a model fit, however, will not quite have the properties of a white noise sequence and the variance of $\widehat{\rho}_e(h)$ can be much less than $1/n$. Details can be found in Box and Pierce (1970) and McLeod (1978). This part of the diagnostics can be viewed as a visual inspection of $\widehat{\rho}_e(h)$, with the main concern being the detection of obvious departures from the independence assumption.

In addition to plotting $\widehat{\rho}_e(h)$, we can perform a general or ***portmanteau*** test that takes into consideration the magnitudes of $\widehat{\rho}_e(h)$ as a group. For example, it may be the case that, individually, each $\widehat{\rho}_e(h)$ is small in magnitude, say, each one is just slightly less that $2/\sqrt{n}$ in magnitude, but, collectively, the values are large. The ***Ljung–Box–Pierce statistic*** given by

$$Q = n(n+2) \sum_{h=1}^{H} \frac{\widehat{\rho}_e^2(h)}{n-h} \tag{2.135}$$

can be used to perform such a test. The value $H$ in (2.135) is chosen somewhat arbitrarily, typically, $H = 20$. Under the null hypothesis of model adequacy, asymptotically $(n \to \infty)$, $Q \sim \chi^2_{H-p-q}$. Thus, we would reject the null hypothesis at level $\alpha$ if the value of $Q$ exceeds the $(1-\alpha)$-quantile of the $\chi^2_{H-p-q}$ distribution. Details can be found in Box and Pierce (1970), Ljung and Box (1978), and Davies et al (1977).

**Example 2.33 Diagnostics for GNP Growth Rate Example**

We will focus on the MA(2) fit from Example 2.32; the analysis of the AR(3) residuals is similar. First, an inspection of the time plot of the unstandardized residuals, Figure 2.16, shows no obvious patterns. An outlier does appear, however, at $t = 13$. In this case, the value of the unstandardized residual is .0051, which is about 3.7 standard deviations (recall $\widehat{\sigma}_w = .0014$) from zero.

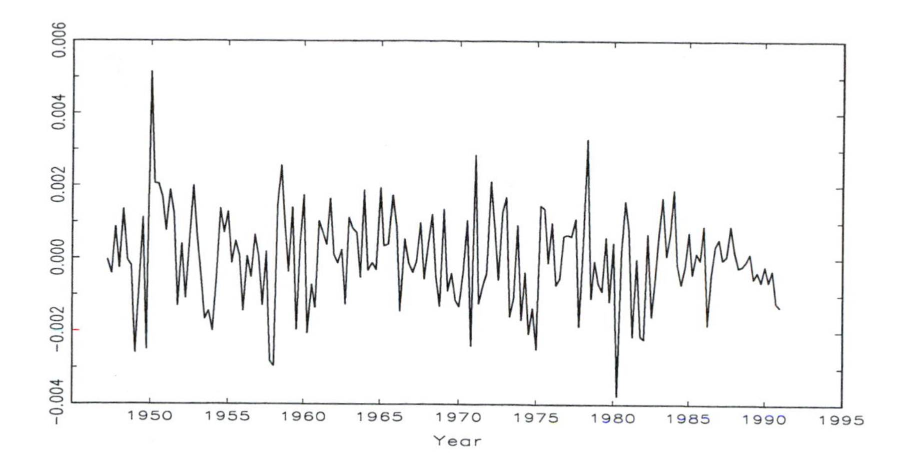


**Figure 2.16:** Residuals from MA(2) fit on GNP growth rate.

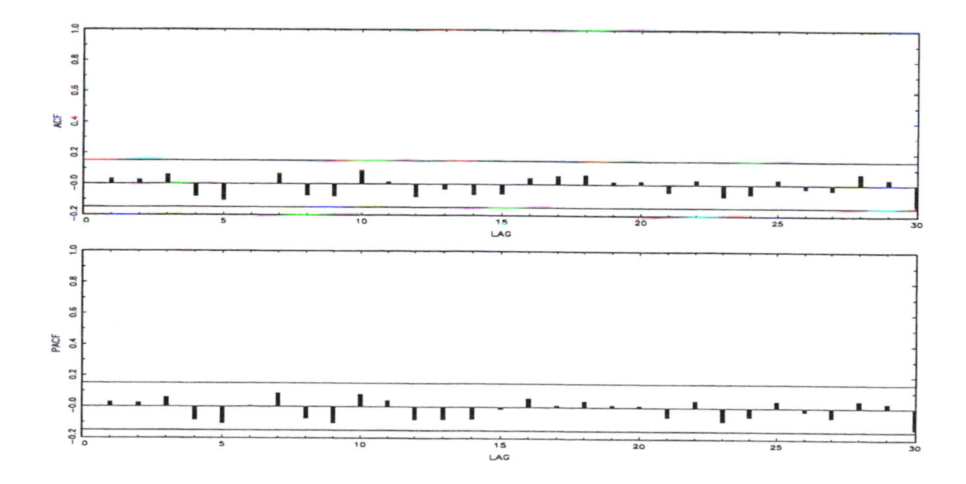


**Figure 2.17:** Sample ACF and PACF of the residuals shown in Figure 2.16.

Next, Figure 2.17 shows the ACF of the residuals, to lag 36, along with the appropriate error limits $\pm 2/\sqrt{173} = 0.15$. In this case, all of the autocorrelations are within the white noise limits.

The Ljung–Box–Pierce statistic, (2.135), for $H = 20$, was $Q = 13.63$, which, under the white noise null hypothesis has a chi-squared distribution with 18 degrees of freedom. This value of $Q$ corresponds to a $p$-value

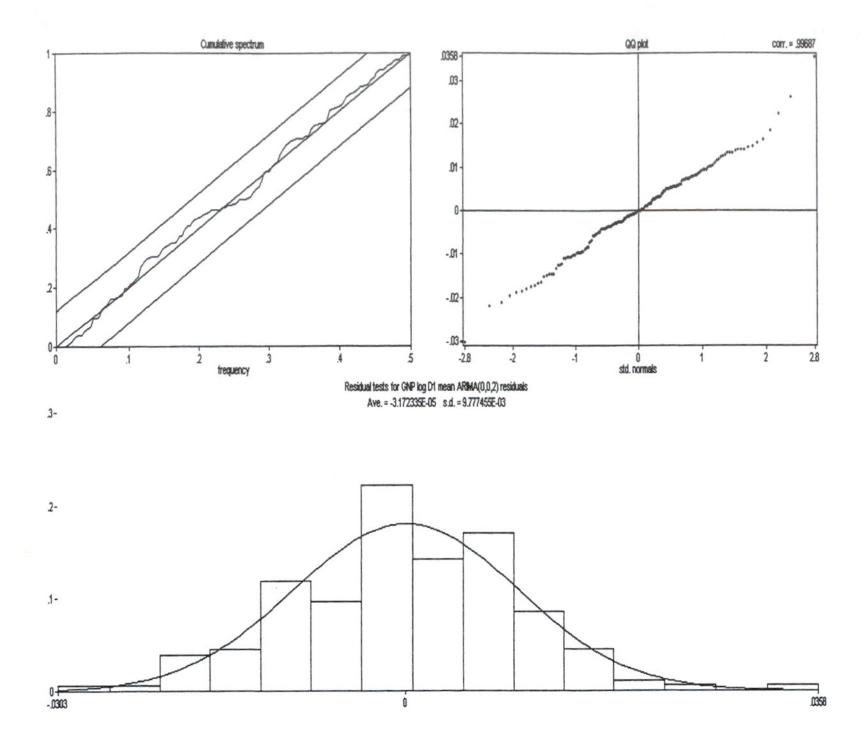

**Figure 2.18:** Further residual diagnostics: Cumulative spectral distribution (top left), Q-Q plot (top right), and Histogram (bottom).

of 0.75, which supports the white noise hypothesis. A runs test (around zero) of the residuals shows 87 runs observed with the expected number of runs, under the assumption of independence, being about 89; this outcome also strongly supports the white noise null hypothesis. Finally, Figure 2.18 shows the results of some additional diagnostics. The top left graph compares the empirical spectral distribution of the residuals with the theoretical spectral distribution of white noise. We will discuss this procedure in more detail in Chapter 3, but we note the empirical results for these residuals are very close to what would be expected for white noise. The top right graph of Figure 2.18 is the Q-Q plot of the residuals. In this case, there is evidence of a strong linear relationship, and the correlation between $e_{(j)}$ and $q_{(j)}$ is about 99.7%; this result strongly supports the null hypothesis of normality. The lower plot in Figure 2.18 shows a histogram of the residuals, with a normal density having the same mean and variance as the sample. This graph also supports the normality of the residuals.

**Example 2.34 Diagnostics for the Glacial Varve Series**

In Example 2.28, we fit an ARIMA(0,1,1) model to the logarithms of the glacial varve data. For this model, the Ljung–Box–Pierce statistic was $Q = 38.48$ when $H = 20$. Comparing this with a $\chi^2_{19}$ distribution, we find that the $p$-value is approximately 0.005, and hence, we would reject the white noise hypothesis. Further inspection of the residuals, $e_t = x_t - \widehat{x}_t^{t-1}$, shows that $\widehat{\rho}_e(1) = 0.121$, $\widehat{\rho}_e(3) = -0.090$, $\widehat{\rho}_e(12) = -0.102$, and $\widehat{\rho}_e(19) = -0.082$ all exceed the white noise limits, $\pm 2/\sqrt{632} = \pm 0.078$, for an ACF. In addition, the PACF of the residuals shows significant values at these lags at about the same magnitude. This result suggests the fitting of at least one additional parameter; this possibility was not evident in the initial modeling phase of the analysis. Given that both the ACF and PACF are not cutting off, according to Table 2.1, we should try fitting an ARIMA(1,1,1) model to the logarithms of the glacial varve data. In this case, $Q = 20.55$, which, when compared to a $\chi^2_{18}$ distribution, is not significant and supports the white noise hypothesis. The ARIMA(1,1,1) parameter estimates and their standard errors were $\widehat{\phi} = .235$ (.047), $\widehat{\theta} = -.888$ (.022), and $\widehat{\sigma}^2_w = .230$. All other diagnostic tests were favorable to this model.

In Example 2.32, we have two competing models, an AR(3) and an MA(2) on the GNP growth rate, that each appear to fit the data well. In addition, we might also consider that an AR(4) or an MA(3) might do better for forecasting. Perhaps combining both models, that is, fitting an ARMA(2,3) to the GNP growth rate, would be the best. As previously mentioned, we have to be concerned with ***overfitting*** the model; it is not always the case that more is better. Overfitting leads to less-precise estimators, and adding more parameters may fit the data better but may also lead to bad forecasts. This result is illustrated in the following example.

**Example 2.35 A Problem with Overfitting**

Figure 2.19 shows the U.S. population by official census, every 10 years from 1910 to 1990, as points. If we use these nine observations to predict the future population of the U.S., we can use an eight-degree polynomial so the fit to the nine observations is perfect. The model in this case is

$$x_t = \beta_0 + \beta_1 t + \beta_2 t^2 + \cdots + \beta_8 t^8 + w_t.$$

The fitted model, which is plotted through the year 2010 as a line, passes through the nine observations. The model predicts that the population of the U.S. to be close to zero in the year 2000, and will cross zero sometime in the year 2002!

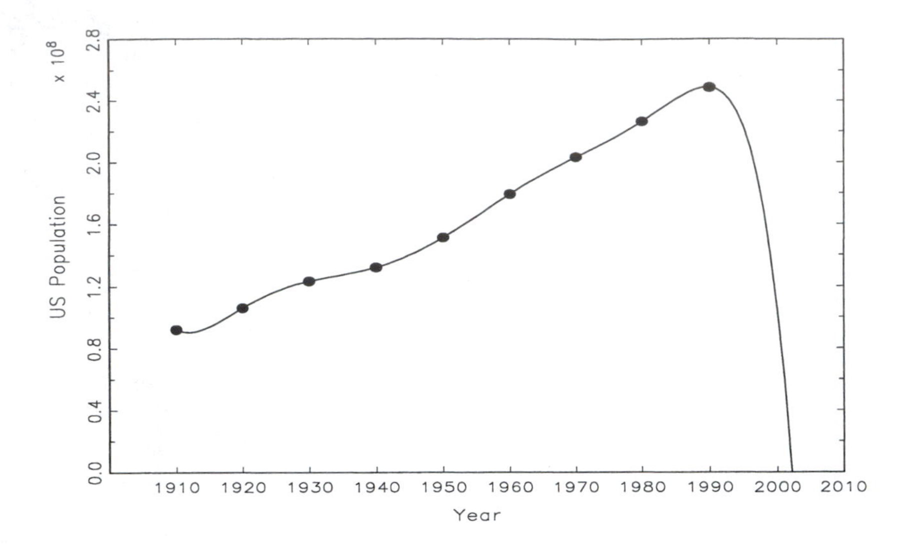


**Figure 2.19:** A perfect fit and a terrible forecast.

The final step of model fitting is ***model choice*** or ***model selection***. That is, we must decide which model we will retain for forecasting. The most popular techniques, AIC, AICc, and SIC, were described in Section 1.8 in the context of regression models. A discussion of AIC based on Kullback–Leibler distance is given in Problems 1.29 and 1.30. Although there are many ways to think about these techniques, one particularly interesting way is that of ***cross-validation***. For example, one way to validate a model is to collect more data and see how well the model fits to the new data. This technique, however, is frequently not viable. A compromise to this method is to leave out some of the data, fit the model to the remaining data, and see how well it fits to the data that was left out. The problem with this technique is that we are not using all of the information available to us to fit the model. The Akaike (1973) approach to model selection can also be viewed as a cross-validation method using an imaginary data set. For example, suppose we fit an ARMA$(p, q)$ model to our data, $\{x_1, ..., x_n\}$, and the estimates are $\widehat{\sigma}_w^2$, and $\widehat{\boldsymbol{\beta}} = (\widehat{\phi}_1, ..., \widehat{\phi}_p, \widehat{\theta}_1, ..., \widehat{\theta}_q)'$. Denote the corresponding likelihood by $L_x(\widehat{\boldsymbol{\beta}}, \widehat{\sigma}_w^2)$. Now, suppose we can get another set of data, $\{y_1, ..., y_n\}$, independent of our data, but with the same dynamics. Denote the likelihood of this data set (which we cannot evaluate because we do not have this data) by $L_y(\widehat{\boldsymbol{\beta}}, \widehat{\sigma}_w^2)$. It makes sense that if we could evaluate this quantity, we would choose the model that maximizes the

**Table 2.2:** Model Selection for the U.S. GNP Series

| $p$ | $q$ | $\widehat{\sigma}_w^2 \times 10^4$ | SIC | AICc |
|---|---|---|---|---|
| 0 | 1 | 1.033 | -9.149 | -8.155 |
| 0 | 2† | 0.962 | -9.191* | -8.215* |
| 0 | 3 | 0.955 | -9.169 | -8.210 |
| 2 | 0 | 0.984 | -9.168 | -8.191 |
| 3 | 0† | 0.973 | -9.149 | -8.191 |
| 4 | 0 | 0.975 | -9.118 | -8.177 |
| 3 | 1 | 0.971 | -9.122 | -8.181 |
| 1 | 2 | 0.964 | -9.158 | -8.200 |

†Preliminary models *Minimum value

likelihood of the new data set. Akaike showed that

$$-2 \ln L_y(\widehat{\boldsymbol{\beta}}, \widehat{\sigma}_w^2) \approx -2 \ln L_x(\widehat{\boldsymbol{\beta}}, \widehat{\sigma}_w^2) + 2(p+q).$$

Hence, we would choose the model that minimizes $-2 \ln L_x(\widehat{\boldsymbol{\beta}}, \widehat{\sigma}_w^2) + 2(p+q)$, which consists of two parts, one measuring model fit and one penalizing for the addition of parameters. Dividing $-2 \ln L_x(\widehat{\boldsymbol{\beta}}, \widehat{\sigma}_w^2) + 2(p+q)$ by $n$, writing $k = p+q$, and ignoring constants and terms involving initial conditions, we obtain AIC as given in Section 1.8. In addition, the SIC is derived from a Bayesian model choice point of view using Bayes factors (see Schwarz, 1978).

**Example 2.36 Model Choice for the U.S. GNP Series**

Returning to the analysis of the U.S. GNP data presented in Examples 2.32 and 2.33, recall that two models, an ARIMA(3,1,0) and an ARIMA(0,1,2), fit the logarithms of the data well. To choose the final model, we considered eight models close to the two preliminary models. These models are ARIMA$(p, 1, 0)$ for $p = 2, 3, 4$, ARIMA$(0, 1, q)$ for $q = 1, 2, 3$, an ARIMA$(3, 1, 1)$ and an ARIMA$(1, 1, 2)$. Table 2.2 displays the values of of $\widehat{\sigma}_w^2$, SIC, and AICc obtained for each model. The ARIMA(0,1,2) model has the smallest value of SIC and AICc, and, hence, would be the model of choice.

## 2.9 Multiplicative Seasonal ARIMA Models

In this section, we introduce several modifications made to the ARIMA model to account for seasonal and nonstationary behavior. In Section 1.7, we noted cases in which the sample ACF exhibited slow decay as the lag increased. One particular example related to the ACF of the global temperature series shown in Figure 1.15. Such seasonality and stationarity can often be incorporated into the model with special multiplicative components that generate the behavior of interest.

Often, the dependence on the past tends to occur most strongly at multiples of some underlying seasonal lag $s$. For example, with monthly economic data, there is a strong yearly component occurring at lags that are multiples of $s = 12$, because of the strong connections of all activity to the calendar year. Data taken quarterly will exhibit the yearly repetitive period at $s = 4$ quarters. Natural phenomena such as temperature also have strong components corresponding to seasons. Hence, the natural variability of many physical, biological, and economic processes tends to match with seasonal fluctuations. Because of this, it is natural to introduce autoregressive and moving average polynomials that identify with the seasonal lags. The resulting ***pure seasonal autoregressive moving average model***, say, ARMA$(P, Q)_s$, then takes the form

$$\Phi_P(B^s)x_t = \Theta_Q(B)w_t, \tag{2.136}$$

where the operators

$$\Phi_P(B^s) = 1 - \Phi_1 B^s - \Phi_2 B^{2s} - \cdots - \Phi_P(B^{Ps}) \tag{2.137}$$

and

$$\Theta_Q(B^s) = 1 + \Theta_1 B^s + \Theta_2 B^{2s} + \cdots + \Theta_Q B^{Qs} \tag{2.138}$$

are seasonal autoregressive and seasonal moving average components of orders $P$ and $Q$, respectively, with seasonal period $s$. Analogous to the properties of nonseasonal ARMA models, the pure seasonal ARMA$(P, Q)_s$ is ***causal*** only when the roots of $\Phi_P(z^s)$ lie outside the unit circle, and it is ***invertible*** only when the roots of $\Theta_Q(z^s)$ lie outside the unit circle.

### Example 2.37 A Seasonal ARMA Series

A first-order seasonal autoregressive moving average series that might run over months could be written as

$$(1 - \Phi B^{12})x_t = (1 + \Theta B^{12})w_t$$

or

$$x_t = \Phi x_{t-12} + w_t + \Theta w_{t-12}.$$

This model exhibits the series $x_t$ in terms of past lags at the multiple of the yearly seasonal period $s = 12$ months. It is clear from the above form that estimation and forecasting for such a process involves only straightforward modifications of the unit lag case already treated. In particular, the causal condition requires $|\Phi| < 1$, and the invertible condition requires $|\Theta| < 1$.

For the first-order seasonal ($s = 12$) MA model, $x_t = w_t + \Theta w_{t-12}$, it is easy to verify that

$$\begin{aligned} \gamma(0) &= (1+\Theta^2)\sigma^2 \\ \gamma(\pm 12) &= \Theta\sigma^2 \\ \gamma(h) &= 0, \quad \text{otherwise.} \end{aligned}$$

Thus, the only nonzero correlation, aside from lag zero, is

$$\rho(\pm 12) = \Theta/(1+\Theta^2).$$

For the first-order seasonal ($s = 12$) AR model, using the techniques of the nonseasonal AR(1), we have

$$\begin{aligned} \gamma(0) &= \sigma^2/(1-\Phi^2) \\ \gamma(\pm 12k) &= \sigma^2\Phi^k/(1-\Phi^2) \quad k = 1, 2, \ldots \\ \gamma(h) &= 0, \quad \text{otherwise.} \end{aligned}$$

In this case, the only non-zero correlations are

$$\rho(\pm 12k) = \Phi^k, \quad k = 0, 1, 2, \ldots .$$

These results can be verified using the general result that $\gamma(h) = \Phi\gamma(h-12)$, for $h \geq 1$. For example, when $h = 1$, $\gamma(1) = \Phi\gamma(11)$, but when $h = 11$, we have $\gamma(11) = \Phi\gamma(1)$, which implies that $\gamma(1) = \gamma(11) = 0$. In addition to these results, the PACF have the analogous extensions from nonseasonal to seasonal models.

As an initial diagnostic criterion, we can use the properties for the pure seasonal autoregressive and moving average series listed in Table 2.3. These properties may be considered as generalizations of the properties for nonseasonal models that were presented in Table 2.1.

In general, we combine the seasonal and nonseasonal operators into the overall ***multiplicative seasonal autoregressive moving average model***, denoted by ARMA$(p, q) \times (P, Q)_s$, of Box and Jenkins (1970) and write

$$\Phi_P(B^s)\phi(B)x_t = \Theta_Q(B^s)\theta(B)w_t \tag{2.139}$$

as the overall model. Although the diagnostic properties in Table 2.3 are not strictly true for the overall mixed model, the behavior of the ACF and PACF tends to show rough patterns of the indicated form. In fact, for mixed models, we tend to see a mixture of the facts listed in Tables 2.1 and 2.3. In fitting such models, focusing on the seasonal autoregressive and moving average components first generally leads to more satisfactory results.

**Table 2.3** Behavior of the ACF and PACF for Causal and Invertible Pure Seasonal ARMA Models

| | $\text{AR}(P)_s$ | $\text{MA}(Q)_s$ | $\text{ARMA}(P,Q)_s$ |
|---|---|---|---|
| ACF* | Tails off at lags $ks$, $k = 1, 2, ...,$ | Cuts off after lag $Qs$ | Tails off at lags $ks$ |
| PACF* | Cuts off after lag $Ps$ | Tails off at lags $ks$ $k = 1, 2, ...,$ | Tails off at lags $ks$ |

*The values at nonseasonal lags $h \neq ks$, for $k = 1, 2, ...,$ are zero.

**Example 2.38 A Mixed Seasonal Model**

Consider the $\text{ARMA}(0, 1) \times (1, 0)_{12}$ model

$$x_t = \Phi x_{t-12} + w_t + \theta w_{t-1},$$

where $|\Phi| < 1$ and $|\theta| < 1$. Then, because $x_{t-12}$, $w_t$, and $w_{t-1}$ are uncorrelated, and $x_t$ is stationary, $\gamma(0) = \Phi^2\gamma(0) + \sigma_w^2 + \theta^2\sigma_w^2$, or

$$\gamma(0) = \frac{1+\theta^2}{1-\Phi^2}\,\sigma_w^2.$$

In addition, multiplying the model by $x_{t-h}$, $h > 0$, and taking expectations, we have $\gamma(1) = \Phi\gamma(11) + \theta\sigma_w^2$, and $\gamma(h) = \Phi\gamma(h-12)$, for $h \geq 2$. Thus, the ACF for this model is

$$\begin{aligned} \rho(12h) &= \Phi^h \quad h = 1, 2, ... \\ \rho(12h-1) &= \rho(12h+1) = \frac{\theta}{1+\theta^2}\Phi^h \quad h = 0, 1, 2, ..., \\ \rho(h) &= 0, \quad \text{otherwise.} \end{aligned}$$

The ACF and PACF for this model, with $\Phi = 0.8$ and $\theta = -0.5$, is shown in Figure 2.20. These type of correlation relationships, although idealized here, are typically seen with seasonal data.

Seasonal nonstationarity can occur, for example, when the process is nearly periodic in the season. For example, with average monthly temperatures over the years, each January would be approximately the same, each February would be approximately the same, and so on. In this case, we might think of average monthly temperature $x_t$ as being modeled as

$$x_t = S_t + w_t,$$

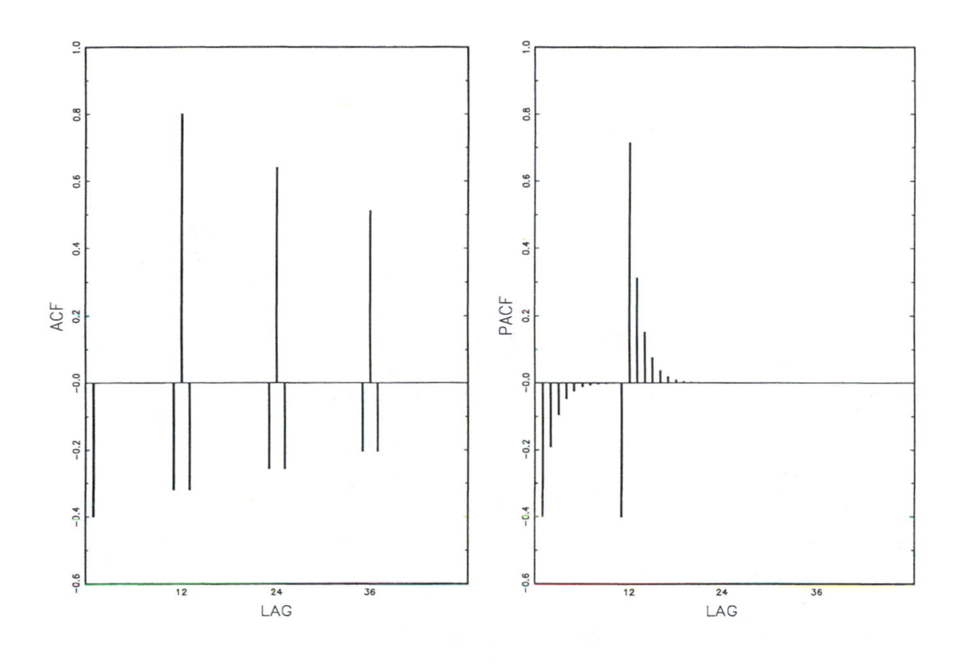


**Figure 2.20:** ACF and PACF of the mixed seasonal ARMA model $x_t = 0.8x_{t-12} + w_t - 0.5w_{t-1}$.

where $S_t$ is a seasonal component that varies slowly from one year to the next, according to a random walk,

$$S_t = S_{t-12} + v_t.$$

In this model, $w_t$ and $v_t$ are uncorrelated white noise processes. The tendency of data to follow this type of model will be exhibited in a sample ACF that is large and decays very slowly at lags $h = 12k$, for $k = 1, 2, \dots$ . If we subtract the effect of successive years from each other, we find that

$$(1 - B^{12})x_t = x_t - x_{t-12} = v_t + w_t - w_{t-12}.$$

This model is a stationary $\text{MA}(1)_{12}$, and its ACF will have a peak only at lag 12. In general, seasonal differencing can be indicated when the ACF decays slowly at multiples of some season $s$, but is negligible between the periods. Then, a ***seasonal difference of order D*** is defined as

$$\nabla_s^D x_t = (1 - B^s)^D x_t, \tag{2.140}$$

where $D = 1, 2, \dots$ takes integer values. Typically, $D = 1$ is sufficient to obtain seasonal stationarity.

Incorporating these ideas into a general model leads to the ***multiplicative seasonal autoregressive integrated moving average model*** of Box and Jenkins (1970) in its most general form. We write the overall model as

$$\Phi_P(B^s)\phi(B)\nabla_s^D\nabla^d x_t = \alpha + \Theta_Q(B^s)\theta(B)w_t, \tag{2.141}$$

and denote it by ***ARIMA(p, d, q) × (P, D, Q)$_s$***. In the above equations and notational expression, the ordinary autoregressive and moving average components are represented by polynomials $\phi(B)$ and $\theta(B)$ of orders $p$ and $q$ respectively [see (2.6) and (2.19)] the seasonal autoregressive and moving average components by $\Phi_P(B^s)$ and $\Theta_Q(B^s)$ [see (2.137) and (2.138)] of orders $P$ and $Q$ and ordinary and seasonal difference components by $\nabla^d = (1-B)^d$ and $\nabla_s^D = (1-B^s)^D$.

**Example 2.39 A Typical Seasonal Multiplicative ARIMA Model.**

Consider the following model, which often provides a reasonable representation for seasonal, nonstationary, economic time series. We exhibit the equations for the model, denoted by ARIMA$(0,1,1) \times (0,1,1)_{12}$ in the notation given above, where the seasonal fluctuations occur every 12 months. Then, the model (2.141) becomes

$$(1-B^{12})(1-B)x_t = (1+\Theta_1 B^{12})(1+\theta_1 B)w_t. \tag{2.142}$$

Expanding both sides of (2.142) leads to the representation

$$(1-B-B^{12}+B^{13})x_t = (1+\theta B+\Theta B^{12}+\Theta\theta B^{13})w_t,$$

or in difference equation form

$$x_t = x_{t-1} + x_{t-12} - x_{t-13} + w_t + \theta w_{t-1} + \Theta w_{t-12} + \Theta\theta w_{t-13}.$$

Selecting the appropriate model for a given set of data from all of those represented by the general form (2.141) is a daunting task, and we usually think first in terms of finding difference operators that produce a roughly stationary series and then in terms of finding a set of simple autoregressive moving average or multiplicative seasonal ARMA to fit the resulting residual series. Any fitted model in the above general form will have a residual, say, $\widehat{w}_t$ that can be computed by substituting successively into (2.141). Differencing operations are applied first, and then the residuals are constructed from a series of reduced length. These residuals should appear to be white noise when a reasonable model has been fitted, so autocorrelation and partial autocorrelation functions computed for these residuals should not have many significant peaks beyond $h = 0$. Peaks that appear in these functions can often be eliminated by fitting an autoregressive or moving average component in accordance with the general properties of Tables 2.1 and 2.3. In considering whether the model is satisfactory, the diagnostic techniques discussed in Section 2.8 still apply.

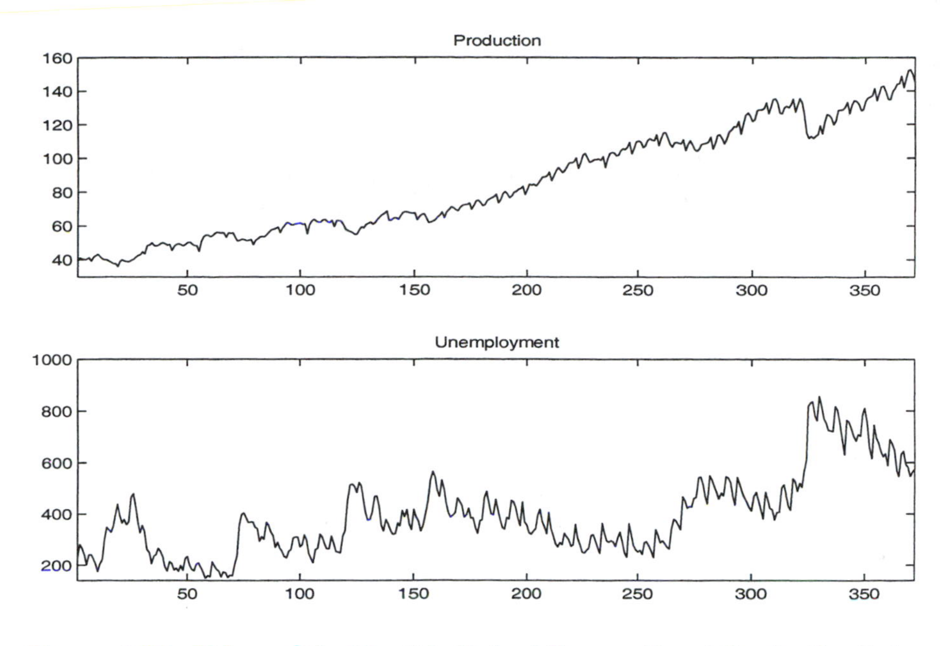


**Figure 2.21:** Values of the Monthly Federal Reserve Board Production Index and Unemployment (1948-1978, $n = 372$ months).

**Example 2.40 Analysis of the Federal Reserve Board Production Index.**

A problem of great interest in economics involves first identifying a model within the Box–Jenkins class for a given time series and then producing forecasts based on the model. For example, we might consider applying this methodology to the Federal Reserve Board Production Index shown in Figure 2.21. The ACF's and PACF's for this series are shown in Figure 2.22, and we note the slow decay in the ACF and the peak at lag $h = 1$ in the PACF, indicating nonstationary behavior.

Following the recommended procedure, a first difference was taken, and the ACF and PACF of the first difference $\nabla x_t = x_t - x_{t-1}$ are shown in Figure 2.23. Noting the peaks at $12, 24, 36$, and 48 with relatively slow decay suggested a seasonal difference and Figure 2.24 shows the seasonal difference of the differenced production, say, $\nabla_{12}\nabla x_t = (1 - B^{12})(1 - B)x_t$. Characteristics of the ACF and PACF of this series tend to show a peak at $h = 12$ in the autocorrelation function, combined with peaks at $12, 24, \ldots$ in the partial autocorrelation function. Using Table 2.3, this suggests either a seasonal moving average of order $Q = 1$ or a seasonal autoregression of possible order $P = 2$. There is also a substantial peak in the PACF at lag $h = 1$, indicating a possible autoregressive series of order $p = 1$ by Table 2.1. Fitting the two models suggested by these observations,

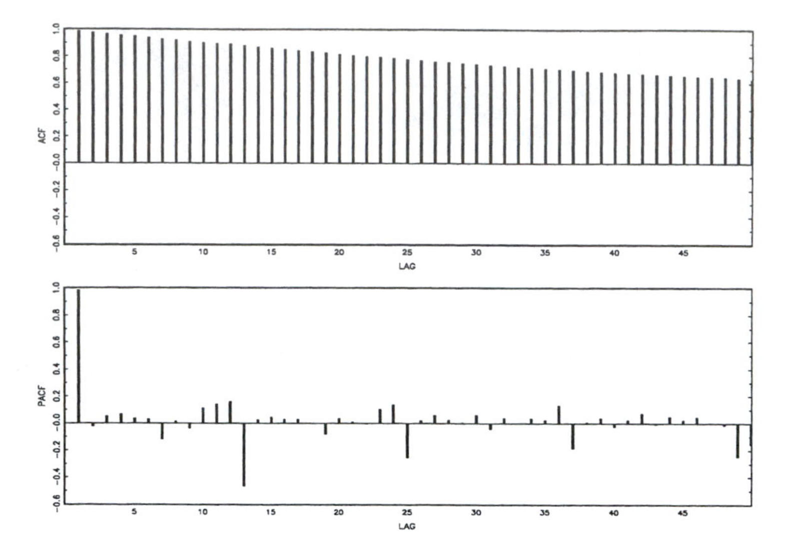


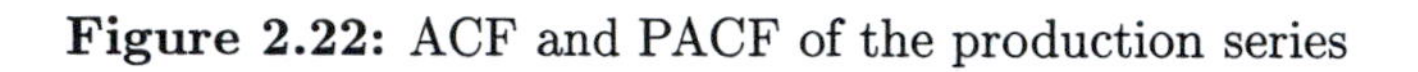

**Figure 2.22:** ACF and PACF of the production series

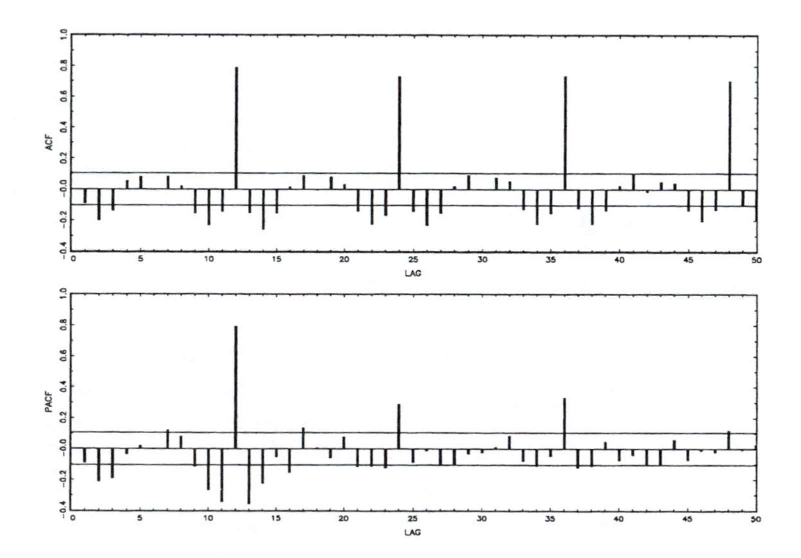


**Figure 2.23:** ACF and PACF of differenced production, $(1 - B)x_t$.

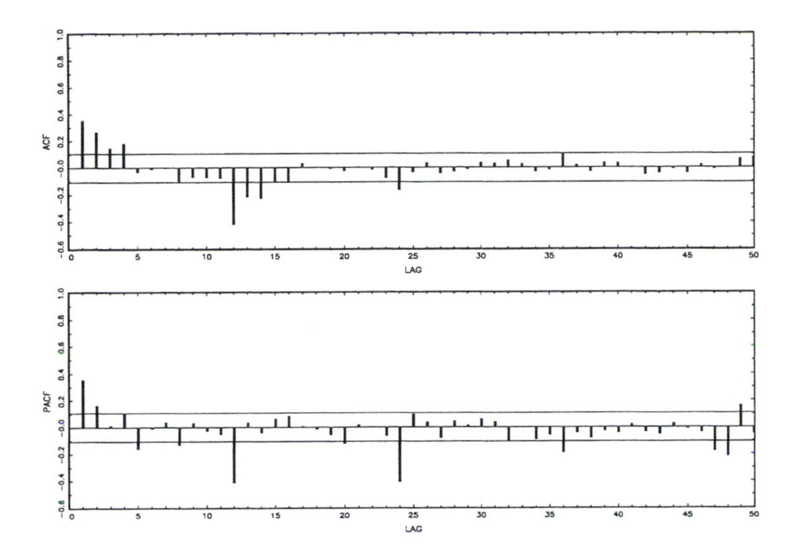


**Figure 2.24:** ACF and PACF of first differenced and then seasonally differenced production, $(1 - B)(1 - B^{12})x_t$.

namely, ARIMA$(1,1,0) \times (0,1,1)_{12}$ and ARIMA$(1,1,0) \times (2,1,0)_{12}$, lead to adjusted AICc values of 1.401 and 1.449, respectively. The value of AICc for the simpler ARIMA$(1,1,0) \times (0,1,0)_{12}$ model was 1.809. On the basis of this behavior, we tend to prefer the ARIMA$(1,1,0) \times (0,1,1)_{12}$ model. Figure 2.25 shows the ACF and PACF of the ARIMA$(1,1,0) \times (0,1,0)_{12}$ model residuals, and we note the continuing presence of the seasonal peaks.

The ACF and PACF of the residuals from the ARIMA$(1,1,0) \times (0,1,1)_{12}$ model shown in Figure 2.26 do not show patterns, and the AICc value is minimized over the class of models searched. The value of the Ljung–Box–Pierce statistic was $Q = 13.9$ when $H = 12$ and comparing this with a $\chi^2_{10}$, the $p$-value is about 0.08; when $H = 24$, $Q = 36.3$, which, when compared with a $\chi^2_{22}$ leads to a $p$-value of 0.03. This result suggests the possibility that there is still some slight seasonal regularity in the residuals, but the addition of another seasonal MA component or another seasonal AR component does not change this outcome. In addition, there are a few isolated outliers in the residuals, but other than these, the residuals behave as normal residuals. Based on these observations, we obtain as the final model, the ARIMA$(1,1,0) \times (0,1,1)_{12}$ form, with estimated parameters given by $\widehat{\phi} = 0.329$, $\widehat{\Theta} = -0.696$, and $\widehat{\sigma}^2_w = 1.468$,

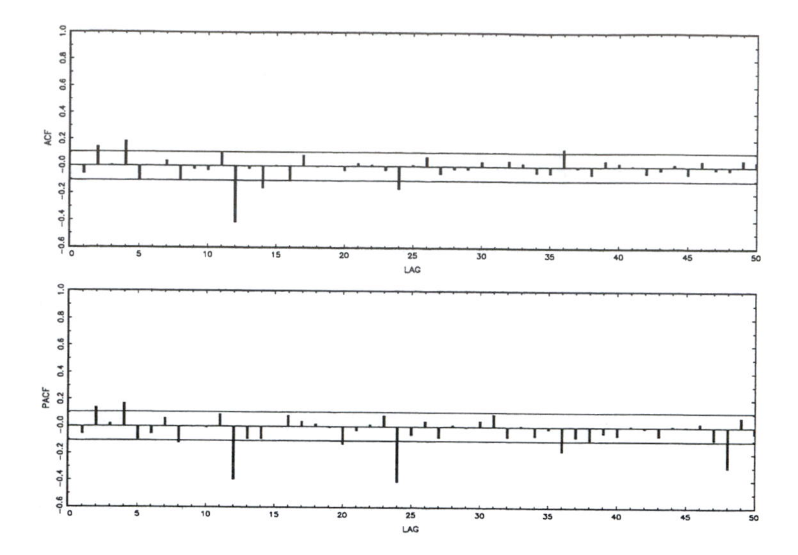


**Figure 2.25:** ACF and PACF of production residuals: ARIMA$(1,1,0) \times (0,1,0)_{12}$ model.

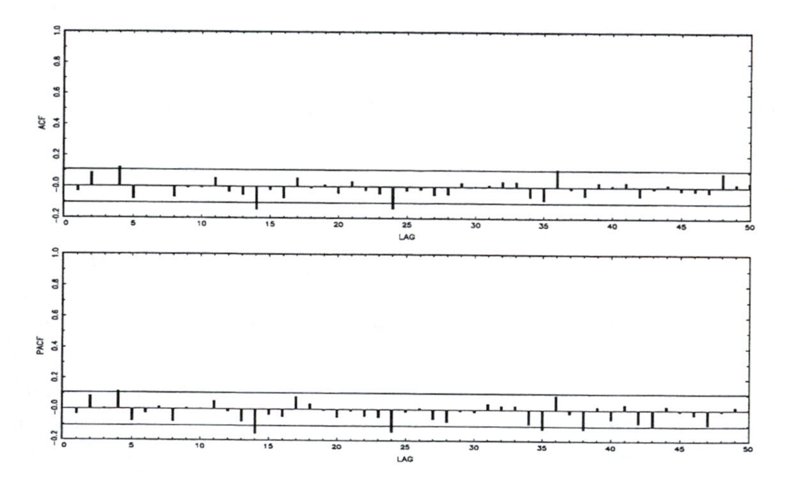


**Figure 2.26:** ACF and PACF of production residuals: ARIMA$(1,1,0) \times (0,1,1)_{12}$ model.

implying the estimated model

$$(1 - 0.329B)(1 - B^{12})(1 - B)x_t = (1 - 0.696B^{12})\widehat{w}_t,$$

where $\widehat{w}_t \sim$ iid N(0, 1.468). Equivalently, we can write the estimated model as

$$\begin{aligned} x_t &= 1.329x_{t-1} - 0.329x_{t-2} + x_{t-12} - 1.329x_{t-13} \\ &\quad +0.329x_{t-14} + \widehat{w}_t - 0.696\widehat{w}_{t-12}, \end{aligned}$$

which is the appropriate form for forecasting.

Although the fitted model is not stationary, it is invertible, and hence, the rules for truncated prediction, (2.80), apply. For example, if we wish to forecast the next 12 months, the estimated forecasts for time $n+m$, where $n = 372$ and $m = 1, 2, ..., 12$, are of the form

$$\begin{aligned} \widehat{x}^n_{n+m} &= 1.329\widehat{x}^n_{n+m-1} - 0.329\widehat{x}^n_{n+m-2} + \widehat{x}^n_{n+m-12} \\ &- 1.329\widehat{x}^n_{n+m-13} + 0.329\widehat{x}^n_{n+m-14} - 0.696\widehat{w}^n_{n+m-12}. \end{aligned}$$

We have substituted the parameter estimates for the true parameters in (2.80) and denoted the estimated truncated forecast by $\widehat{x}^n_{n+m}$.

For the estimated forecast variances, we may equate coefficients of $B^k$ in

$$(1 - 0.329B)(1 - B^{12})(1 - B)(1 + \widehat{\psi}_1 B + \widehat{\psi}_2 B^2 + \cdots) = (1 - 0.696B^{12}),$$

which leads to $\widehat{\psi}_1 = (1 + 0.329)$ and

$$\widehat{\psi}_k = (1 + 0.329)\widehat{\psi}_{k-1} - 0.329\widehat{\psi}_{k-2}$$

for $k = 2, 3, \ldots, 11$ months. Figure 2.27 shows the estimates forecast values with the limits, computed by $\widehat{x}^n_{n+m} \pm 1.96\sqrt{\widehat{P}^n_{n+m}}$ with

$$\widehat{P}^n_{n+m} = \widehat{\sigma}^2_w \sum_{k=0}^{m-1} \widehat{\psi}^2_k,$$

as in (2.78). The resulting forecast and 95% lower and upper prediction limits are shown in Figure 2.27 for a 12-month period. The future values are forecasted as a relatively linear extension of the current series that essentially repeats the last 12-month period. The upper and lower prediction limits are broad, as is customary for most forecasts.

Because the operator $(1 - B)(1 - B^{12})$ has roots on the unit circle, the usual series expansion, (2.25), will not converge in mean square and the representation (2.78) for the estimation error of the finite approximation to the forecast based on the infinite past will be poor. In such cases, it would be more appropriate, for example, to use the innovations algorithm, Property P2.6, which gives exact forecasts and forecast error

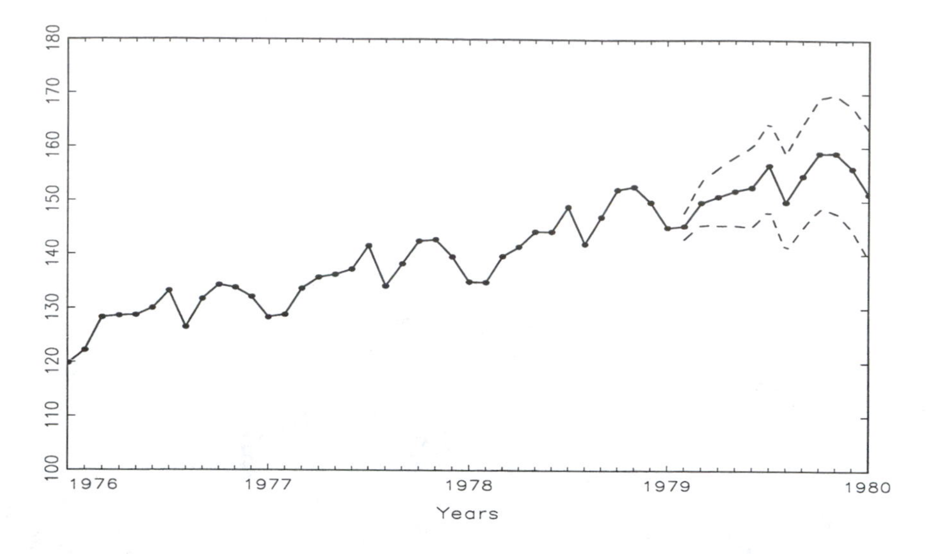


**Figure 2.27:** Forecasts and limits for production index.

variances, and can apply in the case of nonstationarity. Brockwell and Davis (1991, Section 9.5) discuss this approach. In these cases, it is also convenient to put the ARIMA model in ***state-space*** form and generate the forecasts using the Kalman filter, as we do in Chapter 4.

## 2.10 Long Memory ARMA and Fractional Differencing

The conventional seasonal ARMA$(p,q)\times(P,Q)_s$ process is often referred to as a short memory process because the coefficients in the representation

$$x_t = \sum_{j=0}^{\infty} \psi_j w_{t-j},$$

obtained by solving

$$\Phi_P(B^s)\phi(B)\psi(B) = \Theta_Q(B^s)\theta(B),$$

are dominated by exponential decay. As pointed out in Section 2.3, this result implies the ACF of the short memory process $\rho(h)\to 0$ exponentially fast as $h\to\infty$. When the sample ACF of a time series decays slowly, the advice given in the previous sections has been to difference the series until it seems stationary. Following this advice with the glacial varve series first presented in Example 2.28 leads to the first difference of the logarithms of the data being represented as a first-order moving average. Further analysis of the residuals leads to fitting an ARIMA$(1,1,1)$ model,

$$\nabla x_t = \phi \nabla x_{t-1} + w_t + \theta w_{t-1},$$

where we understand $x_t$ is the log-transformed varve series. In particular, the estimates of the parameters (and the standard errors) are $\widehat{\phi} = 0.236$ (0.046), $\widehat{\theta} = -0.890$ (0.021), and $\widehat{\sigma}_w^2 = 0.229$. The use of the first difference $\nabla x_t = (1-B)x_t$ can be too severe a modification in the sense that the nonstationary model might represent an overdifferencing of the original process.

Long memory time series were considered in Hosking (1981) and Granger and Joyeux (1980) as intermediate compromises between the short memory ARMA type models and the fully integrated nonstationary processes in the Box–Jenkins class. The easiest way to generate a long memory series is to think of using the difference operator $(1-B)^d$ for fractional values of $d$, say, $-.5 < d < .5$, so a typical long memory series gets generated as

$$(1-B)^d x_t = w_t, \tag{2.143}$$

where $w_t$ still denotes white noise with variance $\sigma_w^2$. Now, $d$ becomes a parameter to be estimated along with $\sigma_w^2$. Differencing the original process, as in the Box–Jenkins approach, may be thought of as simply assigning a value of $d = 1$. Long memory processes may occur in hydrology (see Hurst, 1951, and McLeod and Hipel, 1978) or in environmental series, such as the varve data we have previously analyzed. Long memory time series data tend to exhibit sample autocorrelations that are not necessarily large (as in the case of $d = 1$), but persist for a long time. Figure 2.28 shows the sample ACF of the log-transformed varve series, which exhibits classic long memory behavior, to lag 100.

To investigate the properties of the fractionally differenced series (2.143), consider the binomial expansion

$$\nabla^d = (1-B)^d = \sum_{j=0}^{\infty} \pi_j B^j, \tag{2.144}$$

where

$$\pi_j = \frac{\Gamma(j-d)}{\Gamma(j+1)\Gamma(-d)}, \tag{2.145}$$

with $\Gamma(x+1) = x\Gamma(x)$ being the gamma function. This, implies the alternate form for (2.143)

$$\sum_{j=0}^{\infty} \pi_j x_{t-j} = w_t \tag{2.146}$$

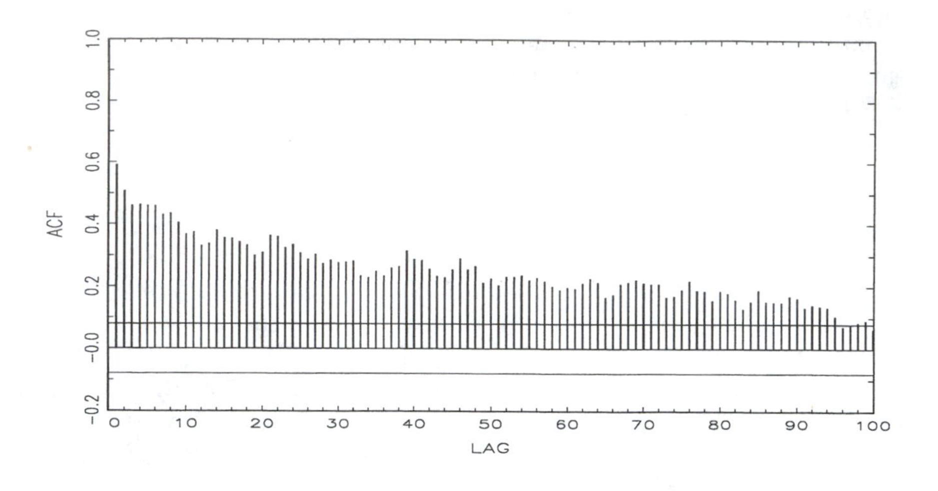


**Figure 2.28:** Sample ACF of the log transformed varve series.

and allows computation of the noise values $w_t$ given the input series $x_t$. It also turns out that (see Brockwell and Davis, 1991) that a mean square convergent representation exists

$$x_t = \sum_{j=0}^{\infty} \psi_j w_{t-j} \tag{2.147}$$

for such a process, where

$$\psi_j = \frac{\Gamma(j+d)}{\Gamma(j+1)\Gamma(d)} \tag{2.148}$$

$j = 0, 1, \ldots$, and $\sum \psi_j^2 < \infty$. The ACF is shown to be of the form

$$\rho(h) = \frac{\Gamma(h+d)\Gamma(1-d)}{\Gamma(h-d+1)\Gamma(d)} \tag{2.149}$$

for $h = 1, 2, \ldots$.

In order to examine a series such as the varve series for a possible long memory pattern, it is convenient to look at ways of estimating $d$. It is easy to derive the recursions

$$\pi_{j+1}(d) = \frac{(j-d)\pi_j(d)}{(j+1)}, \tag{2.150}$$

with $\pi_0(d) = 1$, as in (1.45) of Chapter 1, where we made the dependence on $d$ explicit in this form. Maximizing the joint likelihood of the errors, say, $w_t(d)$, will involve minimizing the sum of squared errors

$$Q(d) = \sum w_t^2(d).$$

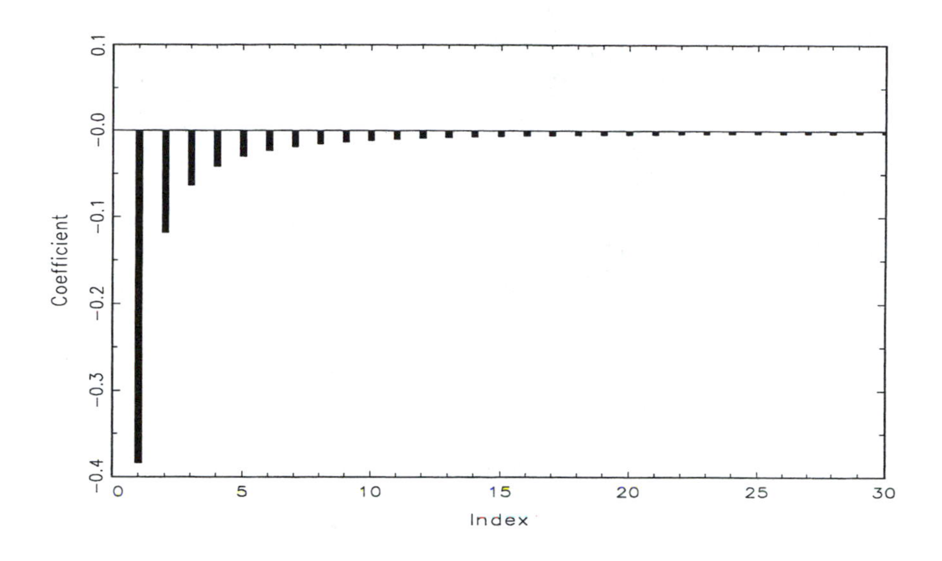


**Figure 2.29:** Coefficients $\pi_j(0.384), j = 1, 2, \ldots, 30$ in the representation (2.150).

The usual Gauss–Newton method, described in Section 2.6, leads to the expansion

$$w_t(d) = w_t(d_0) + w_t'(d_0)(d - d_0),$$

where

$$w_t'(d_0) = \left.\frac{\partial w_t}{\partial d}\right|_{d=d_0}.$$

Setting up the usual regression leads to

$$d = d_0 - \frac{\sum_t w_t'(d_0) w_t(d_0)}{\sum_t w_t'(d_0)^2}.$$

The derivatives are computed recursively by differentiating (2.150) successively with respect to $d$. The errors are computed from an approximation to (2.146), namely,

$$w_t(d) = \sum_{j=0}^{t} \pi_j(d) x_{t-j}(d). \tag{2.151}$$

It is advisable to omit a number of initial terms from the computation and start the sum at some fairly large value of $t$ to have a reasonable approximation. In the next example, omitting $t = 30$ points seems to be reasonable.

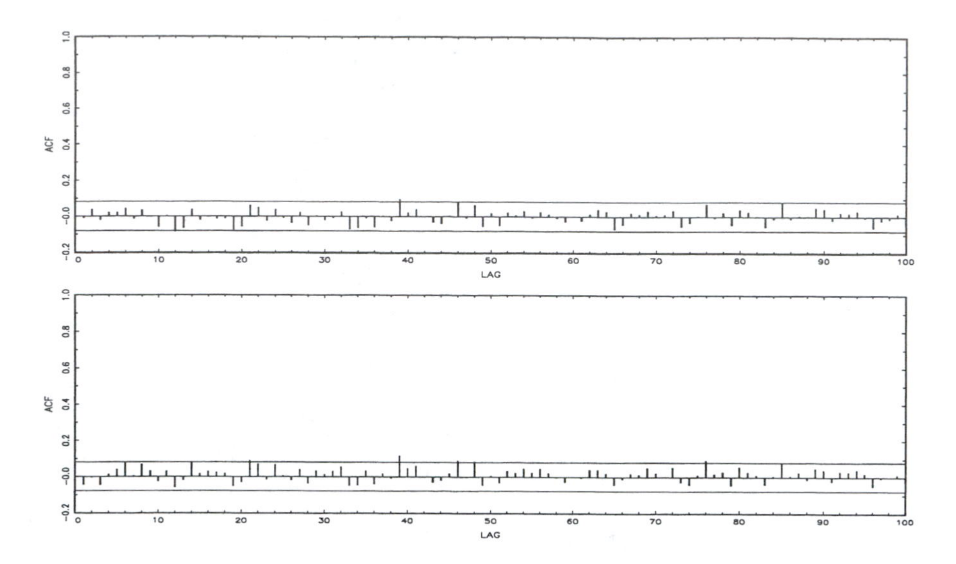


**Figure 2.30:** ACF's of residuals from ARIMA$(1,1,1)$ series (top) and long memory model, $(1-B)^d x_t = w_t$, with $d = .384$ (bottom).

**Example 2.41 Long Memory Fitting of the Glacial Varve Series**

We consider analyzing the glacial varve series discussed in Examples 1.24 and 2.28. Figure 1.16 shows the original and log-transformed series (which we denote by $x_t$). We have noted at the beginning of this section that the first differences of such a series satisfies an ARMA$(1,1)$ process. Next, we fit the fractionally differenced model, (2.143), to the mean-adjusted series, $x_t - \bar{x}$. Applying the Gauss–Newton iterative procedure previously described, starting with $d = .1$ and omitting the first 30 points from the computation, leads to a final value of $d = .384$, which implies the set of coefficients $\pi_j(.384)$, as given in Figure 2.29 with $\pi_0(.384) = 1$. We can compare roughly the performance of the fractional difference operator with the ARIMA model by examining the autocorrelation functions of the two residual series as shown in Figure 2.30. The ACF's of the two residual series are roughly comparable with the white noise model.

Although there is no obvious short memory ARMA-type component in the residuals from the fractionally differenced series, it is natural that cases will exist in which substantial short memory-type components will be left in the ACF and PACF of the residuals. Hence, it is natural to define the general ***fractionally integrated ARIMA***$(p,d,q), -.5 < d < .5$ ***process*** as

$$\phi(B)\nabla^d (x_t - \mu) = \theta(B) w_t, \tag{2.152}$$

where $\phi(B)$ and $\theta(B)$ are the same operators as in the general case given before. The model is sometimes termed an ARFIMA model. Writing the model in the form

$$\phi(B)\pi_d(B)(x_t - \mu) = \theta(B)w_t \tag{2.153}$$

makes it clear how we go about estimating the parameters for the more general model.

Forecasting for the ARIMA$(p, d, q)$ long memory series can be easily done, noting that we may equate coefficients in

$$\phi(B)\psi(B) = (1 - B)^{-d}\theta(B) \tag{2.154}$$

and

$$\theta(B)\pi(B) = (1 - B)^{d}\phi(B) \tag{2.155}$$

to obtain the representations

$$x_t = \mu + \sum_{j=0}^{\infty} \psi_j w_{t-j}$$

and

$$w_t = \sum_{j=0}^{\infty} \pi_j (x_{t-j} - \mu).$$

We then can proceed as for conventional ARMA estimators.

In closing this brief discussion (a comprehensive treatment is Beran, 1994), it should be noted that several other techniques for estimating the parameters, especially, the long memory parameter, can be developed in the frequency domain, as will be shown in Chapter 3. In addition, the Splus procedure `arima.fracdiff` can be used to fit fractionally differenced ARIMA models to data using a Gaussian maximum likelihood technique on the truncated process (2.151).

## 2.11 Threshold Models

In Section 2.6, we discussed the fact that, for a stationary time series, best linear prediction forward in time is the same as best linear prediction backward in time. This result followed from the fact that the variance–covariance matrix of $\boldsymbol{x}_{1:n} = (x_1, x_2, ..., x_n)'$, say, $\Gamma = \{\gamma(i - j)\}_{i,j=1}^{n}$, is the same as the variance–covariance matrix of $\boldsymbol{x}_{n:1} = (x_n, x_{n-1}, ..., x_1)'$. In addition, if the process is Gaussian, the distributions of $\boldsymbol{x}_{1:n}$ and $\boldsymbol{x}_{n:1}$ are identical. In this case, a time plot of $\boldsymbol{x}_{1:n}$ (that is, the data plotted forward in time) should look similar to a time plot of $\boldsymbol{x}_{n:1}$ (that is, the data plotted backward in time).

There are, however, many series that do not fit into this category. For example, Figure 2.31 shows a plot of monthly pneumonia and influenza deaths

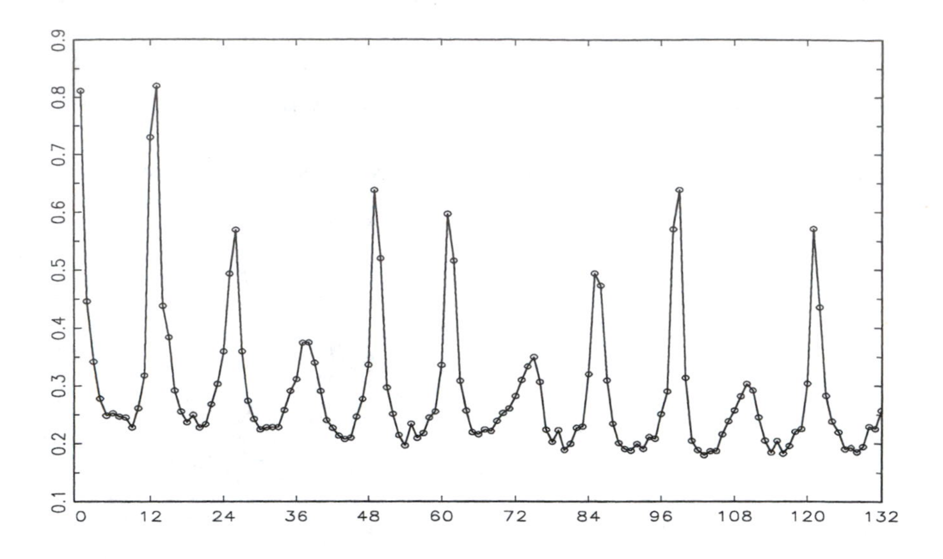


**Figure 2.31:** U.S. monthly pneumonia and influenza deaths per 1,000 over 11 years from 1968 to 1978.

per 1,000 in the U.S., for 11 years, 1968 to 1978. Typically, the number of deaths tends to increase slower than it decreases. Thus, if the data were plotted backward in time, the backward series would tend to increase faster than it decreases. Also, if monthly pneumonia and influenza deaths followed a linear Gaussian process, we would not expect to see such large bursts of positive and negative changes that occur periodically in this series. Moreover, although the number of deaths is typically largest during the winter months, the data are not perfectly seasonal. That is, although the peak of the series often occurs in January, in other years, the peak occurs in December, February, or March.

If our goal is to predict flu epidemics, then it should be clear that a Gaussian linear model would not be appropriate. Many approaches to modeling nonlinear series exist that could be used (see Priestley, 1988); here, we focus on the class of ***threshold autoregressive models*** presented in Tong (1983, 1990). The basic idea of these models is that of fitting local linear AR($p$) models, and their appeal is that we can use the intuition from fitting global linear AR($p$) models. Suppose we know $p$, and given the vectors $\boldsymbol{x}_{t-1} = (x_{t-1}, ..., x_{t-p})'$, we can identify $r$ mutually exclusive and exhaustive regions for $\boldsymbol{x}_{t-1}$, say, $R_1, ..., R_r$, where the dynamics of the system changes. The threshold model is then written as $r$, AR($p$) models,

$$x_t = \alpha^{(j)} + \phi_1^{(j)} x_{t-1} + \cdots + \phi_p^{(j)} x_{t-p} + w_t^{(j)}, \quad \boldsymbol{x}_{t-1} \in R_j, \tag{2.156}$$

for $j = 1, ..., r$. In (2.156), the $w_t^{(j)}$ are independent white noise series, each with variance $\sigma_j^2$, for $j = 1, ..., r$. Model estimation, identification, and diagnostics proceed as in the case in which $r = 1$.

**Example 2.42 Threshold Modeling of the Influenza Series**

As previously discussed, examination of Figure 2.31 leads us to believe that the monthly pneumonia and influenza deaths time series is not linear. It is also evident from Figure 2.31 that there is a slight negative trend in the data. We have found that the most convenient way to fit a threshold model to this data set, while removing the trend, is to work with the first difference of the data. The differenced data, which we call $x_t$, is exhibited in Figure 2.32 as the dark solid line with circles representing observations. The dashed line with squares in Figure 2.32 are the one-month-ahead predictions, and we will discuss this series later.

The nonlinearity of the data is more pronounced in the plot of the first differences, $x_t$. Clearly, the change in the numbers of deaths, $x_t$, slowly rises for some months and, then, sometime in the winter, has a possibility of jumping to a large number once $x_t$ exceeds about 0.5. If the processes does make a large jump, then a subsequent significant decrease occurs in flu deaths. As an initial analysis, we fit the following threshold model

$$\begin{aligned} x_t &= \alpha^{(1)} + \sum_{j=1}^{p} \phi_j^{(1)} x_{t-j} + w_t^{(1)}, \quad x_{t-1} < 0.5 \\ x_t &= \alpha^{(2)} + \sum_{j=1}^{p} \phi_j^{(2)} x_{t-j} + w_t^{(2)}, \quad x_{t-1} \geq 0.5, \end{aligned} \tag{2.157}$$

with $p = 6$, assuming this would be larger than necessary.

Model (2.157) is easy to fit using two linear regression runs. That is, let $\delta_t^{(1)} = 1$ if $x_{t-1} < 0.5$, and zero otherwise, and let $\delta_t^{(2)} = 1$ if $x_{t-1} \geq 0.5$, and zero otherwise. Then, using the notation of Section 1.8, for $t = p+1, ..., n$, either equation in (2.157) can be written as

$$y_t = \boldsymbol{\beta}' \boldsymbol{z}_t + w_t$$

where, for $i = 1, 2$,

$$y_t = \delta_t^{(i)} x_t, \quad \boldsymbol{z}_t', = \delta_t^{(i)} (1, x_{t-1}, ..., x_{t-p}), \quad w_t = \delta_t^{(i)} w_t^{(i)},$$

and

$$\boldsymbol{\beta}' = (\alpha^{(i)}, \phi_1^{(i)}, \phi_2^{(i)}, ..., \phi_p^{(i)}).$$

Parameter estimates can then be obtained using the regression techniques of Section 1.8 twice, once for $i = 1$ and again for $i = 2$.

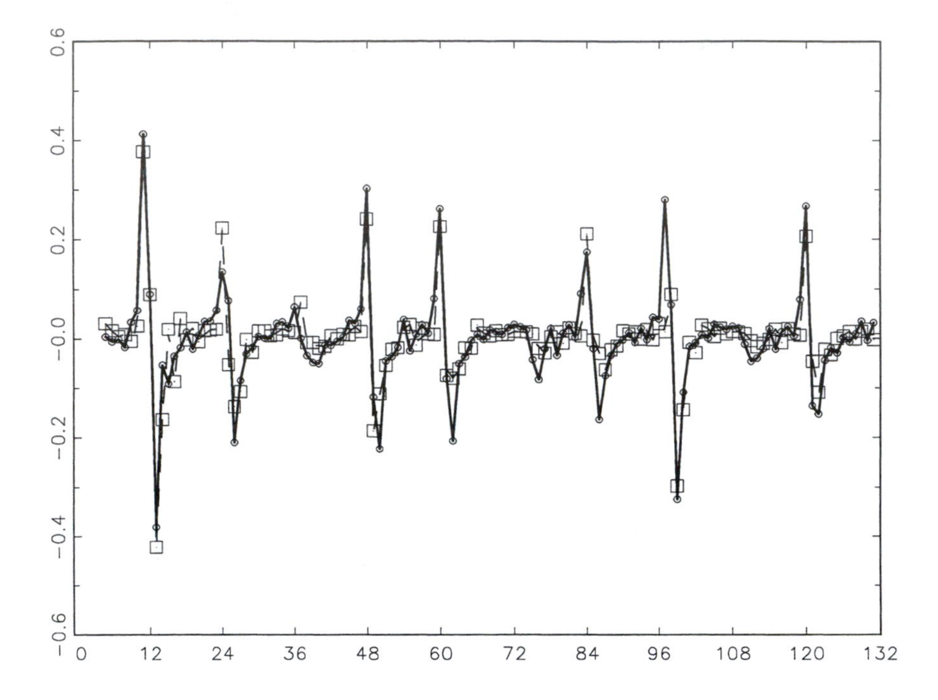


**Figure 2.32:** First differenced U.S. monthly pneumonia and influenza deaths per 1,000 (solid line - circles); one-month-ahead predictions (dashed line - squares).

For each model, an order $p = 4$ model was finally selected. The final model was

$$\begin{aligned}\widehat{x}_t &= 0.51_{(.08)}x_{t-1} - 0.20_{(.06)}x_{t-2} + 0.12_{(.05)}x_{t-3} \\ &\quad -0.11_{(0.5)}x_{t-4} + \widehat{w}_t^{(1)}, \qquad \text{when } x_{t-1} < 0.5\end{aligned}$$

$$\begin{aligned}\widehat{x}_t &= 0.40 - 0.75_{(.17)}x_{t-1} - 1.03_{(.21)}x_{t-2} - 2.05_{(1.05)}x_{t-3} \\ &\quad -6.71_{(1.25)}x_{t-4} + \widehat{w}_t^{(2)}, \qquad \text{when } x_{t-1} \geq 0.5,\end{aligned}$$

where $\widehat{\sigma}_1 = 0.05$ and $\widehat{\sigma}_2 = 0.07$. The threshold of 0.5 was exceeded 17 times. Using the final model, one-month-ahead predictions can be made, and these are shown in Figure 2.32 as a dashed line with squares. Except for one instance around the end of the eighth year ($t = 96$), the model does extremely well in predicting a flu epidemic; the peak at $t = 96$, however, was missed by this model. When we fit a model with a smaller threshold of 0.4, flu epidemics were somewhat underestimated, but the flu epidemic in the eighth year was predicted one month early. We chose the model with a threshold of 0.5 because the residual diagnostics showed no obvious departure from the model assumption (except for one outlier at $t = 96$); the model with a threshold of 0.4 still had some correlation left in the residuals and there were more than one outliers. Finally, prediction beyond one-month-ahead for this model is very complicated, but some approximate techniques exist (see Tong, 1983).

## 2.12 Regression with Autocorrelated Errors

In Section 1.8, we covered the classical regression model with uncorrelated errors $w_t$. In this section, we discuss the modifications that might be considered when the errors are correlated. That is, consider the regression model

$$y_t = \boldsymbol{\beta}' \boldsymbol{z}_t + x_t, \tag{2.158}$$

$t = 1, \ldots, n$, where $x_t$ is a process with some covariance function $\gamma(s,t)$. Then, we have the matrix form

$$\boldsymbol{y} = Z\boldsymbol{\beta} + \boldsymbol{x}, \tag{2.159}$$

where $\boldsymbol{x} = (x_1, \ldots, x_n)'$ is a $n \times 1$ vector with $n \times n$ covariance matrix $\Gamma = \{\gamma(s,t)\}$. Note that $Z = [\boldsymbol{z}_1, \boldsymbol{z}_2, \ldots, \boldsymbol{z}_n]'$ is the $n \times q$ matrix of input variables, as before. If we know the covariance matrix $\Gamma$, it is possible to find a transformation matrix $A$, such that $A\Gamma A' = \sigma^2 I$, where $I$ denotes the $n \times n$ identity matrix. Then, the underlying model can be transformed into

$$\begin{aligned} A\boldsymbol{y} &= AZ\boldsymbol{\beta} + A\boldsymbol{x} \\ &= U\boldsymbol{\beta} + \boldsymbol{w}, \end{aligned}$$

where $U = AZ$ and $\boldsymbol{w}$ is a white noise vector with covariance matrix $\sigma^2 I$ as at the beginning of this chapter. Then, applying least squares or maximum likelihood to the vector $A\boldsymbol{y}$ gives

$$\begin{aligned} \widehat{\boldsymbol{\beta}}_w &= (U'U)^{-1}U'\boldsymbol{y} \\ &= (Z'A'AZ)^{-1}Z'A'A\boldsymbol{y} \\ &= (Z'\Gamma^{-1}Z)^{-1}Z'\Gamma^{-1}\boldsymbol{y} \end{aligned} \tag{2.160}$$

because

$$\sigma^2\Gamma^{-1} = A'A.$$

The difficulty in applying (2.160) always is that we do not know the form of the matrix $\Gamma$.

It may be possible, however, in the time series case, to assume a stationary covariance structure for the error process $x_t$ that corresponds to a linear process and try to find an ARMA representation for $x_t$. For example, if we have a pure AR($p$) error, then

$$\phi(B)x_t = w_t,$$

and $\phi(B)$ is the linear transformation that, when applied to the error process, produces the white noise $w_t$. Regarding this transformation as the appropriate matrix $A$ of the preceding paragraph produces the transformed regression equation

$$\phi(B)y_t = \boldsymbol{\beta}'\phi(B)\boldsymbol{z}_t + w_t,$$

and we are back to the same model as before. Defining $u_t = \phi(B)y_t$ and $\boldsymbol{v}_t = \phi(B)\boldsymbol{z}_t$ leads to the simple regression problem

$$u_t = \boldsymbol{\beta}'\boldsymbol{v}_t + w_t \tag{2.161}$$

considered before. The preceding discussion suggests an algorithm, due to Cochrane and Orcutt (1949), for fitting a regression model with autocorrelated errors.

(i) First, run an ordinary regression of $y_t$ on $z_t$ (acting as if the errors are uncorrelated). Retain the residuals.

(ii) Fit an ARMA model to the residuals $\widehat{x}_t = y_t - \widehat{\boldsymbol{\beta}}'\boldsymbol{z}_t$, say,

$$\widehat{\phi}(B)\widehat{x}_t = \widehat{\theta}(B)w_t \tag{2.162}$$

(iii) Then, apply the ARMA transformation to both sides (2.158), that is,

$$u_t = \frac{\widehat{\phi}(B)}{\widehat{\theta}(B)}y_t$$

and

$$\boldsymbol{v}_t = \frac{\widehat{\phi}(B)}{\widehat{\theta}(B)}\boldsymbol{z}_t,$$

to obtain the transformed regression model (2.161).

(iv) Run an ordinary least squares regression model assuming uncorrelated errors on the transformed regression model (2.161), obtaining

$$\widehat{\boldsymbol{\beta}}_w = (V'V)^{-1}V'\boldsymbol{u}, \tag{2.163}$$

where $V = [\boldsymbol{v}_1, \ldots, \boldsymbol{v}_n]'$ and $\boldsymbol{u} = (u_1, \ldots, u_n)'$ are the corresponding transformed components.

The above procedure can be repeated until convergence and will approach the maximum likelihood solution under normality of the errors.

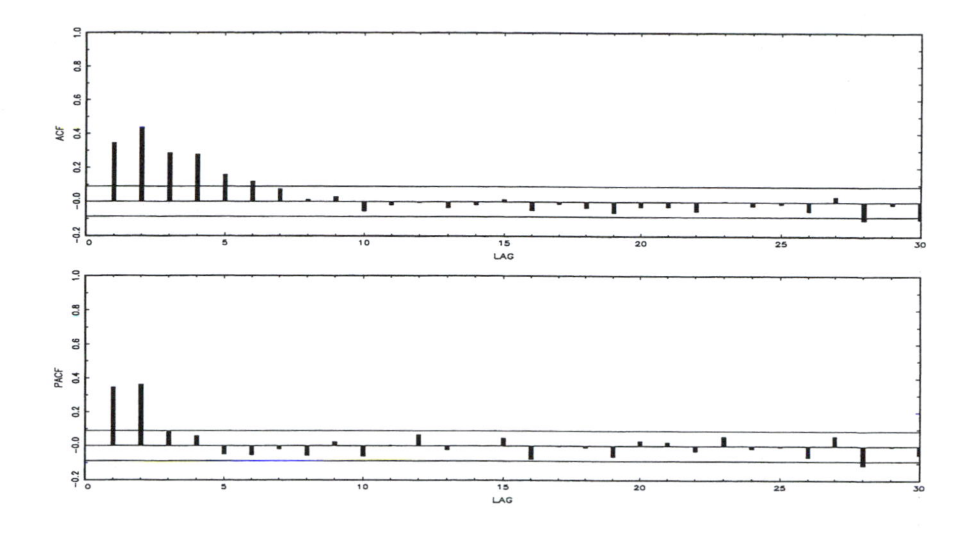


**Figure 2.33:** Sample ACF and PACF of the mortality residuals indicating an AR(2) process.

**Example 2.43 Pollution, Temperature, Mortality with Correlated Errors**

We consider further the best regression obtained in Example 1.27 of Chapter 1, relating adjusted temperature $T_t - T_\cdot$, $(T_t - T_\cdot)^2$ and particulate levels $P_t$ to cardiovascular mortality $M_t$. Identifying the vectors

$$z_t = (1, t, (T_t - T_\cdot), (T_t - T_\cdot)^2, P_t)'$$

leads to a model of the form (2.158). Taking the residuals from the least squares regression, as described in Step (i), the sample ACF and PACF, shown in Figure 2.33, suggest an AR(2) model for the residuals. Note, $\widehat{\sigma}^2 = 40.77, R^2 = .59$ for this model.

For the residuals, we obtain a second-order autoregressive model with operator

$$\phi(B) = 1 - .2207B - .3627B^2$$

which is applied to both sides of the defining equation (2.160) to produce the transformed equation (2.161), as in Step (ii) above. Running the regression, as in Step (iii), yields the model

$$\begin{aligned} \widehat{M_t} &= 83.54 - .028_{(.004)}t - .196_{(.039)}(T_t - 74.6) + .017_{(.002)}(T_t - 74.6)^2 \\ &\quad + .229_{(.023)}P_t \end{aligned}$$

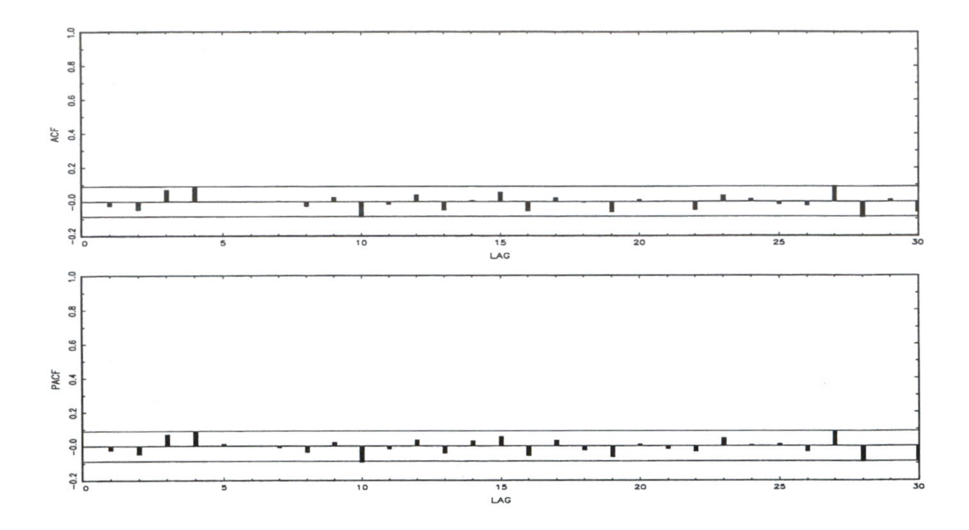


**Figure 2.34:** Sample ACF and PACF of the mortality residuals after fitting an AR(2) model.

as the model for transformed mortality, where the coefficients and estimated variances have changed slightly because of the transformation. The linear temperature component has decreased in magnitude from $-.473$ to $-.196$, whereas the other components stayed almost the same. The new residuals from the transformed model have sample ACF and PACF in Figure 2.34 that show no prominent peaks and can probably be taken as white noise.

## 2.13 Lagged Regression: Transfer Function Modeling

In the previous section, we looked at autocorrelated errors but, still regarded the input series $z_t$ as being fixed unknown functions of time. This consideration made sense for the time argument $t$, but was less satisfactory for the other inputs, which are probably stochastic processes. For example, consider SOI and the Recruitment series that were presented in Example 1.4. The series are displayed in Figure 1.4. In this case, the interest is in predicting the output Recruitment series, say, $y_t$, from the input SOI, say $x_t$. We might consider the

***lagged regression model***

$$y_t = \sum_{j=0}^{\infty} \alpha_j x_{t-j} + \eta_t = \alpha(B)x_t + \eta_t, \tag{2.164}$$

where $\sum_j |\alpha_j| < \infty$. We assume the input process $x_t$ and noise process $\eta_t$ in are both stationary and mutually independent. The coefficients $\alpha_0, \alpha_1, \dots$ describe the weights assigned to past values of $x_t$ used in predicting $y_t$ and we have used the notation

$$\alpha(B) = \sum_{j=0}^{\infty} \alpha_j B^j. \tag{2.165}$$

In the Box and Jenkins (1970) formulation, we assign ARIMA models, say, ARIMA$(p, d, q)$ and ARIMA$(p_\eta, d_\eta, q_\eta)$, to the series $x_t$ and $\eta_t$, respectively. The components of (2.164) in backshift notation, for the case of simple ARMA$(p, q)$ modeling of the input and noise, would have the representation

$$\phi(B)x_t = \theta(B)w_t \tag{2.166}$$

and

$$\phi_\eta(B)\eta_t = \theta_\eta(B)z_t, \tag{2.167}$$

where $w_t$ and $z_t$ are independent white noise processes with variances $\sigma_w^2$ and $\sigma_z^2$, respectively. Box and Jenkins (1970) proposed that systematic patterns often observed in the coefficients $\alpha_j$, for $j = 1, 2, ...$, could often be expressed as a ratio of polynomials involving a small number of coefficients, along with a specified delay, $d$, so

$$\alpha(B) = \frac{\delta(B)B^d}{\omega(B)}, \tag{2.168}$$

where

$$\omega(B) = 1 - \omega_1 B - \omega_2 B^2 - \cdots - \omega_r B^r \tag{2.169}$$

and

$$\delta(B) = \delta_0 + \delta_1 B + \cdots + \delta_s B^s \tag{2.170}$$

are the indicated operators; in this section, we find it convenient to represent the inverse of an operator, say, $[\omega(B)]^{-1}$, as $1/\omega(B)$.

Determining a parsimonious model involving a simple form for $\alpha(B)$ and estimating all of the parameters in the above model are the main tasks in the transfer function methodology. Because of the large number of parameters, it is necessary to develop a sequential methodology. Suppose we focus first on finding the ARIMA model for the input $x_t$ and apply this operator to both sides of (2.164), obtaining the new model

$$\tilde{y}_t \;=\; \frac{\phi(B)}{\theta(B)} y_t$$

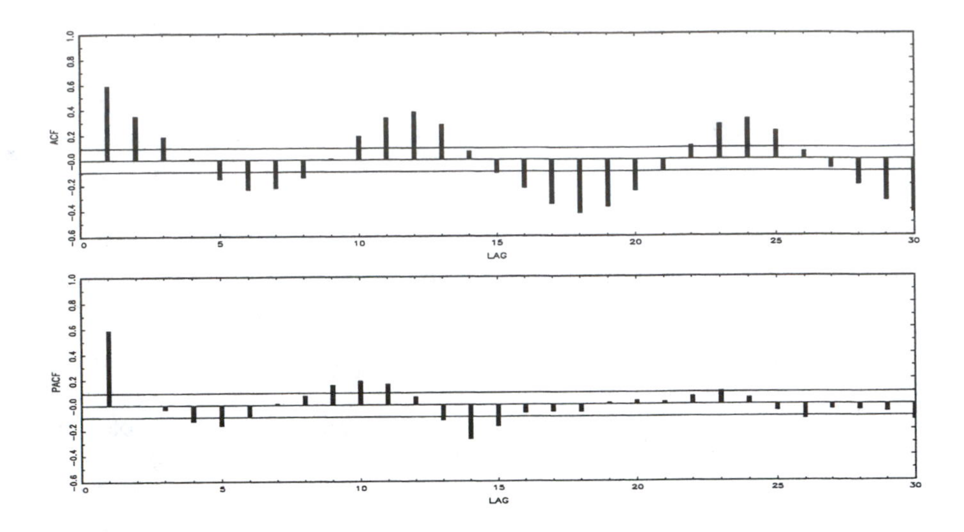


**Figure 2.35:** Sample ACF and PACF of SOI.

$$
\begin{aligned}
&= \alpha(B)w_t + \frac{\phi(B)}{\theta(B)}\eta_t \\
&= \alpha(B)w_t + \tilde{\eta}_t,
\end{aligned}
$$

where $w_t$ and the transformed noise $\tilde{\eta}_t$ are independent.

The series $w_t$ is a ***prewhitened*** version of the input series, and its cross-correlation with the transformed output series $\tilde{y}_t$ will be just

$$
\begin{aligned}
\gamma_{\tilde{y}w}(h) &= E[\tilde{y}_{t+h}w_t] \\
&= E[\sum_{j=0}^{\infty} \alpha_j w_{t+h-j} w_t] \\
&= \sigma_w^2 \alpha_h, \qquad (2.171)
\end{aligned}
$$

because the autocovariance function of white noise will be zero except when $j = h$ in (2.171). Hence, computing the cross-correlation between the prewhitened input series and the transformed output series should yield a rough estimate of the behavior of $\alpha(B)$.

**Example 2.44 Relating the Prewhitened SOI to the Transformed Recruitment Series**

We give a simple example of the suggested procedure for the SOI and the Recruitment series. Figure 2.35 shows the sample ACF and PACF of the detrended SOI index, and it is clear, from the PACF, that an

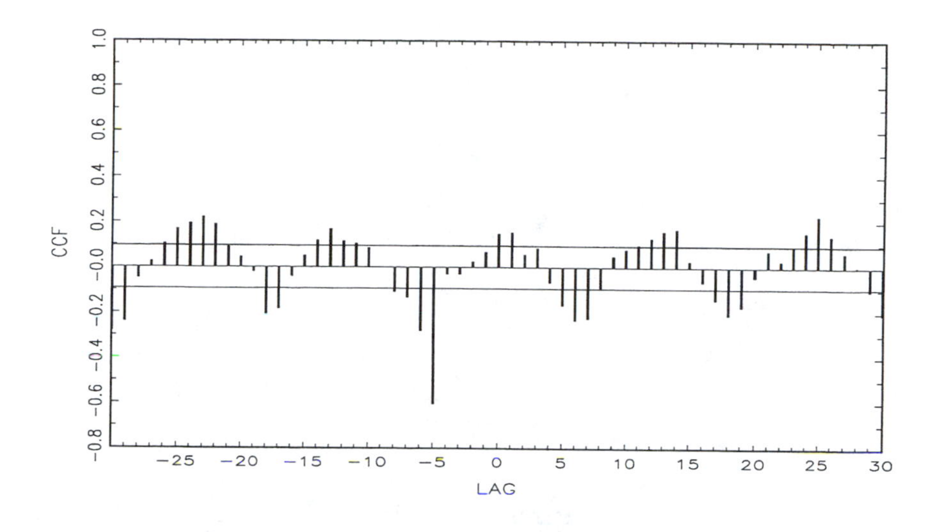


**Figure 2.36:** Sample CCF of the prewhitened, detrended SOI and the similarly transformed Recruitment series; negative lags indicate that SOI leads Recruitment.

autoregressive series with $p = 1$ will do a reasonable job. Fitting the series gave $\widehat{\phi} = 0.589, \widehat{\sigma}_w^2 = .092$, and we applied the operator $(1 - 0.589B)$ to both $x_t$ and $y_t$ and computed the cross-correlation function, which is shown in Figure 2.36. Noting the apparent shift of $d = 5$ months and the exponential decrease thereafter, it seems plausible to hypothesize a model of the form

$$\begin{aligned} \alpha(B) &= B^5(1 + \omega_1 B + \omega_1 B^2 + \cdots) \\ &= \frac{B^5}{1 - \omega_1 B} \end{aligned}$$

for the transfer function. In this case, we would expect $\omega_1$ to be negative.

In some cases, we may postulate the form of the separate components $\delta(B)$ and $\omega(B)$, so we might write the equation

$$y_t = \frac{\delta(B)B^d}{\omega(B)} x_t + \eta_t$$

as

$$\omega(B)y_t = \delta(B)B^d x_t + \omega(B)\eta_t,$$

or in regression form

$$y_t = \sum_{k=1}^{r} \omega_k y_{t-k} + \sum_{k=0}^{s} \delta_k x_{t-d-k} + u_t, \tag{2.172}$$

where

$$u_t = \omega(B)\eta_t. \tag{2.173}$$

The form of (2.172) suggests doing a regression on the lagged versions of both the input and output series to determine the $(r+s) \times 1$ regression vector

$$\widehat{\boldsymbol{\beta}} = (\omega_1, \ldots \omega_r, \delta_0, \delta_1, \ldots, \delta_s)'.$$

The residuals from the regression above, say,

$$\widehat{u}_t = y_t - \widehat{\boldsymbol{\beta}}' \boldsymbol{z}_t,$$

where

$$\boldsymbol{z}_t = (y_{t-1}, \ldots, y_{t-r}, x_{t-d}, \ldots, x_{t-d-s})'$$

denotes the usual vector of independent variables, could be used to approximate the best ARMA model for the noise process $\eta_t$, because we can compute an estimator for that process from the (2.173), using $\widehat{u}_t$ and $\widehat{\omega}(B)$ and applying the moving average operator to get $\widehat{\eta}_t$. Fitting an ARMA$(p_\eta, q_\eta)$ model to the this estimated noise then completes the specification. The preceding suggests the following sequential procedure for fitting the transfer function model to data.

(i) Fit an ARMA model to the input series $x_t$ to estimate the parameters $\phi_1, \ldots, \phi_p, \theta_1, \ldots, \theta_q, \sigma_w^2$ in the specification (2.166). Retain ARMA coefficients for use in Step (ii) and the fitted residuals $\widehat{w}_t$ for use in Step (iii).

(ii) Apply the operator determined in Step (i), that is,

$$\widehat{\phi}(B) y_t = \widehat{\theta}(B) \tilde{y}_t,$$

to determine the transformed output series $\tilde{y}_t$.

(iii) Use the cross-correlation function between $\tilde{y}_t$ and $\widehat{w}_t$ in (i) and (ii) to suggest a form for the components of the polynomial

$$\alpha(B) = \frac{\delta(B) B^d}{\omega(B)}$$

and the estimated time delay $d$.

(iv) Fit a linear regression of the form (2.172) to estimate $\widehat{\omega}_1, \ldots, \widehat{\omega}_r, \widehat{\delta}_0, \widehat{\delta}_1, \ldots, \widehat{\delta}_s$. Retain the residuals $\widehat{u}_t$ for use in Step (v).

(v) Apply the moving average transformation (2.173) to the residuals $\widehat{u}_t$ to find the noise series $\widehat{\eta}_t$, and fit an ARMA model to the noise, obtaining the estimated coefficients in $\widehat{\phi}_\eta(B)$ and $\widehat{\theta}_\eta(B)$.

The above procedure is fairly reasonable, but does not have any recognizable overall optimality. Simultaneous least squares estimation, based on the observed $x_t$ and $y_t$, can be accomplished by noting that the transfer function model can be written as

$$y_t = \frac{\delta(B)B^d}{\omega(B)}x_t + \frac{\theta_\eta(B)}{\phi_\eta(B)}z_t,$$

which can be put in the form

$$\omega(B)\phi_\eta(B)y_t = \phi_\eta(B)\delta(B)B^d x_t + \omega(B)\theta_\eta(B)z_t, \tag{2.174}$$

and it is clear that we may use least squares to minimize $\sum_t z_t^2$, as in earlier sections. We may also express the transfer function in *state-space form* (see Brockwell and Davis, 1991, Chapter 12). It is often easier to fit a transfer function model in the spectral domain, and we will revisit the examples presented in this section in Chapter 3.

**Example 2.45 Transfer Function Model for the SOI and Recruitment Series**

We illustrate the procedure for fitting a transfer function model of the form suggested in Example 2.44 to the detrended SOI series ($x_t$) and the detrended Recruitment series ($y_t$). Note first that Steps (i)-(iii). have already been applied to determine the ARMA model

$$(1 - 0.589B)x_t = w_t,$$

where $\widehat{\sigma}_w^2 = 0.092$. Using the model determined in Example 2.44, we run the regression

$$y_t = \omega_1 y_{t-1} + \delta_0 x_{t-5} + u_t,$$

yielding $\widehat{\omega}_1 = .848, \widehat{\delta}_0 = -20.54$, where the residuals satisfy

$$\widehat{u}_t = (1 - 0.848B)\eta_t.$$

This completes Step (iv). To complete the specification, we apply the moving average operator above to estimate the original noise series $\eta_t$ and fit a second-order autoregressive model, based on the ACF and PACF shown in Figure 2.37. We obtain

$$(1 - 1.255B + 0.410B^2)\eta_t = z_t,$$

with $\widehat{\sigma}_z^2 = 52.46$ as the estimated error variance.

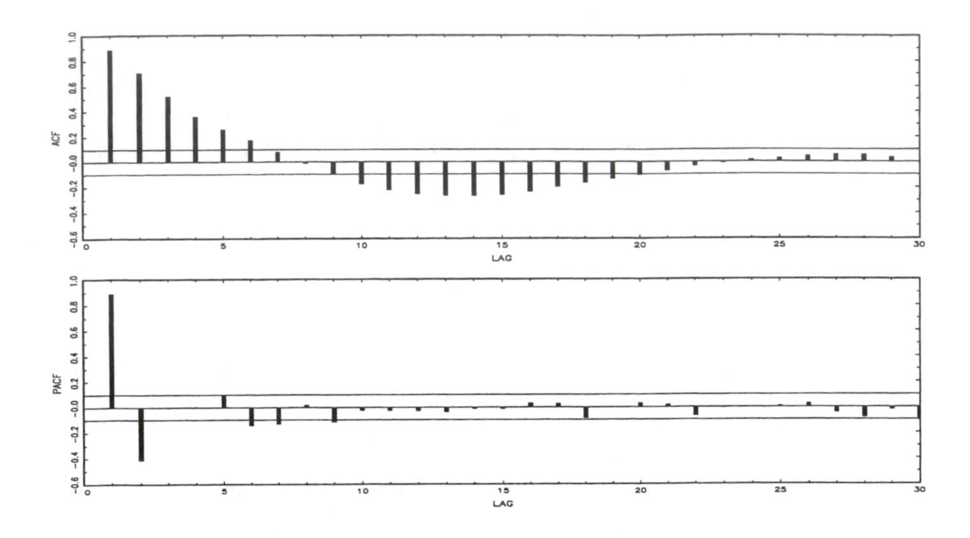


**Figure 2.37:** ACF and PACF of the estimated noise $\widehat{\eta}_t$ departures from the transfer function model.

## 2.14 ARCH Models

Although the focus of this chapter has been on analyzing the mean behavior of a time series, recent problems in finance have motivated the study of the ***volatility***, or variability, of a time series. Although ARMA models assume a constant variance, models such as the ***autoregressive conditionally heteroscedastic (ARCH)*** model, first introduced by Engle (1982), were developed to model changes in volatility. These models were later extended to generalized ARCH, or ***GARCH*** models by Bollerslev (1986).

In Section 2.8, we discussed the return or growth rate of a series. For example, if $x_t$ is the value of a stock at time $t$, then the return or relative gain, $y_t$, of the stock at time $t$ is

$$y_t = \frac{x_t - x_{t-1}}{x_{t-1}}. \tag{2.175}$$

Definition (2.175) implies that $x_t = (1 + y_t)x_{t-1}$. Thus, based on the discussion in Section 2.8, if the return represents a small (in magnitude) percentage change then

$$\nabla[\ln(x_t)] \approx y_t. \tag{2.176}$$

Either value, $\nabla[\ln(x_t)]$ or $(x_t - x_{t-1})/x_{t-1}$, will be called the return, and will be denoted by $y_t$. It is the study of $y_t$ that is the focus of ARCH, GARCH, and other volatility models. Recently there has been interest in ***stochastic***

***volatility*** models and we will discuss these models in Chapter 4 because they are state-space models.

Typically, for financial series, the return $y_t$, does not have a constant variance, and highly volatile periods tend to be clustered together. In other words, there is a strong dependence of sudden bursts of variability in a return on the series own past. For example, Figure 2.38 shows the monthly returns of a stock dividend yield starting from January 1947 to May 1993 (557 observations) taken from Hamilton and Lin (1996). In this case, as is typical, the return $y_t$ is fairly stable, except for short-term bursts of high volatility.

The most simple ARCH model, the ***ARCH(1)***, models the return as

$$\begin{aligned} y_t &= \sigma_t \epsilon_t & (2.177) \\ \sigma_t^2 &= \alpha_0 + \alpha_1 y_{t-1}^2, & (2.178) \end{aligned}$$

where $\epsilon_t$ is standard Gaussian white noise; that is, $\epsilon_t \sim$ iid N$(0,1)$. As with ARMA models, we must impose some constraints on the model parameters to obtain desirable properties. One obvious constraint is that $\alpha_1$ must not be negative, or else $\sigma_t^2$ may be negative.

As we shall see, the ARCH(1) models return as a white noise process with nonconstant conditional variance, and that conditional variance depends on the previous return. First, notice that conditional on $y_{t-1}$, $y_t$ is Gaussian:

$$y_t \mid y_{t-1} \sim \mathrm{N}(0, \alpha_0 + \alpha_1 y_{t-1}^2). \tag{2.179}$$

In addition, it is possible to write the ARCH(1) model as a non-Gaussian AR(1) model in the square of the returns $y_t^2$. To do this, rewrite (2.177)-(2.178) as

$$\begin{aligned} y_t^2 &= \sigma_t^2 \epsilon_t^2 \\ \alpha_0 + \alpha_1 y_{t-1}^2 &= \sigma_t^2, \end{aligned}$$

and subtract the two equations to obtain

$$y_t^2 - (\alpha_0 + \alpha_1 y_{t-1}^2) = \sigma_t^2 \epsilon_t^2 - \sigma_t^2.$$

Now, write this equation as

$$y_t^2 = \alpha_0 + \alpha_1 y_{t-1}^2 + v_t, \tag{2.180}$$

where $v_t = \sigma_t^2(\epsilon_t^2 - 1)$. Because $\epsilon_t^2$ is the square of a N$(0,1)$ random variable, $\epsilon_t^2 - 1$ is a shifted (to have mean-zero), $\chi_1^2$ random variable.

To explore the properties of ARCH, we define $Y_s = \{y_s, y_{s-1}, ...\}$. Then, using (2.179), we immediately see that $y_t$ has a zero mean:

$$E(y_t) = EE(y_t \mid Y_{t-1}) = EE(y_t \mid y_{t-1}) = 0. \tag{2.181}$$

Because $E(y_t \mid Y_{t-1}) = 0$, the process $y_t$ is said to be a martingale difference.

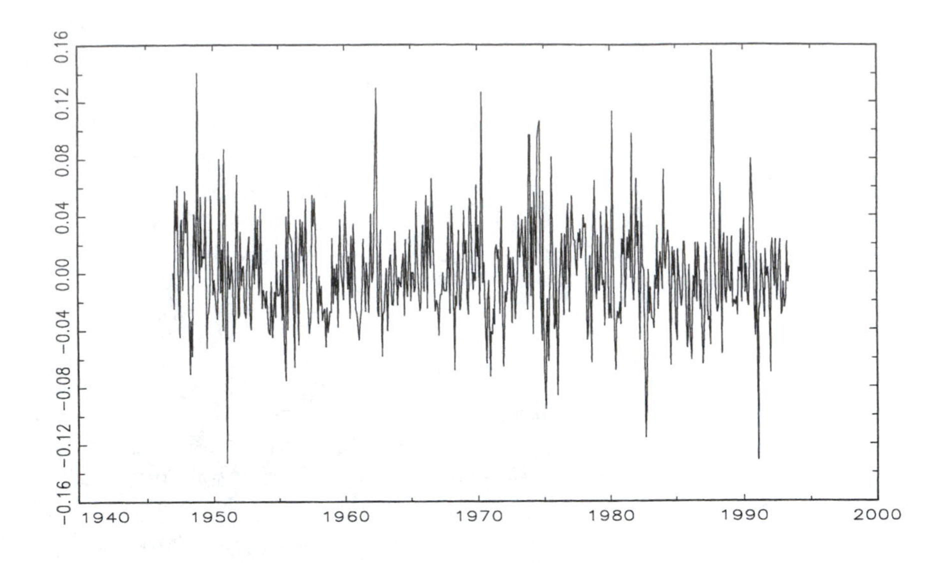


**Figure 2.38:** Monthly returns of a stock dividend yield; January 1947 through May 1993.

The error process $v_t$ in (2.180) is also a martingale difference and, consequently, an uncorrelated sequence. To exhibit this, we write

$$\begin{aligned} E(v_t) &= EE(v_t \mid Y_{t-1}) = EE(v_t \mid y_{t-1}) \\ &= E\left\{\sigma_t^2 E(\epsilon_t^2 - 1)\right\} = 0, \end{aligned} \tag{2.182}$$

and, for $h > 0$, using (2.182)

$$\begin{aligned} \operatorname{cov}(v_{t+h}, v_t) &= E(v_t v_{t+h}) = EE(v_t v_{t+h} \mid Y_{t+h-1}) \\ &= E\left\{v_t E(v_{t+h} \mid Y_{t+h-1})\right\} = 0. \end{aligned} \tag{2.183}$$

The last line of (2.183) follows because $v_t = y_t^2 - (\alpha_0 + \alpha_1 y_{t-1}^2)$ belongs to the information set $Y_{t+h-1}$ for $h > 0$, and, $E(v_{t+h} \mid Y_{t+h-1}) = 0$, as determined in (2.182).

An argument similar to (2.183) will establish the fact that $y_t$ is also an uncorrelated sequence. Such a possibility was discussed in Section 2.8, below equation (2.134), where bilinear models were discussed. That is, the returns, $\{y_t\}$ are uncorrelated, whereas their squares $y_t^2$ follow an autoregressive process, as shown in (2.180).

If the variance of $v_t$ is finite and constant with respect to time, and $0 \leq \alpha_1 < 1$, then based on the Property P2.1, (2.180) specifies a causal AR(1) process for $y_t^2$. Therefore, $E(y_t^2)$ and $\text{var}(y_t^2)$ must be constant with respect to time $t$. This, implies that

$$E(y_t^2) = \text{var}(y_t) = \frac{\alpha_0}{1-\alpha_1} \tag{2.184}$$

and, after some manipulations,

$$\text{var}(y_t^2) = E(y_t^4) = \frac{3\alpha_0^2}{(1-\alpha_1)^2}\frac{1-\alpha_1^2}{1-3\alpha_1^2}, \tag{2.185}$$

provided $3\alpha_1^2 < 1$. These results imply that the kurtosis, $\kappa$, of $y_t$ is

$$\kappa = \frac{E(y_t^4)}{[E(y_t^2)]^2} = 3\frac{1-\alpha_1^2}{1-3\alpha_1^2}, \tag{2.186}$$

which is always larger than 3, the kurtosis of the normal distribution. Thus, the marginal distribution of the returns, $y_t$, is *leptokurtic*, or has "fat tails".

In summary, an ARCH(1) process, $y_t$, as given by (2.177)-(2.178), or equivalently (2.179), is characterized by the following properties.

- If $\alpha_1 < 1$, the process $y_t$ itself is white noise and its unconditional distribution is symmetrically distributed around zero; this distribution is leptokurtic.

- If, in addition, $3\alpha_1^2 < 1$, the square of the process, $y_t^2$, follows a causal AR(1) model with ACF given by $\rho_{y^2}(h) = \alpha_1^h \geq 0$, for all $h > 0$. If $3\alpha_1 \geq 1$, but $\alpha_1 < 1$, then $y_t^2$ is strictly stationary with infinite variance.

Estimation of the parameters $\alpha_0$ and $\alpha_1$ of the ARCH(1) model is typically accomplished by conditional MLE. The conditional likelihood of the data $y_2, ...., y_n$ conditional on $y_1$, is given by

$$L(\alpha_0, \alpha_1 \mid y_1) = \prod_{t=2}^{n} f_{\alpha_0,\alpha_1}(y_t \mid y_{t-1}), \tag{2.187}$$

where the density $f_{\alpha_0,\alpha_1}(y_t \mid y_{t-1})$ is the normal density specified in (2.179). Hence, the criterion function to be minimized, $l(\alpha_0, \alpha_1) \propto -\ln L(\alpha_0, \alpha_1 \mid y_1)$ is given by

$$l(\alpha_0, \alpha_1) = \frac{1}{2}\sum_{t=2}^{n} \ln(\alpha_0 + \alpha_1 y_{t-1}^2) + \frac{1}{2}\sum_{t=2}^{n}\left(\frac{y_t^2}{\alpha_0 + \alpha_1 y_{t-1}^2}\right). \tag{2.188}$$

Estimation is accomplished by numerical methods, as described in Section 2.6. In this case, analytic expressions for the gradient vector, $l^{(1)}(\alpha_0, \alpha_1)$, and Hessian matrix, $l^{(2)}(\alpha_0, \alpha_1)$, as described in Example 2.26, can be obtained by straight-forward calculations. For example, the $2 \times 1$ gradient vector, $l^{(1)}(\alpha_0, \alpha_1)$, is given by

$$\begin{pmatrix} \partial l/\partial\alpha_0 \\ \partial l/\partial\alpha_1 \end{pmatrix} = \sum_{t=2}^{n}\begin{pmatrix} 1 \\ y_{t-1}^2 \end{pmatrix} \times \frac{\alpha_0 + \alpha_1 y_{t-1}^2 - y_t^2}{2\left(\alpha_0 + \alpha_1 y_{t-1}^2\right)^2}. \tag{2.189}$$

The calculation of the Hessian matrix is left as an exercise (Problem 2.46). The likelihood of the ARCH model tends to be flat unless $n$ is very large. A discussion of this problem can be found in Shepard (1996).

**Example 2.46 Analysis of the U.S. GNP Residuals**

Figure 2.16 shows the residuals from the MA(2) fit on the U.S. GNP series. In Example 2.33 we concluded that the residuals appeared to behave like a white noise process. It has been suggested that the U.S. GNP series has ARCH errors, and in this example, we will investigate this claim. Because the values of the residuals are small in magnitude, we prefer to work with the standardized residuals $e_t$, as defined in (2.134). If the $e_t$ are ARCH(1), their squares should behave like a non-Gaussian AR(1) process, as pointed out in (2.180). Figure 2.39 shows the ACF and PACF of $e_t^2$; the ACF and PACF are consistent with data from an AR(1) process.

Using Newton–Raphson to maximize (2.188) for this data set, we obtained the estimates (and standard errors) $\widehat{\alpha}_0 = 0.82$ (0.11) and $\widehat{\alpha}_1 = 0.18$ (0.10). Because $0.18/0.10 = 1.80$, the approximate test of $\text{H}_0 : \alpha_1 = 0$ versus $\text{H}_1 : \alpha_1 > 0$ yields a $p$-value of 0.04, indicating the ARCH(1) behavior of $e_t$. The fact that the estimated standard error of $\widehat{\alpha}_1$ is so large is because, as previously mentioned, the likelihood, (2.188), is relatively flat.

The ARCH(1) model can be extended to the general ARCH($m$) model in an obvious way. That is, (2.177) is retained, but (2.178) is extended:

$$\sigma_t^2 = \alpha_0 + \alpha_1 y_{t-1}^2 + \cdots + \alpha_m y_{t-m}^2. \tag{2.190}$$

Estimation for ARCH($m$) also follows in an obvious way from the discussion of estimation for ARCH(1) models. It is also possible to combine a regression or ARMA model for the mean, with an ARCH model for the errors. For example, a regression with ARCH(1) errors model would have the observations $x_t$ as linear function of $p$ regressors, $\boldsymbol{z}_t = (z_{t1}, ..., z_{tp})'$, and ARCH(1) noise $y_t$, say,

$$x_t = \boldsymbol{\beta}' \boldsymbol{z}_t + y_t,$$

where $y_t$ satisfies (2.177)-(2.178), but, in this case, is unobserved. Similarly, an AR(1) model for data $x_t$ exhibiting ARCH(1) errors would be

$$x_t = \phi x_{t-1} + y_t;$$

these type of models were explored by Weiss (1984). Another extension of ARCH is the generalized ARCH (GARCH) model (Bollerslev, 1986). Briefly, a GARCH(1,1) model retains (2.177), but extends (2.178) as follows:

$$\sigma_t^2 = \alpha_0 + \alpha_1 y_{t-1}^2 + \beta_1 \sigma_{t-1}^2. \tag{2.191}$$

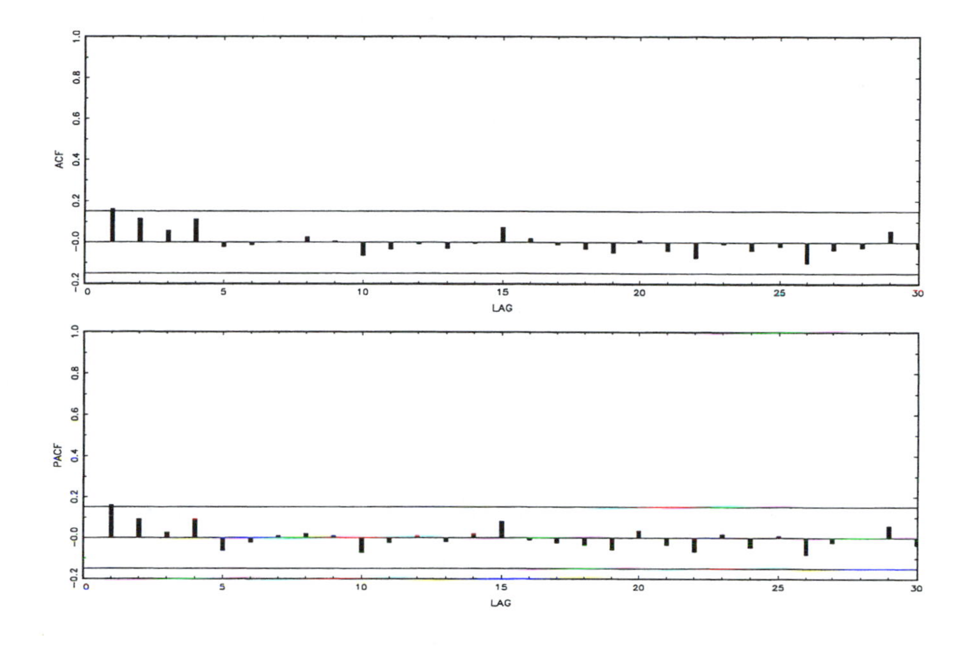


**Figure 2.39:** ACF and PACF of the squares of the standardized residuals from the MA(2) fit on U.S. GNP.

Under the condition that $\alpha_1+\beta_1 < 1$, using similar manipulations as in (2.180), the GARCH(1,1) model, (2.177)-(2.190), admits a non-Gaussian ARMA(1,1) model for the squared process

$$y_t^2 = \alpha_0 + (\alpha_1 + \beta_1)y_{t-1}^2 + v_t - \beta_1 v_{t-1}, \tag{2.192}$$

where $v_t$ is as defined in (2.180). Representation (2.192) follows by writing (2.177) as

$$\begin{aligned} y_t^2 - \sigma_t^2 &= \sigma_t^2(\epsilon_t^2 - 1) \\ \beta_1(y_{t-1}^2 - \sigma_{t-1}^2) &= \beta_1\sigma_{t-1}^2(\epsilon_{t-1}^2 - 1), \end{aligned}$$

subtracting the second equation from the first, and using the fact that, from (2.191), $\sigma_t^2 - \beta_1\sigma_{t-1}^2 = \alpha_0 + \alpha_1 y_{t-1}^2$, on the left-hand side of the result. The GARCH$(m, r)$ model retains (2.177) and extends (2.191) to

$$\sigma_t^2 = \alpha_0 + \sum_{j=1}^{m} \alpha_j y_{t-j}^2 + \sum_{j=1}^{r} \beta_j \sigma_{t-j}^2.$$

In fact, there are many different extensions to the basic ARCH model that were developed to handle the various situations noticed in practice, such as EGARCH (exponential GARCH) for nonsymmetric returns, and IGARCH (integrated GARCH) to model long memory, or persistence, to mention a few. Interested readers might find the general discussions in Bollerslev et al (1994) and Shepard (1996) worthwhile reading. Also, Gouriéroux (1997) gives a detailed presentation of ARCH and related models with financial applications and contains an extensive bibliography.

## T2.15 Hilbert Spaces and the Projection Theorem

Most of the material on mean square estimation and regression can be imbedded in a more general setting involving an inner product space that is also complete (that is, satisfies the Cauchy condition). Two examples of inner products are $E(xy^*)$, where the elements are random variables, and $\sum x_i y_i^*$, where the elements are sequences. These examples include the possibility of complex elements, in which case, $^*$ denotes conjugation. We denote an inner product, in general, by the notation $\langle x, y \rangle$. Now, define an ***inner product space*** by its properties, namely,

(i) $\langle x, y \rangle = \langle y, x \rangle^*$

(ii) $\langle x + y, z \rangle = \langle x, z \rangle + \langle y, z \rangle$

(iii) $\langle \alpha x, y \rangle = \alpha \langle x, y \rangle$

(iv) $\langle x, x \rangle = ||x||^2 \geq 0$

(v) $\langle x, x \rangle = 0$ iff $x = 0$.

We introduced the notation $|| \cdot ||^2$ for the ***norm*** or distance in property (iv). The norm satisfies the ***triangle inequality***

$$||x + y|| \leq ||x|| + ||y|| \tag{2.193}$$

and the ***Cauchy–Schwarz inequality***

$$|\langle x, y \rangle|^2 \leq ||x||^2 ||y||^2, \tag{2.194}$$

which we have seen before for random variables in (1.64). Now, a ***Hilbert space***, $\mathcal{H}$, is defined as an inner product space with the Cauchy property. In other words, $\mathcal{H}$ is a ***complete inner product space***. This means that every Cauchy sequence converges in norm; that is, $x_n \to x$ if an only if $||x_n - x_m|| \to 0$ as $m, n \to \infty$. This is just the $L^2$ completeness Theorem 1.1 for random variables.

For a broad overview of Hilbert space techniques that are useful in statistical inference and in probability, see Small and McLeish (1994). Also, Brockwell and Davis (1991, Chapter 2) is a nice summary of Hilbert space techniques that are useful in time series analysis. In our discussions, we mainly use the ***projection theorem*** (Theorem 2.1) and the associated ***orthogonality principle*** as a means for solving various kinds of linear estimation problems.

**Theorem 2.1:** *Let $\mathcal{M}$ be a closed subspace of the Hilbert space $\mathcal{H}$ and let $y$ be an element in $\mathcal{H}$. Then, $y$ can be uniquely represented as*

$$y = \widehat{y} + z, \tag{2.195}$$

*where $\widehat{y}$ belongs to $\mathcal{M}$ and $z$ is orthogonal to $\mathcal{M}$; that is, $\langle z, w\rangle = 0$ for all $w$ in $\mathcal{M}$. Furthermore, the point $\widehat{y}$ is closest to $y$ in the sense that, for any $w$ in $\mathcal{M}$, $||y - w|| \geq ||y - \widehat{y}||$, where equality holds if and only if $w = \widehat{y}$.*

We note that (2.195) and the statement following it yield the ***orthogonality property***

$$\langle y - \widehat{y}, w\rangle = 0 \tag{2.196}$$

for any $w$ belonging to $\mathcal{M}$, which can sometimes be used easily to find an expression for the projection. The norm of the error can be written as

$$\begin{aligned} ||y - \widehat{y}||^2 &= \langle y - \widehat{y}, y - \widehat{y}\rangle \\ &= \langle y - \widehat{y}, y\rangle - \langle y - \widehat{y}, \widehat{y}\rangle \\ &= \langle y - \widehat{y}, y\rangle \end{aligned} \tag{2.197}$$

because of orthogonality.

***Proof of Theorem 2.1:***
First, $\mathcal{M}$ is itself a Hilbert space, and the ***projection of*** $y$ ***onto*** $\mathcal{M}$, say $\widehat{y} \in \mathcal{M}$, is defined as

$$||y - \widehat{y}|| = \inf\{||y - w||, w \in \mathcal{M}\}.$$

To prove the existence of $\widehat{y}$, by the definition of infimum, there is a sequence $w_n \in \mathcal{M}$ such that

$$||y - w_n|| \to \delta = \inf\{||y - w||, w \in \mathcal{M}\}.$$

From this fact, it is easy to show that the sequence $w_n$ is Cauchy and thus converges to some point $w_0 \in \mathcal{M}$ because $\mathcal{M}$ is closed. Furthermore,

$$\delta \leq ||y - w_0|| \leq ||y - w_n|| + ||w_n - w_0||,$$

so that, taking $n \to \infty$, we must have $||y - w_0|| = \delta$. This result proves the existence of an element in $\mathcal{M}$ that we call the projection (that is, put $\widehat{y} = w_0$). To prove uniqueness of the projection, we assume that $y \notin \mathcal{M}$, otherwise, set $\widehat{y} = y$. Suppose there are two projections, say, $y_1$ and $y_2$ of $y$ onto $\mathcal{M}$. Then, putting $\tilde{y} = (y_1 + y_2)/2$, and noting that $\tilde{y} \in \mathcal{M}$, by the triangle inequality, (2.193), we have

$$\delta \leq ||y - \tilde{y}|| = ||\frac{1}{2}(y - y_1 + y - y_2)|| \leq \frac{1}{2}||y - y_1|| + \frac{1}{2}||y - y_2|| = \delta.$$

Thus, we have equality in the triangle inequality, which implies $(y - y_1) = c(y - y_2)$ for some constant $c$ (that is, for $u, v \in \mathcal{H}$, $||u + v|| = ||u|| + ||v||$ implies that $u$ and $v$ are linearly dependent). If $c \neq 1$ then $y$ is a linear combination of $y_1$ and $y_2$, which implies $y \in \mathcal{M}$, contradicting the assumption that $y \notin \mathcal{M}$. Thus, we must have $c = 1$, in which case, $y_1 = y_2$.

Next, we address the "if" statement of the theorem. In view of (2.196), suppose that $\widehat{y} \in \mathcal{M}$ and $\langle y - \widehat{y}, w \rangle = 0$ for all $w \in \mathcal{M}$. Then, for any $w \in \mathcal{M}$,

$$\begin{aligned} ||y - \widehat{y} + w||^2 &= ||y - \widehat{y}||^2 + 2\langle y - \widehat{y}, w \rangle + ||w||^2 \\ &= ||y - \widehat{y}||^2 + ||w||^2 \\ &\geq ||y - \widehat{y}||^2. \end{aligned}$$

That is, $||y - \widehat{y}|| = \inf\{||y - w||, w \in \mathcal{M}\}$.

To address the "only if" part, suppose that $\widehat{y} \in \mathcal{M}$ but there is a $w \in \mathcal{M}$ for which $\langle y - \widehat{y}, w \rangle = \beta \neq 0$. Then, for any scalar $\lambda$,

$$||y - \widehat{y} + \lambda w||^2 = ||y - \widehat{y}||^2 + 2\lambda\beta + \lambda^2||w||^2.$$

Setting $\lambda = -\beta/||w||^2$, we have

$$||y - \widehat{y} + \lambda w||^2 = ||y - \widehat{y}||^2 - \beta^2/||w||^2 < ||y - \widehat{y}||^2,$$

which means $\widehat{y} + \beta w/||w||^2$ is an element in $\mathcal{M}$ that is closer to $y$ than $\widehat{y}$. □

Using the notation of Theorem 2.1, we call the mapping $P_{\mathcal{M}} y = \widehat{y}$, for $y \in \mathcal{H}$, the ***projection mapping of $\mathcal{H}$ onto $\mathcal{M}$***. In addition, the ***closed span*** of a finite set $\{x_1, ..., x_n\}$ of elements in a Hilbert space, $\mathcal{H}$, is defined to be the set of all linear combinations $w = a_1 x_1 + \cdots + a_n x_n$, where $a_1, ..., a_n$ are scalars. This subspace of $\mathcal{H}$ is denoted by $\mathcal{M} = \overline{\text{sp}}\{x_1, ..., x_n\}$. By the projection theorem, the projection of $y \in \mathcal{H}$ onto $\mathcal{M} = \overline{\text{sp}}\{x_1, ..., x_n\}$ is unique and given by

$$P_{\mathcal{M}} y = a_1 x_1 + \cdots + a_n x_n,$$

where $\{a_1, ..., a_n\}$ are found using the orthogonality principle

$$\langle y - P_{\mathcal{M}} y, x_i \rangle = 0 \quad j = 1, ..., n.$$

Evidently, $\{a_1, ..., a_n\}$ can be obtained by solving

$$\sum_{i=1}^{n} a_i \langle x_i, x_j \rangle = \langle y, x_j \rangle \quad j = 1, ..., n. \tag{2.198}$$

When the elements of $\mathcal{H}$ are vectors, this problem is the linear regression problem.

**Example 2.47 Linear Regression Analysis**

For the regression model introduced in Section 1.8, we want to find the regression coefficients $\beta_i$ that minimize the residual sum of squares. Consider the vectors $\boldsymbol{y} = (y_1, \ldots, y_n)'$ and $\tilde{\boldsymbol{z}}_i = (z_{1i}, \ldots, z_{ni})'$, for $i = 1, ..., q$ and the inner product

$$\langle \tilde{\boldsymbol{z}}_i, \boldsymbol{y} \rangle = \sum_{t=1}^{n} z_{ti} y_t = \tilde{\boldsymbol{z}}_i' \, \boldsymbol{y}.$$

We solve the problem of finding a projection of the observed $\boldsymbol{y}$ on the linear space spanned by $\beta_1 \tilde{\boldsymbol{z}}_1 + \cdots + \beta_q \tilde{\boldsymbol{z}}_q$, that is, linear combinations of the $\tilde{\boldsymbol{z}}_i$. The orthogonality principle gives

$$\langle \boldsymbol{y} - \sum_{i=1}^{q} \beta_i \tilde{\boldsymbol{z}}_i \ , \ \tilde{\boldsymbol{z}}_j \rangle = 0$$

for $j = 1, \ldots, q$. Writing the orthogonality condition, as in (2.198), in vector form gives

$$\boldsymbol{y}' \, \tilde{\boldsymbol{z}}_j = \sum_{i=1}^{q} \beta_i \tilde{\boldsymbol{z}}_i' \, \tilde{\boldsymbol{z}}_j \quad j = 1, \ldots, q, \tag{2.199}$$

which can be written in the usual matrix form by letting $Z = (\tilde{\boldsymbol{z}}_1, \ldots, \tilde{\boldsymbol{z}}_q)$ in the notation of this section and Section 1.8. That is, (2.199) can be written as

$$\boldsymbol{y}' Z = \boldsymbol{\beta}'(Z'Z), \tag{2.200}$$

where $\boldsymbol{\beta} = (\beta_1, ..., \beta_q)'$. Transposing both sides of (2.200) yields (1.53), which provides the solution for the coefficients,

$$\widehat{\boldsymbol{\beta}} = (Z'Z)^{-1} Z' \boldsymbol{y}.$$

The mean square error in this case would be

$$\begin{aligned} \|\boldsymbol{y} - \sum_{i=1}^{q} \widehat{\beta}_i \tilde{\boldsymbol{z}}_i\|^2 &= \langle \boldsymbol{y} - \sum_{i=1}^{q} \widehat{\beta}_i \tilde{\boldsymbol{z}}_i \ , \ \boldsymbol{y} \rangle \\ &= \langle \boldsymbol{y}, \boldsymbol{y} \rangle - \sum_{i=1}^{q} \widehat{\beta}_i \langle \tilde{\boldsymbol{z}}_i \ , \ \boldsymbol{y} \rangle \\ &= \boldsymbol{y}'\boldsymbol{y} - \widehat{\boldsymbol{\beta}}' Z' \boldsymbol{y}, \end{aligned}$$

which is in agreement with Section 1.8.

The extra generality in the above approach hardly seems necessary in the-finite dimensional case, where differentiation works perfectly well. It is convenient, however, in many cases to regard the elements of $\mathcal{H}$ as infinite dimensional, so that the orthogonality principle becomes of use. For example, the projection of the process $y_t, t = 0 \pm 1, \pm 2, \ldots$ on the linear manifold spanned by all filtered convolutions of the form

$$\widehat{x}(t) = \sum_{k=-\infty}^{\infty} a_k x_{t-k}$$

would be in this form.

There are some useful results, that we state without proof, pertaining to projection mappings.

**Theorem 2.2:** *Under the established notation and conditions:*

(i) $P_{\mathcal{M}}(ax + by) = aP_{\mathcal{M}}x + bP_{\mathcal{M}}y$, *for* $x, y \in \mathcal{H}$, *where* $a$ *and* $b$ *are scalars.*

(ii) *If* $||y_n - y|| \to 0$, *then* $P_{\mathcal{M}}y_n \to P_{\mathcal{M}}y$, *as* $n \to \infty$.

(iii) $w \in \mathcal{M}$ *if and only if* $P_{\mathcal{M}}w = w$. *Consequently, a projection mapping can be characterized by the property that* $P_{\mathcal{M}}^2 = P_{\mathcal{M}}$, *in the sense that, for any* $y \in \mathcal{H}$, $P_{\mathcal{M}}(P_{\mathcal{M}}y) = P_{\mathcal{M}}y$.

(iv) *Let* $\mathcal{M}_1$ *and* $\mathcal{M}_2$ *be closed subspaces of* $\mathcal{H}$. *Then,* $\mathcal{M}_1 \subseteq \mathcal{M}_2$ *if and only if* $P_{\mathcal{M}_1}(P_{\mathcal{M}_2}y) = P_{\mathcal{M}_1}y$ *for all* $y \in \mathcal{H}$.

(v) *Let* $\mathcal{M}$ *be a closed subspace of* $\mathcal{H}$ *and let* $\mathcal{M}_\perp$ *denote the orthogonal complement of* $\mathcal{M}$. *Then,* $\mathcal{M}_\perp$ *is also a closed subspace of* $\mathcal{H}$, *and for any* $y \in \mathcal{H}$, $y = P_{\mathcal{M}}y + P_{\mathcal{M}_\perp}y$.

Part (iii) of Theorem 2.2 leads to the well-known result, often used in linear models, that a square matrix $M$ is a projection matrix if and only if it is symmetric and idempotent (that is, $M^2 = M$). For example, using notation of Example 2.47 for linear regression, the projection of $\boldsymbol{y}$ onto $\overline{\text{sp}}\{\tilde{\boldsymbol{z}}_1, ..., \tilde{\boldsymbol{z}}_q\}$, the space generated by the columns of $Z$, is $P_Z(\boldsymbol{y}) = Z\widehat{\boldsymbol{\beta}} = Z(Z'Z)^{-1}Z'\boldsymbol{y}$. The matrix $M = Z(Z'Z)^{-1}Z'$ is an $n \times n$, symmetric and idempotent matrix of rank $q$ (which is the dimension of the space that $M$ projects $\boldsymbol{y}$ onto). Parts (iv) and (v) of Theorem 2.2 are useful for establishing recursive solutions for estimation and prediction.

By imposing extra structure, ***conditional expectation*** can be defined as a projection mapping for random variables in $L^2$ with the equivalence relation that, for $x, y \in L^2$, $x = y$ if $\Pr(x = y) = 1$. In particular, for $y \in L^2$, if $\mathcal{M}$ is a closed subspace of $L^2$ containing 1, the conditional expectation of $y$ given $\mathcal{M}$ is defined to be the projection of $y$ onto $\mathcal{M}$, namely, $E_{\mathcal{M}}y = P_{\mathcal{M}}y$. This means that conditional expectation, $E_{\mathcal{M}}$, must satisfy the orthogonality principle of the Projection Theorem and that the results of Theorem 2.2 remain valid (the most widely used tool in this case is item (iv) of the theorem). If we let $\mathcal{M}(x)$ denote the closed subspace of all random variables in $L^2$ that can be written as a (measurable) function of $x$, then we may define, for $x, y \in L^2$, the ***conditional expectation of*** $y$ ***given*** $x$ as $E(y|x) = E_{\mathcal{M}(x)}y$. This idea may be generalized in an obvious way to define the conditional expectation of $y$ given $\boldsymbol{x} = (x_1, ..., x_n)$; that is $E(y|\boldsymbol{x}) = E_{\mathcal{M}(\boldsymbol{x})}y$. Of particular interest to us is the following result which states that, in the Gaussian case, conditional expectation and linear prediction are equivalent.

**Theorem 2.3:** *Under the established notation and conditions, if* $(y, x_1, ..., x_n)$ *is multivariate normal, then*

$$E(y \mid x_1, ..., x_n) = P_{\overline{\text{sp}}\{1, x_1, ..., x_n\}}y.$$

***Proof.*** First, by the projection theorem, the conditional expection of $y$ given $\boldsymbol{x} = \{x_1, ..., x_n\}$ is the unique element $E_{\mathcal{M}(\boldsymbol{x})}y$ that satisfies the orthogonality principle,

$$E\left\{\left(y - E_{\mathcal{M}(\boldsymbol{x})}y\right) w\right\} = 0 \quad \text{for all } w \in \mathcal{M}(\boldsymbol{x}).$$

We will show that $\widehat{y} = P_{\overline{\text{sp}}\{1, x_1, ..., x_n\}}y$ is that element. In fact, by the projection theorem, $\widehat{y}$ satisfies

$$\langle y - \widehat{y}, x_i \rangle = 0 \quad \text{for } i = 0, 1, ..., n,$$

where we have set $x_0 = 1$. But $\langle y - \widehat{y}, x_i \rangle = \text{cov}(y - \widehat{y}, x_i) = 0$, implying that $y - \widehat{y}$ and $(x_1, ..., x_n)$ are independent because the vector $(y - \widehat{y}, x_1, ..., x_n)'$ is multivariate normal. Thus, if $w \in \mathcal{M}(\boldsymbol{x})$, then $w$ and $y - \widehat{y}$ are independent and, hence, $\langle y - \widehat{y}, w \rangle = E\{(y - \widehat{y})w\} = E(y - \widehat{y})E(w) = 0$, recalling that $0 = \langle y - \widehat{y}, 1 \rangle = E(y - \widehat{y})$. □

In the Gaussian case, conditional expectation has the explicit form

$$\begin{aligned} E(y \mid \boldsymbol{x}) &= \mu_y + \Sigma_{yx}\Sigma_{xx}^{-1}(\boldsymbol{x} - \boldsymbol{\mu}_x) \\ \text{var}(y \mid \boldsymbol{x}) &= \sigma_{yy} - \Sigma_{yx}\Sigma_{xx}^{-1}\Sigma_{xy}, \end{aligned} \tag{2.201}$$

where $\mu_y = E(y)$ and $\sigma_{yy} = \text{var}(y)$ are scalars, $\boldsymbol{\mu}_x = E(\boldsymbol{x})$ is an $n \times 1$ vector, $\Sigma_{yx} = \Sigma_{xy}' = \text{cov}(y, \boldsymbol{x})$ is $1 \times n$, and $\Sigma_{xx} = \text{var}(\boldsymbol{x})$ is an $n \times n$ matrix, assumed to be nonsingular.

# T2.16 Causal Conditions for ARMA Models

In this section, we prove Property P2.1 of Section 2.2 pertaining to the causality of ARMA models. The proof of Property P2.2, which pertains to invertibility of ARMA models, is similar.

***Proof of Property P2.1:***
Suppose first that the roots of $\phi(z)$, say, $z_1, ..., z_p$, lie outside the unit circle. We write the roots in the following order, $1 < |z_1| \leq |z_2| \leq \cdots \leq |z_p|$, noting that $z_1, ..., z_p$ are not necessarily unique, and put $|z_1| = 1 + \epsilon$, for some $\epsilon > 0$.

Thus, $\phi(z) \neq 0$ as long as $|z| < |z_1| = 1 + \epsilon$ and, hence, $\phi^{-1}(z)$ exists and has a power series expansion,

$$\frac{1}{\phi(z)} = \sum_{j=0}^{\infty} a_j z^j, \quad |z| < 1 + \epsilon.$$

Now, choose a value $\delta$ such that $0 < \delta < \epsilon$, and set $z = 1 + \delta$, which is inside the radius of convergence. It then follows that

$$\phi^{-1}(1+\delta) = \sum_{j=0}^{\infty} a_j (1+\delta)^j < \infty. \tag{2.202}$$

Thus, we can bound each of the terms in the sum in (2.202) by constant, say, $|a_j(1+\delta)^j| < c$, for $c > 0$. In turn, $|a_j| < c(1+\delta)^{-j}$, from which it follows that

$$\sum_{j=0}^{\infty} |a_j| < \infty. \tag{2.203}$$

Recalling the results from Chapter 1 on time-invariant linear filters, Section T1.10, equations (1.70) and (1.71), we may apply $\phi^{-1}(B)$ to both sides of the ARMA model $\phi(B)x_t = \theta(B)w_t$ to obtain

$$x_t = \phi^{-1}(B)\phi(B)x_t = \phi^{-1}(B)\theta(B)w_t,$$

which, in view of (2.203), is a well-defined process. Thus, putting $\psi(B) = \phi^{-1}(B)\theta(B)$, we have

$$x_t = \psi(B)z_t = \sum_{j=0}^{\infty} \psi_j w_{t-j},$$

where the (absolutely summable) $\psi$-weights are determined by $\psi(z) = \phi^{-1}(z)\theta(z)$, for $|z| \leq 1$.

Now, suppose $x_t$ is a causal process; that is, it has the representation

$$x_t = \sum_{j=0}^{\infty} \psi_j w_{t-j}, \qquad \sum_{j=0}^{\infty} |\psi_j| < \infty.$$

In this case, we write

$$x_t = \psi(B)w_t,$$

and premultiplying by $\phi(B)$ yields

$$\phi(B)x_t = \phi(B)\psi(B)w_t. \tag{2.204}$$

In addition to (2.204), the model is ARMA, and can be written as

$$\phi(B)x_t = \theta(B)w_t. \tag{2.205}$$

From (2.204) and (2.205), we see that

$$\phi(B)\psi(B)w_t = \theta(B)w_t. \tag{2.206}$$

Now, let

$$a(z) = \phi(z)\psi(z) = \sum_{j=0}^{\infty} a_j z^j \quad |z| \le 1$$

and, hence, we can write (2.206) as

$$\sum_{j=0}^{\infty} a_j w_{t-j} = \sum_{j=0}^{q} \theta_j w_{t-j}. \tag{2.207}$$

Next, multiply both sides of (2.207) by $w_{t-h}$, for $h = 0, 1, 2, ...$, and take expectation. In doing this, we obtain

$$\begin{aligned} a_h &= \theta_h, \quad h = 0, 1, ..., q \\ a_h &= 0, \quad h > q. \end{aligned} \tag{2.208}$$

From (2.208), we conclude that

$$\phi(z)\psi(z) = a(z) = \theta(z), \quad |z| \le 1. \tag{2.209}$$

If there is a complex number in the unit circle, say $z_0$, for which $\phi(z_0) = 0$, then by (2.209), $\theta(z_0) = 0$. But, if there is such a $z_0$, then $\phi(z)$ and $\theta(z)$ have a common factor which is not allowed. Thus, we may write $\psi(z) = \theta(z)/\phi(z)$. In addition, by hypothesis, we have that $|\psi(z)| < \infty$ for $|z| \le 1$, and hence

$$|\psi(z)| = \left| \frac{\theta(z)}{\phi(z)} \right| < \infty, \quad \text{for} \quad |z| \le 1. \tag{2.210}$$

Finally, (2.210) implies $\phi(z) \neq 0$ for $|z| \le 1$; that is, the roots of $\phi(z)$ lie outside the unit circle. □

## T2.17 Large Sample Distribution of AR Estimators

In Section 2.6, we alluded to the procedure for estimating the parameters $\phi_1, \phi_2, \ldots, \phi_p$ and $\sigma_w^2$ in the AR($p$) model

$$x_t = \sum_{k=1}^{p} \phi_k x_{t-k} + w_t.$$

Using the regression setup discussed in Section 1.8 of Chapter 1 (we assume $\mu = 0$, for convenience),

$$x_t = \boldsymbol{\phi}' \boldsymbol{x}_{t-1} + w_t, \tag{2.211}$$

where $\boldsymbol{x}_{t-1} = (x_{t-1}, x_{t-2}, \ldots, x_{t-p})'$ is the stacked $p \times 1$ vector that takes the place of the independent vector $\boldsymbol{z}_t$ in (1.50) and $\boldsymbol{\phi} = (\phi_1, \phi_2, \ldots, \phi_p)'$ replaces the regression coefficient vector $\boldsymbol{\beta}$. Assuming observations are available at $x_1, \ldots, x_n$ means that we might only use (2.211) for $t = p+1, \ldots, n$, obtaining ***least squares estimators*** of the form

$$\widehat{\boldsymbol{\phi}} = \left( \sum_{t=p+1}^{n} \boldsymbol{x}_{t-1} \boldsymbol{x}_{t-1}' \right)^{-1} \sum_{t=p+1}^{n} \boldsymbol{x}_{t-1} x_t \tag{2.212}$$

for the regression vector $\boldsymbol{\phi}$ and

$$\widehat{\sigma}_w^2 = \frac{1}{n-p} \sum_{t=p+1}^{n} \left( x_t - \widehat{\boldsymbol{\phi}}' \boldsymbol{x}_{t-1} \right)^2 . \tag{2.213}$$

In addition, as pointed out following (2.102), Yule–Walker estimators and least squares estimators are approximately the same in that the estimators differ only by inclusion or exclusion of terms involving the endpoints of the data. Hence, it is easy to show the asymptotic equivalence of the two estimators; this is why, for AR($p$) models, (2.91) and (2.115), are equivalent. Details on the asymptotic equivalence can be found in Brockwell and Davis (1991, Chapter 8).

Here, we use the same approach as in Chapter 1, replacing the lower limits of the sums in (2.212) and (2.213) by one and noting the asymptotic equivalence of the estimators

$$\widetilde{\boldsymbol{\phi}} = \left( \sum_{t=1}^{n} \boldsymbol{x}_{t-1} \boldsymbol{x}_{t-1}' \right)^{-1} \sum_{t=1}^{n} \boldsymbol{x}_{t-1} x_t \tag{2.214}$$

and

$$\widetilde{\sigma}_w^2 = \frac{1}{n} \sum_{t=1}^{n} \left( x_t - \widetilde{\boldsymbol{\phi}}' \boldsymbol{x}_{t-1} \right)^2 \tag{2.215}$$

to those two estimators. In (2.214) and (2.215), we are acting as if we are able to observe $x_{1-p}, \ldots, x_0$ in addition to $x_1, \ldots, x_n$. The asymptotic equivalence is then seen by arguing that for $n$ sufficiently large, it makes no difference whether or not we observe $x_{1-p}, \ldots, x_0$. In the case of (2.214) and (2.215), we obtain the following theorem.

**Theorem 2.4:** *Let $x_t$ be a causal AR(p) series with white noise $w_t$ satisfying $E(w_t^4) = \eta \sigma_w^4$. Then,*

$$\widetilde{\boldsymbol{\phi}} \sim \mathrm{AN}\Big( \boldsymbol{\phi},\ n^{-1} \sigma_w^2 \Gamma_p^{-1} \Big), \tag{2.216}$$

*where $\Gamma_p = \{\gamma(i-j)\}_{i,j=1}^{p}$ is the $p \times p$ autocovariance matrix of the vector $\boldsymbol{x}_{t-1}$. We also have, as $n \to \infty$,*

$$n^{-1} \sum_{t=1}^{n} \boldsymbol{x}_{t-1} \boldsymbol{x}_{t-1}' \xrightarrow{p} \Gamma_p \tag{2.217}$$

*and*

$$\widetilde{\sigma}_w^2 \xrightarrow{p} \sigma_w^2. \tag{2.218}$$

***Proof.*** First, (2.217) follows from the fact that $E(\boldsymbol{x}_{t-1}\boldsymbol{x}_{t-1}') = \Gamma_p$, recalling that from Theorem 1.6, second-order sample moments converge in probability to their population moments for linear processes in which $w_t$ has a finite fourth moment. To show (2.216), we can write

$$\begin{aligned}
\widetilde{\boldsymbol{\phi}} &= \left(\sum_{t=1}^{n} \boldsymbol{x}_{t-1}\boldsymbol{x}_{t-1}'\right)^{-1} \sum_{t=1}^{n} \boldsymbol{x}_{t-1}(\boldsymbol{x}_{t-1}'\boldsymbol{\phi} + w_t) \\
&= \boldsymbol{\phi} + \left(\sum_{t=1}^{n} \boldsymbol{x}_{t-1}\boldsymbol{x}_{t-1}'\right)^{-1} \sum_{t=1}^{n} \boldsymbol{x}_{t-1}w_t,
\end{aligned}$$

so that

$$\begin{aligned}
n^{1/2}(\widetilde{\boldsymbol{\phi}} - \boldsymbol{\phi}) &= \left(n^{-1}\sum_{t=1}^{n} \boldsymbol{x}_{t-1}\boldsymbol{x}_{t-1}'\right)^{-1} n^{-1/2}\sum_{t=1}^{n} \boldsymbol{x}_{t-1}w_t \\
&= \left(n^{-1}\sum_{t=1}^{n} \boldsymbol{x}_{t-1}\boldsymbol{x}_{t-1}'\right)^{-1} n^{-1/2}\sum_{t=1}^{n} \boldsymbol{u}_t,
\end{aligned}$$

where $\boldsymbol{u}_t = \boldsymbol{x}_{t-1}w_t$. We use the fact that $w_t$ and $\boldsymbol{x}_{t-1}$ are independent to write $E\boldsymbol{u}_t = E\boldsymbol{x}_{t-1}Ew_t = \boldsymbol{0}$, because the errors have zero means. Also,

$$\begin{aligned}
E\boldsymbol{u}_t\boldsymbol{u}_t' &= E\boldsymbol{x}_{t-1}w_tw_t\boldsymbol{x}_{t-1}' \\
&= E\boldsymbol{x}_{t-1}\boldsymbol{x}_{t-1}'Ew_t^2 \\
&= \sigma_w^2\Gamma_p.
\end{aligned}$$

In addition, we have, for $h > 0$,

$$\begin{aligned}
E\boldsymbol{u}_{t+h}\boldsymbol{u}_t' &= E\boldsymbol{x}_{t+h-1}w_{t+h}w_t\boldsymbol{x}_{t-1}' \\
&= E\boldsymbol{x}_{t+h-1}w_t\boldsymbol{x}_{t-1}'Ew_{t+h} \\
&= 0.
\end{aligned}$$

A similar computation works for $h < 0$.

Next, consider the mean square convergent approximation

$$x_t^m = \sum_{j=0}^{m} \psi_j w_{t-j}$$

for $x_t$, and define the $(m+p)$-dependent process $\boldsymbol{u}_t^m = w_t(x_{t-1}^m, x_{t-2}^m, \ldots, x_{t-p}^m)'$. Note that we need only look at a central limit theorem for the sum

$$y_{nm} = n^{-1/2}\sum_{t=1}^{n} \boldsymbol{\lambda}'\boldsymbol{u}_t^m,$$

for arbitrary vectors $\boldsymbol{\lambda} = (\lambda_1, \dots, \lambda_p)'$, where $y_{nm}$ is used as an approximation to

$$S_n = n^{-1/2} \sum_{t=1}^{n} \boldsymbol{\lambda}' \boldsymbol{u}_t.$$

First, apply the the $m$-dependent central limit theorem to $y_{nm}$ as $n \to \infty$ for fixed $m$ to establish (i) of Theorem 1.2. This result shows $y_{nm} \xrightarrow{d} y_m$, where $y_m$ is asymptotically normal with covariance $\boldsymbol{\lambda}' \Gamma_p^{(m)} \boldsymbol{\lambda}$, where $\Gamma_p^{(m)}$ is the covariance matrix of $\boldsymbol{u}_t^m$. Then, we have $\Gamma_p^{(m)} \to \Gamma_p$, so that $y_m$ converges in distribution to a normal random variable with mean zero and variance $\boldsymbol{\lambda}' \Gamma_p \boldsymbol{\lambda}$ and we have verified part (ii) of Theorem 1.2. We verify part (iii) of Theorem 1.2 by noting that

$$E[(S_n - y_{nm})^2] = n^{-1} \sum_{t=1}^{n} \boldsymbol{\lambda}' E[(\boldsymbol{u}_t - \boldsymbol{u}_t^m)(\boldsymbol{u}_t - \boldsymbol{u}_t^m)'] \boldsymbol{\lambda}$$

clearly converges to zero as $n, m \to \infty$ because

$$x_t - x_t^m = \sum_{j=m+1}^{\infty} \psi_j w_{t-j}$$

form the components of $\boldsymbol{u}_t - \boldsymbol{u}_t^m$.

Now, the form for $\sqrt{n}(\widetilde{\boldsymbol{\phi}} - \boldsymbol{\phi})$ contains the premultiplying matrix

$$\left( n^{-1} \sum_{t=1}^{n} \boldsymbol{x}_{t-1} \boldsymbol{x}_{t-1}' \right)^{-1} \xrightarrow{p} \Gamma_p^{-1},$$

because (1.93) can be applied to the function that defines the inverse of the matrix. Then, applying (1.92), shows that

$$n^{1/2} \left( \widetilde{\boldsymbol{\phi}} - \boldsymbol{\phi} \right) \xrightarrow{d} \mathrm{N} \left( 0, \sigma_w^2 \Gamma_p^{-1} \Gamma_p \Gamma_p^{-1} \right),$$

so we may regard it as being multivariate normal with mean zero and covariance matrix $\sigma_w^2 \Gamma_p^{-1}$.

To investigate $\widetilde{\sigma}_w^2$, note

$$\begin{aligned} \widetilde{\sigma}_w^2 &= n^{-1} \sum_{t=1}^{n} \left( x_t - \widetilde{\boldsymbol{\phi}}' \boldsymbol{x}_{t-1} \right)^2 \\ &= n^{-1} \sum_{t=1}^{n} x_t^2 - n^{-1} \sum_{t=1}^{n} \boldsymbol{x}_{t-1}' x_t \left( n^{-1} \sum_{t=1}^{n} \boldsymbol{x}_{t-1} \boldsymbol{x}_{t-1}' \right)^{-1} n^{-1} \sum_{t=1}^{n} \boldsymbol{x}_{t-1} x_t \\ &\xrightarrow{p} \gamma(0) - \boldsymbol{\gamma}_p' \Gamma_p^{-1} \boldsymbol{\gamma}_p \\ &= \sigma_w^2, \end{aligned}$$

and we have that the sample estimator converges in probability to $\sigma_w^2$, which is written in the form of (2.60). □

The arguments above imply that, for sufficiently large $n$, we may consider the estimator $\widehat{\boldsymbol{\phi}}$ in (2.212) as being approximately multivariate normal with mean $\boldsymbol{\phi}$ and variance–covariance matrix $\sigma_w^2 \Gamma_p^{-1}/n$. Inferences about the parameter $\boldsymbol{\phi}$ are obtained by replacing the $\sigma_w^2$ and $\Gamma_p$ by their estimates given by (2.213) and

$$\widehat{\Gamma}_p = n^{-1} \sum_{t=p+1}^{n} \boldsymbol{x}_{t-1} \boldsymbol{x}_{t-1}',$$

respectively. In the case of a nonzero mean, the data $x_t$ are replaced by $x_t - \bar{x}$ in the estimates and the results of Theorem 2.4 remain valid.

# Problems

*Section 2.2*

**2.1** For an MA(1), $x_t = w_t + \theta w_{t-1}$, show that $|\rho_x(1)| \leq 1/2$ for any number $\theta$. For which values of $\theta$ does $\rho_x(1)$ attain its maximum and minimum?

**2.2** Let $w_t$ be white noise with variance $\sigma_w^2$ and let $|\phi| < 1$ be a constant. Consider the process

$$\begin{aligned} x_1 &= w_1 \\ x_t &= \phi x_{t-1} + w_t \quad t = 2, 3, \ldots . \end{aligned}$$

(a) Find the mean and the variance of $\{x_t,\ t = 1, 2, \ldots\}$. Is $x_t$ stationary?

(b) Show

$$\operatorname{corr}(x_t, x_{t-h}) = \phi^h \left[ \frac{\operatorname{var}(x_{t-h})}{\operatorname{var}(x_t)} \right]^{1/2}$$

for $h \geq 0$.

(c) Argue that for large $t$,

$$\operatorname{var}(x_t) \approx \frac{\sigma_w^2}{1 - \phi^2}$$

and

$$\operatorname{corr}(x_t, x_{t-h}) \approx \phi^h, \quad h \geq 0,$$

so in a sense, $x_t$ is "asymptotically stationary."

(d) Comment on how you could use these results to simulate $n$ observations of a stationary Gaussian AR(1) model from simulated iid N(0,1) values.

(e) Now suppose $x_1 = w_1/\sqrt{1 - \phi^2}$. Is this process stationary?

**2.3** Identify the following models as ARMA$(p, q)$ models (watch out for parameter redundancy), and determine whether they are causal and/or invertible:

(a) $x_t = 0.80x_{t-1} - 0.15x_{t-2} + w_t - 0.30w_{t-1}$.

(b) $x_t = x_{t-1} - 0.50x_{t-2} + w_t - w_{t-1}$.

**2.4** Verify the causal conditions for an AR(2) model given in (2.28). That is, show that an AR(2) is causal if and only if (2.28) holds.

*Section 2.3*

**2.5** For the AR(2) model given by $x_t = -0.9x_{t-2} + w_t$, find the roots of the autoregressive polynomial, and then sketch the ACF, $\rho(h)$.

**2.6** For the AR(2) autoregressive series shown below, determine a set of difference equations that can be used to find $\psi_j, j = 0, 1, \ldots$ in the representation (2.25) and the autocorrelation function $\rho(h), h = 0, 1, \ldots$. Solve for the constants in the ACF using the known initial conditions, and plot the first eight values.

(a) $x_t + 1.6x_{t-1} + .64x_{t-2} = w_t$.

(b) $x_t - .40x_{t-1} - .45x_{t-2} = w_t$.

(c) $x_t - 1.2x_{t-1} + .85x_{t-2} = w_t$.

*Section 2.4*

**2.7** Verify the calculations for the autocorrelation function of an ARMA(1, 1) process given in Example 2.11. Compare the form with that of the ACF for the ARMA(1, 0) and the ARMA(0, 1) series. Plot the ACF's of the three series on the same graph for $\phi = .6, \theta = .9$, and comment on the diagnostic capabilities of the ACF in this case.

**2.8** Generate $n = 100$ observations from each of the three models discussed in Problem 2.7. Compute the sample ACF for each model and compare it to the theoretical values. Compute the sample PACF for each of the generated series and compare the sample ACFs and PACFs with the general results given in Table 2.1.

*Section 2.5*

**2.9** Consider the MA(1) series

$$x_t = w_t + \theta w_{t-1},$$

where $w_t$ is white noise with variance $\sigma_w^2$.

(a) Derive the minimum mean square error one-step forecast based on the infinite past, and determine the mean square error of this forecast.

(b) Let $\widetilde{x}_{n+1}^n$ be the truncated one-step-ahead forecast as given in (2.81). Show that

$$E\left[(x_{n+1} - \widetilde{x}_{n+1}^n)^2\right] = \sigma^2(1 + \theta^{2+2n}).$$

Compare the result with (a), and indicate how well the finite approximation works in this case.

**2.10** In the context of equation (2.57), show that, if $\gamma(0) > 0$ and $\gamma(h) \to 0$ as $h \to \infty$, then $\Gamma_n$ is positive definite.

**2.11** Suppose $x_t$ is stationary with zero mean and recall the definition of the PACF given by (2.50) and (2.51). That is, let

$$\epsilon_t = x_t - \sum_{i=1}^{h-1} a_k x_{t-i}$$

and

$$\delta_{t-h} = x_{t-h} - \sum_{j=1}^{h-1} b_j x_{t-j}$$

be the two residuals where $\{a_1, ..., a_{h-1}\}$ and $\{b_1, ..., b_{h-1}\}$ are chosen so that they minimize the mean-squared errors

$$E[\epsilon_t^2] \quad \text{and} \quad E[\delta_{t-h}^2].$$

The PACF at lag $h$ was defined as the cross-correlation between $\epsilon_t$ and $\delta_{t-h}$; that is,

$$\phi_{hh} = \frac{E(\epsilon_t \delta_{t-h})}{\sqrt{E(\epsilon_t^2)E(\delta_{t-h}^2)}}.$$

Let $R_h$ be the $h \times h$ matrix with elements $\rho(i-j), i, j = 1, \dots, h$, and let $\boldsymbol{\rho}_h = (\rho(1), \rho(2), \dots, \rho(h))'$ be the vector of lagged autocorrelations, $\rho(h) = \text{corr}(x_{t+h}, x_t)$. Let $\widetilde{\boldsymbol{\rho}}_h = (\rho(h), \rho(h-1), \dots, \rho(1))'$ be the reversed vector. In addition, let $x_t^h$ denote the BLP of $x_t$ given $\{x_{t-1}, \dots, x_{t-h}\}$:

$$x_t^h = \alpha_{h1} x_{t-1} + \cdots + \alpha_{hh} x_{t-h},$$

as described in Property P2.3. Prove

$$\phi_{hh} = \frac{\rho(h) - \widetilde{\boldsymbol{\rho}}_{h-1}' R_{h-1}^{-1} \boldsymbol{\rho}_h}{1 - \widetilde{\boldsymbol{\rho}}_{h-1}' R_{h-1}^{-1} \widetilde{\boldsymbol{\rho}}_{h-1}} = \alpha_{hh}.$$

In particular, this result proves Property P2.4.

*Hint:* Divide the prediction equations [see (2.57)] by $\gamma(0)$ and write the matrix equation in the partitioned form as

$$\begin{pmatrix} R_{h-1} & \widetilde{\boldsymbol{\rho}}_{h-1} \\ \widetilde{\boldsymbol{\rho}}'_{h-1} & \rho(0) \end{pmatrix} \begin{pmatrix} \boldsymbol{\alpha}_1 \\ \alpha_{hh} \end{pmatrix} = \begin{pmatrix} \boldsymbol{\rho}_{h-1} \\ \rho(h) \end{pmatrix},$$

where the $h \times 1$ vector of coefficients $\boldsymbol{\alpha} = (\alpha_{h1}, ..., \alpha_{hh})'$ is partitioned as $\boldsymbol{\alpha} = (\boldsymbol{\alpha}'_1, \alpha_{hh})'$.

**2.12** Let $M_t$ represent the cardiovascular mortality series discussed in Chapter 1, Example 1.27. An AR(2) model was fit to the data resulting in the following model:

$$M_t = 11.45 + .43M_{t-1} + .44M_{t-2} + w_t,$$

where $\text{var}(w_t) = 32.5$. Assuming this is the true model, find the forecasts over a four-month horizon, $x^n_{n+m}$, for $m = 1, 2, 3, 4$, and the corresponding 95% prediction intervals.

**2.13** Suppose we wish to find a prediction function $g(x)$ that minimizes

$$MSE = E[(y - g(x))^2],$$

where $x$ and $y$ are jointly distributed random variables with density function $f(x, y)$.

(a) Show that MSE is minimized by the choice

$$g(x) = E(y \mid x).$$

*Hint:*

$$MSE = \int \left[ \int (y - g(x))^2 f(y|x) dy \right] f(x) dx.$$

(b) Apply the above result to the model

$$y = x^2 + z,$$

where $x$ and $z$ are independent zero-mean normal variables with variance one. Show that $MSE = 1$.

(c) Suppose we restrict our choices for the function $g(x)$ to linear functions of the form

$$g(x) = a + bx$$

and determine $a$ and $b$ to minimize $MSE$. Show that $a = 1$ and

$$b = \frac{E(xy)}{E(x^2)} = 0$$

and $MSE = 3$. What do you interpret this to mean?

**2.14** Write out the model for an ARMA(1,0) series. Determine the $m$-step-ahead forecast $x_{t+m}^t$ and show

$$E[(x_{t+m} - x_{t+m}^t)^2] = \sigma_w^2 \frac{1-\phi^{2m}}{1-\phi^2}.$$

**2.15** Consider the ARMA(1,1) model discussed in Example 2.6, equation (2.27); that is, $x_t = 0.9x_{t-1} + 0.5w_{t-1} + w_t$. Show that truncated prediction as defined in (2.80) is equivalent to truncated prediction using the recursive formula (2.81).

**2.16** Verify statement (2.79), that for a fixed sample size, the ARMA prediction errors are correlated.

*Section 2.6*

**2.17** Let $M_t$ represent the cardiovascular mortality series discussed in Chapter 1, Example 1.27. Fit an AR(2) model to the data using linear regression and using Yule–Walker.

(a) Compare the parameter estimates obtained by the two methods.

(b) Compare the estimated standard errors of the coefficients obtained by linear regression with their corresponding asymptotic approximations, as given in Property P2.9.

**2.18** Suppose $x_1, \ldots, x_n$ are observations from an AR(1) process with $\mu = 0$.

(a) Show the backcasts can be written as $x_t^n = \phi^{1-t}x_1$, for $t \leq 1$.

(b) In turn, show, for $t \leq 1$, the backcasted errors are $\widehat{w}_t(\phi) = x_t^n - \phi x_{t-1}^n = \phi^{1-t}(1-\phi^2)x_1$.

(c) Use the result of (b) to show $\sum_{t=-\infty}^{1} \widehat{w}_t^2(\phi) = (1-\phi^2)x_1^2$.

(d) Use the result of (c) to verify the unconditional sum of squares, $S(\phi)$, can be written in the innovations form as $\sum_{t=-\infty}^{n} \widehat{w}_t^2(\phi)$.

(e) Find $x_t^{t-1}$ and $r_t^{t-1}$, and show that $S(\phi)$ can also be written as $\sum_{t=1}^{n}(x_t - x_t^{t-1})^2 \,/\, r_t^{t-1}$.

**2.19** Generate 10 realizations of length $n = 50$ standard Gaussian white noise observations, and fit an ARMA(1,1) model to the simulated data in each case. What happened and how do you explain the results?

**2.20** Generate 10 realizations of length $n = 200$ of a series from an ARMA(1,1) model with $\phi_1 = .90, \theta_1 = .2$ and $\sigma^2 = .25$. Fit the model by nonlinear least squares in each case and compare the estimators to the true values.

**2.21** Generate $n = 25$ observations from a Gaussian AR(1) model with $\phi = 0.99$ and $\sigma_w = 1$. Using an estimation technique of your choice, compare the approximate asymptotic distribution of your estimate (the one you would use for inference) with the results of a bootstrap experiment (use $B = 200$).

**2.22** Using Example 2.27 as your guide, find the Gauss–Newton procedure for estimating the autoregressive parameter, $\phi$, from the AR(1) model, $x_t = \phi x_{t-1} + w_t$, given data $x_1, ..., x_n$. Does this procedure produce the unconditional or the conditional estimator? *Hint:* Write the model as $w_t(\phi) = x_t - \phi x_{t-1}$; your solution should work out to be a non-recursive procedure.

**2.23** Consider the stationary series generated by

$$x_t = \alpha + \phi x_{t-1} + w_t + \theta w_{t-1},$$

where $E(x_t) = \mu$, $|\theta| < 1, |\phi| < 1$ and the $w_t$ are iid random variables with zero mean and variance $\sigma_w^2$.

(a) Determine the mean as a function of $\alpha$ for the above model. Find the covariance and ACF of the process $x_t$, and show that the process is weakly stationary. Is the process strictly stationary? *Hint:* See Problem T1.19.

(b) Prove the limiting distribution as $n \to \infty$ of the sample mean,

$$\bar{x} = n^{-1} \sum_{t=1}^{n} x_t,$$

is normal, and find its limiting mean and variance in terms of $\alpha$, $\phi$, $\theta$, and $\sigma_w^2$.

**2.24** A problem of interest in the analysis of geophysical time series involves a simple model for observed data containing a signal and a reflected version of the signal with unknown amplification factor $a$ and unknown time delay $\delta$. For example, the depth of an earthquake is proportional to the time delay $\delta$ for the P wave and its reflected form pP on a seismic record. Assume the signal is white and Gaussian with variance $\sigma_s^2$, and consider the generating model

$$x_t = s_t + a s_{t-\delta}.$$

(a) Prove the process $x_t$ is stationary. If $|a| < 1$, show that

$$s_t = \sum_{j=0}^{\infty} (-a)^j x_{t-\delta j}$$

is a mean square convergent representation for the signal $s_t$, for $t = 1, \pm 1, \pm 2, \ldots$.

(b) If the time delay $\delta$ is assumed to be known, suggest an approximate computational method for estimating the parameters $a$ and $\sigma_s^2$ using maximum likelihood and the Gauss–Newton method.

(c) If the time delay $\delta$ is an unknown integer, specify how we could estimate the parameters including $\delta$. Generate a $n = 500$ point series with $a = .9$, $\sigma_w^2 = 1$ and $\delta = 5$. Estimate the integer time delay $\delta$ by searching over $\delta = 3, 4, \ldots, 7$.

**2.25** *Forecasting with estimated parameters:* Let $x_1, x_2, \ldots, x_n$ be a sample of size $n$ from a causal AR(1) process, $x_t = \phi x_{t-1} + w_t$. Let $\widehat{\phi}$ be the Yule–Walker estimator of $\phi$.

(a) Show $\widehat{\phi} - \phi = O_p(n^{-1/2})$. See Section T1.10 for the definition of $O_p(\cdot)$.

(b) Let $x_{n+1}^n$ be the one-step-ahead forecast of $x_{n+1}$ given the data $x_1, ..., x_n$, based on the known parameter, $\phi$, and let $\widehat{x}_{n+1}^n$ be the one-step-ahead forecast when the parameter is replaced by $\widehat{\phi}$. Show $x_{n+1}^n - \widehat{x}_{n+1}^n = O_p(n^{-1/2})$.

*Section 2.7*

**2.26** Suppose

$$y_t = \beta_0 + \beta_1 t + \cdots \beta_q t^q + x_t, \quad \beta_q \neq 0,$$

where $x_t$ is stationary. First, show that $\nabla^k x_t$ is stationary for any $k = 1, 2, ...,$ and then show that $\nabla^k y_t$ is not stationary for $k < q$, but is stationary for $k \geq q$.

**2.27** Verify that the IMA(1,1) model given in (2.128) can be inverted and written as (2.129).

**2.28** For the logarithm of the glacial varve data, say, $x_t$, presented in Example 2.28, use the first 100 observations and calculate the EWMA, $\widetilde{x}_{t+1}^t$, given in (2.131) for $t = 1, ..., 100$, using $\theta = 0.25, 0.50$, and $0.75$, and plot the EWMAs and the data superimposed on each other. Comment on the results.

*Section 2.8*

**2.29** In Example 2.34, we summarized the diagnostics for an ARIMA fit to the glacial varve series. Using that example as a guide, verify the results of the diagnostic analyses.

**2.30** Using the gas price series described in Problem 1.19 fit an ARIMA$(p, d, q)$ model to the data, performing all necessary diagnostics. Comment.

**2.31** One of the series collected along with particulates, temperature, and mortality described in Example 1.27 is the sulfur dioxide series. Fit an ARIMA$(p, d, q)$ model to the sulfur dioxide data, performing all of the necessary diagnostics. After deciding on an appropriate model, forecast the data into the future four time periods ahead (about one month) and calculate 95% prediction intervals for each of the four forecasts.

*Section 2.9*

**2.32** Consider the ARIMA model

$$x_t = w_t + \Theta w_{t-2}.$$

(a) Identify the model using the notation ARIMA$(p, d, q) \times (P, D, Q)_s$.

(b) Show that the series is invertible for $|\Theta| < 1$, and find the coefficients in the representation

$$w_t = \sum_{k=0}^{\infty} \pi_k x_{t-k}.$$

(c) Develop equations for the $m$-step ahead forecast, $\widetilde{x}_{n+m}$, and its variance based on the infinite past, $x_n, x_{n-1}, \dots$ .

**2.33** Sketch the ACF of the seasonal ARIMA$(0, 1) \times (1, 0)_{12}$ model with $\Phi = 0.8$ and $\theta = 0.5$.

**2.34** Fit a seasonal ARIMA model of your choice to the U.S. Live Birth Series.

**2.35** Fit an appropriate seasonal ARIMA model to the log-transformed Johnson and Johnson earnings series of Example 1.1. Use the corrected AICc criterion to aid in model selection.

*Section 2.10*

**2.36** The data set labeled `fracdiff.dat` is $n = 1000$ simulated observations from a fractionally differenced ARIMA$(1, 1, 0)$ model with $\phi = 0.75$ and $d = .4$.

(a) Do a time plot of the data, and comment.

(b) Plot the ACF and PACF of the data, and comment.

(c) Estimate the parameters, and test for the significance of the estimates $\widehat{\phi}$ and $\widehat{d}$.

(d) Explain why, using the results of part (a) and (b), it would seem reasonable to difference the data prior to the analysis. That is, if $x_t$ represents the data, explain why we might choose to fit an ARMA model to $\nabla x_t$.

(e) Plot the ACF and PACF of $\nabla x_t$, and comment.

(f) Fit an ARMA model to $\nabla x_t$, and comment.

**2.37** Fit a fractionally differenced ARIMA to the global temperature series displayed in Figure 1.2.

*Section 2.11*

**2.38** The sunspot data are plotted in Chapter 3, Figure 3.20. From a time plot of the data, discuss why is it reasonable to fit a threshold model to the data, and then fit a threshold model.

*Section 2.12*

**2.39** Let $S_t$ represent the monthly sales data listed in `sales.dat` ($n = 150$), and let $L_t$ be the leading indicator listed in `lead.dat`. Fit the regression model $S_t = \beta_0 + \beta_1 L_{t-3} + x_t$, where $x_t$ is an ARMA process.

**2.40** Consider the correlated regression model, defined in the text by (2.192), say,

$$\boldsymbol{y} = Z\boldsymbol{\beta} + \boldsymbol{x},$$

where $\boldsymbol{x}$ has mean zero and covariance matrix $\Gamma$. In this case, we know that the weighted least squares estimator is (2.93), namely,

$$\widehat{\boldsymbol{\beta}}_w = (Z'\Gamma^{-1}Z)^{-1}Z'\Gamma^{-1}\boldsymbol{y}.$$

Now, a problem of interest in spatial series can be formulated in terms of this basic model. Suppose $y_i = y(\sigma_i), i = 1, 2, \dots, n$ is a function of the spatial vector coordinates $\sigma_i = (s_{i1}, s_{i2}, \dots, s_{ir})'$, the error is $x_i = x(\sigma_i)$, and the rows of $Z$ are defined as $\boldsymbol{z}(\sigma_i)', i = 1, 2, \dots, n$. The ***Kriging estimator*** is defined as the best spatial predictor of $y_0 = \boldsymbol{z}_0'\boldsymbol{\beta} + x_0$ using the estimator

$$\widehat{y}_0 = \boldsymbol{a}'\boldsymbol{y},$$

subject to the unbiased condition $E\widehat{y}_0 = Ey_0$, and such that the mean square prediction error

$$\text{MSE} = E[(y_0 - \widehat{y}_0)^2]$$

is minimized.

(a) Prove the estimator is unbiased when $Z'\boldsymbol{a} = \boldsymbol{z}_0$.

(b) Show the MSE is minimized by solving the equations

$$\Gamma\boldsymbol{a} + Z\boldsymbol{\lambda} = \boldsymbol{\gamma}_0$$

and

$$Z'\boldsymbol{a} = \boldsymbol{\gamma}_0,$$

where $\boldsymbol{\gamma}_0 = E[\boldsymbol{x}x_0]$ represents the vector of covariances between the error vector of the observed data and the error of the new point the vector $\boldsymbol{\lambda}$ is a $q \times 1$ vector of LaGrangian multipliers.

(c) Show the predicted value can be expressed as

$$\widehat{y}_0 = \boldsymbol{z}_0'\widehat{\boldsymbol{\beta}}_w + \boldsymbol{\gamma}_0'\Gamma^{-1}(\boldsymbol{y} - Z\widehat{\boldsymbol{\beta}}_w),$$

so the optimal prediction is a linear combination of the usual predictor and the least squares residuals.

*Section 2.13*

**2.41** The file labeled `clim-hyd` has 454 months of measured values for the climatic variables air temperature, dew point, cloud cover, wind speed, precipitation ($p_t$), and inflow ($i_t$), at Shasta Lake. We would like to look at possible relations between the weather factors and the inflow to Shasta Lake.

(a) Fit ARIMA$(0,0,0) \times (0,1,1)_{12}$ models to (i) transformed precipitation $P_t = \sqrt{p_t}$ and (ii) transformed inflow $I_t = \log i_t$.

(b) Apply the ARIMA model fitted in part (a) for transformed precipitation to the flow series to generate the prewhitened flow residuals assuming the precipitation model. Compute the cross-correlation between the flow residuals using the precipitation ARIMA model and the precipitation residuals using the precipitation model and interpret. Use the coefficients from the ARIMA model to construct the transformed flow residuals.

**2.42** Consider predicting the transformed flows $I_t = \log i_t$ from transformed precipitation values $P_t = \sqrt{p_t}$ using a transfer function model of the form

$$(1 - B^{12})I_t = \alpha(B)(1 - B^{12})P_t + n_t,$$

where we assume that seasonal differencing is a reasonable thing to do. The data are the 454 monthly values of precipitation and inflow from the Shasta Lake reservoir in the file *clim-hyd*. You may think of it as fitting

$$y_t = \alpha(B)x_t + n_t,$$

where $y_t$ and $x_t$ are the seasonally differenced transformed flows and precipitations.

(a) Argue that $x_t$ can be fitted by a first-order seasonal moving average, and use the transformation obtained to prewhiten the series $x_t$.

(b) Apply the transformation applied in (a) to the series $y_t$, and compute the cross-correlation function relating the prewhitened series to the transformed series. Argue for a transfer function of the form

$$\alpha(B) = \frac{\delta_0}{1 - \omega_1 B}.$$

(c) Write the overall model obtained in regression form to estimate $\delta_0$ and $\omega_1$. Note that you will be minimizing the sums of squared residuals for the transformed noise series $(1 - \widehat{\omega}_1 B)n_t$. Retain the residuals for further modeling involving the noise $n_t$. The observed residual is $u_t = (1 - \widehat{\omega}_1 B)n_t$.

(d) Fit the noise residuals obtained in (c) with an ARMA model, and give the final form suggested by your analysis in the previous parts.

(e) Discuss the problem of forecasting $y_{t+m}$ using the infinite past of $y_t$ and the present and infinite past of $x_t$. Determine the predicted value and the forecast variance.

*Section 2.14*

**2.43** Investigate whether the monthly returns of a stock dividend yield (the data are listed in `sdyr.dat`; see Figure 2.38) exhibit ARCH behavior. If so, fit an appropriate model to the returns.

**2.44** Investigate whether the growth rate of the monthly Oil Prices exhibit ARCH behavior. If so, fit an appropriate model to the growth rate.

**2.45** Fit an ARCH model to the NYSE returns (the data are listed in `nyse.dat` for Chapter 4).

**2.46** In Section 2.14, the $2 \times 1$ gradient vector, $l^{(1)}(\boldsymbol{a}_0, \boldsymbol{a}_1)$, given for an ARCH(1) model was displayed in (2.189). Verify (2.189) and then use the result to calculate the $2 \times 2$ Hessian matrix

$$l^{(2)}(\boldsymbol{a}_0, \boldsymbol{a}_1) = \begin{pmatrix} \partial^2 l/\partial \boldsymbol{a}_0^2 & \partial^2 l/\partial \boldsymbol{a}_0 \partial \boldsymbol{a}_1 \\ \partial^2 l/\partial \boldsymbol{a}_0 \partial \boldsymbol{a}_1 & \partial^2 l/\partial \boldsymbol{a}_1^2 \end{pmatrix}.$$

*Section T2.15*

**2.47** Suppose $x_t = \sum_{j=1}^{p} \phi_j x_{t-j} + w_t$, where $\phi_p \neq 0$ and $w_t$ is white noise such that $w_t$ is uncorrelated with $\{x_k; k < t\}$. Use the Projection Theorem to show that, for $n > p$, the BLP of $x_{n+1}$ on $\overline{\text{sp}}\{x_k, k \leq n\}$ is

$$\widehat{x}_{n+1} = \sum_{j=1}^{p} \phi_j x_{n+1-j}.$$

**2.48** Use the Projection Theorem to derive the Innovations Algorithm, Property P2.6, equations (2.69)-(2.71). Then, use Theorem 2.2 to derive the $m$-step-ahead forecast results given in (2.72) and (2.73).

**2.49** Consider the series $x_t = w_t - w_{t-1}$, where $w_t$ is a white noise process with mean zero and variance $\sigma_w^2$. Suppose we consider the problem of predicting $x_n$, based on only $x_0, x_1, \ldots x_t$, for $t < n$. Use the Projection Theorem to answer the questions below.

(a) Show the best linear predictor is

$$x_n^t = -\frac{1}{n+1} \sum_{k=0}^{t} (k+1) x_k.$$

(b) Prove the mean square error is

$$E[(x_n - x_n^t)^2] = \frac{n+2}{n+1} \sigma_w^2.$$

**2.50** Use Theorems 2.2 and 2.3 to verify (2.103).

**2.51** Prove Theorem 2.2.

*Section T2.16*

**2.52** Prove Property P2.2.

# CHAPTER 3

# Spectral Analysis and Filtering

## 3.1 Introduction

The notion that a time series exhibits repetitive or regular behavior over time is of fundamental importance because it distinguishes time series analysis from classical statistics which assumes complete independence over time. We have seen in Chapters 1 and 2 how dependence over time can be introduced through models that describe in detail the way certain empirical data behaves, even to the extent of producing forecasts based on the models. It is natural that models based on predicting the present as a regression on the past such as are provided by the celebrated ARIMA or state-space forms, will be attractive to statisticians, who are trained to view nature in terms of linear models. In fact, the difference equations used to represent these kinds of models are simply the discrete versions of linear differential equations that may, in some instances, provide the ideal physical model for a certain phenomenon. An alternate version of the way nature behaves exists, however, based on a decomposition of an empirical series into its regular components.

In this chapter, we argue, the concept of regularity of a series can best be expressed in terms of ***periodic*** variations of the underlying phenomenon that produced the series, expressed as ***Fourier frequencies*** being driven by sines and cosines. From a regression point of view, we may imagine a system responding to various driving frequencies by producing linear combinations of sine and cosine functions. Expressed in these terms, the distinction between a ***time domain approach*** and a ***frequency domain approach*** becomes one between regression on the past, as favored in time domain approaches or regressions on periodic sines and cosines, as embodied in the frequency domain approaches. The frequency domain approaches are the focus of this chapter and Chapter 5. To illustrate the two methods for generating series with a single primary periodic component, consider Figure 1.8, which was generated from a simple second-order autoregressive model and the bottom panel of Figure 1.9, which was generated by adding a sine wave with a period of 20 points to white noise Both series exhibit strong periodic fluctuations, illustrating that both models can generate time series with regular behavior. In this case, it is also obvious that the rates of oscillation or ***frequencies*** of these two series are different; the length of a single cycle for the autoregressive series is about six points, whereas the length of the primary cycle of the sine wave embedded in noise is about 20 points. In most cases, mixtures of driving frequencies exist and a fundamental objective of ***spectral analysis*** is to identify these dominant frequencies and to find an explanation of the system from which the measurements were derived.

Of course, the primary justification for any alternate model must lie in its potential for explaining the behavior of some empirical phenomenon. In this sense, an explanation involving only a few kinds of primary oscillations becomes simpler and more physically meaningful than a collection of parameters estimated for some selected difference equation. It is the tendency of observed data to show periodic kinds of fluctuations that justify the use of frequency domain methods. As examples of time series representing real phenomena that are driven by periodic components, we mention Examples 1.3-1.6 of Chapter 1. The speech recording of the syllable aa...hh contains a complicated mixture of frequencies related to the opening and closing of the glottis. Figure 1.4 shows the monthly SOI, which we find later explain as a combination of two kinds of periodicities, a seasonal periodic component of 12 months and an El Niño component of about 72 months. Of fundamental interest is the return period of the El Niño phenomenon, which can have profound effects on local climate. Also of interest is whether the different periodic components of the new fish population depend on corresponding seasonal and El Niño-type oscillations. We introduce the ***coherence*** as a tool for relating the common periodic behavior of two series. Seasonal periodic components are often pervasive in economic time series; this phenomenon can be seen in the quarterly earnings series shown in Figure 1.1. In Figure 1.5, we see the extent to which various parts of the brain will respond to a periodic stimulus generated by having the subject do alternate left and right finger tapping. Figure 1.6 shows series from an earthquake and a nuclear explosion. The relative amounts of energy at various frequencies for the two phases can produce statistics, useful for discriminating between earthquakes and explosions.

In this chapter, we summarize an approach to handling correlation generated in stationary time series that begins by transforming the series to the frequency domain. This simple linear transformation essentially matches sines and cosines of various frequencies against the underlying data and serves two purposes. First, the transformation can be thought of as producing a kind of partition into ***principal components***, in which the principal components are arranged according to the variances of the periodic contributors. The variances of these periodic components, arranged by frequency, define the ***power spectrum*** and the evaluation of the contributions of these periodic components is just what is done in spectral analysis. The second purpose is more one of statistical convenience, because the periodic components are nearly uncorrelated. This property facilitates writing likelihoods based on classical statistical methods applicable to independent random variables.

An important part of the analyzing data in the frequency domain, as well as the time domain, is the investigation and exploitation of the properties of the time-invariant ***linear filter***. This special linear transformation is used similarly to linear regression in conventional statistics, and we use many of the same terms in the time series context. We have previously mentioned the coherence as a measure of the relation between two series at a given frequency, and we show later that this coherence also measures the performance of the best linear filter relating the two series. Linear filtering can also be an important step in isolating a signal embedded in noise. For example, in Figure 1.9, the lower panel contains a signal contaminated with an additive noise, whereas the upper panel contains the pure signal. It might also be appropriate to ask whether a linear filter transformation exists that could be applied to the lower panel to produce a series closer to the signal in the upper panel. The use of filtering for reducing noise will also be a part of the presentation in this chapter. We emphasize, throughout, the analogy between filtering techniques and conventional linear regression.

## 3.2 Cyclical Behavior and Periodicity

We have already implicitly encountered the notion of periodicity in our example involving the SOI and Recruitment series in Figure 1.4. The rather regular oscillations of the series can also be noted by observing the periodicities in the autocorrelation function, as shown by Figure 1.13.

The general notion of periodicity can be made more precise by introducing some terminology. In order to define the rate at which a series oscillates, we first define a ***cycle*** as one complete period of a sine or cosine function defined over a time interval of length $2\pi$. For purposes of illustration, consider the periodic process

$$x_t = A \sin(2\pi\nu t + \phi) \tag{3.1}$$

for $t = 0, \pm 1, \pm 2, \ldots$, where $\nu$ is a frequency index, defined in cycles per unit time, and $A$ and $\phi$ are constants called parameters, with $A$ determining the height or ***amplitude*** of the function and $\phi$, called the ***phase***, determining the start point of the sine function. We can introduce random variation in this time series by allowing the amplitude and phase to vary randomly; a set of realizations will have different amplitudes, and the zero point of the sine function will vary. An alternate form of 3.1 is more convenient for time series modeling. Using the trigonometric identity

$$\sin(\alpha+\beta) = \sin(\alpha)\cos(\beta) + \cos(\alpha)\sin(\beta),$$

we obtain the alternate form

$$x_t = u_1 \sin(2\pi\nu t) + u_2 \cos(2\pi\nu t), \tag{3.2}$$

where $u_1 = A\cos\phi$ and $u_2 = A\sin\phi$ are transformed independent random variables, often taken to be normally distributed. Then, the amplitude and phase are defined as $A = \sqrt{u_1^2 + u_2^2}$ and $\phi = \tan^{-1}(u_2/u_1)$, respectively (see Problem 3.1).

The above random process is also a function of its ***frequency***, defined by the parameter $\nu$. The frequency is measured in cycles per unit time, or in cycles per point in the above illustration. For $\nu = 1$, the series makes one cycle per time unit; for $\nu = .50$, the series makes a cycle every two time units; for $\nu = .25$, every four units, and so on. In general, data that occurs at discrete time points will need at least two points to determine a cycle, so the highest frequency of interest is .5 cycles per point. This frequency is called the ***folding frequency*** and defines the highest frequency that can be seen using one point as the defining time unit. Higher frequencies sampled this way will appear at lower frequencies, called aliases; an example is the way a camera samples a rotating wheel on a moving automobile in a television commercial, in which the wheel appears to be rotating at a different rate.

Consider a generalization of (3.2) that allows mixtures of periodic series, with multiple frequencies and amplitudes.

$$x_t = \sum_{k=1}^{q} [u_{1k} \sin(2\pi\nu_k t) + u_{2k} \cos(2\pi\nu_k t)], \tag{3.3}$$

where $u_{k1}, u_{k2}$ are independent zero-mean random variables with variances $\sigma_k^2$ and frequencies $\nu_k$ for $k = 1, 2, \ldots, q$ component processes. Notice that (3.3) exhibits the process as a sum of independent components, with variance $\sigma_k^2$ for frequency $\nu_k$. The autocovariance function of the process is easily shown to be

$$\gamma(h) = \sum_{k=1}^{q} \sigma_k^2 \cos(2\pi\nu_k h), \tag{3.4}$$

and we note the autocovariance function is the sum of periodic components with weights proportional to the variances $\sigma_k^2$. Also, the mean square error $\gamma(0) = Ex_t^2 = \sum \sigma_k^2$ exhibits the overall variance as a sum of variances of each of the component parts.

**Example 3.1 A Periodic Random Series**

To this end, consider Figure 3.1, which shows the mixture (3.3) with $q = 2$, where $u_{11} = -1.67$, $u_{21} = -.43$, and $u_{12} = .29$, $u_{22} = .13$

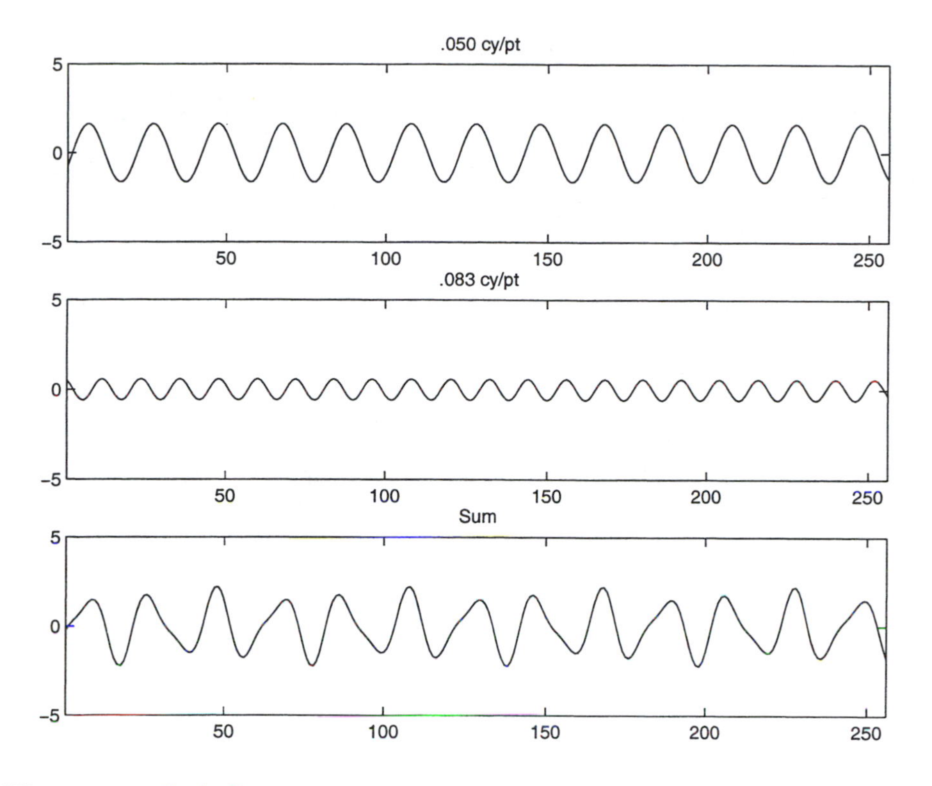


**Figure 3.1:** Periodic components with periods 20 and 12 points, respectively, and linear combination (bottom panel) corresponding to the model (3.3) with $q = 2$.

have been drawn from independent normal distributions with zero means and standard deviations $\sigma_1 = 1, \sigma_2 = .5$. The frequencies chosen were $\nu_1 = 1/20$ and $\nu_2 = 1/12$ cycles per point, respectively. Examining the plot shows that the first series makes a cycle every 20 points and the second series makes a cycle every 12 points; these latter values are the periods of the two components. Adding the two components together produces a sum in the bottom panel that begins to take on the character of an observed time series. Also, the lower amplitude of the higher frequency component, shown in the middle panel, causes the higher frequency to be obscured in the sum. The systematic sorting out of the essential frequency components in a time series, including their relative contributions, constitutes one of the main objectives of spectral analysis.

In order to illustrate different time scales, consider some of the examples given in the plots of Chapter 1. In Figure 1.1, the sampling rate is one point per quarter, so the seasonal fluctuation is at a frequency of .25 cycles per quarter or one cycle per year. The yearly average global temperature deviations of Figure

1.2 show no obvious frequencies, although we might argue for a low frequency cycle of about 50 years by looking at the detrended version in Figure 1.15. The speech recording in Figure 1.3 is sampled at 10,000 points per second. The SOI Index and fish populations, shown in Figure 1.4, are sampled monthly. For this data, we are primarily interested in a frequency scale over years, so a seasonal effect is at one cycle per year and the El Niño frequency is $\nu = 1/72$ cycles per month or $12/72 = .17$ cycles per year. In Figure 1.5, we have fMRI imaging data sampled at .5 points per second and the frequency of the stimulus is $1/32$ cycles per seconds and the process makes about eight cycles in 128 points, i.e., eight cycles in 256 seconds.

Clearly, many frequency scales will often coexist, depending on the nature of the problem. For simplicity, we keep the frequency at cycles per point and discuss the implications of certain frequencies in terms of the problem context. Of descriptive interest is the ***period*** of a time series, defined as the number of points in a cycle, i.e.,

$$T = \frac{1}{\nu}. \tag{3.5}$$

Hence, the period of the SOI index will be 72 or $72/12 = 6$ years if the estimated frequency is correct. The period of the earnings data of Figure 1.1 is 4 quarters, because the seasonal series makes a complete cycle in one year. If we are examining monthly data, a seasonal period of 12 months will often be present corresponding to the seasonal frequency of $\nu = 1/12$ cycles per month.

The representations of the process $x_t$ and autocovariance in (3.3) and (3.4) suggest the possibility of representing those two functions as linear combinations of periodic components with coefficients proportional to the variances of the separate components. We introduce the generalization of this notion in the next section and show how it relates to the spectral analysis of weakly stationary time series.

## 3.3 Power Spectrum and Cross-Spectrum

The idea that a time series is composed of periodic components, appearing in proportion to their underlying variances, is fundamental in the ***spectral representation*** of the autocovariance function, as given in Theorem 3.1 of Section T3.11. That result is applied to a weakly stationary process $x_t$, with autocovariance $\gamma(h) = E[(x_{t+h} - \mu)(x_t - \mu)]$ by noting that a monotone non-decreasing function $F(\nu)$ exists, called the ***spectral distribution function***, that is bounded for $-1/2 \le \nu \le 1/2$ with $F(-1/2) = 0, F(1/2) = \gamma(0)$ such that

$$\gamma(h) = \int_{-1/2}^{1/2} e^{2\pi i\nu h}\, dF(\nu). \tag{3.6}$$

We call $F(\nu)$ the spectral distribution function, by analogy with the conventional probability distribution function, even though the integral (for $h = 0$)

is $\gamma(0)$ rather than one. The spectral representation becomes less mysterious by noting the similar representation of the characteristic function in terms of the probability density in (1.118) of Chapter 1.

**Example 3.2 A Periodic Stationary Process**

For example, consider the periodic stationary random process given in (3.2), at a particular frequency $\nu_0$, say,

$$x_t = u_1 \sin(2\pi\nu_0 t) + u_2 \cos(2\pi\nu_0 t),$$

where $u_1$ and $u_2$ are independent zero-mean random variables with equal variance $\sigma^2$. The number of time periods needed for the above series to complete one cycle is exactly $1/\nu_0$, and the process makes exactly $\nu_0$ cycles per point for $t = 0, \pm 1, \pm 2, \ldots$. It is easily shown that

$$\begin{aligned} \gamma_x(h) &= \sigma^2 \cos(2\pi\nu_0 h) \\ &= \frac{\sigma^2}{2} e^{-2\pi i \nu_0 h} + \frac{\sigma^2}{2} e^{2\pi i \nu_0 h} \\ &= \int_{-1/2}^{1/2} e^{2\pi i \nu h} dF_x(\nu) \end{aligned}$$

using a Riemann–Stieltjes integration, where $F_x(\nu)$ is the function defined by

$$F_x(\nu) = \begin{cases} 0 & \nu < -\nu_0 \\ \sigma^2/2, & -\nu_0 \leq \nu < \nu_0 \\ \sigma^2, & \nu \geq \nu_0 \end{cases}$$

Clearly, defining the proper step function shows that the representation (3.6) holds in this case.

A more important situation we use repeatedly is the one covered by Theorem 3.2, where it is shown that, subject to absolute summmability of the autocovariance ($\sum |\gamma(h)| < \infty$), the spectral distribution function is absolutely continuous with $dF(\nu) = f(\nu)\, d\nu$, and the representation (3.6) becomes the motivation for the property given below.

***Property P3.1: Spectral Representation the Autocovariance Function of a Stationary Process***

*Any stationary process with autocovariance function $\gamma(h)$ satisfying*

$$\sum_{h=-\infty}^{\infty} |\gamma(h)| < \infty \tag{3.7}$$

*has the representation*

$$\gamma(h) = \int_{-1/2}^{1/2} e^{2\pi i\nu h} f(\nu)\, d\nu \quad h = 0, \pm 1, \pm 2, \ldots \tag{3.8}$$

*as the inverse transform of the* ***spectral density****, which has the representation*

$$f(\nu) = \sum_{h=-\infty}^{\infty} \gamma(h) e^{-2\pi i\nu h} \quad -1/2 \le \nu \le 1/2. \tag{3.9}$$

This spectral density is the analogue of the probability density function; the fact that $\gamma(h)$ is non-negative definite ensures $f(\nu) \ge 0$ for all $\nu$ (see Section T3.11, Theorem 3.1). In the case of a stationary process, it is easy to show $f(\nu) = f(-\nu)$ and $f(\nu + 1) = f(\nu)$, verifying the spectral density is an even function of period one. Also, at this point, we are focusing on the frequency $\nu$, expressed in cycles per point rather than the more common (in statistics) alternative $\lambda = 2\pi\nu$ that would give radians per point. Finally, the absolute summability condition is not satisfied by (3.4), the example that we have used to introduce the idea of a spectral representation.

The use of (3.8)and (3.9) as ***Fourier transform pairs*** is fundamental in the study of stationary discrete time processes. For a general function $a_t$ satisfying the absolute summability condition (3.7), a Fourier transform pair of the form

$$A(\nu) = \sum_{t=-\infty}^{\infty} a_t e^{-2\pi i\nu t} \tag{3.10}$$

and

$$a_t = \int_{-1/2}^{1/2} A(\nu) e^{2\pi i\nu t}\, d\nu \tag{3.11}$$

will exist and this relation is unique.

One immediate motivation for identifying the spectral density function with the variance of the process, $x_t$, at frequency $\nu$ is provided by noting that, from (3.8) with $h = 0$,

$$\gamma(0) = \text{var}(x_t) = \int_{-1/2}^{1/2} f(\nu)\, d\nu,$$

which expresses the total variance as the integrated spectral density over all of the frequencies. We show later on a linear transformation can isolate the variance in certain frequency intervals or ***bands***.

It is illuminating to examine the spectral density, as defined above, for the series that we have looked at in earlier discussions. In particular, Figure 3.2 shows sample realizations from the white noise of Example 1.7, the three-point moving average of Example 1.8, and the autoregressive model of Example 1.9.

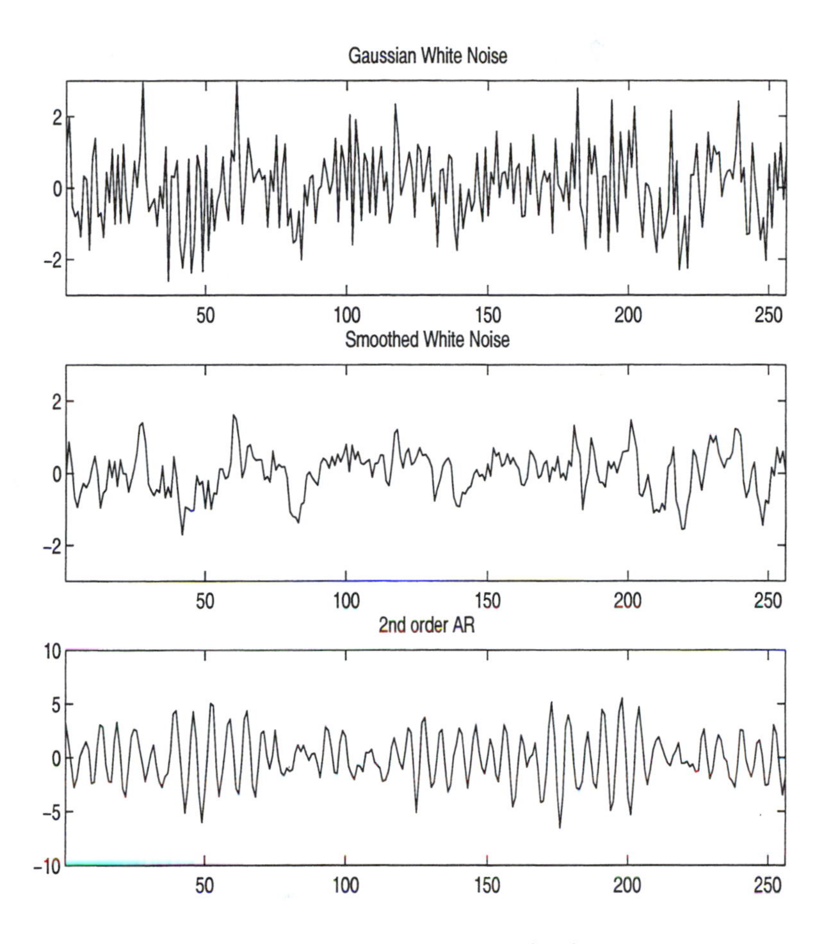


**Figure 3.2:** Sample realizations of white noise (top), smoothed white noise (middle), and a second order autoregressive process (bottom).

### Example 3.3 White Noise Series

As a simple example, consider the theoretical power spectrum of a sequence of independent, identically distributed random variables $w_t, t = 1, \ldots 256$, with zero means and equal variances $\sigma_w^2$. Because the autocovariance function was computed in Example 1.15 as $\gamma_w(h) = \sigma_w^2$ for $h = 0$ and zero, otherwise, it follows from (3.9) that

$$f_w(\nu) = \sigma_w^2$$

for $-1/2 \leq \nu \leq 1/2$ with the resulting equal power at all frequencies. This property is seen in the realization, which seems to contain all different frequencies in a roughly equal mix. In fact, the name ***white noise*** comes from the analogy to white light which contains all frequencies in the color spectrum. Figure 3.3 shows a plot of the white noise spectrum for $\sigma_w^2 = 1$.

### Example 3.4 A Simple Moving Average

A series that does not have an equal mix of frequencies is the smoothed white noise series shown in the middle panel of Figure 3.2. Specifically, we construct the three-point moving average series, defined by

$$y_t = \frac{1}{3}\big(w_{t-1} + w_t + w_{t+1}\big).$$

It is clear from the sample realization that the series has less of the higher or faster frequencies, and we calculate its power spectrum to verify this modification. We have previously computed the autocovariance of this process in Example 1.16, obtaining

$$\gamma_y(h) = \frac{\sigma_w^2}{9}\Big(3 - |h|\Big)$$

for $|h| \leq 2$ and $\gamma_y(h) = 0$ for $|h| > 2$. Then, using (3.8) gives

$$\begin{aligned} f_y(\nu) &= \sum_{h=-2}^{2} \gamma_y(h) \exp\{-2\pi\nu h\} \\ &= \frac{\sigma_w^2}{9}\big(e^{-4\pi i\nu} + e^{4\pi i\nu}\big) + \frac{2\sigma_w^2}{9}\big(e^{-2\pi i\nu} + e^{2\pi\nu}\big) + \frac{3\sigma_w^2}{9} \\ &= \frac{\sigma_w^2}{9}\big[3 + 4\cos(2\pi\nu) + 2\cos(4\pi\nu)\big]. \end{aligned}$$

Plotting the spectrum for $\sigma_w^2 = 1$, as in Figure 3.3, shows the lower frequencies near zero have greater power and the higher or faster frequencies, say, $\nu > .2$, tend to have less power.

### Example 3.5 A Second-Order Autoregressive Series

As a final example, we consider the spectrum of an AR(2) series of the form

$$x_t - \phi_1 x_{t-1} - \phi_2 x_{t-2} = w_t,$$

for the special case $\phi_1 = 1, \phi_2 = -.9, \sigma_w^2 = 1$ given in Example 1.9. The third panel in Figure 3.2 shows a sample realization of such a process, and a strong periodic component exists that makes a cycle about every five points. First, computing the autocovariance function of the left side and equating it to the autocovariance on the right yields

$$\begin{aligned}\gamma_w(h) &= E[(x_{t+h} - \phi_1 x_{t+h-1} - \phi_2 x_{t+h-2})(x_t - \phi_1 x_{t-1} - \phi_2 x_{t-2})] \\ &= [1 + \phi_1^2 + \phi_2^2]\gamma_x(h) + (\phi_1\phi_2 - \phi_1)[\gamma_x(h+1) + \gamma_x(h-1)] \\ &\quad -\phi_2[\gamma_x(h+2) + \gamma_x(h-2)] \\ &= 2.81\gamma_x(h) - 1.90[\gamma_x(h+1) + \gamma_x(h-1)] \\ &\quad +.90[\gamma_x(h+2) + \gamma_x(h-2)],\end{aligned}$$

where we have substituted the values of $\phi_1$ and $\phi_2$ in the equation. Now, substituting the spectral representation (3.8) in the above equation yields

$$\begin{aligned}\gamma_w(h) &= \int_{-1/2}^{1/2} [2.81 - 1.90(\mathrm{e}^{2\pi i\nu} + \mathrm{e}^{-2\pi i\nu}) \\ &\qquad +.90(\mathrm{e}^{4\pi i\nu} + \mathrm{e}^{-4\pi i\nu})]\ \mathrm{e}^{2\pi i\nu h} f_x(\nu) d\nu \\ &= \int_{-1/2}^{1/2} [2.81 - 3.80\cos(2\pi\nu) + 1.80\cos(4\pi\nu)]\ \mathrm{e}^{2\pi i\nu h} f_x(\nu)\ d\nu.\end{aligned}$$

The spectrum of the white noise process is just $\sigma_w^2$, and the uniqueness of the Fourier transform allows us to write

$$f_x(\nu) = \frac{\sigma_w^2}{2.81 - 3.80\cos(2\pi\nu) + 1.80\cos(4\pi\nu)}$$

as the spectrum of the autoregressive series. Figure 3.3 shows a strong power component at about $\nu = .16$ cycles per point or a period between six and seven cycles per point and very little power at other frequencies. In this case, modifying the white noise series by applying the second order AR operator has concentrated the power or variance of the resulting series in a very narrow frequency band.

The above examples have been given primarily to motivate the use of the power spectrum for describing the theoretical variance fluctuations of a stationary time series. Indeed, the interpretation of the spectral density function as the variance of the time series over a given frequency band gives us the intuitive explanation for its physical meaning. The plot of the function $f(\nu)$ over the frequency argument $\nu$ can even be thought of as an ***analysis of variance***, in which the columns or block effects are the frequencies, indexed by $\nu$.

The notion of analyzing frequency fluctuations using classical statistical ideas extends to the case in which there are several jointly stationary series, for example, $x_t$ and $y_t$, In this case, we can introduce the idea of a correlation indexed by frequency, called the ***coherence***. The results in Section T3.11 imply the covariance function

$$\gamma_{xy}(h) = E[(x_{t+h} - \mu_x)(y_t - \mu_y)]$$

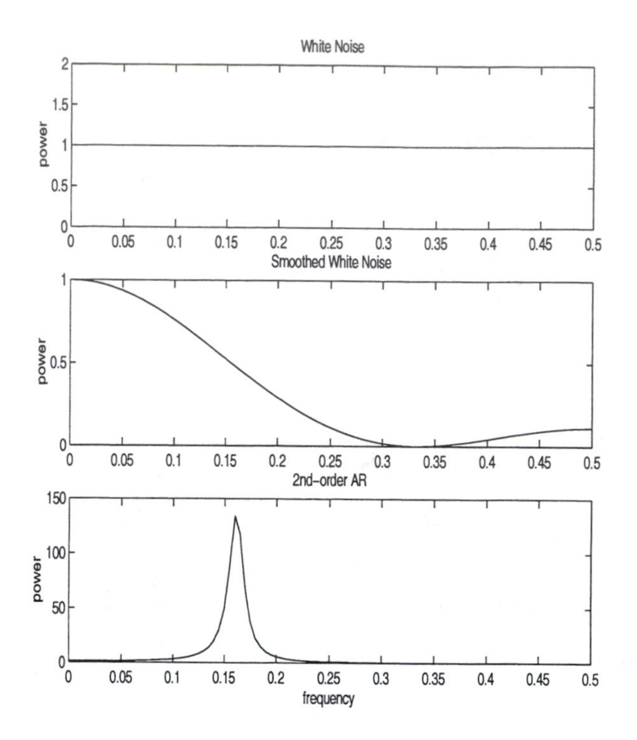


**Figure 3.3:** Theoretical spectra of white noise (top), smoothed white noise (middle), and a second-order autoregressive process (bottom).

has the representation

$$\gamma_{xy}(h) = \int_{-1/2}^{1/2} f_{xy}(\nu) e^{2\pi i\nu h} \, d\nu \quad h = 0, \pm 1, \pm 2, ..., \tag{3.12}$$

where the ***cross-spectrum*** is defined as the Fourier transform

$$f_{xy}(\nu) = \sum_{h=-\infty}^{\infty} \gamma_{xy}(h) \; e^{-2\pi i\nu h} \qquad -1/2 \leq \nu \leq 1/2, \tag{3.13}$$

assuming that the cross-covariance function is absolutely summable, as was the case for the autocovariance. The cross-spectrum is generally a complex-valued function, and writing out the exponential part using the identity

$$e^{-ix} = \cos(x) - i\sin(x)$$

yields

$$f_{xy}(\nu) = c_{xy}(\nu) - iq_{xy}(\nu), \tag{3.14}$$

where

$$c_{xy}(\nu) = \sum_{h=-\infty}^{\infty} \gamma_{xy}(h) \; \cos(2\pi\nu h) \tag{3.15}$$

and

$$q_{xy}(\nu) = \sum_{h=-\infty}^{\infty} \gamma_{xy}(h) \ \sin(2\pi\nu h) \tag{3.16}$$

are defined as the ***cospectrum*** and ***quadspectrum***, respectively. Because $\gamma_{yx}(h) = \gamma_{xy}(-h)$, it follows, by substituting into (3.13) and rearranging, that

$$f_{yx}(\nu) = \overline{f_{xy}(\nu)}, \tag{3.17}$$

where $\overline{z}$ denotes the complex conjugate; that is, $z = x + iy, \overline{z} = x - iy$. This result, in turn, implies that the cospectrum and quadspectrum satisfy

$$c_{yx}(\nu) = c_{xy}(\nu) \tag{3.18}$$

and

$$q_{yx}(\nu) = -q_{xy}(\nu). \tag{3.19}$$

An important example of the application of the cross-spectrum is to the problem of predicting an output series $y_t$ from some input series $x_t$ through a linear filter relation such as the three-point moving average considered below. A measure of the strength of such a relation is the ***squared coherence*** function, defined as

$$\rho^2_{y\cdot x}(\nu) = \frac{|f_{yx}(\nu)|^2}{f_x(\nu) f_y(\nu)}. \tag{3.20}$$

Although we consider a more general form of this that applies to multiple inputs later, it is instructive to display the single input case as (3.20) to emphasize the analogy with conventional squared correlation, which takes the form

$$\rho^2_{yx} = \frac{\sigma^2_{yx}}{\sigma^2_x \sigma^2_y},$$

for random variables with variances $\sigma^2_x$ and $\sigma^2_y$ and covariance $\sigma_{yx} = \sigma_{xy}$. This motivates the interpretation of squared coherence and the squared correlation between two time series at frequency $\nu$.

### Example 3.6 Cross-Spectrum and Coherence of a Process and a Three-point Moving Average

As a simple example, we compute the cross-spectrum between $x_t$ and the three-point moving average $y_t = (x_{t-1} + x_t + x_{t+1})/3$, where $x_t$ is a stationary input process with spectral density $f_x(\nu)$. First,

$$\begin{aligned} \gamma_{xy}(h) &= E[x_{t+h} y_t] \\ &= \frac{1}{3} E[x_{t+h}(x_{t-1} + x_t + x_{t+1})] \\ &= \frac{1}{3}\Big(\gamma_x(h+1) + \gamma_x(h) + \gamma_x(h-1)\Big) \end{aligned}$$

$$= \frac{1}{3} \int_{-1/2}^{1/2} (e^{2\pi i\nu} + 1 + e^{-2\pi i\nu}) f_x(\nu) \, d\nu$$
$$= \frac{1}{3} \int_{-1/2}^{1/2} [1 + 2\cos(2\pi\nu)] f_x(\nu) e^{2\pi i\nu h} \, d\nu.$$

Using the uniqueness of the Fourier transform we argue from the spectral representation (3.12) that the above must be the transform of $f_{xy}(\nu)$, implying that

$$f_{xy}(\nu) = \frac{1}{3} \, [1 + \cos(2\pi\nu)] \, f_x(\nu)$$

so that the cross-spectrum is real in this case. From Example 3.4, the spectral density of $y_t$ is

$$\begin{aligned} f_y(\nu) &= \frac{1}{9}[3 + 4\cos(2\pi\nu) + 2\cos(4\pi\nu)] f_x(\nu) \\ &= \frac{1}{9} \, [1 + 2\cos(2\pi\nu)]^2 \, f_x(\nu), \end{aligned}$$

using the identity $\cos(2\alpha) = 2\cos^2(\alpha) - 1$ in the last step. Substituting into (3.20) yields the squared coherence between $x_t$ and $y_t$ as unity over all frequencies. This is a characteristic inherited by more general linear filters, as will be shown in Problem 3.22. However, if some noise is added to the three-point moving average, the coherence is not unity; these kinds of models will be considered in detail later.

***Property P3.2: Spectral Representation of a Vector Stationary Process***

*Any $p \times 1$ stationary process, $\boldsymbol{x}_t = (x_{t1}, x_{t2}, \ldots, x_{tp})'$, with the elements of the autocovariance matrix*

$$\Gamma(h) = E[(\boldsymbol{x}_{t+h} - \boldsymbol{\mu})(\boldsymbol{x}_t - \boldsymbol{\mu})']$$

*satisfying*

$$\sum_{h=-\infty}^{\infty} |\gamma_{jk}(h)| < \infty \tag{3.21}$$

*for all $j, k = 1, \ldots, p$ has the representation*

$$\Gamma(h) = \int_{-1/2}^{1/2} e^{2\pi i\nu h} \, f(\nu) \, d\nu \quad h = 0, \pm1, \pm2, \ldots, \tag{3.22}$$

*as the inverse transform of the **spectral density matrix**, $f(\nu) = \{f_{jk}(\nu)\}, j, k = 1, \ldots, p$, with elements equal to the cross-spectral components. The matrix $f(\nu)$ has the representation*

$$f(\nu) = \sum_{h=-\infty}^{\infty} \Gamma(h) e^{-2\pi i\nu h} \quad -1/2 \le \nu \le 1/2. \tag{3.23}$$

**Example 3.7 Spectral Matrix of a Bivariate Process**

Consider a jointly stationary bivariate process $(x_t, y_t)$. We arrange the autocovariances in the matrix

$$\Gamma(h) = \begin{pmatrix} \gamma_x(h) & \gamma_{xy}(h) \\ \gamma_{yx}(h) & \gamma_y(h) \end{pmatrix},$$

where, for simplicity of notation, we will often suppress the second subscript, as when we write $\gamma_x(h)$ instead of $\gamma_{xx}(h)$. The spectral matrix would be given by

$$f(\nu) = \begin{pmatrix} f_x(\nu) & f_{xy}(\nu) \\ f_{yx}(\nu) & f_y(\nu) \end{pmatrix},$$

where the Fourier transform (3.22) and (3.23) relate the autocovariance and spectral matrices.

## 3.4 Linear Filters

Some of the examples of the previous section have hinted at the possibility the distribution of power or variance in a time series can be modified by making a linear transformation. In this section, we explore that notion further by defining a ***linear filter*** and showing how it can be used to extract signals from a time series. The linear filter modifies the spectral characteristics of a time series in a predictable way, and the systematic development of methods for taking advantage of the special properties of linear filters is an important topic in time series analysis.

A linear filter uses a set of specified coefficients $a_t$, for $t = 0, \pm 1, \pm 2 \ldots$, to smooth a stationary ***input series***, $x_t$, producing an ***output series***, $y_t$, of the form

$$y_t = \sum_{r=-\infty}^{\infty} a_r x_{t-r}. \tag{3.24}$$

The form (3.24) is also called a ***convolution*** in some statistical contexts. The coefficients, collectively called the ***impulse response function***, are required to satisfy absolute summability

$$\sum_{t=-\infty}^{\infty} |a_t| < \infty, \tag{3.25}$$

so (3.24) exists as a limit in mean square and the infinite Fourier transform

$$A(\nu) = \sum_{t=-\infty}^{\infty} a_t \exp\{-2\pi i \nu t\}, \tag{3.26}$$

called the ***frequency response function*** , is well defined. We have already encountered a simple linear filter in Example 3.4. For example, the simple three-point moving average can be put into the form of (3.24) by letting $a_{-1} = a_0 = a_1 = 1/3$ and taking $a_t = 0$ for $|t| \geq 2$.

The importance of the linear filter stems from its ability to enhance certain parts of the spectrum of the input series. To see this, the autocovariance function of the filtered output (3.24) can be derived as

$$\begin{aligned}
\gamma_y(h) &= E[(y_{t+h} - Ey_{t+h})(y_t - Ey_t)] \\
&= E\left[\sum_r \sum_s a_r(x_{t+h-r} - \mu)(x_{t-s} - \mu)a_s\right] \\
&= \sum_r \sum_s a_r \gamma_x(h - r + s)a_s \\
&= \sum_r \sum_s a_r \left[\int_{-1/2}^{1/2} e^{2\pi i\nu(h-r+s)} f_x(\nu) d\nu\right] a_s \\
&= \int_{-1/2}^{1/2} \left(\sum_r a_r e^{-2\pi i\nu r}\right)\left(\sum_s a_s e^{2\pi i\nu s}\right) e^{2\pi i\nu h} f_x(\nu)\, d\nu \\
&= \int_{-1/2}^{1/2} e^{2\pi i\nu h} |A(\nu)|^2 f_x(\nu)\, d\nu,
\end{aligned}$$

where we have first replaced $\gamma_x(\cdot)$ by its representation (3.8) and then substituted $A(\nu)$ from (3.26). The computation is one we do repeatedly, exploiting the uniqueness of the Fourier transform. Now, because the left-hand side is the Fourier transform of the spectral density of the output, say, $f_y(\nu)$, we get the important multivariate filtering property as follows.

***Property P3.3: Output Spectrum of a Linearly Filtered Stationary Series***

*The spectrum of the filtered output $y_t$ in (3.24) is related to the spectrum of the input $x_t$ by*

$$f_y(\nu) = |A(\nu)|^2 \; f_x(\nu), \tag{3.27}$$

*where the frequency response function $A(\nu)$ is defined in (3.26).*

The result (3.27) enables us to calculate the exact effect on the spectrum of any given filtering operation. This important property shows the spectrum of the input series is changed by filtering and the effect of the change can be characterized as a frequency-by-frequency multiplication by the squared magnitude of the frequency response function. Again, an obvious analogy to a property of the variance in classical statistics holds, namely, if $x$ is a random variable with variance $\sigma_x^2$, $y = ax$ will have variance $\sigma_y^2 = a^2\sigma_x^2$, so the variance of the linearly transformed random variable is changed by multiplication by $a^2$ in much the same way as the linearly filtered spectrum is changed in (3.27).

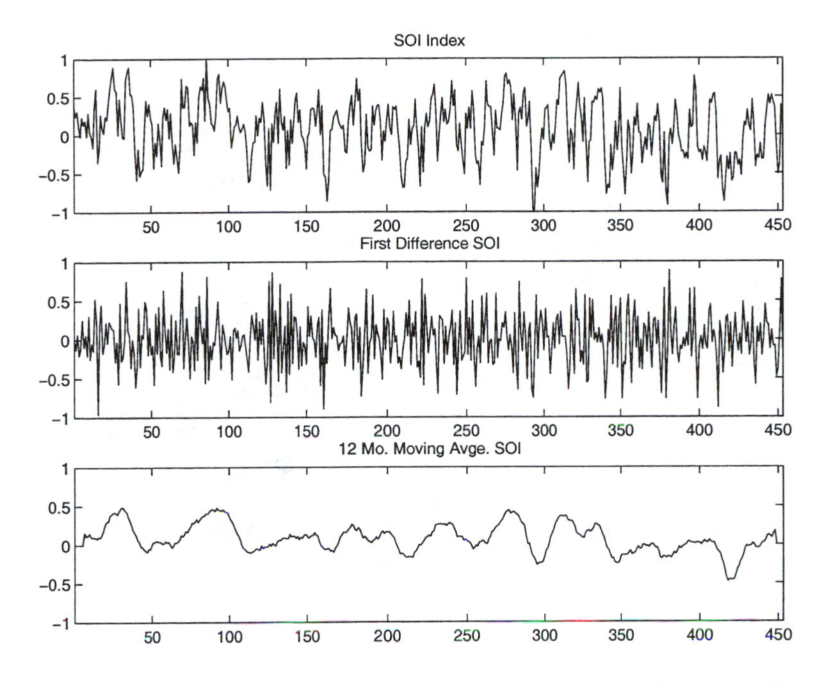


**Figure 3.4:** SOI Index (top) compared to the differenced SOI (middle) and a centered 12-month moving average (bottom).

### Example 3.8 First Difference and Moving Average Filters

We illustrate the effect of filtering with two common examples, the first difference filter

$$\nabla x_t = x_t - x_{t-1}$$

and the symmetric moving average filter

$$y_t = \frac{1}{24}\big(x_{t-6} + x_{t+6}\big) + \frac{1}{12}\sum_{r=-5}^{5} x_{t-r}.$$

We take this form of the moving average filter because it gives equal weight to both sides of the center. The results of filtering the SOI series, first discussed in Example 1.4, using the two filters are shown in the middle and bottom panels of Figure 3.4. Notice that the effect of differencing is to roughen the series because it tends to retain the higher or faster frequencies. The centered moving average smoothes the series because it retains the lower frequencies and tends to attenuate the higher frequencies. In general, differencing is an example of a ***high-pass filter*** because it retains or passes the higher frequencies, whereas the moving average is a ***low-pass filter*** because it passes the lower or slower frequencies. Notice that 72-month periods are enhanced in the symmetric moving average and the seasonal or yearly frequencies are attenuated. The 72-month period is associated with El Ninõ, and the moving average filter tends to enhance or ***extract*** that signal.

Now, having done the filtering, it is essential to determine the exact way in which the filters change the input spectrum. We shall use (3.26) and (3.27) for this purpose. The first difference filter can be written in the form (3.24) by letting $a_0 = 1, a_1 = -1$, and $a_r = 0$ otherwise. This implies that

$$A(\nu) = 1 - e^{-2\pi i\nu},$$

and the squared frequency response becomes

$$\begin{aligned} |A(\nu)|^2 &= (1 - e^{-2\pi i\nu})(1 - e^{2\pi i\nu}) \\ &= 2[1 - \cos(2\pi\nu)]. \end{aligned} \tag{3.28}$$

The top panel of Figure 3.5 shows that the first difference filter will attenuate the lower frequencies and enhance the higher frequencies since the multiplier of the spectrum, say $|A(\nu)|^2$, is large for the higher frequencies and small for the lower frequencies. Generally, the slow rise of this kind of filter does not particularly recommend it as a procedure for retaining only the high frequencies.

For the centered 12-month moving average, we can take $a_{-6} = a_6 = 1/24$, $a_k = 1/12$ for $-5 \leq k \leq 5$ and $a_k = 0$ elsewhere. Substituting and recognizing the cosine terms gives

$$A(\nu) = \frac{1}{12}[1 + \cos(12\pi\nu) + 2\sum_{k=1}^{5}\cos(2\pi\nu k)]. \tag{3.29}$$

Plotting the squared frequency response of this function as in Figure 3.5 shows that we can expect this filter to cut most of the frequency content above .05 cycles per point. This corresponds to eliminating periods shorter than $T = 1/.05 = 20$ points. In particular, this drives down the yearly components with periods of $T = 12$ months and enhances the El Niño frequency, which is somewhat lower. The filter is not completely efficient at attenuating high frequencies; some power contributions are left at higher frequencies, as shown in the function $|A(\nu)|^2$ and in the filtered series in Figure 3.4. The question arises as to whether or not it is possible to develop a filter capable of making a sharper cutoff is answered in the affirmative later in the next section.

The two filters discussed in the previous example were slightly different in that the frequency response function of the first difference was complex-valued, whereas the frequency response of the moving average was purely real.

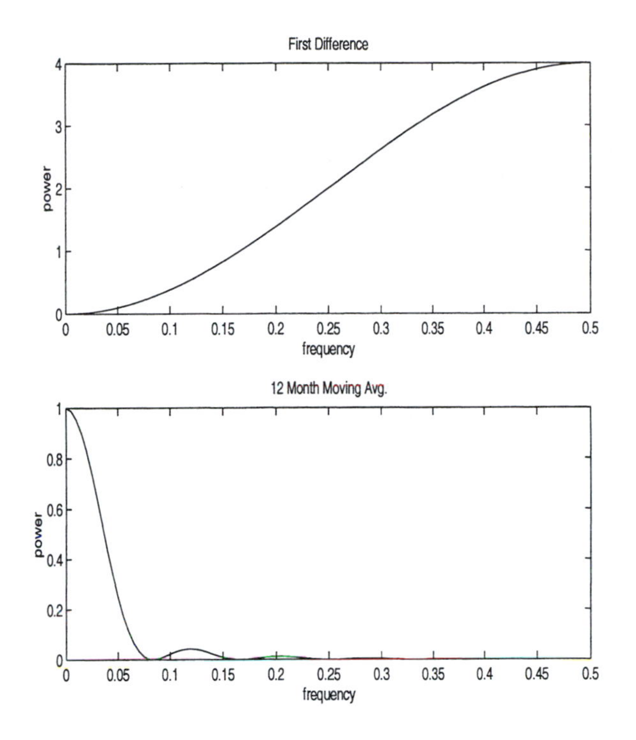


**Figure 3.5:** Squared frequency response functions of the first difference and 12-month moving average filters.

A short derivation similar to that used to verify (3.27) shows, when $x_t$ and $y_t$ are related by the linear filter relation (3.24), the cross-spectrum satisfies

$$f_{yx}(\nu) = A(\nu) f_x(\nu),$$

so the frequency response is of the form

$$A(\nu) = \frac{f_{yx}(\nu)}{f_x(\nu)} \tag{3.30}$$

$$= \frac{c_{yx}(\nu)}{f_x(\nu)} - i\frac{q_{yx}(\nu)}{f_x(\nu)}, \tag{3.31}$$

where we have used (3.14) to get the last form. Then, we may write (3.31) in complex form as

$$A(\nu) = |A(\nu)| \ \exp\{-i \ \phi_{yx}(\nu)\}, \tag{3.32}$$

where the ***amplitude*** and ***phase*** of the filter are defined by

$$|A(\nu)| = \frac{\sqrt{c_{yx}^2(\nu) + q_{yx}^2(\nu)}}{f_x(\nu)} \tag{3.33}$$

and

$$\phi_{yx}(\nu) = \tan^{-1}\left(-\frac{q_{yx}(\nu)}{c_{yx}(\nu)}\right). \tag{3.34}$$

A simple interpretation of the phase of a linear filter is that it represents the time delays as a function of frequency in the same way as the spectrum is a measure of the variance as a function of frequency. Additional insight can be gained by considering the simple delaying filter

$$y_t = Ax_{t-D},$$

where the series gets replaced by a version, amplified by multiplying by $A$ and delayed by $D$ points. For this case,

$$f_{yx}(\nu) = A\mathrm{e}^{-2\pi i\nu D} f_x(\nu),$$

and the amplitude is $|A|$, and the phase is

$$\phi_{yx}(\nu) = -2\pi\nu D,$$

or just a linear function of frequency $\nu$. For this case, applying a simple time delay causes frequency delays that depend on the frequency of the periodic component being delayed. Interpretation is further enhanced by setting $x_t = \cos(2\pi\nu t)$, in which case $y_t = A\cos(2\pi\nu t - 2\pi\nu D)$. Thus, the output series, $y_t$, has the same period as the input series, $x_t$, but the amplitude of the output has increased by a factor of $|A|$ and the phase has been changed by a factor of $-2\pi\nu D$.

### Example 3.9 Amplitude and Phase of Difference and Moving Average

We consider calculating the amplitude and phase of the two filters discussed in Example 3.8. The case for the moving average is easy since $A(\nu)$ given in (3.29) is purely real. So, amplitude is just $|A(\nu)|$ and the phase is $\phi_{yx}(\nu) = 0$; the symmetric ($a_t = a_{-t}$) filters always have zero phase. The first difference, however, changes this, as we might expect from the example above involving the time delay filter. In this case, the squared amplitude is given in (3.28). To compute the phase, we write

$$\begin{aligned}
A(\nu) &= 1 - \mathrm{e}^{-2\pi i\nu} \\
&= \mathrm{e}^{-i\pi\nu}(e^{i\pi\nu} - e^{-i\pi\nu}) \\
&= 2i\mathrm{e}^{-i\pi\nu}\sin(\pi\nu) \\
&= 2\sin^2(\pi\nu) + 2i\cos(\pi\nu)\sin(\pi\nu) \\
&= c_{yx}(\nu) - iq_{yx}(\nu),
\end{aligned}$$

so

$$\phi_{yx}(\nu) = \tan^{-1}\left(-\frac{q_{yx}(\nu)}{c_{yx}(\nu)}\right) = \tan^{-1}\left(\frac{\cos(\pi\nu)}{\sin(\pi\nu)}\right).$$

Noting that

$$\cos(\pi\nu) = \sin(-\pi\nu + \pi/2)$$

and that

$$\sin(\pi\nu) = \cos(-\pi\nu + \pi/2),$$

we get

$$\phi_{yx}(\nu) = -\pi\nu + \pi/2,$$

and the phase is again a linear function of frequency.

The above tendency of the frequencies to arrive at different times in the filtered version of the series remains as one of two annoying features of the difference type filters. The other weakness is the gentle increase in the frequency response function. If low frequencies are really unimportant and high frequencies are to be preserved, we would like to have a somewhat sharper response than is obvious in Figure 3.5. Similarly, if low frequencies are important and high frequencies are not, the moving average filters are also not very efficient at passing the low frequencies and attenuating the high frequencies. Improvement is possible by using longer filters, obtained by approximations to the infinite inverse Fourier transform. From the transform pair (3.10) and (3.11), the relationship

$$a_t = \int_{-1/2}^{1/2} A(\nu)\mathrm{e}^{2\pi i\nu t}d\nu \quad t = 0, \pm1, \pm2, ... \tag{3.35}$$

shows if (3.35) can be evaluated in closed form, we know exactly what the sequence $\{a_t\}$ should be for a given desired $A(\nu)$. Unfortunately, we cannot extend the data indefinitely to compute the exact filter $\{a_t\}$, and the integral (3.35) will rarely be computable in closed form. The construction of useful finite approximations to the filter output is a problem in ***filter design*** which we discuss further in Sections 3.8 and 3.9.

We will occasionally use results for multivariate series $\boldsymbol{x}_t = (x_{t1}, \dots, x_{tp})'$ that are comparable to the simple property shown in (3.27). Consider the ***matrix filter***

$$\boldsymbol{y}_t = \sum_{r=-\infty}^{\infty} A_r \boldsymbol{x}_{t-r}, \tag{3.36}$$

where $\{A_r\}$ denotes a sequence of $q \times p$ matrices such that $\sum_{r=-\infty}^{\infty} ||A_r|| < \infty$, $\boldsymbol{x}_t = (x_{t1}, \dots, x_{tp})'$ is a $p \times 1$ stationary vector process with mean vector $\boldsymbol{\mu}_x$

and $p \times p$, matrix covariance function $\Gamma_x(h)$ and spectral matrix $f_x(\nu)$, and $\boldsymbol{y}_t$ is the $q \times 1$ vector output process. Then, we can obtain the following property.

***Property P3.4: Output Spectral Matrix of a Linearly Filtered Stationary Vector Series***
*The spectral matrix of the filtered output $\boldsymbol{y}_t$ in (3.36) is related to the spectrum of the input $\boldsymbol{x}_t$ by*

$$f_y(\nu) = \mathcal{A}(\nu) f_x(\nu) \mathcal{A}^*(\nu), \tag{3.37}$$

*where the matrix frequency response function $\mathcal{A}(\nu)$ is defined by*

$$\mathcal{A}(\nu) = \sum_{t=-\infty}^{\infty} A_t \exp(-2\pi i \nu t). \tag{3.38}$$

We will often use the notation $\mathcal{A}^*$ to denote the ***complex conjugate transpose*** $\overline{\mathcal{A}}'$, that is, the result of replacing each element of $\mathcal{A}$ by its complex conjugate and transposing the resulting matrix.

## 3.5 Discrete Fourier Transform, Periodogram

The theory that lead to the spectral density as the Fourier transform of the autocovariance function and to its interpretation as variance components depending on frequency suggests two possible paths for dealing with sample data. One suggested approach, developed in early references, such as Blackman and Tukey (1959), uses the representation (3.9) to suggest an estimator of the form

$$\widehat{f}(\nu) = \sum_{h=-(n-1)}^{(n-1)} \widehat{\gamma}(h) \exp\{-2\pi i \nu h\}, \tag{3.39}$$

where $\widehat{\gamma}(h)$ is just the sample autocovariance function defined in Chapter 1, namely,

$$\widehat{\gamma}(h) = n^{-1} \sum_{t=1}^{n-h} (x_{t+h} - \bar{x})(x_t - \bar{x}), \tag{3.40}$$

with $\widehat{\gamma}(-h) = \widehat{\gamma}(h)$. Replacing the autocovariance function by a tapered version, obtained by multiplying $\widehat{\gamma}(h)$ point by point by some weight function or ***taper*** $w(h)$ was used to improve the properties of the spectral estimator.

An alternative but closely related way of thinking about estimating the spectral density uses the idea that the spectrum is essentially the variance at a given frequency so that we might get useful information about the magnitude of that variance by isolating the frequency component. Hence, we might propose enhancing the periodic component in a time series at frequency $\nu$ by matching or correlating the series against periodic sine and cosine functions at some frequency $\nu$ of interest that we will term the ***probe frequency***. In fact, the ***sine and cosine transforms*** at frequency $\nu_k$

$$X_c(\nu_k) = n^{-1/2} \sum_{t=1}^{n} x_t \cos(2\pi\nu_k t) \tag{3.41}$$

and

$$X_s(\nu_k) = n^{-1/2} \sum_{t=1}^{n} x_t \sin(2\pi\nu_k t) \tag{3.42}$$

should be large when the series contains probe frequency $\nu_k$ and should be small otherwise. It will be seen later that the best choice for the frequency scale means choosing frequencies of the form $\nu_k = k/n$ for $k = 0, 1, \ldots, n-1$ in (3.41) and (3.42). Because of their special role, frequencies of the form $\nu_k = k/n$ are called ***fundamental*** or ***Fourier frequencies***. As it turns out, both the sine and cosine transforms are needed to detect frequencies arriving at different delays. In addition, the quantities (3.41) and (3.42) will not be strictly positive, so a squaring operation seems to make sense. These two features suggest measuring the power or variance in a series in terms of a squared function, called the ***periodogram***, that was introduced by Schuster (1906) for studying the periodicities in the sunspot series (shown in Figure 3.20). The periodogram

$$I(\nu_k) = X_c^2(\nu_k) + X_s^2(\nu_k) \tag{3.43}$$

measures the sample variance or power at the frequency $\nu_k$.

### Example 3.10 Periodogram of the Periodic Random Series

As an example, consider the periodic random series of Example 3.1, where random sines and cosines with frequencies $\nu = 1/20$, $1/12$ cycles per point were mixed and added together. In Figure 3.6, we show the cosine transforms, (3.41), the sine transforms, (3.42), and the periodograms, (3.43), as a function of the probe frequencies $\nu_k = k/256$ for $k = 0, 1, \ldots, 64$. The cosine transform enhances the primary cycle at 20 points whereas the sine transform enhances both primary cycle and the secondary 12-point cycle. The periodogram shows both kinds of cycles and has peaks at $\nu = .0508$ (13/256) and $\nu = .0820$ (21/256) cycles per point, or at periods of $T = 19.69$ and $T = 12.19$ points, which are the closest frequencies of the form $\nu_k = k/256$ to the input values. The peak values in the periodogram are 149 and 14, respectively, so the power of the primary periodic component at 20 points is about 10 times that of the secondary one at 12 points. Clearly, the periodogram shows the small secondary component, which is well hidden in the original series. Some

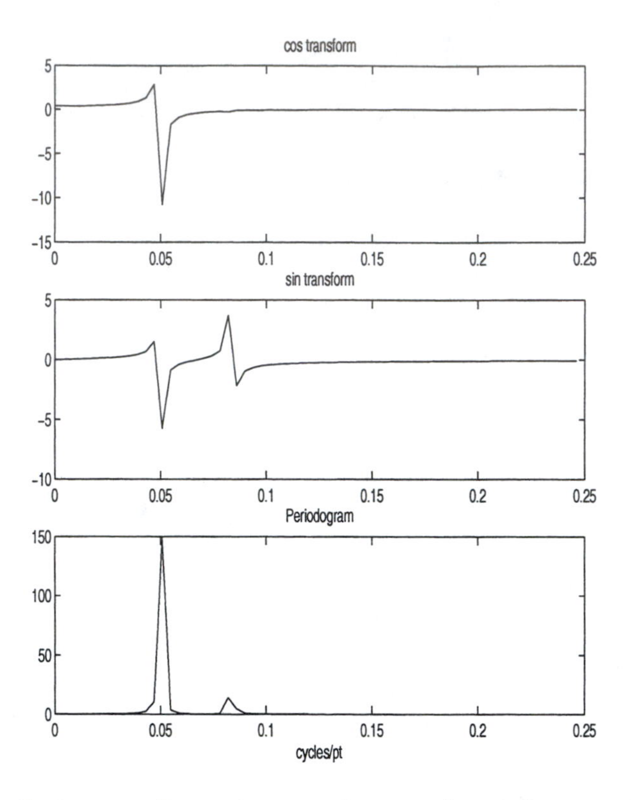


**Figure 3.6:** Cosine transform, sine transform, and periodogram of a periodic random series.

variance is evident at adjacent frequencies; in particular at $T = 21.33$ points, the value of the periodogram is 10 and at $T = 11.64$ points, the value is around five. Other values outside the immediate neighborhood of the input frequencies are essentially zero.

Now, it will be convenient to write the periodogram in terms of the ***discrete Fourier transform (DFT)***, defined as

$$X(\nu_k) = n^{-1/2} \sum_{t=1}^{n} x_t e^{-2\pi i \nu_k t} \tag{3.44}$$

with $\nu_k = k/n$ for $k = 0, 1, \ldots, n-1$. Because $e^{-ix} = \cos(x) - i\sin(x)$, it is immediate that

$$X(\nu_k) = X_c(\nu_k) - iX_s(\nu_k), \tag{3.45}$$

so the DFT is a complex random variable, with real and imaginary parts proportional to the sine and cosine transforms of the original series, as defined by (3.41) and (3.42). It is then possible to write the periodogram in the form

$$I(\nu_k) = |X(\nu_k)|^2. \tag{3.46}$$

A further simple calculation (see Problem 3.12) shows also that $I(\nu_k)$ is equal to the estimator (3.39), based on the spectral representation results.

Sometimes it is helpful to exploit the inversion result for DFTs which shows the linear transformation is one-to-one. We have

$$x_t = n^{-1/2} \sum_{k=1}^{n} X(\nu_k) e^{2\pi i \nu_k t} \tag{3.47}$$

for $t = 1, \ldots, n$. Because $X(1/2 + \nu_k) = \overline{1/2 - X(1 - \nu_k)}$, the transformation is one-to one, relating $x_1, x_2, \ldots x_n$ to $X_c(0), X_c(\nu_1), \ldots, X_c(1/2), X_s(1), \ldots, X_s(1/2 - 1/n)$. The inversion formula can be shown by replacing $X(\nu_k)$ in (3.47) by the basic definition in (3.44) and then using the orthogonality result

$$\sum_{t=1}^{n} e^{\pm 2\pi i k t/n} = \begin{cases} n, & k = \ell n;\ \ell = 0, \pm 1, \pm 2, \ldots, \\ 0, & \text{otherwise} \end{cases} \tag{3.48}$$

which follows from the finite sum result

$$\sum_{t=1}^{n} z^t = \begin{cases} \frac{z(1-z^n)}{(1-z)}, & z \neq 1 \\ n, & z = 1. \end{cases} \tag{3.49}$$

Working with the discrete Fourier transform offers some distinct advantages from both the computational and statistical points of view. For example, there are extremely fast computer algorithms (Cooley and Tukey, 1965) available for calculating $X(\nu_k)$ for all values of $\nu_k$. Such algorithms are known as ***fast Fourier transforms (FFT's)***.

From the standpoint of estimating the spectrum $f(\nu)$, we tend to focus on the periodogram (3.43) form rather than the Fourier transform of the autocovariance function given by (3.39), because the random variables $X_c(\nu_k)$ and $X_s(\nu_k)$ have some convenient statistical properties, which we derive in Section 3.11. In the first place, if $x_t$ is a normal time series, the sine and cosine transforms will also be jointly normal, because they are just linear combinations of the jointly normal random variables $x_1, x_2, \ldots, x_n$. In that case, the assumption that the covariance function satisfies the condition

$$\theta = \sum_{h=-\infty}^{\infty} |h||\gamma(h)| < \infty \tag{3.50}$$

is enough to obtain simple large sample approximations for the variances and covariances. First, the variances and covariances of the sine and cosine transforms at two different frequencies $\nu_k$ and $\nu_\ell$ can be derived as

$$\text{cov}[X_c(\nu_k), X_c(\nu_\ell)] = n^{-1} \sum_{s=1}^{n} \sum_{t=1}^{n} \gamma(s-t) \cos(2\pi \nu_k s) \cos(2\pi \nu_\ell t), \tag{3.51}$$

$$\text{cov}[X_c(\nu_k), X_s(\nu_\ell)] = n^{-1} \sum_{s=1}^{n} \sum_{t=1}^{n} \gamma(s-t) \cos(2\pi\nu_k s) \sin(2\pi\nu_\ell t), \tag{3.52}$$

and

$$\text{cov}[X_s(\nu_k), X_s(\nu_\ell)] = n^{-1} \sum_{s=1}^{n} \sum_{t=1}^{n} \gamma(s-t) \sin(2\pi\nu_k s) \sin(2\pi\nu_\ell t), \tag{3.53}$$

where the variance terms are obtained by setting $\nu_k = \nu_\ell$ in (3.51) and (3.53). In Section T3.12, we show the terms in (3.51)-(3.53) have interesting properties under assumption (3.50), namely,

$$\text{cov}[X_c(\nu_k), X_c(\nu_\ell)] = \begin{cases} f(\nu_k)/2 + \epsilon_n, & \nu_k = \nu_\ell \\ \epsilon_n, & \nu_k \neq \nu_\ell \end{cases} \tag{3.54}$$

$$\text{cov}[X_s(\nu_k), X_s(\nu_\ell)] = \begin{cases} f(\nu_k)/2 + \epsilon_n, & \nu_k = \nu_\ell \\ \epsilon_n, & \nu_k \neq \nu_\ell \end{cases} \tag{3.55}$$

and

$$\text{cov}[X_c(\nu_k), X_s(\nu_\ell)] = \epsilon_n, \tag{3.56}$$

where the error term $\epsilon_n$ in the approximations can be bounded,

$$|\epsilon_n| \leq \theta/n, \tag{3.57}$$

and $\theta$ is given by (3.50). If $\nu_k = 0$ or $1/2$ in (3.54) or (3.55), the multiplier $1/2$ disappears.

**Example 3.11 Covariance of Sines and Cosines for Moving Average Process**

For the three-point moving average series of Example 3.4, the theoretical spectrum is shown in Figure 3.3. For $n = 256$ points, the theoretical covariance matrix of the vector

$$\boldsymbol{X} = (X_c(\nu_{26}), X_s(\nu_{26}), X_c(\nu_{27}), X_s(\nu_{27}))'$$

is

$$\text{cov}(\boldsymbol{X}) = \begin{pmatrix} .3752 & -.0009 & -.0022 & -.0010 \\ -.0009 & .3777 & -.0009 & .0003 \\ -.0022 & -.0009 & .3667 & -.0010 \\ -.0010 & .0003 & -.0010 & .3692 \end{pmatrix}.$$

The diagonal elements can be compared with the theoretical spectral values of .3774 for the cosine transforms at frequency $\nu_{26} = .102$, and of .3689 for the two transforms at $\nu_{27} = .105$. Hence, the DFT produces nearly uncorrelated variables with variances nearly equal to the theoretical spectrum. For this particular case, the uniform bound is determined from $\theta = 8/9$, yielding $|\epsilon_{256}| \leq .0035$ for the bound on the approximation error.

The bounds specified by (3.54)-(3.57) show the DFT defines a transformation of the stationary time series whose values are almost independent at adjacent frequencies of $\nu_k = k/n$ for $k = 0, 1, \ldots, n-1$. The relation $X(1/2+\nu_k) = \overline{X(1/2-\nu_k)}$ means the values of the DFT between the frequencies of $1/2$ and one or between the frequencies of $-1/2$ and 0 are redundant. If $x_t$ is a normal series, the DFTs will also have a ***large-sample normal distribution***, although the variances are still unequal because the spectrum will vary as a function of $\nu$. If $x_t$ is not a normal time series, we can still get approximate normality for long series by assuming $x_t$ is a linear process with well-behaved coefficients, as in Theorem 3.5 of Section T3.12. Other approaches to large sample normality are in terms of cumulants, as in Brillinger (1981), or in terms of mixing conditions, such as in Rosenblatt (1956). We adopt the approach here used by Hannan (1970), Fuller (1995), and Brockwell and Davis (1991).

The asymptotic ($n \to \infty$) results show $X_c(\nu_k^n)$ and $X_s(\nu_k^n)$, jointly, tend to independent normals with zero means and variances $f(\nu)/2$, where $\nu_k^n$ denotes a frequency close to $\nu$ for an given $n$. It follows that

$$\frac{2\ I(\nu_k^n)}{f(\nu)} = \frac{2X_c^2(\nu_k^n)}{f(\nu)} + \frac{2X_s^2(\nu_k^n)}{f(\nu)}$$

will tend in distribution toward the sum of two independent, squared normal random variables and will have approximately a ***chi-squared distribution*** with two degrees of freedom. Denoting the chi-squared distribution with $m$ degrees of freedom by $\chi_m^2$, we may write approximately, for large $n$,

$$\frac{2\ I(\nu_k^n)}{f(\nu)} \sim \chi_2^2. \tag{3.58}$$

The distributional result (3.58) can be used to derive an approximate ***confidence interval for the spectrum*** in the usual way. Let $\chi_m^2(\alpha)$ denote the upper $\alpha$ probability tail for the chi-squared distribution; that is,

$$\Pr\{\chi_m^2 > \chi_m^2(\alpha)\} = \alpha. \tag{3.59}$$

Then, an approximate $100(1-\alpha)\%$ confidence interval for the spectral density function would be of the form

$$\frac{2\ I(\nu_k^n)}{\chi_2^2(\alpha/2)} \le f(\nu) \le \frac{2I\ (\nu_k^n)}{\chi_2^2(1-\alpha/2)} \tag{3.60}$$

Often, ***nonstationary trends*** are present that should be eliminated before computing the periodogram. Trends introduce extremely low frequency components in the periodogram that tend to obscure the appearance at higher frequencies. For this reason, it is usually conventional to do spectral analysis using either ***mean-adjusted data*** of the form $x_t - \bar{x}_t$ to eliminate the zero or d-c component or to use ***detrended data*** of the form $x_t - \widehat{\beta}_1 - \widehat{\beta}_2 t$ to eliminate the term that will be considered a half cycle by the spectral analysis. Note that ***higher order polynomial regressions in*** $t$ or ***nonparametric smoothing*** (linear filtering) could be used in cases where the trend is nonlinear. A further modification, improving the estimator is ***tapering***, which replaces each adjusted point $x_t$ by $w_t x_t$, where $w_t$ is a weight function, often a cosine bell, that is largest in the center and tapers off to zero at the endpoints. Tapering is useful when large fluctuations are present at the beginning or end of the time series or when a frequency component with very high power or variance obscuring an adjacent frequency with lower power. We discuss tapering in the next section.

It is often convenient to use a ***power of two*** fast Fourier transform algorithm in spectral estimation, and extending the length of $x_t, t = 1, 2, \ldots, n$ by adding zeros, i.e., setting $x_{n+1} = x_{n+2} = \cdots = x_{n'} = 0$, where $n'$ is the next highest power of two simply replaces the frequency ordinates by $\nu'_k = k/n'$ and doesn't change the estimated spectrum. We illustrate by considering the periodogram of the SOI and Recruitment series, as has been given in Figure 1.4 of Chapter 1.

**Example 3.12 Periodogram of SOI and Recruitment Series**

In Figure 3.4, we noticed a lower frequency corresponding to the possible El Niño effect, and we can look for a similar component in the periodogram. In order to get the periodogram, the series of $n = 453$ months can be extended to $n' = 2^9 = 512$ months, so the periodogram will be computed at frequencies of the form $\nu'_k = k/512$ for $k = 0, 1, \ldots, 256$. These frequencies can be expressed in cycles per month, and the folding frequency is .5 cycles per month or six cycles per year. The periodogram, shown in Figure 3.7, has a large (8.57) peak at a frequency corresponding to a period of 11.91 months, obviously the yearly seasonal frequency. The smaller peaks are split between periods of 73.14, 51.20, and 42.67 months, that is, between four and six years; these peaks are probably reflecting the El Niño frequencies. Other possible secondary peaks appear at .17 and .25 cycles per month. We need to verify these peaks are statistically significant by computing confidence intervals of the form given in (3.60). Noting $\chi^2_2(.025) = 7.3778$ and $\chi^2_2(.975) = .0506$, an approximate 95% confidence interval for the yearly frequency is

$$[2(8.57)/7.3778\ ,\ 2(8.57)/.0506] = [2.3\ ,\ 338.7],$$

which is wide. In the lower band, there is the peak $I(.02) = 1.0$ at about 50 months, which leads to the interval $[.27, 39.53]$ for that frequency and the lower value barely exceeds the neighboring noise levels. Hence, we are unable to establish either the statistical significance nor the frequency of the presumed El Niño frequency for the SOI series. The periodogram of the Recruitment series, shown in the lower panel of Figure 3.7, has power

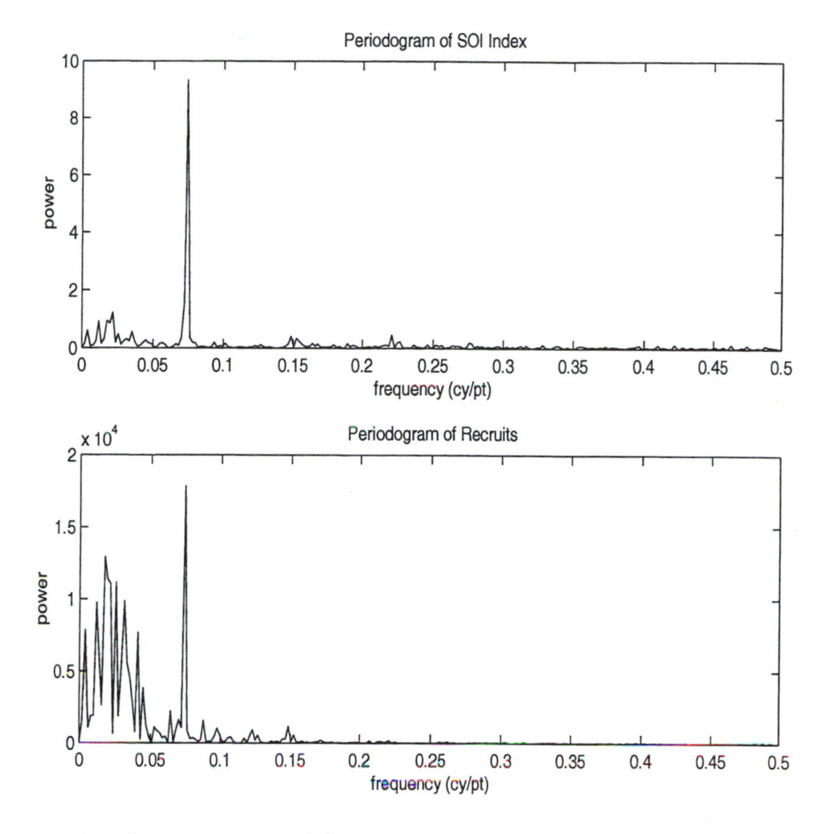


**Figure 3.7:** Periodogram of SOI and Recruitment, $n = 453$ ($n' = 512$), showing common peaks at $\nu = .023$ and $\nu = .084$ cycles/month.

at the seasonal frequency and even more power $1.333 \times 10^4$ at the lower frequency of $\nu = .02$ cycles per month. The approximate 95% confidence interval here will be of the form

$$[2(1.33 \times 10^4)/7.3778 \ , \ 2(1.33 \times 10^4)/.0506] = [.36 \times 10^4 \ , \ 52.57 \times 10^4],$$

and the interval again is broad and difficult to distinguish from neighboring frequencies. It is interesting, however, that the same frequencies persist in both bands, and we will examine this phenomenon further in Section 3.6 using the coherence.

The example above makes it fairly clear the periodogram as an estimator is susceptible to large uncertainties, and we need to find a way to reduce the variance. Not surprisingly, this result follows if we think about (3.43) as an estimator and realize that it is the sum of squares of only two random variables for any sample size. The solution to this dilemma is suggested by the analogy with classical statistics where we look for independent random variables with the same variance and average the squares of these common variance observations. Independence and equality of variance does not hold in the time series case, but the covariance structure of the two adjacent estimators given in Example 3.11 suggests that for neighboring frequencies, these assumptions are approximately true. In the next section, we discuss smoothed estimators for the spectra and cross-spectra that accumulate degrees of freedom for the purpose of reducing the uncertainty in the estimated spectra and cross-spectra.

## 3.6 Nonparametric Spectral Estimation

To continue the discussion that ended the last section, we define a ***frequency band***, $B$, of contiguous fundamental frequencies centered around $\nu_k = k/n$ that is close to the frequency of interest, $\nu$, as

$$B = \left\{ \nu;\ \nu_k - \frac{L}{2n} \le \nu \le \nu_k + \frac{L}{2n} \right\}, \tag{3.61}$$

where $L << n$ is an odd number, chosen such that the spectral values

$$f(\nu_k + \ell/n), \quad \ell = -\frac{L-1}{2}, \ldots, 0, \ldots, \frac{L-1}{2}$$

are approximately equal to $f(\nu)$ in the interval $B$. This structure can be realized for large sample sizes, as shown formally in Section T3.12. Values of the spectrum in this band should be relatively constant, as well, for the smoothed spectra defined below to be good estimators. The length of the interval defined by (3.61) is obviously

$$B_w = \frac{L}{n} \tag{3.62}$$

and will be called the ***bandwidth***.

Using the above band, we may now define the ***smoothed spectral estimator*** as the average of the periodogram values, say,

$$\begin{aligned} \widehat{f}(\nu) &= \frac{1}{L} \sum_{\ell=-(L-1)/2}^{(L-1)/2} I(\nu_k + \ell/n) \\ &= \frac{1}{L} \sum_{\ell=-(L-1)/2}^{(L-1)/2} |X(\nu_k + \ell/n)|^2, \end{aligned} \tag{3.63}$$

as the average over the band $B$. We omit the dependence on $n$ for simplicity and write $\nu_k$ from now on instead of $\nu_k^n$. Now, we know from Section T3.12 that, for large $n$, the variances of the cosine and sine transforms are each approximately equal to $f(\nu)$ as long as we keep $L$ fairly small relative to $n$. In this case, we will have

$$\widehat{f}(\nu) = \frac{1}{L} \sum_{\ell=-(L-1)/2}^{(L-1)/2} [X_c^2(\nu_k + \ell/n) + X_s^2(\nu_k + \ell/n)]$$

approximately distributed as the average of $2L$ independent chi-squared random variables with one degree of freedom each. It follows that, for large $n$,

$$\frac{2L\widehat{f}(\nu_k)}{f(\nu)} \sim \chi^2_{2L}; \tag{3.64}$$

that is, $2L\widehat{f}(\nu_k)/f(\nu)$ has an approximate chi-squared distribution with $2L$ degrees of freedom. Note (3.62) implies the degrees of freedom can be expressed as

$$2L = 2B_w n, \tag{3.65}$$

or twice the ***time-bandwidth product***. The result (3.64) can be rearranged to obtain an approximate $100(1-\alpha)\%$ confidence interval of the form

$$\frac{2L\widehat{f}(\nu_k)}{\chi^2_{2L}(\alpha/2)} \leq f(\nu) \leq \frac{2L\widehat{f}(\nu_k)}{\chi^2_{2L}(1-\alpha/2)} \tag{3.66}$$

for the true spectrum, $f(\nu)$.

Many times, the visual impact of a spectral density plot will be improved by plotting the logarithm of the spectrum instead of the spectrum. This phenomenon can occur when regions of the spectrum exist with peaks of interest much smaller than some of the main power components. For the log spectrum, we obtain an interval of the form

$$\left[\ln \widehat{f}(\nu_k) + \ln 2L - \ln \chi^2_{2L}(\alpha/2),\ \ln \widehat{f}(\nu_k) + \ln 2L - \ln \chi^2_{2L}(1-\alpha/2)\right]. \tag{3.67}$$

We can also test hypotheses relating to the equality of spectra using the fact that the distributional result (3.64) implies that the ratio of spectra based on roughly independent samples will have an approximate $F_{2L,2L}$ distribution. The independent estimators can either be from different frequency bands or from different series.

If zeros are appended before computing the spectral estimators, we need to adjust the degrees of freedom and an approximation is to replace $2L$ by $2Ln/n'$. Hence, we define the ***adjusted degrees of freedom*** as

$$df = \frac{2Ln}{n'} \tag{3.68}$$

and use it instead of $2L$ in the confidence intervals (3.66) and (3.67). For example, (3.67) becomes

$$\frac{df\,\widehat{f}(\nu_k)}{\chi^2_{df}(\alpha/2)} \leq f(\nu) \leq \frac{df\,\widehat{f}(\nu_k)}{\chi^2_{df}(1-\alpha/2)}. \tag{3.69}$$

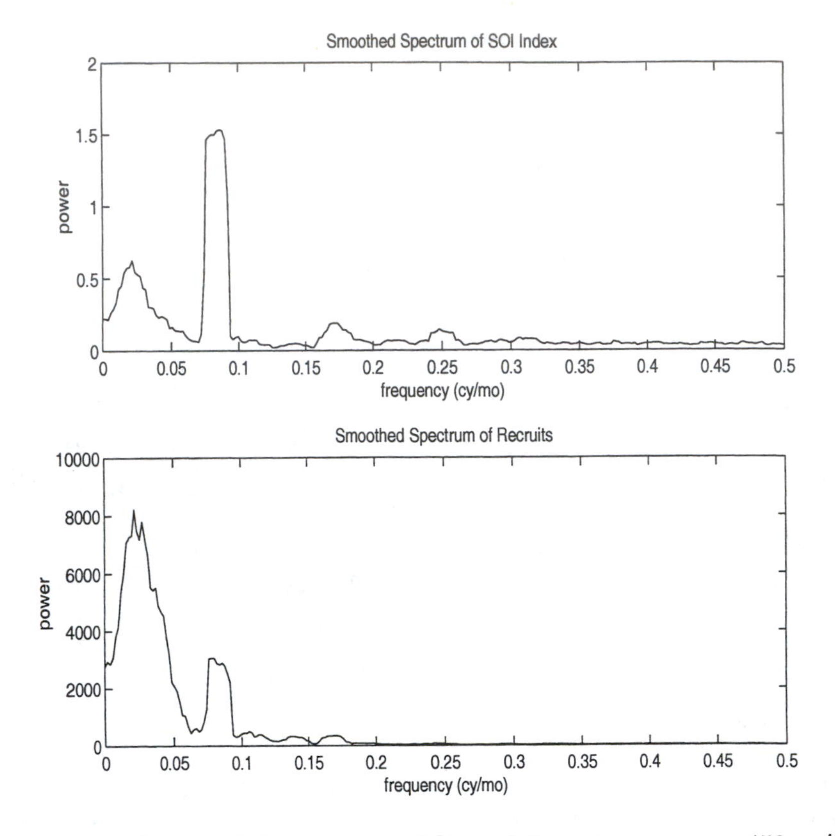


**Figure 3.8:** Smoothed Spectrum of SOI and Recruitment $n = 453$, $n' = 512$, $L = 9$, $df = 16$, showing common peaks at $\nu = .023$ and $.084$ cycles/month.

A number of assumptions are made in computing the approximate confidence intervals given above, which may not hold in practice. In such cases, it may be reasonable to employ resampling techniques such as the ***local bootstrap*** proposed by Hurvich and Zeger (1987) and investigated by Paparoditis and Politis (1999). To develop the bootstrap distributions, we assume that the contiguous DFTs in a frequency band of the form (3.61) all came from a time series with identical spectrum $f(\nu)$. This, in fact, is exactly the same assumption made in deriving the large-sample theory. We may then simply resample the $L$ DFTs in the band, with replacement, calculating a spectral estimate from each bootstrap sample. The sampling distribution of the bootstrap estimators approximates the distribution of the nonparametric spectral estimator. For further details, including the theoretical properties of such estimators, see Paparoditis and Politis (1999).

Before proceeding further, we pause to consider computing the smoothed spectrum of the SOI and Recruitment series, shown in Figure 3.8.

**Table 3.1:** Spectral Analysis of SOI and Recruitment Series

| Series | $\nu$ | Period | Power | Lower | Upper |
|---|---|---|---|---|---|
| SOI | .0215 | 46.5 | .62 | .35 | 1.45 |
| | .0800 | 12.5 | 1.50 | 83 | 3.53 |
| Recruits | .0215 | 46.5 | 8.23 | 4.56 | 19.06 |
| $\times 10^{-3}$ | .0781 | 12.8 | 3.05 | 1.69 | 7.07 |

**Example 3.13 Smoothed Spectra of SOI and Recruitment Series**

Generally, it is a good idea to try several bandwidths that seem to be compatible with the general overall shape of the spectrum, as suggested by the periodogram. The SOI and Recruitment series periodograms, previously computed in Figure 3.7, suggests the power in the lower El Niño frequency needs smoothing to identify the predominant overall period. Trying values of $L$ leads to the choice $L = 9$ as a reasonable value, leading to a bandwidth of $B = 9/512 = .018$ cycles per month for the spectral estimator. This bandwidth means we are assuming a relatively constant spectrum over about $.018/.5 = .036$ or about $1/30$ of the interval. The smoothed spectra, shown in Figure 3.8, provide a sensible compromise between the noisy version, shown in Figure 3.7, and a more heavily smoothed spectrum, which might lose some of the peaks. The adjusted degrees of freedom are $df = 2(9)(453)/512 \approx 16$, and we use this value for the 95% confidence intervals, with $\chi^2_{16}(.975) = 6.9077$, $\chi^2_{16}(.025) = 28.8454$. Substituting into (3.69) gives the intervals in Table 3.1 for the two frequency bands identified as having the maximum power.

To examine the two peak power possibilities, we may look at the 95% confidence intervals and see whether the lower limits are substantially larger than adjacent baseline spectral levels. For example, the El Niño frequency of about 46.5 months has lower limits that exceed the values the spectrum would have if there were simply a smooth underlying spectral function without the peaks. The relative distribution of power over frequencies is different, with the SOI index having less power at the lower frequency, relative to the seasonal periods, and the recruit series having relatively more power at the lower or El Niño frequency.

The example points out the necessity for having some relatively systematic procedure for deciding whether peaks are significant. The question of deciding whether a single peak is significant usually rests on establishing what we might think of as a ***baseline level*** for the spectrum, defined rather loosely as the shape that one would expect to see if no spectral peaks were present. This profile can usually be guessed by looking at the overall shape of the spectrum that includes the peaks; usually, a kind of baseline level will be apparent, with the peaks seeming to emerge from this baseline level. If the lower confidence limit for the spectral value is still greater than the baseline level at some predetermined level of significance, we may claim that frequency value as a statistically significant peak. To maintain an $\alpha$ that is consistent with our stated indifference to the upper limits, we might use a one-sided confidence interval.

An important aspect of interpreting the significance of confidence intervals and tests involving spectra is that almost always, more than one frequency will be of interest, so that we will potentially be interested in ***simultaneous statements*** about a whole collection of frequencies. For example, it would be unfair to claim in Table 3.1 the two frequencies of interest as being statistically significant and all other potential candidates as nonsignificant at the overall level of $\alpha = .05$. In this case, we follow the usual statistical approach, noting that if $K$ statements $S_1, S_1, \ldots, S_k$ are made at significance level $\alpha$, i.e., $P\{S_k\} = 1 - \alpha$, then the overall probability all statements are true satisfies the ***Bonferroni inequality***

$$P\{\text{all } S_k \text{ true}\} \geq 1 - K\alpha. \tag{3.70}$$

For this reason, it is desirable to set the significance level for testing each frequency at $\alpha/K$ if there are $K$ potential frequencies of interest. If, *a priori*, potentially $K = 10$ frequencies are of interest, setting $\alpha = .01$ would give an overall significance level of bound of .10.

The use of the confidence intervals and the necessity for smoothing requires that we make a decision about the bandwidth $B_w$ over which the spectrum will be essentially constant. Taking too broad a band will tend to smooth out valid peaks in the data when the constant variance assumption is not met over the band. Taking too narrow a band will lead to confidence intervals so wide that peaks are no longer statistically significant. Thus, we note that there is a conflict here between variance properties or ***bandwidth stability***, which can be improved by increasing $B_w$ and ***resolution***, which can be improved by decreasing $B_w$. A common approach is to try a number of different bandwidths and to look qualitatively at the spectral estimators for each case.

The problem of ***resolution*** is related to the fact that the smoothed estimator (3.63) does not produce the value of the theoretical spectrum $f(\nu)$ at any given point on average, but estimates a smoothed version of the true spectrum in a neighborhood of the center frequency $\nu$. For example, it is a homework problem to verify that replacing the original series by the tapered series

$$y_t = h_t x_t, \tag{3.71}$$

for $t = 1, 2, \ldots, n$, and using the modified DFT

$$Y(\nu_k) = n^{-1/2} \sum_{t=1}^{n} h_t x_t e^{-2\pi i \nu_k t} \tag{3.72}$$

leads to a spectral estimator with approximate expectation

$$E[\widehat{f}_y(\nu_k)] \approx \int_{-1/2}^{1/2} W_n(\nu_k - \nu)\; f_x(\nu)\; d\nu, \tag{3.73}$$

where

$$W_n(\nu) = \frac{1}{L} \sum_{\ell=-(L-1)/2}^{(L-1)/2} |H_n(\nu + \ell/n)|^2 \tag{3.74}$$

and

$$H_n(\nu) = n^{-1/2} \sum_{t=1}^{n} h_t e^{-2\pi i \nu t} \tag{3.75}$$

In the case of the standard estimator, sometimes called the Bartlett window, the weight function, $h_t$, is unity for all $t$, we have

$$W_n(\nu) = \frac{1}{nL} \sum_{\ell=-(L-1)/2}^{(L-1)/2} \frac{\sin^2[\pi(\nu + \ell/n)(n+1)]}{\sin^2[\pi(\nu + \ell/n)]} \tag{3.76}$$

Note that (3.49) is used in the evaluation. Tapers generally have a shape that enhances the center of the data relative to the extremities, such as a cosine bell of the form

$$h_t = .5\left[1 + \cos\left(\frac{2\pi(t - \bar{t})}{n}\right)\right], \tag{3.77}$$

where $\bar{t} = (n + 1)/2$, favored by Blackman and Tukey (1959). Alternative approaches exist based on nonparametric ***kernel estimators***, as discussed in Section 1.9, equations (1.77) and (1.78), that smooth the periodogram with weight functions, chosen to have certain optimal properties (for details, see Parzen, 1961, Hannan, 1970, Brillinger, 1981, or Brockwell and Davis, 1991 for example). In Figure 3.9, we have plotted the shapes of the two windows, $W_n(\nu)$, when (i) $h_t \equiv 1$, in which case, (3.76) applies, and (ii) $h_t$ is the cosine taper in (3.77). In both cases, $n = 512$ and $L = 9$, so the predicted bandwidth should be $B_w = .018$ cycles per point. Both windows produce an integrated average spectrum over this band but the untapered window in the top panel shows ripples over the band and outside the band. This behavior tends to introduce frequencies from outside the interval that may contaminate the desired spectral estimate within the band. For example, a large dynamic range for the values in the spectrum introduces spectra in contiguous frequency intervals several orders of magnitude greater than the value in the interval of interest. In this case, a relatively small peak outside the frequency band, called a ***side lobe***, may introduce a considerable distortion; this effect is sometimes called ***leakage***. The shape of the window also affects the degrees of freedom, although the effect in this case is clearly negligible. We can calculate the approximate effect by noting that the mean and variance of a $\chi^2_m$ random variable are $m$ and $2m$ respectively, so twice the square of the mean divided by the variance is an estimator for the degrees of freedom. For our purposes, a simpler method is to plot the window as in Figure 3.9 and then simply estimate the degrees of freedom using the graphically estimated equivalent bandwidth, $B_w$, the width over which the function is essentially constant, and then take $df = 2B_w n$. Further details on the chi-squared approximation and other windows can be found in Brockwell and Davis (1991).

**Example 3.14 Spectra of P and S Components for Earthquake and Explosion**

Figure 3.10 shows the spectra computed separately from the two phases of the earthquake and explosion in Figure 1.6 of Chapter 1. Because the sampling rate is 40 points per second, the folding frequency is 20 cycles per second or 20 Hertz (Hz). Hence, the highest frequency shown in the plots is .25 cycles per point or 10 Hz. A fundamental problem in the analysis of seismic data is discriminating between earthquakes and explosions using the kind of close monitoring instruments that might be

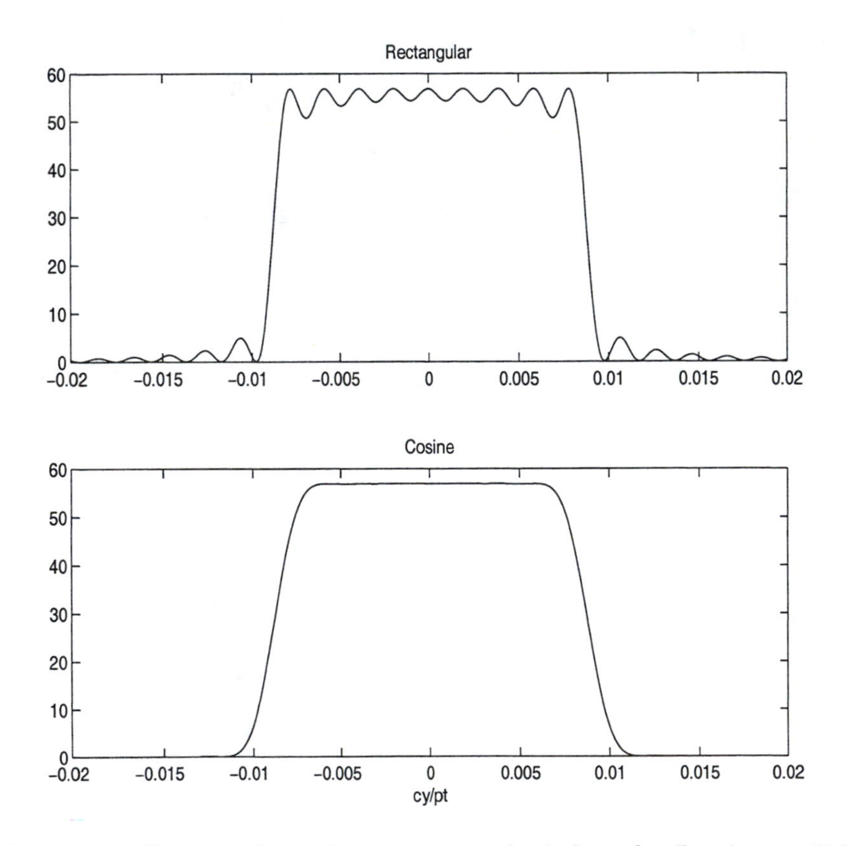


**Figure 3.9:** Rectangular and cosine spectral windows for $L = 9$, $n = 512$.

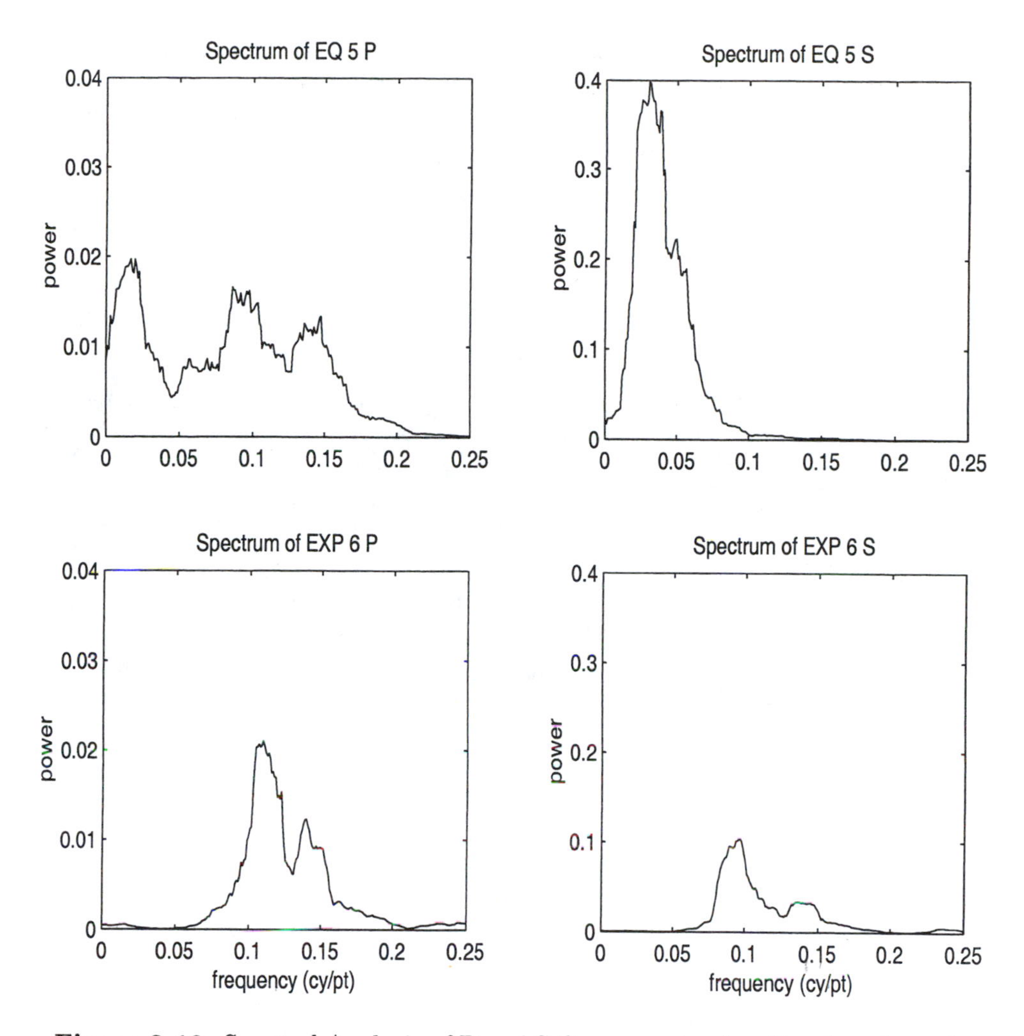


**Figure 3.10:** Spectral Analysis of P and S Components of an Earthquake and an Explosion $n = 1024$, $L = 21$, $df = 42$. Multiply frequency by 10 to convert to Hertz (cycles/second).

used in monitoring a nuclear test ban treaty. If we plot an ensemble of earthquakes and explosions comparable to Figure 1.6, some gross features appear that may lead to discrimination. The most common differences that we look for are subtle differences between the spectra of the two classes of events. In this case, note the strong frequency components of the P and S components of the explosion are at frequencies .07 and .15 cycles/pt or between .7 and 1.5 Hz. On the other hand, the spectral content of the earthquakes tends to occur along a broader frequency band and at lower frequencies for both components. Often, we assume that the ratio of P to S power is in different proportions at different frequencies, and this distinction can form a basis for discriminating between the two classes. In Section 5.7, we test formally for discrimination using a random effects analysis of variance approach.

The extension of spectral estimation to vector series is fairly obvious because we can take DFTs of any two components of the vector, say $x_t$, $y_t$, and use

$$\widehat{f}_{xy}(\nu) = L^{-1} \sum_{\ell=-(L-1)/2}^{L-1)/2} X(\nu_k + \ell/n)\overline{Y(\nu_k + \ell/n)}. \tag{3.78}$$

For the vector series $\boldsymbol{x}_t = x_{t1}, x_{t2}, \ldots, x_{tp})'$, we may use the vector of DFTs, say $\boldsymbol{X}(\nu_k) = (X_1(\nu_k), X_2(\nu_k), \ldots, X_p(\nu_k))'$, and estimate the spectral matrix by

$$\widehat{f}(\nu) = L^{-1} \sum_{\ell=-(L-1)/2}^{L-1)/2} \boldsymbol{X}(\nu_k + \ell/n)\boldsymbol{X}^*(\nu_k + \ell/n). \tag{3.79}$$

Again, the series may be tapered before the DFT is taken in (3.79).

If the theoretical values of the spectra and cross-spectra in the squared coherence (3.20) are replaced by sample estimators of the spectra and cross-spectrum, under the hypothesis that $\rho^2_{y\cdot x}(\nu) = 0$ , we have that the statistic

$$F_{2,2L-2} = \frac{\widehat{\rho}^2_{y\cdot x}(\nu)}{(1 - \widehat{\rho}^2_{y\cdot x}(\nu))}(L-1) \tag{3.80}$$

has an approximate ***F-distribution*** with two and $2L-2$ degrees of freedom, where

$$\widehat{\rho}^2_{y\cdot x}(\nu) = \frac{|\widehat{f}_{yx}(\nu)|^2}{\widehat{f}_x(\nu)\widehat{f}_y(\nu)} \tag{3.81}$$

is the estimated sample squared coherence. When the series have been extended to length $n'$, we replace $2L-2$ by $df-2$, where $df$ is defined in (3.68). Solving (3.80) for a particular significance level $\alpha$ leads to

$$C_\alpha = \frac{F_{2,2L-2}(\alpha)}{L-1+F_{2,2L-2}(\alpha)} \tag{3.82}$$

as the approximate value which, must be exceeded for the original squared coherence to be able to reject $\rho^2_{y\cdot x}(\nu) = 0$ at an *a priori* specified frequency $\nu$.

**Example 3.15 Coherence Between SOI and Recruitment Series**

Figure 3.11 shows the squared coherence between the SOI and Recruitment series over a wider band than was used for the spectrum. In this case, we used $L = 19$, $df = 2(19)(453/512) = 26.5$ and $F_{2,24}(.01) = 5.61$

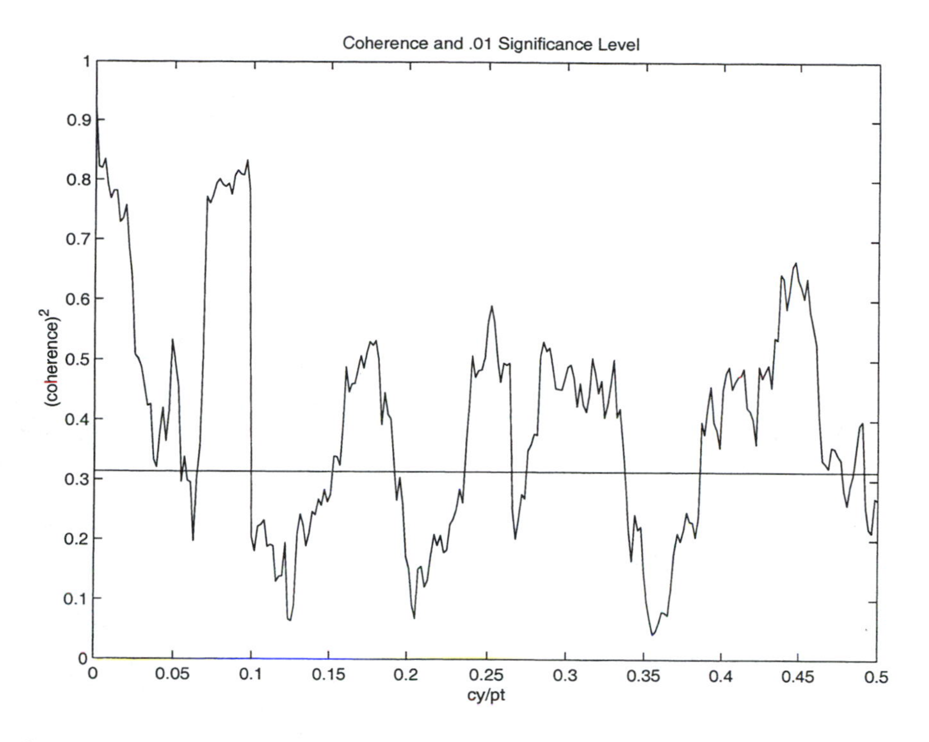


**Figure 3.11:** Coherence function relating the SOI to the number of new fish. $L = 19,\ n = 453, n' = 512$, and $\alpha = .01$.

at the significance level $\alpha = .01$. Hence, we may reject the hypothesis of no coherence for values of $C_{.01} > .32$. We emphasize that this method is crude because, in addition to the fact that the $F$-statistic is approximate, we are examing the squared coherence across all frequencies with the Bonferroni inequality, (3.70), in mind.

In the above case, the El Niño and seasonal frequencies are strongly coherent. Other frequencies are also strongly coherent, although the strong coherence is less impressive because the underlying power spectrum at these higher frequencies is fairly small. Besides the main components at about 46 months and at 12.8 months, significant activity occurs at six months, four months, 3.5 months, and three months. Again, these can be seasonal variations that persist both series.

## 3.7 Parametric Spectral Estimation

The methods of the previous sections lead to estimators, generally referred to as ***nonparametric spectra*** because they only involve choosing a bandwidth and do not depend on any parametric model. In Example 3.5, we derived the spectrum of a second-order autoregressive series and we might consider basing a spectral estimator on this function, using the estimated parameters $\phi_1, \phi_2$ and $\sigma^2$. Then, substituting the parameter estimates into the spectral density $f_x(\nu)$ determined in that example would lead to a parametric estimator for the spectrum. Similarly, we might fit a $p$-th order autoregression, with the order $p$ determined by one of the model selection criteria, such as AIC, AICc, o5 SIC, defined in (1.66)-(1.68) for the regression model. Parametric autoregressive spectral estimators will often have superior resolution in problems when several closely spaced narrow spectral peaks are present, and are preferred by engineers for a broad variety of problems (see Kay, 1988). The development of autoregressive spectral estimators has been summarized by Parzen (1983).

To be specific, consider the equation determining the order $p$ autoregressive model (2.1), written in the form

$$x_t - \sum_{k=1}^{p} \phi_k x_{t-k} = w_t, \tag{3.83}$$

where $w_t$ is a white noise process with mean zero and variance $\sigma_w^2$. Then, note the linear filter Property 3.3, combined with equating the spectra of the left- and right-hand sides of the defining equation above can be equated to yield

$$|\phi(\mathrm{e}^{-2\pi i\nu})|^2 f_x(\nu) = \sigma_w^2, \tag{3.84}$$

where

$$\phi(\mathrm{e}^{-2\pi i\nu}) = 1 - \sum_{k=1}^{p} \phi_k \mathrm{e}^{-2\pi i\nu k}. \tag{3.85}$$

Then, denoting the maximum likelihood or least squares estimators of the model parameters by $\widehat{\phi}_1, \widehat{\phi}_2, \ldots, \widehat{\phi}_p$ and $\widehat{\sigma}_w^2$, we may substitute them into the form of the spectrum implied by (3.84), obtaining

$$\widehat{f}_x(\nu) = \frac{\widehat{\sigma}_w^2}{|\widehat{\phi}(\mathrm{e}^{-2\pi i\nu})|^2}. \tag{3.86}$$

The asymptotic distribution of the autoregressive spectral estimator has been obtained by Berk (1974) under the conditions ($p \to \infty$, $p^3/n \to 0$) as $p$, $n \to \infty$, which may be too severe for most applications. The limiting results imply a confidence interval of the form

$$\frac{\hat{f}(\nu)}{(1 + Cz_{\alpha/2})} \le f(\nu) \le \frac{\hat{f}(\nu)}{(1 - Cz_{\alpha/2})}, \tag{3.87}$$

where

$$C = \sqrt{2p/T} \tag{3.88}$$

and $z_{\alpha/2}$ is ordinate corresponding to the upper $\alpha/2$ probability of the standard normal distribution. If the sampling distribution is to be checked, we suggest

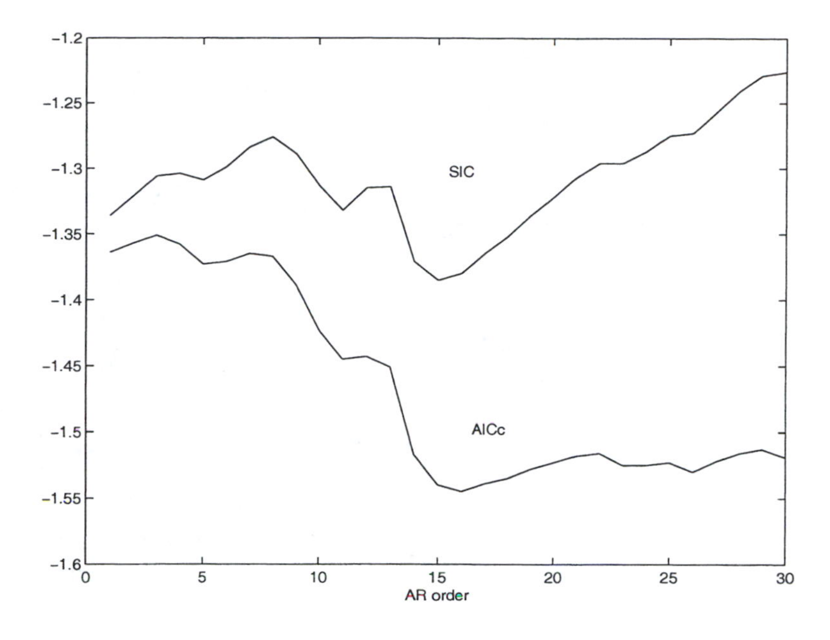


**Figure 3.12:** Model selection criteria AICc and SIC as a function of order $p$ for autoregressive models fitted to the SOI series.

applying the bootstrap estimator to get the sampling distribution of $\widehat{f}_x(\nu)$ using a procedure similar to the one used for $p = 1$ in Example 2.30. An alternative for higher order autoregressive series is to put the AR($p$) in state-space form and use the bootstrap procedure discussed in Section 4.7.

**Example 3.16 Autoregressive Spectral Estimator of the SOI Series**

Consider obtaining results comparable to the nonparametric estimators shown in Figure 3.8 for the SOI series. Fitting successively higher order models for $p = 1, 2, \ldots, 30$ yields a minimum SIC at $p = 15$ and a minimum AICc at $p = 16$, as shown in Figure 3.12. The parameter estimates are (.41,.09,.16,.08,-.05, -.08,-.08,-.08,.01,.12,.18,.16,.02,-.20,-.15) and $\widehat{\sigma}_w^2 = .07545$. The spectra of the two cases are almost identical, as shown in Figure 3.13, and we note the strong peaks at 51 months and 12 months corresponding to the nonparametric estimators, which showed broad peaks (Table 3.1) at 46.5 months and 12.5 months

Also, it would be possible to define an autoregressive moving average spectral estimator using the spectrum implied by the defining equation (3.83) but the most useful approach seems to be to look at long autoregressions as approximations to the mixed case.

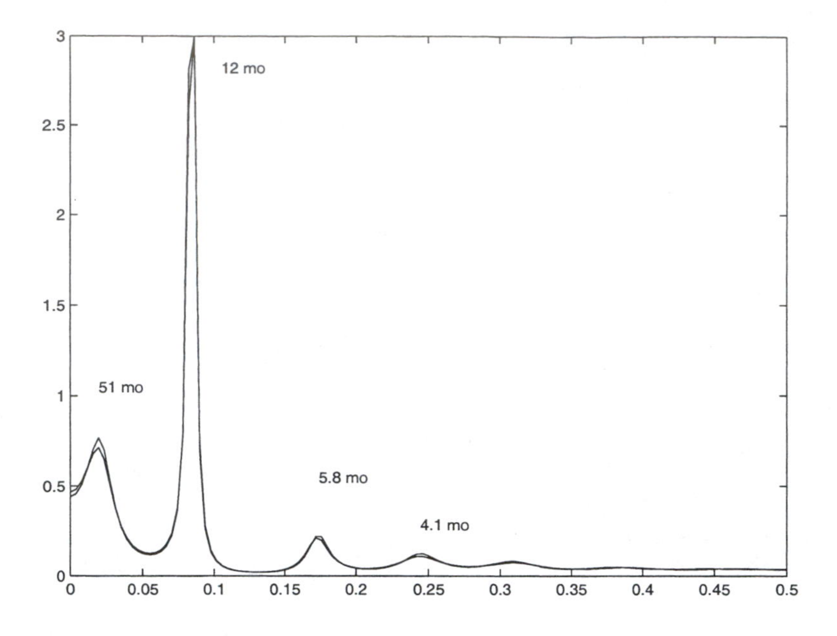


**Figure 3.13:** Autoregressive spectral estimators for SOI series using models selected by AICc and SIC.

Finally, it should be mentioned that any parametric spectrum, say $f(\nu;\boldsymbol{\theta})$, depending on the vector parameter $\boldsymbol{\theta}$ can be estimated via the approximate ***Whittle likelihood***, see Whittle (1961), using the approximate properties of the discrete Fourier transform derived later in this chapter. We have that the DFTs, $X(\nu_k)$, are approximately complex normally distributed with mean zero and variance $f(\nu_k;\boldsymbol{\theta})$ and are approximately independent for $\nu_k \neq \nu_\ell$. This implies that an approximate log likelihood can be written in the form

$$\ln L(\boldsymbol{x};\boldsymbol{\theta}) \approx - \sum_{0<\nu_k<1/2} \left( \ln f_x(\nu_k;\boldsymbol{\theta}) + \frac{|X(\nu_k)|^2}{f_x(\nu_k;\boldsymbol{\theta})} \right), \tag{3.89}$$

where the sum often ignores the frequencies $\nu_k = 0, 1/2$. If the form with the two additional frequencies is used, the multiplier of the sum will be unity, except for the purely real points at $\nu_k = 0, 1/2$ for which the multipler is $1/2$. For a discussion of applying the Whittle approximation to the problem of estimating parameters in the autoregressive moving average (ARMA) spectrum, see Anderson (1978). Although this yields valid answers, it seems more involved than simply using the time domain methods discussed in Chapter 2.

For cases close to nonstationarity, it may be useful to reconsider the frequency domain version of the fractionally differenced long memory process long memory process (2.143). In this case, we may think of the equations as generated by an infinite order autoregressive series with coefficients $\pi_j$ given by (2.146). Using the same approach as before, we might obtain

$$f_x(\nu) = \frac{\sigma_w^2}{|\sum_{k=0}^{\infty} \pi_k e^{-2\pi i k \nu}|^2} \tag{3.90}$$

$$= \sigma_w^2 |1 - e^{-2\pi i \nu}|^{-2d} \tag{3.91}$$

$$= [4\sin^2(\pi\nu)]^{-d} \sigma_w^2 \tag{3.92}$$

as equivalent representations of the spectrum of a long memory process. The long memory spectrum approaches infinity as the frequency $\nu \to 0$. The long memory model seems to offer a reasonable compromise to complete nonstationarity, which would be implied by taking $d = 1$. Actually, the process is non-stationary for $.5 < d \leq 1$, but can be transformed by a first difference to a long memory process.

The main reason for defining the Whittle approximation to the log likelihood is to propose its use for estimating the parameter $d$ in the long memory case as an alternative to the time domain method employed in Chapter 2. The time domain approach, that has already been suggested in Section 2.10 of Chapter 2, is useful because of its simplicity and easily computed standard errors. One may also use an exact likelihood approach by developing an innovations form of the likelihood as in Brockwell and Davis (1991).

For the approximate approach using the Whittle likelihood (3.96), we consider using the approach of Fox and Taqqu (1986) who showed that maximizing the Whittle log likelihood leads to a consistent estimator with the usual asymptotic normal distribution that would be obtained by treating (3.96) as a conventional log likelihood (see also Dahlhaus, 1989, Robinson, 1995, Hurvich et al, 1998). Unfortunately, the periodogram ordinates are not asymptotically independent (Hurvich and Beltrao, 1993) although a quasi-likelihood in the form of the Whittle approximation works well and has good asymptotic properties.

To see how this would work for the purely long memory case, write the long memory spectrum as

$$f_x(\nu_k;\ d, \sigma_w^2) = \sigma_w^2 g_k^{-d}, \tag{3.93}$$

where

$$g_k = 4\sin^2(\pi\nu_k). \tag{3.94}$$

Then, differentiating the log likelihood, say,

$$\ln L(\boldsymbol{x}; d, \sigma_w^2) \approx -m \ln \sigma_w^2 + d \sum_{k=1}^{m} \ln g_k - \frac{1}{\sigma_w^2} \sum_{k=1}^{m} g_k^d |X(\nu_k)|^2 \tag{3.95}$$

at $m = n/2 - 1$ frequencies and solving for $\sigma_w^2$ yields

$$\sigma_w^2(d) = \frac{1}{m} \sum_{k=1}^{m} g_k^d |X(\nu_k)|^2 \tag{3.96}$$

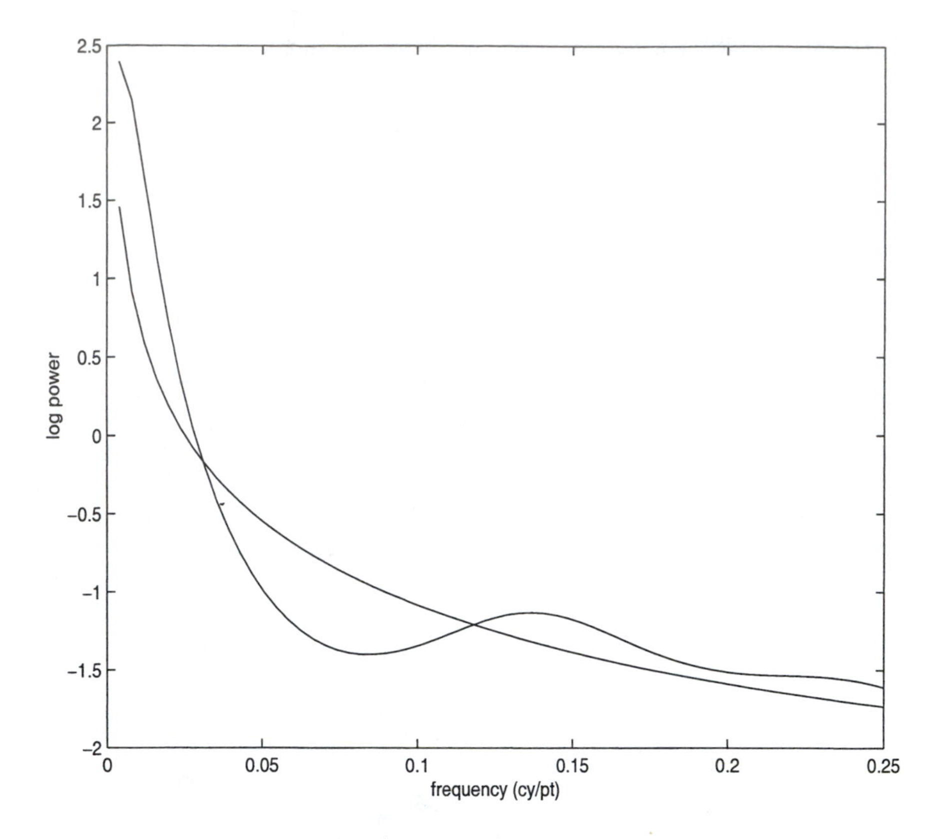


**Figure 3.14:** Long Memory ($d = .394$) and autoregressive AR(8) spectral estimators for the paleoclimatic glacial varve series.

as the approximate maximum likelihood estimator for the variance parameter. To estimate $d$, we use a grid scan of the concentrated log likelihood

$$\ln L(\boldsymbol{x}; d) \approx -m \ln \sigma_w^2(d) - d \sum_{k=1}^{m} \ln g_k - m \tag{3.97}$$

over the interval $(-.5, .5)$, followed by a Newton–Raphson procedure to convergence.

### Example 3.17 Long Memory Spectra for the Varve Series

We have previously examined the fit of the long memory model for the glacial varve data that is thought to be a reasonable surrogate for temperature. Fitting the long memory model using the Whittle approximation above gives $\widehat{d} = .394$, with an estimated standard error of .022. The earlier time domain method in Chapter 2 gave $\widehat{d} = .384$, with a standard error of .030, so the results of the two methods are slightly different. Standard errors for the time domain method follow from the usual regression form of the time domain model and from minus one over the the second derivative of the log likelihood for the frequency domain method. The error variance estimated was $\widehat{\sigma}_w^2 = .2320$. One might also consider fitting an autoregressive model to this data using a procedure similar to that used in Example 3.16. Following this approach gave an autoregressive model with $p = 8$ and $\widehat{\boldsymbol{\phi}} = (.35, .13, .05, .10, .09, .11)'$, with $\widehat{\sigma}_w^2 = .2306$ as the error variance. The two log spectra are plotted in Figure 3.14 for $\nu > 0$, and we note that long memory spectrum is lower for the first frequency estimated ($\nu_1 = 1/512$) but will eventually become infinite, whereas the AR(8) spectrum is higher at that point, but takes a finite value at $\nu = 0$.

It should be noted that there is a strong likelihood that the spectrum will not be purely long memory, as it seemed to be in the example given above. A common situation has the long memory component multiplied by a short memory component, leading to an alternate version of (3.95) of the form

$$f_x(\nu_k;\ d, \theta) = g_k^{-d} f_0(\nu_k; \boldsymbol{\theta}), \tag{3.98}$$

where $f_0(\nu_k; \theta)$ might be the spectrum of an autoregressive moving average process with vector parameter $\boldsymbol{\theta}$, or it might be unspecified. If the spectrum has a parametric form, the Whittle likelihood can be used. However, there is a substantial amount of semiparametric literature that develops the estimators when the underlying spectrum $f_0(\nu; \boldsymbol{\theta})$ is unknown. A class of ***Gaussian semi-parametric*** estimators simply uses the same Whittle likelihood (3.97), evaluated over a sub-band of low frequencies, say $m' = \sqrt{n}$. There is some latitude in selecting a band that is relatively free from low frequency interference due to the short memory component in (3.98).

Geweke and Porter–Hudak (1983) developed an approximate GPH method for estimating $d$ based on a regression model, derived from (3.85). Note that we may write a simple equation for the logarithm of the spectrum as

$$\ln f_x(\nu_k; d) = \ln f_0(\nu_k; \boldsymbol{\theta}) - d \ln[4 \sin^2(\pi \nu_k)], \tag{3.99}$$

with the frequencies $\nu_k = k/n$ restricted to a range $k = 1, 2, \ldots, m'$ near the zero frequency with $m' = \sqrt{n}$ as the recommended value. Relationship (3.99) suggests using a simple linear regression model of the form,

$$\ln I(\nu_k) = \beta_0 - d \ln[4 \sin^2(\pi \nu_k)] + e_k \tag{3.100}$$

for the periodogram to estimate the parameters $\sigma_w^2$ and $d$. In this case, one performs least squares using $\ln I(\nu_k)$ as the dependent variable, and $\ln[4 \sin^2(\pi \nu_k)]$ as the independent variable for $k = 1, 2, \ldots, m$. The resulting slope estimate is then used as an estimate of $-d$. For a good discussion of various alternative methods for selecting $m$, see Hurvich and Deo (1999).

One of the above two procedures works well for estimating the long memory component but there will be cases (such as ARFIMA) where there will be a parameterized short memory component $f_0(\nu_k;\boldsymbol{\theta})$ that needs to be estimated. If the spectrum is highly parameterized, one might estimate using the Whittle log likelihood (3.94) and

$$f_x(\nu_k;\boldsymbol{\theta}) = g_k^{-d} f_0(\nu_k;\boldsymbol{\theta})$$

and jointly estimating the parameters $c$ and $\boldsymbol{\theta}$ using the Newton–Raphson method. If we are interested in a nonparametric estimator, using the conventional smoothed spectral estimator for the periodogram, adjusted for the long memory component, say $g_k^d\, I(\nu_k)$ might be a possible approach.

## 3.8 Lagged Regression Models

One of the intriguing possibilities offered by the coherence analysis of the relation between the SOI and Recruitment series would be extending classical regression to the analysis of lagged regression models of the form

$$y_t = \sum_{r=-\infty}^{\infty} \beta_r x_{t-r} + v_t, \tag{3.101}$$

where $v_t$ is a stationary noise process, $x_t$ is the observed input series, and $y_t$ is the observed output series. We are interested in estimating the filter coefficients $\beta_r$ relating the adjacent lagged values of $x_t$ to the output series $y_t$.

In the case of SOI and Recruitment series, we might identify the El-Niño driving series, SOI, as the input, $x_t$, and $y_t$, the Recruitment series, as the output. In general, there will be more than a single possible input series and we may envision a $q \times 1$ vector of driving series. This multivariate input situation is covered in Chapter 5. The model given by (3.101) is useful under several different scenarios, corresponding to different assumptions that can be made about the components.

Assuming that the inputs and outputs have zero means and are jointly stationary with the $2 \times 1$ vector process $(x_t, y_t)'$ assumed to have a spectral matrix of the form

$$f(\nu) = \begin{pmatrix} f_x(\nu) & f_{xy}(\nu) \\ f_{yx}(\nu) & f_y(\nu) \end{pmatrix}, \tag{3.102}$$

where $f_{xy}(\nu)$ is the cross-spectrum, relating the input $x_t$ to the output $y_t$, and $f_x(\nu)$ and $f_y(\nu)$ are the spectra of the input and output series, respectively. Generally, we observe two series, regarded as input and output and search for regression functions $\{\beta_t\}$ relating the inputs to the outputs. We assume all autocovariance functions satisfy the absolute summability conditions of the form (3.50).

Then, minimizing the mean squared error

$$MSE = E\big[(y_t - \sum_{r=-\infty}^{\infty} \beta_r x_{t-r})^2\big] \tag{3.103}$$

leads to the usual orthogonality conditions

$$E\big[(y_t - \sum_{r=-\infty}^{\infty} \beta_r x_{t-r}) x_{t-s}\big] = 0 \tag{3.104}$$

for all $s = 0, \pm 1, \pm 2, \ldots$. Taking the expectations inside leads to the normal equations

$$\sum_{r=-\infty}^{\infty} \beta_r \ \gamma_x(s-r) = \gamma_{yx}(s) \tag{3.105}$$

for $s = 0, \pm 1, \pm 2, \ldots$. These equations might be solved, with some effort, if the covariance functions were known exactly. If data $(x_t, y_t)$ for $t = 1, ..., n$ are available, we might use a finite approximation to the above equations with $\widehat{\gamma}_x(h)$ and $\widehat{\gamma}_{yx}(h)$ substituted into (3.105). If the regression vectors are essentially zero for $|s| \geq M/2$, and $M < n$, the system (3.105) would be of full rank and the solution would involve inverting an $(M-1) \times (M-1)$ matrix.

A frequency domain approximate solution is easier in this case for two reasons. First, the computations depend on spectra and cross-spectra that can be estimated from sample data using (3.78) and (3.79). In addition, no matrices will have to be inverted, although the frequency domain ratio will have to be computed for each frequency. In order to develop the frequency domain solution, substitute the representation (3.22) into the normal equations, using the convention defined in (3.102). The left side of (3.105) can then be written in the form

$$\int_{-1/2}^{1/2} \sum_{r=-\infty}^{\infty} \beta_r \ e^{2\pi i\nu(s-r)} \ f_x(\nu) \ d\nu = \int_{-1/2}^{1/2} e^{2\pi i\nu s} B(\nu) f_x(\nu) \ d\nu,$$

where

$$B(\nu) = \sum_{r=-\infty}^{\infty} \beta_r \ e^{-2\pi i\nu r} \tag{3.106}$$

is the Fourier transform of the regression coefficients $\beta_t$. Now, because $\gamma_{yx}(s)$ is the inverse transform of the cross-spectrum $f_{yx}(\nu)$, we might write the system of equations in the frequency domain, using the uniqueness of the Fourier transform, as

$$B(\nu) f_x(\nu) = f_{yx}(\nu), \tag{3.107}$$

which then become the analogs of the usual normal equations. Then, we may take

$$\widehat{B}(\nu_k) = \frac{\widehat{f}_{yx}(\nu_k)}{\widehat{f}_x(\nu_k)} \tag{3.108}$$

as the estimator for the Fourier transform of the regression coefficients, evaluated at some subset of fundamental frequencies $\nu_k = k/M$ with $M << n$. Generally, we assume smoothness of $B(\cdot)$ over intervals of the form $\{\nu_k + \ell/n;\ \ell = -(L-1)/2, \ldots, (L-1)/2\}$. The inverse transform of the function $\widehat{B}(\nu)$ would give $\widehat{\beta}_t$, and we note that the discrete time approximation can be taken as

$$\widehat{\beta}_t = M^{-1} \sum_{k=0}^{M-1} \widehat{B}(\nu_k) e^{2\pi i \nu_k t} \tag{3.109}$$

for $t = 0, \pm 1, \pm 2, \ldots, \pm(M/2 - 1)$. In general, the approximation introduces reflections at multiples of the form $t \pm \ell M$, but the relation is exact if $\widehat{\beta}_t = 0$ for $|t| \geq M/2$. Problem 3.21 explores the error resulting from this approximation.

**Example 3.18 Lagged Regression Results for SOI and Recruitment Series**

The high coherence between the SOI and Recruitment series noted in Example 3.15 suggests a lagged regression relation between the two series. A natural direction for the implication in this situation is implied because we feel that the sea surface temperature or SOI should be the input and the Recruitment series should be the output. With this in mind, let $x_t$ be the SOI series and $y_t$ the Recruitment series.

Although we think naturally of the SOI as the input and the Recruitment as the output, two input-output configurations are of interest. With SOI as the input, the model is

$$y_t = \sum_{r=-\infty}^{\infty} a_r x_{t-r}$$

whereas a model that reverses the two roles would be

$$x_t = \sum_{r=-\infty}^{\infty} b_r y_{t-r}.$$

Even though there is no plausible environmental explanation for the second of these two models, displaying both possibilities helps to settle on a parsimonious transfer function model. The two estimated regression or impulse response functions with $M = 32$ and $L = 15$ are shown in Figure 3.15. Note the negative peak at a lag of five points in the first of the two situations where the SOI series is assumed to be the input. The fall-off after lag five seems to be approximately exponential. A possible model for this situation is

$$y_t = -22x_{t-5} - 15x_{t-4} - 12x_{t-3} - 10x_{t-4} - 9x_{t-10} - \ldots.$$

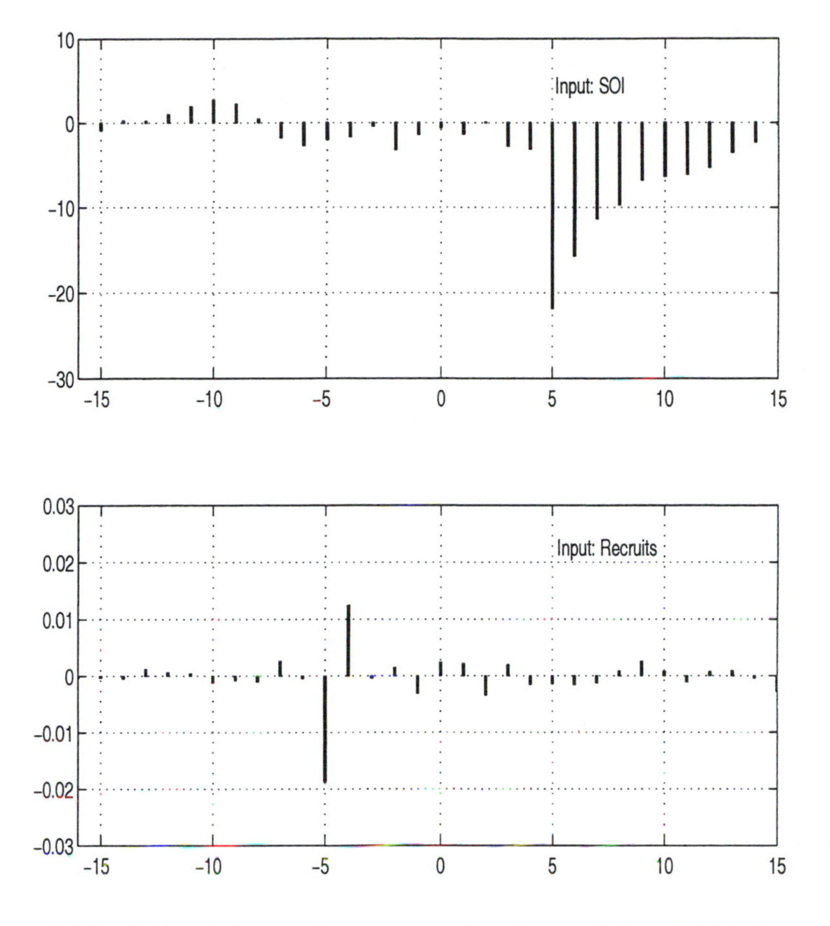


**Figure 3.15:** Estimated impulse response functions relating SOI to Recruitment (top) and Recruitment to SOI (bottom) $L = 15, M = 32$.

If we examine the inverse relation, namely, a regression model with the Recruitment series $y_t$ as the input, we get a much simpler model that seems to depend on only two coefficients, namely,

$$x_t = .012y_{t+4} - .018y_{t+5},$$

or, shifting by five points and transposing,

$$y_t = .667y_{t-1} - 56x_{t-5},$$

which suggests immediately the transfer function model considered in Example 2.45 of Chapter 2. In the notation of that chapter

$$(1 - .667B)y_t = -56B^5x_t,$$

and we may add a noise term for convenience. The exponential decaying component shows more clearly than in the prewhitening approach that lead to the time domain version shown in Example 2.45. Furthermore, computing the regression both ways allows us immediately to arrive at the more economical model that involves just two regression parameters rather than the 12-15 coefficients implied by regressing $y_t$ on $x_t$.

The example shows we can get a clean estimator for the transfer functionsrelating the two series if the coherence $\widehat{\rho}^2_{xy}(\nu)$ is large. The reason is that we can write the minimized mean squared error (3.103) as

$$MSE = E\left[\left(y_t - \sum_{r=-\infty}^{\infty} \beta_r x_{t-r}\right) y_t\right] = \gamma_y(0) - \sum_{r=-\infty}^{\infty} \beta_r \gamma_{xy}(-r),$$

using the result about the orthogonality of the data and error term in the Projection theorem. Then, substituting the spectral representations autocovariance and cross-covariance functions and identifying the Fourier transform (3.106) in the result leads to

$$\begin{aligned} MSE &= \int_{-1/2}^{1/2} [f_y(\nu) - B(\nu) f_{xy}(\nu)]\, d\nu \\ &= \int_{-1/2}^{1/2} f_y(\nu)[1 - \rho^2_{yx}(\nu)] d\nu, \end{aligned} \tag{3.110}$$

where $\rho^2_{yx}(\nu)$ is just the squared coherence given by (3.20). The similarity of (3.110) to the usual mean square error that results from predicting $y$ from $x$ is obvious. In that case, we would have

$$E[(y - \beta x)^2] = \sigma^2_y (1 - \rho^2_{xy})$$

for jointly distributed random variables $x$ and $y$ with zero means, variances $\sigma^2_x$ and $\sigma^2_y$, and covariance $\sigma_{xy} = \rho_{xy}\sigma_x\sigma_y$. Because the mean squared error in (3.110) satisfies $MSE \geq 0$ with $f_y(\nu)$ a non-negative function, it follows that the coherence satisfies

$$0 \leq \rho^2_{xy}(\nu) \leq 1$$

for all $\nu$. Furthermore, Problem 3.22 shows the squared coherence is one when the output are linearly related by the filter relation (3.101), and there is no noise, i.e., $v_t = 0$. Hence, the multiple coherence gives a measure of the association or correlation between the input and output series as a function of frequency.

The matter of verifying that the $F$-distribution claimed for (3.80) will hold when the sample coherence values are substituted for theoretical values still remains. Again, the form of the $F$-statistic is exactly analogous to the usual $t$-test for no correlation in a regression context. We give an argument leading to this conclusion later using the results in Section T3.13. Another question that has not been resolved in this section is the extension to the case of multiple inputs $x_{t1}, x_{t2}, \ldots, x_{tq}$. Often, more than just a single input series is present that can possibly form a lagged predictor of the output series $y_t$. An example is the cardiovascular mortality series that depended on possibly a number of pollution series and temperature. We discuss this particular extension as a part of the multivariate time series techniques considered in Chapter 5.

## 3.9 Signal Extraction and Optimum Filtering

A model closely related to regression can be developed by assuming that (3.101) still holds, but that the convolving regression function is fixed and known the time series $x_t$ is some unknown random ***signal***, uncorrelated with the ***noise*** process $v_t$. In this case, we observe only $y_t$ and are interested in an estimator for the signal $x_t$ of the form

$$\widehat{x}_t = \sum_{r=-\infty}^{\infty} a_r y_{t-r}. \tag{3.111}$$

In the frequency domain, it is convenient to make the additional assumptions that the series $x_t$ and $v_t$ are both mean-zero stationary series with spectra $f_x(\nu)$ and $f_v(\nu)$, often referred to as the ***signal spectrum*** and ***noise spectrum***, respectively. Often, the special case $\beta_t = \delta_t$, in which $\delta_t$ is the Kronecker delta, is of interest because (3.101) reduces to the simple ***signal plus noise*** model

$$y_t = x_t + v_t \tag{3.112}$$

in that case. In general, we seek the set of filter coefficients $a_t$ that minimize the mean squared error of estimation, say,

$$MSE = E[(x_t - \sum_{r=-\infty}^{\infty} a_r y_{t-r})^2]. \tag{3.113}$$

This problem was originally solved by Kolmogorov (1941) and by Wiener (1949), who derived the result in 1941 and published it in classified reports during World War II.

Again, we can apply the orthogonality principle to write

$$E[(x_t - \sum_{r=-\infty}^{\infty} a_r y_{t-r}) y_{t-s}] = 0$$

for $s = 0, \pm 1, \pm 2, \ldots$, which leads to

$$\sum_{r=-\infty}^{\infty} a_r \gamma_y(s-r) = \gamma_{xy}(s),$$

to be solved for the filter coefficients. Substituting the spectral representations for the autocovariance functions into the above and identifying through the uniqueness of the Fourier transform produces an equation nearly the same as (3.107), namely,

$$A(\nu)f_y(\nu) = f_{xy}(\nu), \tag{3.114}$$

where $A(\nu)$ and the optimal filter $a_t$ are Fourier transform pairs, as in (3.106) for $B(\nu)$ and $\beta_t$. Now, a special consequence of the model is that (see Problem 3.9)

$$f_{xy}(\nu) = \overline{B(\nu)} f_x(\nu) \tag{3.115}$$

and

$$f_y(\nu) = |B(\nu)|^2 f_x(\nu) + f_v(\nu), \tag{3.116}$$

implying the optimal filter would be Fourier transform of

$$A(\nu) = \frac{\overline{B(\nu)}}{\left(|B(\nu)|^2 + \frac{f_v(\nu)}{f_x(\nu)}\right)}, \tag{3.117}$$

where the second term in the denominator is just the inverse of the ***signal to noise ratio***, say,

$$SNR(\nu) = \frac{f_x(\nu)}{f_v(\nu)}. \tag{3.118}$$

The result shows the optimum filters can be computed for this model if the signal and noise spectra are both known or if we can assume knowledge of the signal-to-noise ratio $SNR(\nu)$ as function of frequency. In Chapter 5, we show some methods for estimating these two parameters in conjunction with random effects analysis of variance models, but we assume here that it is possible to specify the signal-to-noise ratio *a priori*. If the signal-to-noise ratio is known, the optimal filter can be computed by the inverse transform of the function $A(\nu)$. It is more likely that the inverse transform will be intractable and a finite filter approximation like that used in the previous section can be applied to the data. In this case, we will have

$$a_t^M = M^{-1} \sum_{k=0}^{M-1} A(\nu_k) e^{2\pi i \nu_k t} \tag{3.119}$$

as the estimated filter function. It will often be the case that the form of the specified frequency response will have some rather sharp transitions between regions where the signal-to-noise ratio is high and regions where there is little signal. In these cases, the shape of the frequency response function will have ripples that can introduce frequencies at different amplitudes. An aesthetic solution to this problem is to introduce tapering as was done with spectral estimation in (3.71)-(3.77). We use below the tapered filter $\tilde{a}_t = h_t a_t$ where

$h_t$ is the cosine taper given in (3.77). The squared frequency response of the resulting filter will be $|\tilde{A}(\nu)|^2$, where

$$\tilde{A}(\nu) = \sum_{t=-\infty}^{\infty} a_t h_t e^{-2\pi i \nu t}. \tag{3.120}$$

The results are illustrated in the example below that extracts the El Niño component of the sea surface temperature series.

**Example 3.19 Estimating the El Niño Signal Using Optimal Filters**

Figure 3.8 shows the spectrum of the SOI series, and we note that essentially two components have power, the El Niño frequency of about .02 cycles per month and a yearly frequency of about .08 cycles per month. We assume, for this example, that we wish to preserve the lower frequency as signal and to eliminate the higher order frequencies. In this case, we assume the simple signal plus noise model

$$y_t = x_t + v_t,$$

so that there is no convolving function $\beta_t$. Furthermore, the signal-to-noise ratio is assumed to be high to about .06 cycles per month and zero thereafter. The optimal frequency response was assumed to be unity to .05 cycles per point and then to decay linearly to zero in several steps. Figure 3.16 shows the Fourier (3.119) transform at $M = 64$ frequencies, say, $a_t^M$ and the tapered version $h_t a_t^M$. The estimated squared frequency response, approximated as a long (256 point) transform of the form (3.120), has ripples when tapering is not applied and is relatively smooth for the tapered filter. Figure 3.16 shows both positive and negative frequencies. Figure 3.17 shows the original and filtered SOI index, and we see a smooth extracted signal that conveys the essence of the underlying El Niño signal. The frequency response of the designed filter can be compared with that of the symmetric 12-month moving average applied to the same series in Example 3.8. The filtered series, shown in Figure 3.4, shows a good deal of higher frequency chatter riding on the smoothed version, which has been introduced by the higher frequencies that leak through in the squared frequency response, as in Figure 3.5.

The design of finite filters with a specified frequency response requires some experimentation with various target frequency response functions and we have only touched on the methodology here. The filter designed here, sometimes called a low-pass filter reduces the high frequencies and keeps or passes the low frequencies. Alternately, we could design a high-pass filter to keep high frequencies if that is where the signal is located. An example of a simple

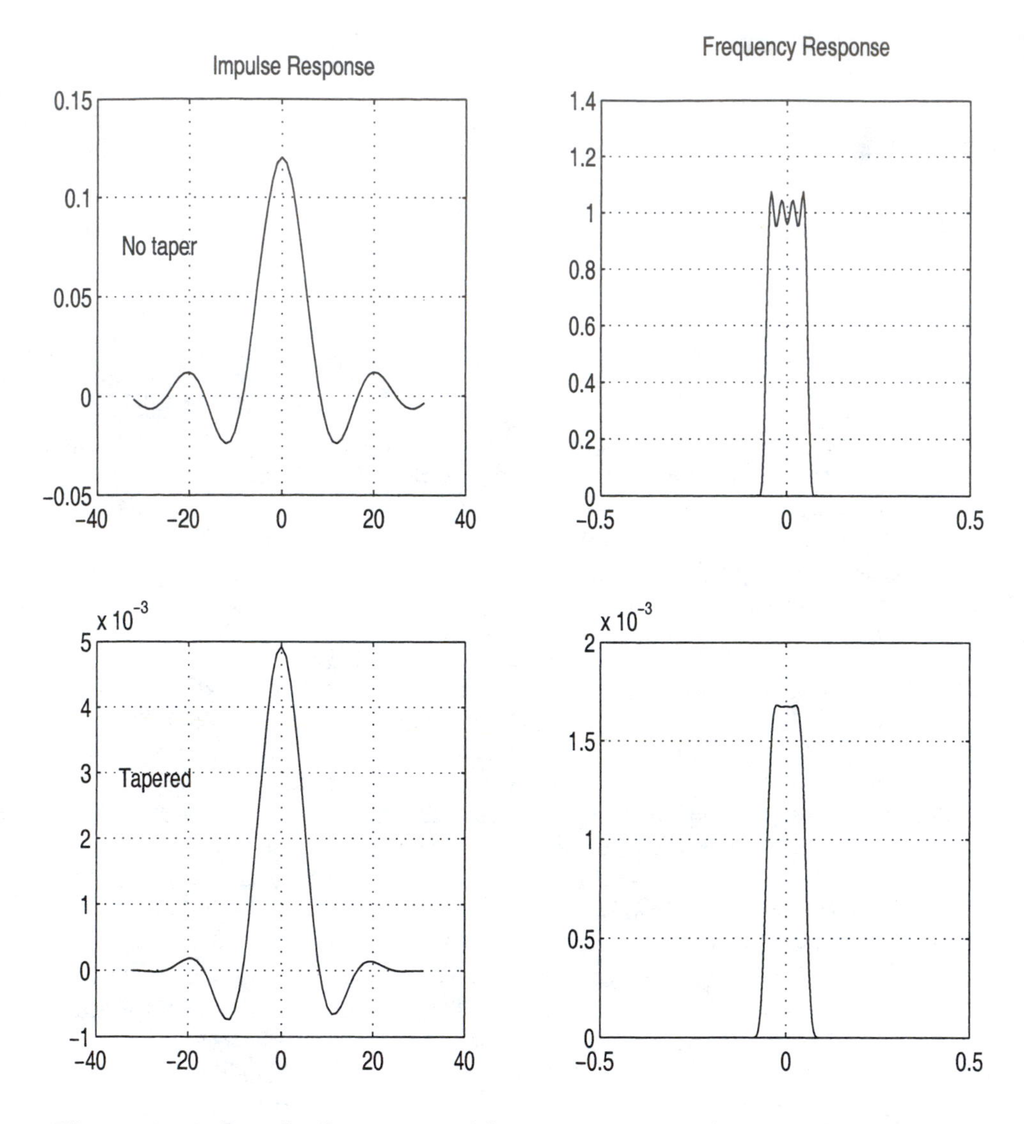


**Figure 3.16:** Impulse Response and frequency response functions for designed SOI filters. Note the ripples in the top panel frequency response of the untapered filter.

high-pass filter is the first difference with a frequency response that is shown in Figure 3.5. We can also design band-pass filters that keep frequencies in specified bands. For example, seasonal adjustment filters are often used in economics to reject seasonal frequencies while keeping both high frequencies, lower frequencies, and trend (see, for example, Grether and Nerlove, 1970).

The filters we have discussed here are all symmetric two-sided filters, since

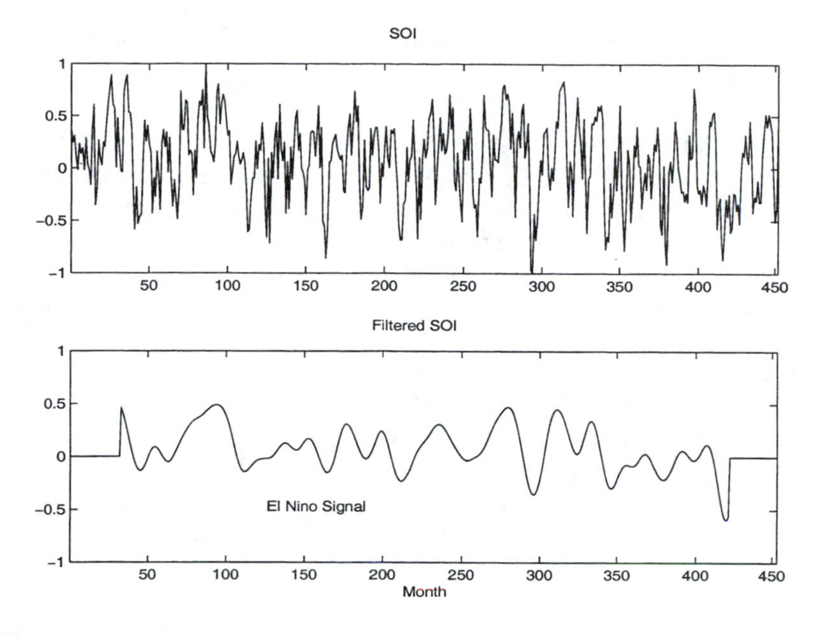


**Figure 3.17:** Original SOI series (top) compared to filtered version showing the estimated El Niño temperature signal (bottom).

the designed frequency response functions were purely real. Alternatively, we may design ***recursive filters*** to produce a desired response. An example of a recursive filter is one that replaces the input $x_t$ by the filtered output

$$y_t = \sum_{k=1}^{p} \phi_k y_{t-k} + x_t - \sum_{k=1}^{q} \theta_k x_{t-k}. \tag{3.121}$$

Note the similarity between (3.121) and the ARIMA(1,0,1) model, in which the white noise component is replaced by the input. Transposing the terms involving $y_t$ and using the basic linear filter result in Property 3.3 leads to

$$f_y(\nu) = \frac{|\theta(\mathrm{e}^{-2\pi i\nu})|^2}{|\phi(\mathrm{e}^{-2\pi i\nu})|^2} f_x(\nu), \tag{3.122}$$

where

$$\phi(\mathrm{e}^{-2\pi i\nu}) = 1 - \sum_{k=1}^{p} \phi_k \mathrm{e}^{-2\pi ik\nu}$$

and

$$\theta(\mathrm{e}^{-2\pi i\nu}) = 1 - \sum_{k=1}^{q} \theta_k \mathrm{e}^{-2\pi ik\nu}.$$

Recursive filters such as those given by (3.122) distort the phases of arriving frequencies, and we do not consider the problem of designing such filters in any detail.

## 3.10 Spectral Analysis of Multidimensional Series

Multidimensional series of the form $x_{\boldsymbol{s}}$, where $\boldsymbol{s} = (s_1, s_2, \ldots, s_r)'$ is an $r$-dimensional vector of spatial coordinates or a combination of space and time coordinates, were introduced in Section 1.8. The example given there, shown in Figure 1.19, was a collection of temperature measurements taking on a rectangular field. This data would form a two-dimensional process, indexed by row and column in space. In that section, the multidimensional autocovariance function of an $r$-dimensional stationary series was given as $\gamma_x(\boldsymbol{h}) = E[x_{\boldsymbol{s}+\boldsymbol{h}} x_{\boldsymbol{s}}]$, where the multidimensional lag vector is $\boldsymbol{h} = (h_1, h_2, \ldots, h_r)'$.

The multidimensional ***wavenumber spectrum*** is given as the Fourier transform of the autocovariance, namely,

$$f_x(\boldsymbol{\nu}) = \sum_{\boldsymbol{h}} \gamma_x(\boldsymbol{h}) e^{-2\pi i \boldsymbol{\nu}'\boldsymbol{h}}. \tag{3.123}$$

Again, the inverse result

$$\gamma_x(\boldsymbol{h}) = \int_{-1/2}^{1/2} f_x(\boldsymbol{\nu}) e^{2\pi i \boldsymbol{\nu}'\boldsymbol{h}} d\boldsymbol{\nu} \tag{3.124}$$

holds, where the integral is over the multidimensional range of the vector $\boldsymbol{\nu}$. The wavenumber argument is exactly analogous to the frequency argument, and we have the corresponding intuitive interpretation as the cycling rate $\nu_i$ per distance traveled $s_i$ in the $i^{th}$ direction.

Two-dimensional processes occur often in practical applications, and the representations above reduce to

$$f_x(\nu_1, \nu_2) = \sum_{h_1=-\infty}^{\infty} \sum_{h_2=-\infty}^{\infty} \gamma_x(h_1, h_2) e^{-2\pi i(\nu_1 h_1 + \nu_2 h_2)} \tag{3.125}$$

and

$$\gamma_x(h_1, h_2) = \int_{-1/2}^{1/2} \int_{-1/2}^{1/2} f_x(\nu_1, \nu_2) e^{2\pi i(\nu_1 h_1 + \nu_2 h_2)} d\nu_1 \, d\nu_2 \tag{3.126}$$

in the case $r = 2$. The notion of linear filtering generalizes easily to the two-dimensional case by defining the impulse response function $a_{s_1,s_2}$ and the spatial filter output as

$$y_{s_1,s_2} = \sum_{u_1} \sum_{u_2} a_{u_1,u_2} x_{s_1-u_1,s_2-u_2}. \tag{3.127}$$

The spectrum of the output of this filter can be derived as

$$f_y(\nu_1, \nu_2) = |A(\nu_1, \nu_2)|^2 f_x(\nu_1, \nu_2), \tag{3.128}$$

where

$$A(\nu_1, \nu_2) = \sum_{u_1} \sum_{u_2} a_{u_1,u_2} e^{-2\pi i(\nu_1 u_1 + \nu_2 u_2)}. \tag{3.129}$$

These results are analogous to those in the one-dimensional case, described by Property P3.3.

The multidimensional DFT is also a straightforward generalization of the univariate expression (3.44). In the two-dimensional case with data on a rectangular grid, $\{x_{s_1,s_2};\ s_1 = 1, ..., n_1,\ s_2 = 1, ..., n_2\}$, we will write, for $-1/2 \le \nu_1, \nu_2 \le 1/2$,

$$X(\nu_1, \nu_2) = (n_1 n_2)^{-1/2} \sum_{s_1=1}^{n_1} \sum_{s_2=1}^{n_2} x_{s_1,s_2} e^{-2\pi i(\nu_1 s_1 + \nu_2 s_2)} \tag{3.130}$$

as the two-dimensional DFT, where the frequencies $\nu_1, \nu_2$ are evaluated at multiples of $(1/n_1, 1/n_2)$ on the spatial frequency scale. The two-dimensional wavenumber spectrum can be estimated by the smoothed ***sample wavenumber spectrum***

$$\widehat{f}_x(\nu_1, \nu_2) = (L_1 L_2)^{-1} \sum_{\ell_1,\ell_2} |X(\nu_1 + \ell_1/n_1, \nu_2 + \ell_2/n_2)|^2, \tag{3.131}$$

where the sum is taken over the grid $\{-(L_j - 1)/2 \le \ell_j \le (L_j - 1)/2;\ j = 1, 2\}$, where $L_1$ and $L_2$ are odd. The statistic

$$\frac{2 L_1 L_2 \widehat{f}_x(\nu_1, \nu_2)}{f_x(\nu_1, \nu_2)} \sim \chi^2_{2L_1L_2} \tag{3.132}$$

has an approximate chi-squared distribution with $2L_1L_2$ degrees of freedom. As before, this result can be used to set confidence intervals or make approximate tests against a fixed assumed spectrum $f_0(\nu_1, \nu_2)$.

**Example 3.20 Wavenumber Spectrum of Soil Surface Temperatures**

As an example, consider the periodogram of the two-dimensional temperature series shown in Figure 1.25 and analyzed by Bazza et al (1988). We recall the spatial coordinates in this case will be $(s_1, s_2)$, which define the spatial coordinates rows and columns so that the frequencies in the two directions will be expressed as cycles per row and cycles per column. Figure 3.18 shows the periodogram of the two-dimensional temperature series, and we note the ridge of strong spectral peaks running over rows at a column frequency of zero. An obvious periodic component appears at frequencies of .0625 and -.0625 cycles per row, which corresponds to 16 rows or about 272 ft. On further investigation of previous irrigation patterns over this field, treatment levels of salt varied periodically over columns. This analysis is extended in Problem 3.15, where we recover the salt treatment profile over rows and compare it to a signal, computed by averaging over columns.

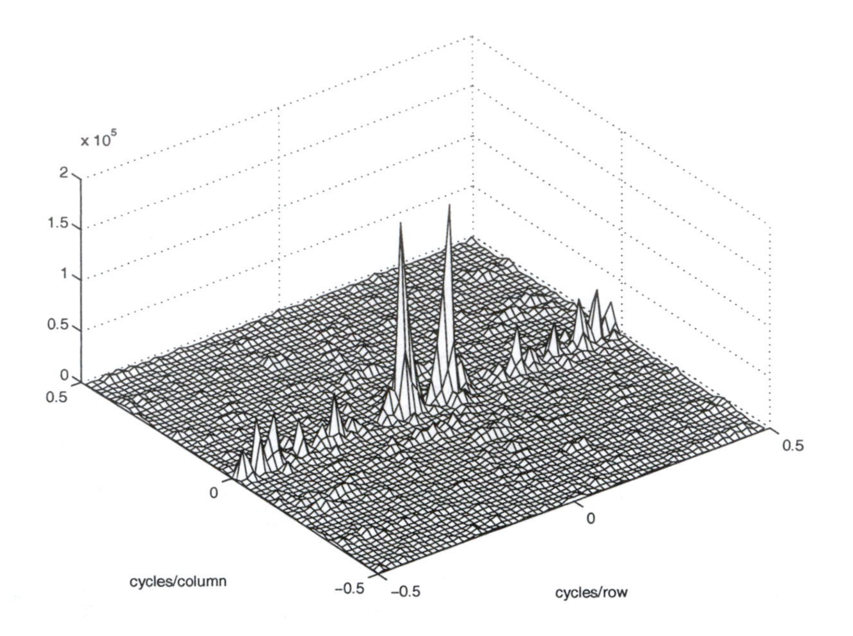


**Figure 3.18:** Two-dimensional periodogram of soil temperature profile showing peak at .0625 cycles/row. The period is 16 rows, and this corresponds to $16 \times 17$ ft $= 272$ ft.

Another application of two-dimensional spectral analysis of agricultural field trials is given in McBratney and Webster (1981), who used it to detect ridge and furrow patterns in yields. The requirement for regular, equally spaced samples on fairly large grids has tended to limit enthusiasm for strict two-dimensional spectral analysis. An exception is when a propagating signal from a given velocity and azimuth is present so predicting the wavenumber spectrum as a function of velocity and azimuth becomes feasible (see Shumway et al, 1999).

## T3.11 Spectral Representation Theorem

We consider in this section some results that justify representing the autocovariance function $\gamma_x(h)$ of the weakly stationary process $x_t$ in terms of a non-negative spectral density function. In addition, we present a spectral representation for the process $x_t$ itself, which allows us to think of a stationary process as a random sum of sines and cosines as described in (3.3). The spectral density function essentially measures the variance or power in a particular kind of periodic oscillation in the function. We denote this spectral density of variance function by $f(\nu)$, where the variance is measured as a function of the frequency of oscillation $\nu$, measured in cycles per unit time.

We consider developing a representation of the same general form as the above for the general stationary, possibly complex, series $x_t$ with zero mean and stationary autocovariance function $\gamma(h) = E(x_{t+h}x_t^*)$. We prove the representation for arbitrary non-negative definite functions $\gamma_x(h)$ and then simply note the autocovariance function is Hermitian non-negative definite, since, for any set of complex constants, $a_t, t = 0 \pm 1, \pm 2, \ldots$, we may write, for any finite subset,

$$E|\sum_{s=1}^{n} a_s^* x_s|^2 = \sum_{s=1}^{n}\sum_{t=1}^{n} a_s^*\gamma(s-t)a_t \geq 0.$$

The representation is stated in terms of non-negative definite functions and a spectral distribution function $F(\nu)$ that is monotone nondecreasing, and continuous from the right, taking the values $F(-1/2) = 0$ and $F(1/2) = \sigma^2 = \gamma_x(0)$ at $\nu = -1/2$ and $1/2$, respectively.

**Theorem 3.1 (a):** *A function $\gamma(h)$, for $h = 0 \pm 1, \pm 2, \ldots$ is Hermitian non-negative definite if and only if it can be expressed as*

$$\gamma(h) = \int_{-1/2}^{1/2} \exp\{2\pi i\nu h\} dF(\nu) \tag{3.133}$$

*where $F(\cdot)$ is monotone non-decreasing. The function $F(\cdot)$ is right continuous, bounded in $[-1/2, 1/2]$, and uniquely determined by the conditions $F(-1/2) = 0, F(1/2) = \gamma(0)$.*

To prove the result, note first if $\gamma(h)$ has the representation above,

$$\begin{aligned}
\sum_{s=1}^{n}\sum_{t=1}^{n} a_s^*\gamma(s-t)a_t &= \int_{-1/2}^{1/2} a_s^*\gamma(s-t)a_t e^{2\pi i\nu(s-t)} dF(\nu) \\
&= \int_{-1/2}^{1/2} \left|\sum_{s=1}^{n} a_s e^{-2\pi i\nu s}\right|^2 dF(\nu) \\
&\geq 0
\end{aligned}$$

and $\gamma(h)$ is non-negative definite. Conversely, suppose $\gamma(h)$ is a non-negative definite function, and define the non-negative function

$$\begin{aligned}
f_n(\nu) &= n^{-1}\sum_{s=1}^{n}\sum_{t=1}^{n} e^{-2\pi i\nu s}\gamma(s-t)e^{2\pi i\nu t} \\
&= n^{-1}\sum_{u=-(n-1)}^{(n-1)} (n-|u|)e^{-2\pi i\nu u}\gamma(u) \\
&\geq 0.
\end{aligned}$$

Now, let $F_n(\nu)$ be the distribution function corresponding to $f_n(\nu)I_{(-1/2,1/2]}$, where $I_{(\cdot)}$ denotes the indicator function of the interval in the subscript. Note that $F_n(\nu) = 0, \nu \le -1/2$ and $F_n(\nu) = F_n(1/2)$ for $\nu \ge 1/2$. Then,

$$\begin{aligned}\int_{-1/2}^{1/2} e^{2\pi i\nu h} dF_n(\nu) &= \int_{-1/2}^{1/2} e^{2\pi i\nu h} f_n(\nu)\, d\nu \\ &= \begin{cases} (1-|u|/n)\gamma_x(u), & |u| < n \\ 0, & \text{elsewhere.}\end{cases}\end{aligned}$$

We also have

$$\begin{aligned}F_n(1/2) &= \int_{-1/2}^{1/2} f_n(\nu)\, d\nu \\ &= \int_{-1/2}^{1/2} \sum_{|u|<n} (1-|u|/n)\gamma(u) e^{-2\pi i\nu u} d\nu \\ &= \gamma(0).\end{aligned}$$

Now, by Helly's first convergence theorem (Bhat, 1985, p.157), there exists a subsequence $F_{n_k}$ converging to $F$, and by the Helly-Bray Lemma (see Bhat, p. 157), this implies

$$\int_{-1/2}^{1/2} e^{2\pi i\nu u} dF_{n_k}(\nu) \to \int_{-1/2}^{1/2} e^{2\pi i\nu u} dF(\nu)$$

and, from the right-hand side of the earlier equation,

$$(1-|u|/n_k)\gamma(u) \to \gamma(u)$$

as $n_k \to \infty$, and the required result follows.

We now present the version of the ***Spectral Representation Theorem*** in terms of a stationary (mean-zero) process, $x_t$ (see Hannan, 1970, Section 2.3 for details). This version allows us to think of a stationary process as being generated (approximately) by a random sum of sines and cosines such as described in (3.3).

**Theorem 3.1 (b):** *If $x_t$ is a mean-zero, stationary process with spectral distribution $F(\nu)$, then there exists a (complex-valued) stochastic process $z(\nu)$, for $-1/2 \le \nu \le 1/2$, having stationary uncorrelated increments, such that $x_t$ can be written as the stochastic integral*

$$x_t = \int_{-1/2}^{1/2} \exp(-2\pi i t\nu) dz(\nu)$$

*where, for $-1/2 \le \nu_1 \le \nu_2 \le 1/2$,*

$$\text{var}\,(z(\nu_2) - z(\nu_1)) = F(\nu_2) - F(\nu_1).$$

An uncorrelated increment process such as $z(\nu)$ is a mean-zero, finite variance, continuous-time stochastic process for which events occurring in non-overlapping intervals are uncorrelated. The integral in this representation is a stochastic integral. To understand its meaning, let $\nu_0, \nu_1, ...., \nu_n$ be a partition of the interval $[-1/2, 1/2]$. Define

$$I_n = \sum_{j=1}^{n} \exp(2\pi it\nu_j)[z(\nu_j) - z(\nu_{j-1})].$$

Then $I = \int_{-1/2}^{1/2} \exp(-2\pi it\nu)dz(\nu)$ is defined to be the mean square limit of $I_n$, that is $I_n \stackrel{ms}{\to} I$ as $n \to \infty$.

In general, the spectral distribution function can be a mixture of discrete and continuous distributions. The special case of greatest interest is the absolutely continuous case, namely, when $dF(\nu) = f(\nu)d\nu$, and the resulting function is the spectral density considered in Section 3.3. In this case, we have the following theorem

**Theorem 3.2:** *If $\gamma(h)$ is a covariance function with*

$$\sum_{h=-\infty}^{\infty} |\gamma(h)| < \infty, \tag{3.134}$$

*we have*

$$f(\nu) = \sum_{h=-\infty}^{\infty} \gamma(h)e^{-2\pi i\nu h}. \tag{3.135}$$

To prove the above, write

$$\begin{aligned} \int_{-1/2}^{1/2} e^{2\pi i\nu h} f(\nu)\, d\nu &= \int_{-1/2}^{1/2} e^{2\pi i\nu h} \sum_{k=-\infty}^{\infty} \gamma(k)e^{-2\pi i\nu k} d\nu \\ &= \sum_{k=-\infty}^{\infty} \gamma(k)e^{2\pi i(h-k)\nu} d\nu \\ &= \gamma(h), \end{aligned}$$

using the Fubini theorem (Bhat, 1985, p.126) and

$$\int_{-1/2}^{1/2} \sum_{h=-\infty}^{\infty} |\gamma(h)||e^{2\pi i(h-k)\nu}|d\nu \leq \sum_{h=-\infty}^{\infty} |\gamma(h)| < \infty.$$

We may extend the representation to the vector case $\boldsymbol{x}_t = (x_{t1}, \ldots, x_{tp})'$ by considering linear combinations of the form

$$y_t = \sum_{j=1}^{p} a_j^* x_{tj},$$

which will be stationary with autocovariance functions of the form

$$\gamma_y(h) = \sum_{j=1}^{p}\sum_{k=1}^{p} a_j^* \gamma_{jk}(h) a_k,$$

where $\gamma_{jk}(h)$ is the usual cross-covariance function between $x_{tj}$ and $x_{tk}$. To develop the spectral representation of $\gamma_{jk}(h)$ from the representations of the univariate series, consider the linear combinations

$$y_{t1} = x_{tj} + x_{tk}$$

and

$$y_{t2} = x_{tj} + i x_{tk},$$

which are both stationary series with respective representations

$$\begin{aligned}\gamma_{y1}(h) &= \gamma_j(h) + \gamma_{jk}(h) + \gamma_{kj}(h) + \gamma_k(h) \\ &= \int_{-1/2}^{1/2} e^{2\pi i\nu h} dG_1(\nu)\end{aligned}$$

and

$$\begin{aligned}\gamma_{y2}(h) &= \gamma_j(h) + i\gamma_{kj}(h) - i\gamma_{jk}(h) + \gamma_k(h) \\ &= \int_{-1/2}^{1/2} e^{2\pi i\nu h} dG_2(\nu).\end{aligned}$$

Introducing the spectral representations for $\gamma_j(h)$ and $\gamma_k(h)$ yields

$$\gamma_{jk}(h) = \int_{-1/2}^{1/2} e^{2\pi i\nu h} dF_{jk}(\nu),$$

with

$$F_{jk}(\nu) = \frac{1}{2}[G_1(\nu) + iG_2(\nu) - (1+i)(F_j(\nu) + F_k(\nu)].$$

Now, under the summability condition

$$\sum_{h=-\infty}^{\infty} |\gamma_{jk}(h)| < \infty,$$

we have the representation

$$\gamma_{jk}(h) = \int_{-1/2}^{1/2} e^{2\pi i\nu h} f_{jk}(\nu) d\nu,$$

where the cross-spectral density function has the inverse Fourier representation

$$f_{jk}(\nu) = \sum_{h=-\infty}^{\infty} \gamma_{jk}(h) e^{-2\pi i \nu h}$$

The cross-covariance function satisfies $\gamma_{jk}(h) = \gamma_{kj}^*(-h)$, which implies $f_{jk}(\nu) = f_{kj}^*(-\nu)$ using the above representation.

Then, defining the autocovariance function of the general vector process $\boldsymbol{x}_t$ as the $p \times p$ matrix

$$\Gamma(h) = E[(\boldsymbol{x}_{t+h} - \boldsymbol{\mu}_x)(\boldsymbol{x}_t - \boldsymbol{\mu}_x)'],$$

and the $p \times p$ spectral matrix as $f(\nu) = \{f_{jk}(\nu), j, k = 1, \ldots, p\}$, we have the representation in matrix form, written as

$$\Gamma(h) = \int_{-1/2}^{1/2} e^{2\pi i \nu h} f(\nu) \, d\nu, \tag{3.136}$$

and the inverse result

$$f(\nu) = \sum_{h=-\infty}^{\infty} \Gamma(h) e^{-2\pi i \nu h}. \tag{3.137}$$

which appears as ***Property 3.2*** in Section 3.3. Theorem 3.1 (b) can also be extended to the multivariate case in an obvious way.

# T3.12 Large Sample Distribution of the Discrete Fourier Transform

We have previously introduced the DFT, for the stationary zero-mean process $x_t$, observed at $t = 1, \ldots, n$ as

$$X(\nu) = n^{-1/2} \sum_{t=1}^{n} x_t \, e^{-2\pi i \nu t}, \tag{3.138}$$

as the result of matching sines and cosines of frequency $\nu$ against the series $x_t$. We will suppose now that $x_t$ has an absolutely continuous spectrum $f_x(\nu)$ corresponding to the autocovariance function $\gamma_x(h)$. Our purpose in this section is to examine the statistical properties of the complex random variables $X(\nu_k), \nu_k = k/n, k = 0, 1, \ldots, n$ in the hope they can provide a basis for estimating $f_x(\nu)$ and for setting limits on the spectral density function. To develop the statistical properties, we need to examine the behavior of

$$
\begin{aligned}
S_n(\nu,\omega) &= E[X(\nu)X^*(\omega)] \\
&= n^{-1}E\left[\sum_{s=1}^{n} x_s\ \mathrm{e}^{-2\pi i\nu s}\sum_{t=1}^{n} x_t\ \mathrm{e}^{2\pi i\omega t}\right] \\
&= n^{-1}\sum_{s=1}^{n}\sum_{t=1}^{n}\mathrm{e}^{-2\pi i\nu s}\mathrm{e}^{2\pi i\omega t}\gamma(s-t). \qquad (3.139)
\end{aligned}
$$

This definition can be motivated by noting for $\omega = \nu$,

$$
\begin{aligned}
S_n(\nu,\nu) &= E[|X(\nu)|^2] \\
&= n^{-1}E\left[\sum_{s=1}^{n} x_s\ \mathrm{e}^{-2\pi i\nu s}\sum_{t=1}^{n} x_t\mathrm{e}^{2\pi i\nu t}\right] \\
&= n^{-1}\sum_{s=1}^{n}\sum_{t=1}^{n}\mathrm{e}^{-2\pi i\nu s}\mathrm{e}^{2\pi i\nu t}\gamma(s-t) \\
&= \sum_{u=-(n-1)}^{(n-1)} (1-|u|/n)\gamma(u)\mathrm{e}^{-2\pi i\nu u},
\end{aligned}
$$

where we have let $u = s - t, v = t$. Using dominated convergence,

$$
S_n(\nu,\nu) \to \sum_{u=-\infty}^{\infty} \gamma(u)\mathrm{e}^{-2\pi i\nu u} = f(\nu),
$$

making the large sample variance of the Fourier transform equal to the spectrum evaluated at $\nu$. For exact bounds it is also convenient to add an absolute summability assumption for the autocovariance function, namely,

$$
\theta = \sum_{h=-\infty}^{\infty} |h||\gamma(h)| \qquad (3.140)
$$

is finite.

**Example 3.21 Condition (3.140) Verified for an AR(1)**

We may write the condition for an AR(1) series as

$$
\theta = \frac{\sigma_w^2}{1-\phi_1^2}\sum_{h=-\infty}^{\infty} |h|\phi_1^{|h|}
$$

being finite. Note the condition is equivalent to summability of

$$\begin{aligned}\sum_{h=1}^{\infty} h\phi_1^h &= \phi \sum_{h=1}^{\infty} h\phi_1^{h-1} \\ &= \phi_1 \frac{\partial}{\partial \phi_1} \sum_{h=1}^{\infty} \phi_1^h \\ &= \frac{\phi_1}{(1-\phi_1)^2},\end{aligned}$$

and

$$\theta = \frac{2\sigma_w^2 \phi_1}{(1-\phi_1)^3(1+\phi_1)}.$$

To elaborate further, we derive two approximation lemmas.

**Lemma 3.1:** *For* $S_n(\nu, \nu)$ *as defined in (3.139) and* $\theta$ *in (3.140) finite, we have*

$$|S_n(\nu,\nu) - f(\nu)| \le \frac{\theta}{n} \tag{3.141}$$

*or*

$$S_n(\nu,\nu) = f(\nu) + O(n^{-1}). \tag{3.142}$$

To prove the above, write

$$\begin{aligned} n|S_n(\nu,\nu) - f_x(\nu)| &= \left| \sum_{|u|<n} (n-|u|)\gamma(u)\mathrm{e}^{-2\pi i\nu u} - n \sum_{u=-\infty}^{\infty} \gamma(u)\mathrm{e}^{-2\pi i\nu u} \right| \\ &= \left| -n \sum_{|u|\ge n} \gamma(u)\mathrm{e}^{-2\pi i\nu u} - \sum_{|u|<n} |u|\gamma(u)\mathrm{e}^{-2\pi i\nu u} \right| \\ &\le \sum_{|u|\ge n} |u||\gamma(u)| + \sum_{|u|<n} |u||\gamma(u)| \\ &= \theta, \end{aligned}$$

and the lemma is proven.

**Lemma 3.2:** *For* $\nu_k = k/n, \nu_\ell = \ell/n, \nu_k - \nu_\ell \ne 0, \pm 1, \pm 2, \pm 3, \ldots,$ *and* $\theta$ *in (3.140), we have*

$$|S_n(\nu_k, \nu_\ell)| \le \frac{\theta}{n}, \tag{3.143}$$

*or*

$$|S_n(\nu_k \nu_\ell)| = O(n^{-1}). \tag{3.144}$$

To prove Lemma 3.2, write

$$\begin{aligned} n|S_n(\nu_k,\nu_\ell)| &= \sum_{u=-(n-1)}^{-1} \gamma(u) \sum_{v=-(u-1)}^{n} e^{-2\pi i(\nu_k-\nu_\ell)v} e^{-2\pi i \nu_k u} \\ &\quad + \sum_{u=0}^{n-1} \gamma(u) \sum_{v=1}^{n-u} e^{-2\pi i(\nu_k-\nu_\ell)v} e^{-2\pi i \nu_k u}. \end{aligned}$$

Now, for the first term, with $u < 0$,

$$\begin{aligned} \sum_{v=-(u-1)}^{n} e^{-2\pi i(\nu_k-\nu_\ell)v} &= \left(\sum_{v=1}^{n} - \sum_{v=1}^{-u}\right) e^{-2\pi i(\nu_k-\nu_\ell)v} \\ &= 0 - \sum_{v=1}^{-u} e^{-2\pi i(\nu_k-\nu_\ell)v}. \end{aligned}$$

For the second term with $u \geq 0$,

$$\begin{aligned} \sum_{v=1}^{n-u} e^{-2\pi i(\nu_k-\nu_\ell)v} &= \left(\sum_{v=1}^{n} - \sum_{v=n-u+1}^{n}\right) e^{-2\pi i(\nu_k-\nu_\ell)v} \\ &= 0 - \sum_{v=n-u+1}^{n} e^{-2\pi i(\nu_k-\nu_\ell)v}. \end{aligned}$$

Consequently,

$$\begin{aligned} n|S_n(\nu_k,\nu_\ell)| &= \Bigg| - \sum_{u=-(n-1)}^{-1} \gamma(u) \sum_{v=1}^{-u} e^{-2\pi i(\nu_k-\nu_\ell)v} e^{-2\pi i \nu_k u} \\ &\qquad - \sum_{u=1}^{n-1} \gamma(u) \sum_{v=n-u+1}^{n} e^{-2\pi i(\nu_k-\nu_\ell)v} e^{-2\pi i \nu_k u} \Bigg| \\ &\leq \sum_{u=-(n-1)}^{0} (-u)|\gamma(u)| + \sum_{u=1}^{n-1} u|\gamma(u)| \\ &= \sum_{u=-(n-1)}^{(n-1)} |u|\, |\gamma(u)|. \end{aligned}$$

Hence, we have

$$S_n(\nu_k,\nu_\ell) \leq \frac{\theta}{n},$$

and the asserted relations of the lemma follow.

Because the DFTs are approximately uncorrelated, say, of order $1/n$, when the frequencies are of the form $\nu_k = k/n$, we shall compute at those frequencies.

The behavior of $f_x(\nu)$ at neighboring frequencies, however, will often be of interest and we shall use Lemma 3.3 below to handle such cases

**Lemma 3.3:** *For $|\nu_k - \nu| \le L/2n$ and $\theta$ in (3.140), we have*

$$|f(\nu_k) - f(\nu)| \le \frac{\pi\theta L}{n} \tag{3.145}$$

*or*

$$f(\nu_k) - f(\nu) = O(L/n). \tag{3.146}$$

To prove Lemma 3.3, we write the difference

$$\begin{aligned}
|f(\nu_k) - f(\nu)| &= \left| \sum_{h=-\infty}^{\infty} \gamma(h) \big( e^{-2\pi i \nu_k h} - e^{-2\pi i \nu h} \big) \right| \\
&\le \sum_{h=-\infty}^{\infty} |\gamma(h)| |e^{-\pi i(\nu_k - \nu)h} - e^{\pi i(\nu_k - \nu)h}| \\
&= 2 \sum_{h=-\infty}^{\infty} |\gamma(h)| |\sin[\pi(\nu_k - \nu)h]| \\
&\le 2\pi|\nu_k - \nu| \sum_{h=-\infty}^{\infty} |h||\gamma(h)| \\
&\le \frac{\pi\theta L}{n}
\end{aligned}$$

because $|\sin x| \le |x|$.

The main use of the properties described by Lemmas 3.1 and 3.2 is in identifying the covariance structure of the DFT, say,

$$\begin{aligned}
X(\nu_k) &= n^{-1/2} \sum_{t=1}^{n} x_t \, e^{-2\pi i \nu_k t} \\
&= X_c(\nu_k) - i X_s(\nu_k),
\end{aligned}$$

where

$$X_c(\nu_k) = n^{-1/2} \sum_{t=1}^{n} x_t \cos(2\pi i \nu_k t)$$

and

$$X_s(\nu_k) = n^{-1/2} \sum_{t=1}^{n} x_t \sin(2\pi i \nu_k t)$$

are the cosine and sine transforms, respectively, of the observed series, defined previously in (3.41) and (3.42). For example, assuming zero means for convenience, we will have

$$E[X_c(\nu_k) X_c(\nu_\ell)] = \frac{1}{4} n^{-1} \sum_{s=1}^{n} \sum_{t=1}^{n} \gamma(s-t) \big( e^{2\pi i \nu_k s} + e^{-2\pi i \nu_k s} \big)$$

$$
\begin{aligned}
& \times\left(e^{2\pi i\nu_\ell t}+e^{-2\pi i\nu_\ell t}\right) \\
= \quad & \frac{1}{4}\big[S_n(-\nu_k,\nu_l)+S_n(\nu_k,\nu_\ell)+S_n(\nu_\ell,\nu_k) \\
& +S_n(\nu_k,-\nu_\ell)\big].
\end{aligned}
$$

Lemmas 3.1 and 3.2 imply, for $k=\ell$,

$$
\begin{aligned}
E[X_c(\nu_k)X_c(\nu_\ell)] &= \frac{1}{4}[O(n^{-1})+f(\nu_k)+O(n^{-1}) \\
&\quad +f(\nu_k)+O(n^{-1})+O(n^{-1})] \\
&= \frac{1}{2}f(\nu_k)+O(n^{-1}). \qquad (3.147)
\end{aligned}
$$

For $k \neq \ell$, all terms are $O(n^{-1})$. Hence, we have

$$
E[X_c(\nu_k)X_c(\nu_\ell)] = \begin{cases} \frac{1}{2}f(\nu_k)+O(n^{-1}), & k=\ell \\ O(n^{-1}), & k\neq\ell. \end{cases} \qquad (3.148)
$$

A similar argument gives

$$
E[X_s(\nu_k)X_s(\nu_\ell)] = \begin{cases} \frac{1}{2}f(\nu_k)+O(n^{-1}), & k=\ell, \\ O(n^{-1}), & k\neq\ell \end{cases} \qquad (3.149)
$$

and we also have $E[X_s(\nu_k)X_c(\nu_\ell)] = O(n^{-1})$ for all $k,\ell$. We may summarize the results of Lemmas 3.1-3.3 as follows.

**Theorem 3.3:** *For a stationary mean zero process with autocovariance function satisfying (3.140) and frequencies $\nu_k$, $|\nu_k^n-\nu|<L/n$ close to some target frequency $\nu$, the cosine and sine transforms (3.41) and (3.42) are approximately uncorrelated with variances equal to $(1/2)f(\nu)$, and the error in the approximation can be uniformly bounded by $\pi\theta L/n$.*

Now, consider estimating the spectrum in a neighborhood of some target frequency $\nu$, using the periodogram estimator

$$
\begin{aligned}
I(\nu_k^n) &= |X(\nu_k^n)|^2 \\
&= X_c^2(\nu_k^n)+X_s^2(\nu_k^n),
\end{aligned}
$$

where we take $|\nu_k^n-\nu|\leq n^{-1}$ for each $n$. In case the series $x_t$ is Gaussian with zero mean,

$$
\begin{pmatrix} X_c(\nu_k) \\ X_s(\nu_k) \end{pmatrix} \xrightarrow{d} N\left\{\begin{pmatrix} 0 \\ 0 \end{pmatrix}, \frac{1}{2}\begin{pmatrix} f(\nu) & 0 \\ 0 & f(\nu) \end{pmatrix}\right\},
$$

and we have that

$$
\frac{2\,I(\nu_k^n)}{f(\nu)} \xrightarrow{d} \chi_2^2,
$$

where $\chi_n^2$ denotes a chi-squared random variable with $n$ degrees of freedom, as usual. Unfortunately, the distribution does not become more concentrated as $n \to \infty$, because the variance of the periodogram estimator does not go to zero.

We may develop a fix for the deficiencies mentioned above by considering the average of the periodogram over a set of frequencies in the neighborhood of $\nu$. For example, we can always find a set of $L$ frequencies of the form $\nu_k^n + \ell/n$ for $\ell = 0, \pm 1, \pm 2, \ldots, \pm(L-1)/2$, for which

$$f(\nu_k^n + \ell/n) = f(\nu) + O(Ln^{-1})$$

by Lemma 3.3. As $n$ increases, the values of the separate frequencies change. Then, consider the smoothed spectral estimator

$$\begin{aligned} \widehat{f}(\nu) &= L^{-1} \sum_{\ell=-(L-1)/2}^{(L-1)/2} |X(\nu_k^n + \ell/n)|^2 \\ &= L^{-1} \sum_{\ell=-(L-1)/2}^{(L-1)/2} I(\nu_k^n + \ell/n) \end{aligned}$$

By the same limiting arguments as before with $O(Ln^{-1})$ replacing $O(n^{-1})$, we have exactly the same limiting distribution as above for $X_c(\nu_k^n + \ell/n), X_s(\nu_k^n + \ell/n)$ for any $\ell$, and the joint distribution is that of independent normal variables. Hence,

$$\frac{2L\widehat{f}(\nu)}{f(\nu)} \xrightarrow{d} \chi^2_{2L}$$

gives a distributional result that can be used to justify the approximate confidence intervals (3.60) and yields an estimator with a variance that decreases as $L$ increases.

We may extend the above arguments to vector series of the form $\boldsymbol{x}_t = (x_{t1}, \ldots, x_{tp})'$, when the cross-spectrum is given by

$$\begin{aligned} f_{ij}(\nu) &= \sum_{h=-\infty}^{\infty} \gamma_{ij}(h) e^{-2\pi i \nu h} \\ &= c_{ij}(\nu) - i q_{ij}(\nu), \end{aligned} \tag{3.150}$$

where

$$c_{ij}(\nu) = \sum_{h=-\infty}^{\infty} \gamma_{ij}(h) \cos(2\pi\nu h) \tag{3.151}$$

and

$$q_{ij}(\nu) = \sum_{h=-\infty}^{\infty} \gamma_{ij}(h) \sin(2\pi\nu h) \tag{3.152}$$

denote the cospectrum and quadspectrum, respectively. We denote the DFT of the series $x_{mt}$ by

$$\begin{aligned} X_j(\nu_k) &= n^{-1/2}\sum_{t=1}^{n} x_{tj}\ e^{-2\pi i\nu_k t} \\ &= X_{cj}(\nu_k) - iX_{sj}(\nu_k), \end{aligned}$$

where $X_{cj}$ and $X_{sj}$ are the cosine and sine transforms of $x_{tj}, j = 1, 2, \ldots p$. We bound the covariance structure as before and summarize the results as follows.

**Theorem 3.4:** *The covariance structure of the multivariate cosine and sine transforms, subject to*

$$\theta_{ij} = \sum_{h=-\infty}^{\infty} |h||\gamma_{ij}(h)| < \infty, \tag{3.153}$$

*is given by*

$$E[X_{ci}(\nu_k)X_{cj}(\nu_\ell)] = \begin{cases} \frac{1}{2}c_{ij}(\nu_k) + O(n^{-1}), & k = \ell \\ O(n^{-1}), & k \neq \ell. \end{cases} \tag{3.154}$$

$$E[X_{ci}(\nu_k)X_{sj}(\nu_\ell)] = \begin{cases} -\frac{1}{2}q_{ij}(\nu_k) + O(n^{-1}), & k = \ell \\ O(n^{-1}), & k \neq \ell \end{cases} \tag{3.155}$$

$$E[X_{si}(\nu_k)X_{cj}(\nu_\ell)] = \begin{cases} \frac{1}{2}q_{ij}(\nu_k) + O(n^{-1}), & k = \ell \\ O(n^{-1}), & k \neq \ell \end{cases} \tag{3.156}$$

$$E[X_{si}(\nu_k)X_{sj}(\nu_\ell)] = \begin{cases} \frac{1}{2}c_{ij}(\nu_k) + O(n^{-1}), & k = \ell \\ O(n^{-1}), & k \neq \ell. \end{cases} \tag{3.157}$$

We may verify the above with manipulations like

$$\begin{aligned} E[X_{ci}(\nu_k)X_{sj}(\nu_k)] &= \frac{1}{4i}\sum_{s=1}^{n}\sum_{t=1}^{n}\gamma_{ij}(s-t)(e^{2\pi i\nu_k s} + e^{-2\pi i\nu_k s}) \\ &\quad \times (e^{2\pi i\nu_k t} - e^{-2\pi i\nu_k t}) \\ &= \frac{1}{4i}\Big[S_n^{ij}(-\nu_k,\nu_k) + S_n^{ij}(\nu_k,\nu_k) \\ &\quad -S_n^{ij}(\nu_k,\nu_k) - S_n^{ij}(\nu_k,-\nu_k)\Big] \\ &= \frac{1}{4i}\Big[c_{ij}(\nu_k) - iq_{ij}(\nu_k) \\ &\quad -(c_{ij}(\nu_k) + iq_{ij}(\nu_k)) + O(n^{-1})\Big] \\ &= -\frac{1}{2}q_{ij}(\nu_k) + O(n^{-1}), \end{aligned}$$

where we have used the definition

$$S_n^{ij}(\nu_k, \nu_\ell) = \sum_{s=1}^{n} \sum_{t=1}^{n} \gamma_{ij}(s-t) e^{-2\pi i \nu_k s} e^{2\pi i \nu_\ell t} \tag{3.158}$$

and the fact that the properties embodied by Lemmas 3.1-3.3 can be verified for the cross-spectral density functions $f_{ij}(\nu), i, j = 1, \ldots, p$.

Now, if the underlying multivariate time series $\boldsymbol{x}_t$ is a normal process, it is clear that the DFTs will be jointly normal and we may define the vector DFT, $\boldsymbol{X}(\nu_k) = (X_1(\nu_k), \ldots, X_p(\nu_k))'$

$$\begin{aligned} \boldsymbol{X}(\nu_k) &= n^{-1/2} \sum_{t=1}^{n} \boldsymbol{x}_t \, e^{-2\pi i \nu_k t} \\ &= \boldsymbol{X}_c(\nu_k) - i\boldsymbol{X}_s(\nu_k), \end{aligned} \tag{3.159}$$

where

$$\boldsymbol{X}_c(\nu_k) = n^{-1/2} \sum_{t=1}^{n} \boldsymbol{x}_t \cos(2\pi i \nu_k t) \tag{3.160}$$

and

$$\boldsymbol{X}_s(\nu_k) = n^{-1/2} \sum_{t=1}^{n} \boldsymbol{x}_t \sin(2\pi i \nu_k t) \tag{3.161}$$

are the cosine and sine transforms, respectively, of the observed vector series $\boldsymbol{x}_t$. Then, constructing the vector of real and imaginary parts $(\boldsymbol{X}_c(\nu_k)', \boldsymbol{X}_s(\nu_k)')$, we may note it has mean zero and $2p \times 2p$ covariance matrix

$$\Sigma(\nu_k) = \frac{1}{2} \begin{pmatrix} C(\nu_k) & -Q(\nu_k) \\ Q(\nu_k) & C(\nu_k) \end{pmatrix} \tag{3.162}$$

to order $n^{-1}$ as long as $\nu_k - \nu = O(n^{-1})$. We have introduced the $p \times p$ matrices $C(\nu_k) = \{c_{ij}(\nu_k)\}$ and $Q = \{q_{ij}(\nu_k)\}$. The complex random variable $\boldsymbol{X}(\nu_k)$ has covariance

$$\begin{aligned} S(\nu_k) &= E[\boldsymbol{X}(\nu_k)\boldsymbol{X}^*(\nu_k)] \\ &= E\Big[\big(\boldsymbol{X}_c(\nu_k) - i\boldsymbol{X}_s(\nu_k)\big)\big(\boldsymbol{X}_c(\nu_k) - i\boldsymbol{X}_s(\nu_k)\big)^*\Big] \\ &= E[\boldsymbol{X}_c(\nu_k)\boldsymbol{X}_c(\nu_k)'] + E[\boldsymbol{X}_s(\nu_k)\boldsymbol{X}_s(\nu_k)'] \\ &\quad -i(E[\boldsymbol{X}_s(\nu_k)\boldsymbol{X}_c(\nu_k)'] - E[\boldsymbol{X}_c(\nu_k)\boldsymbol{X}_s(\nu_k)']) \\ &= C(\nu_k) - iQ(\nu_k). \end{aligned} \tag{3.163}$$

If the process $\boldsymbol{x}_t$ has a multivariate normal distribution, the complex vector $\boldsymbol{X}(\nu_k)$ has approximately the ***complex multivariate normal distribution*** with mean zero and covariance matrix $S(\nu_k) = C(\nu_k) - iQ(\nu_k)$ if the real and imaginary parts have the covariance structure as specified above. In the next section, we work further with this distribution and show how it adapts to the real case. If we wish to estimate the spectral matrix $S(\nu)$, it is natural to take a band of frequencies of the form $\nu_k^n + \ell/n, \ell = -(L-1)/2, \ldots, (L-1)/2$ as before, so that the estimator becomes (3.79) of Section 3.6. A discussion of further properties of the multivariate complex normal distribution is deferred.

It is also of interest to develop a large sample theory for cases in which the underlying distribution is not necessarily normal. If $x_t$ is not necessarily a normal process, some additional conditions are needed to get asymptotic normality. In particular, introduce the notion of a ***generalized linear process***

$$\boldsymbol{y}_t = \sum_{r=-\infty}^{\infty} A_r \boldsymbol{w}_{t-r}, \tag{3.164}$$

where $\boldsymbol{w}_t$ is a $p \times 1$ vector white noise process with $p \times p$ covariance $E[\boldsymbol{w}_t \boldsymbol{w}_t'] = G$ and the $p \times p$ matrices of filter coefficients $A_t$ satisfy

$$\sum_{t=-\infty}^{\infty} \operatorname{tr}\{A_t A_t'\} = \sum_{t=-\infty}^{\infty} \|A_t\|^2 < \infty. \tag{3.165}$$

In particular, stable vector ARMA processes, as introduced in Chapters 2 and 3, satisfy these conditions. For generalized linear processes, we state the following general result from Hannan (1970, p.224).

**Theorem 3.5:** *If $\boldsymbol{x}_t$ is generated by a generalized linear process with a continuous spectrum that is not zero at $\nu$ and $\nu_k^n + \ell/n$ are a set of frequencies within $L/n$ of $\nu$, the joint density of the cosine and sine transforms (3.160) and (3.161) converges to that of $L$ independent $2p \times 1$ normal vectors with covariance matrix $\Sigma(\nu)$ with structure given by (3.162). At $\nu = 0$ or $\nu = 1/2$, the distribution is real with covariance matrix $2\Sigma(\nu)$.*

The above result provides the basis for inference involving the Fourier transforms of stationary series because it justifies approximations to the likelihood function based on multivariate normal theory. We make extensive use of this result in Chapter 5, but will still need a simple form to justify the distributional result for the sample coherence given in (3.80). The next section gives an elementary introduction to the complex normal distribution.

## T3.13 The Complex Multivariate Normal Distribution

The ***multivariate normal distribution*** will be the fundamental tool for expressing the likelihood function and determining approximate maximum likelihood estimators and their large sample probability distributions. A detailed treatment of the multivariate normal distribution can be found in standard texts such as Anderson (1984). We will use the multivariate normal distribution of the $p \times 1$ vector $x = (x_1, x_2, \ldots, x_p)'$, as defined by its density function

$$p(\boldsymbol{x}) = (2\pi)^{-p/2}|\Sigma|^{-1/2} \exp\{-\frac{1}{2}(\boldsymbol{x} - \boldsymbol{\mu})'\Sigma^{-1}(\boldsymbol{x} - \boldsymbol{\mu})\}, \tag{3.166}$$

which can be shown to have mean vector $E[\boldsymbol{x}] = \boldsymbol{\mu} = (\mu_1, \ldots, \mu_p)'$ and covariance matrix

$$\Sigma = E[(\boldsymbol{x} - \boldsymbol{\mu})(\boldsymbol{x} - \boldsymbol{\mu})']. \tag{3.167}$$

We use the notation $\boldsymbol{x} \sim N_p\{\boldsymbol{\mu}, \Sigma\}$ for densities of the form (3.166) and note that linearly transformed multivariate normal variables of the form $\boldsymbol{y} = A\boldsymbol{x}$, with $A$ a $q \times p$ matrix $q \leq p$, will also be multivariate normal with distribution

$$\boldsymbol{y} \sim N_q\{A\boldsymbol{\mu}, A\Sigma A'\}. \tag{3.168}$$

Often, the ***partitioned multivariate normal*** , based on the vector $\boldsymbol{x} = (\boldsymbol{x}_1', \boldsymbol{x}_2')'$, split into to $p_1 \times 1$ and $p_2 \times 1$ components $\boldsymbol{x}_1$ and $\boldsymbol{x}_2$, respectively, will be used where $p = p_1 + p_2$. If the mean vector $\boldsymbol{\mu} = (\boldsymbol{\mu}_1', \boldsymbol{\mu}_2')'$ and covariance matrices

$$\Sigma = \begin{pmatrix} \Sigma_{11} & \Sigma_{12} \\ \Sigma_{21} & \Sigma_{22} \end{pmatrix} \tag{3.169}$$

are also compatibly partitioned, the marginal distribution of any subset of components is multivariate normal, say,

$$\boldsymbol{x}_1 \sim N_{p_1}\{\boldsymbol{\mu}_1, \Sigma_{11}\},$$

and that the conditional distribution $\boldsymbol{x}_2$ given $\boldsymbol{x}_1$ is normal with mean

$$E[\boldsymbol{x}_2|\boldsymbol{x}_1] = \boldsymbol{\mu}_2 + \Sigma_{21}\Sigma_{11}^{-1}(\boldsymbol{x}_1 - \boldsymbol{\mu}_1) \tag{3.170}$$

and conditional covariance

$$\text{cov}[\boldsymbol{x}_2|\boldsymbol{x}_1] = \Sigma_{22} - \Sigma_{21}\Sigma_{11}^{-1}\Sigma_{12}. \tag{3.171}$$

In the previous section, the real and imaginary parts of the DFT had a partitioned covariance matrix as given in (3.55), and we use this result to say the complex $p \times 1$ vector

$$z = \boldsymbol{x}_1 - i\boldsymbol{x}_2 \tag{3.172}$$

has a ***complex multivariate normal distribution***, with mean vector $\boldsymbol{\mu}_z = \boldsymbol{\mu}_1 - i\boldsymbol{\mu}_2$ and $p \times p$ covariance matrix

$$\Sigma_z = C - iQ \tag{3.173}$$

if the real multivariate $2p \times 1$ normal vector $\boldsymbol{x} = (\boldsymbol{x}_1', x_2')'$ has a real multivariate normal distribution with mean vector $\boldsymbol{\mu} = (\boldsymbol{\mu}_1', \boldsymbol{\mu}_2')'$ and covariance matrix

$$\Sigma = \frac{1}{2}\begin{pmatrix} C & -Q \\ Q & C \end{pmatrix}. \tag{3.174}$$

The restrictions $C' = C$ and $Q' = -Q$ are necessary for the matrix $\Sigma$ to be a covariance matrix, and these conditions then imply $\Sigma_z = \Sigma_z^*$ is Hermitian. The probability density function of the complex multivariate normal vector $\boldsymbol{z}$ can be expressed in the concise form

$$p_{\boldsymbol{z}}(\boldsymbol{z}) = \pi^{-p}|\Sigma_z|^{-1}\exp\{-(\boldsymbol{z}-\boldsymbol{\mu}_z)^*\Sigma_z^{-1}(\boldsymbol{z}-\boldsymbol{\mu}_z)\}, \tag{3.175}$$

and this is the form that we will often use in the likelihood. The result follows from showing that $p_{\boldsymbol{x}}(\boldsymbol{x}_1, \boldsymbol{x}_2) = p_{\boldsymbol{z}}(\boldsymbol{z})$ exactly, using the fact that the quadratic and Hermitian forms in the exponent are equal and that $|\Sigma_x| = |\Sigma_z|^2$. The second assertion follows directly from the fact that the matrix $\Sigma_{\boldsymbol{x}}$ has repeated eigenvalues, $\lambda_1, \lambda_2, \ldots, \lambda_p$ corresponding to eigenvectors $(\alpha_1', \alpha_2')'$ and the same set, $\lambda_1, \lambda_2, \ldots, \lambda_p$ corresponding to $(\alpha_2', -\alpha_1')'$. Hence

$$|\Sigma_x| = \prod_{i=1}^{p} \lambda_i^2 = |\Sigma_z|^2.$$

For further material relating to the complex multivariate normal distribution, see Goodman (1963), Giri (1965), or Khatri (1965).

**Example 3.22 A Bivariate Complex Normal Distribution**

Consider the joint distribution of the complex random variables $u_1 = x_1 - ix_2$ and $u_2 = y_1 - iy_2$, where the partitioned vector $(x_1, x_2, y_1, y_2)'$ has a real multivariate normal distribution with mean $(0, 0, 0, 0)'$ and covariance matrix

$$\Sigma = \frac{1}{2}\begin{pmatrix} c_{xx} & 0 & c_{xy} & -q_{xy} \\ 0 & c_{xx} & q_{xy} & c_{xy} \\ c_{xy} & q_{xy} & c_{yy} & 0 \\ -q_{xy} & c_{yx} & 0 & c_{yy} \end{pmatrix}. \tag{3.176}$$

Now, consider the conditional distribution of $\boldsymbol{y} = (y_1, y_2)'$, given $\boldsymbol{x} = (x_1, x_2)'$. Using (3.170), we obtain

$$E[\boldsymbol{y}|\boldsymbol{x}] = \begin{pmatrix} x_1 & -x_2 \\ x_2 & x_1 \end{pmatrix}\begin{pmatrix} b_1 \\ b_2 \end{pmatrix}, \tag{3.177}$$

where

$$(b_1, b_2) = \left(\frac{c_{yx}}{c_{xx}}, \frac{q_{yx}}{c_{xx}}\right). \tag{3.178}$$

It is natural to identify the cross-spectrum

$$f_{xy} = c_{xy} - iq_{xy}, \tag{3.179}$$

so that the complex variable identified with the pair is just

$$\begin{aligned} b &= b_1 - ib_2 \\ &= \frac{c_{yx} - iq_{yx}}{c_{xx}} \\ &= \frac{f_{yx}}{f_x}, \end{aligned}$$

and we identify it as the complex regression coefficient. The conditional covariance follows from (3.171) and simplifies to

$$\text{cov}(\boldsymbol{y}|\boldsymbol{x}) = \frac{1}{2} f_{y\cdot x}\ I_2, \tag{3.180}$$

where $I_2$ denotes the $2 \times 2$ identity matrix and

$$\begin{aligned} f_{y\cdot x} &= c_{yy} - \frac{c_{xy}^2 + q_{xy}^2}{c_{xx}} \\ &= f_y - \frac{|f_{xy}|^2}{f_x} \end{aligned} \tag{3.181}$$

Example 3.20 leads to an approach for justifying the distributional results for the function coherence given in (3.80). That equation suggests that the result can be derived using the regression results that lead to the F-statistics in Section 1.8. Suppose that we consider $L$ values of the since and cosine transforms or the input $x_t$ and output $y_t$, which we will denote by $X_c(\nu_k+\ell/n), X_s(\nu_k+\ell/n), Y_c(\nu_k+\ell/n), Y_s(\nu_k+\ell/n)$, sampled at $L$ frequencies, $\ell = -(L-1)/2, \ldots, (L-1)/2$, in the neighborhood of some target frequency $\nu$ Suppose these cosine and sine transforms are re-indexed and denoted by $X_{cj}, X_{sj}, Y_{cj}, Y_{sj}, j = 1, 2, \ldots, L$, producing $2L$ real random variables with a large sample normal distribution that have limiting covariance matrices of the form (3.176) for each $j$. Then, the conditional distribution of the $2 \times 1$ vector $Y_{cj}, Y_{sj}$ given $X_{cj}, X_{sj}$, given in Example 3.20, shows that we may write, approximately, the regression model

$$\begin{pmatrix} Y_{cj} \\ Y_{sj} \end{pmatrix} = \begin{pmatrix} X_{cj} & -X_{sj} \\ X_{sj} & X_{cj} \end{pmatrix} \begin{pmatrix} b_1 \\ b_2 \end{pmatrix} + \begin{pmatrix} V_{cj} \\ V_{sj} \end{pmatrix},$$

where $V_{cj}, V_{sj}$ are approximately uncorrelated with approximate variances

$$E[V_{cj}^2] = E[V_{sj}^2] = (1/2) f_{y\cdot x}.$$

Now, construct, by stacking, the $2L \times 1$ vectors $\boldsymbol{y}_c = (Y_{c1}, \ldots, Y_{cL})'$, $\boldsymbol{y}_s = (Y_{s1}, \ldots, Y_{sL})'$, $\boldsymbol{x}_c = (X_{c1}, \ldots, X_{cL})'$ and $\boldsymbol{x}_s = (X_{s1}, \ldots, X_{sL})'$, and rewrite the regression model as

$$\begin{pmatrix} \boldsymbol{y}_c \\ \boldsymbol{y}_s \end{pmatrix} = \begin{pmatrix} \boldsymbol{x}_c & -\boldsymbol{x}_s \\ \boldsymbol{x}_s & \boldsymbol{x}_c \end{pmatrix} \begin{pmatrix} b_1 \\ b_2 \end{pmatrix} + \begin{pmatrix} \boldsymbol{v}_c \\ \boldsymbol{v}_s \end{pmatrix}$$

where $\boldsymbol{v}_c$ and $\boldsymbol{v}_s$ are the error stacks. Finally, write the overall model as the regression model in Chapter 1, namely,

$$\boldsymbol{y} = Z\boldsymbol{b} + \boldsymbol{v},$$

making the obvious identifications in the previous equation. Conditional on $Z$, the model becomes exactly the regression model considered in Chapter 1 where there are $q = 2$ regression coefficients and $2L$ observations in the observation vector $\boldsymbol{y}$. To test the hypothesis of no regression for that model, we use an F-Statistic that depends on the difference between the residual sum of squares for the full model, say,

$$RSS = \boldsymbol{y}'\boldsymbol{y} - \boldsymbol{y}'Z(Z'Z)^{-1}Z'\boldsymbol{y} \tag{3.182}$$

and the residual sum of squares for the reduced model, $RSS_0 = \boldsymbol{y}'\boldsymbol{y}$. Then,

$$F_{2,2L-2} = (L-1)\frac{RSS_0 - RSS}{RSS} \tag{3.183}$$

has the F-distribution with 2 and $2L-2$ degrees of freedom. Also, it follows by substitution for $\boldsymbol{y}$ that

$$\begin{aligned} RSS_0 &= \boldsymbol{y}'\boldsymbol{y} \\ &= \boldsymbol{y}_c'\boldsymbol{y}_c + \boldsymbol{y}_s'\boldsymbol{y}_s \\ &= \sum_{j=1}^{L}(Y_{cj}^2 + Y_{sj}^2) \\ &= L\widehat{f}_y(\nu), \end{aligned}$$

which is just the sample spectrum of the output series. Similarly,

$$Z'Z = \begin{pmatrix} L\widehat{f}_x & 0 \\ 0 & L\widehat{f}_x \end{pmatrix}$$

and

$$\begin{aligned} Z'\boldsymbol{y} &= \begin{pmatrix} (\boldsymbol{x}_c'\boldsymbol{y}_c + \boldsymbol{x}_s'\boldsymbol{y}_s) \\ (\boldsymbol{x}_c'\boldsymbol{y}_s - \boldsymbol{x}_s'\boldsymbol{y}_c) \end{pmatrix} \\ &= L\begin{pmatrix} \sum_{j=1}^{L}(X_{cj}Y_{cj} + X_{sj}Y_{sj}) \\ \\ \sum_{j=1}^{L}(X_{cj}Y_{sj} - X_{sj}Y_{cj}) \end{pmatrix} \\ &= \begin{pmatrix} L\widehat{c}_{yx} \\ L\widehat{q}_{yx} \end{pmatrix}. \end{aligned}$$

together imply that

$$\boldsymbol{y}'Z(Z'Z)^{-1}Z'\boldsymbol{y} = L\ |\widehat{f}_{xy}|^2/\widehat{f}_x.$$

Substituting into (3.183) gives

$$F_{2,2L-2} = (L-1)\frac{|\widehat{f}_{xy}|^2/\widehat{f}_x}{\left(\widehat{f}_y - |\widehat{f}_{xy}|^2/\widehat{f}_x\right)},$$

which converts directly into the F-statistic (3.80), using the sample coherence defined in (3.81).

# Problems

*Section 3.2*

**3.1** With reference to equations (3.1) and (3.2), let $u_1$ and $u_2$ be independent, standard normal variables. Consider the polar coordinates of the point $(u_1, u_2)$, that is,

$$A^2 = u_1^2 + u_2^2 \quad \text{and} \quad \phi = \tan^{-1}(u_2/u_1).$$

(a) Find the joint density of $A^2$ and $\phi$, and from the result, conclude that $A^2$ and $\phi$ are independent random variables, where $A^2$ is a chi-squared random variable with 2 df, and $\phi$ is is uniformly distributed on $(0, 2\pi)$.

(b) Going in reverse from polar coordinates to rectangular coordinates, suppose we assume that $A^2$ and $\phi$ are independent random variables, where $A^2$ is chi-squared with 2 df, and $\phi$ is uniformly distributed on $(0, 2\pi)$. With $u_1 = A\cos(\phi)$ and $u_2 = A\sin(\phi)$, where $A$ is the positive square root of $A^2$, show that $u_1$ and $u_2$ are independent, standard normal random variables.

**3.2** Verify (3.4).

*Section 3.3*

**3.3** A time series was generated by first drawing the white noise series $w_t$ from a normal distribution with mean zero and variance one. The observed series $x_t$ was generated from

$$x_t = w_t - \theta_1 w_{t-1}, \quad t = 0, \pm 1, \pm 2, \ldots,$$

where $\theta$ is a parameter.

(a) Derive the theoretical mean value and autocovariance functions for the series $x_t$ and $w_t$. Are the series $x_t$ and $w_t$ stationary? Give your reasons.

(b) Give a formula for the power spectrum of $x_t$, expressed in terms of $\theta$ and $\nu$.

(c) Calculate the cross-spectrum $f_{xw}(\nu)$ in terms of $\theta$ and $\nu$.

(d) Show the squared coherence between $x_t$ and $w_t$ is unity.

**3.4** Suppose $x_t$ and $y_t$ are stationary zero-mean time series with $x_t$ independent of $y_s$ for all $s$ and $t$. Consider the product series

$$z_t = x_t y_t.$$

Prove the spectral density for $z_t$ can be written as

$$f_z(\nu) = \int_{-1/2}^{1/2} f_x(\nu - \omega) f_y(\omega)\, d\omega.$$

**3.5** A first-order autoregressive model is generated from the white noise series $w_t$ using the generating equations

$$x_t = \phi x_{t-1} + w_t,$$

where $\phi, |\phi| < 1$ is a parameter and the $w_t$ are independent random variables with mean zero and variance $\sigma_w^2$.

(a) Show the power spectrum of $x_t$ is given by

$$f_x(\nu) = \frac{\sigma_w^2}{1 + \phi^2 - 2\phi \cos(2\pi\nu)}.$$

(b) Verify the autocovariance function of this process is

$$\gamma_x(h) = \frac{\sigma_w^2\ \phi^{|h|}}{1 - \phi^2},$$

$h = 0, \pm 1, \pm 2, \ldots$. It suffices to verify that the inverse transform of the autocovariance function is the spectrum derived in part (b) using the summation form.

**3.6** In applications, we will often observe series containing a signal that has been delayed by some unknown time $D$, i.e.,

$$x_t = s_t + A s_{t-D} + n_t,$$

where $s_t$ and $n_t$ are stationary and independent with zero means. The delayed signal is multiplied by some unknown constant $A$.

(a) Prove

$$f_x(\nu) = [1 + A^2 + 2A\cos(2\pi\nu D)] f_s(\nu) + f_n(\nu),$$

where the spectra of the signal and noise are $f_s(\nu)$ and $f_n(\nu)$, respectively.

(b) How could the periodicity expected in the spectrum derived in (a) be used to estimate the delay $D$?

(c) Suppose the noise is zero in the model and that the signal is white noise with variance $\sigma_s^2$. Discuss a possible time domain method for estimating $D$ using a seasonal moving average model.

(d) Generate a series $y_t$ using $A = .9$ and $D = 5$. Apply the time domain method to estimating the parameters, and compare it with the known results.

*Section 3.4*

**3.7** Determine the theoretical power spectrum of the series formed by combining the white noise series $w_t$ to form

$$y_t = w_{t-2} + 4w_{t-1} + 6w_t + 4w_{t+1} + w_{t+2}.$$

Determine which frequencies are present by plotting the power spectrum.

**3.8** Let $x_t = \cos(2\pi\nu t)$, and consider the output

$$y_t = \sum_{k=-\infty}^{\infty} a_k x_{t-k},$$

where $\sum_k |a_k| < \infty$. Show

$$y_t = |A(\nu)| \cos(2\pi\nu t + \phi(\nu)),$$

where $A(\nu)$ and $\phi(\nu)$ are the amplitude and phase of the filter, respectively. Interpret the result in terms of the relationship between the input series, $x_t$, and the output series, $y_t$.

**3.9** Suppose $x_t$ is a stationary series, and we apply two filtering operations in succession, say,

$$y_t = \sum_r a_r x_{t-r},$$

and then

$$z_t = \sum_s b_s y_{t-s}.$$

(a) Show the spectrum of the output is

$$f_z(\nu) = |A(\nu)|^2 |B(\nu)|^2 f_x(\nu),$$

where $A(\nu)$ and $B(\nu)$ are the Fourier transforms of the filter sequences $a_t$ and $b_t$, respectively.

(b) What would be the effect of applying the filter

$$u_t = x_t - x_{t-1}$$

followed by

$$v_t = u_t - u_{t-12}$$

to a time series?

(c) Plot the predicted frequency responses of the simple difference filter and of the seasonal difference of the first difference. Filters like these are called seasonal adjustment filters in economics because they tend to attenuate frequencies at multiples of the monthly periods. The difference filter tends to attenuate low-frequency trends.

**3.10** Suppose we are given a stationary zero-mean series $x_t$ with spectrum $f_x(\nu)$ and then construct the derived series

$$y_t = ay_{t-1} + x_t. \quad t = \pm 1, \pm 2, ...,$$

(a) Show how the theoretical $f_y(\nu)$ is related to $f_x(\nu)$.

(b) Plot the function that multiplies $f_x(\nu)$ in part (a) for $a = .1, .8$. This filter is called a recursive filter.

*Section 3.5*

**3.11** Prove the convolution property of the DFT, namely,

$$\sum_{s=1}^{n} a_s x_{t-s} = \sum_{k=1}^{n} A(\nu_k) X(\nu_k) \exp\{2\pi\nu_k t\},$$

for $t = 1, 2, \ldots, n$, where $A(\nu_k)$ and $X(\nu_k)$ are the discrete Fourier transforms of $a_t$ and $x_t$, respectively, and we assume that $x_t = x_{t+n}$ is periodic.

**3.12** Show that we could compute the periodogram estimator of the mean corrected series $x_t - \bar{x}$ as

$$I_x(\nu_k) = \sum_{h=-(n-1)}^{(n-1)} \widehat{\gamma}_x(h) e^{-2\pi i \nu_k h},$$

where

$$\widehat{\gamma}_x(h) = n^{-1} \sum_{t=1}^{n-h} (x_{t+h} - \bar{x})(x_t - \bar{x})$$

is the sample autocovariance function. Blackman and Tukey (1959) used this method before the advent of the fast algorithms for the discrete Fourier transform.

**3.13** Let the observed series $x_t$ be composed of a periodic signal and noise so it can be written as

$$x_t = \beta_1 cos(2\pi\nu_k t) + \beta_2 sin(2\pi\nu_k t) + w_t,$$

where $w_t$ is a white noise process with variance $\sigma_w^2$. The frequency $\nu_k$ is assumed to be an integer multiple of $1/n$ and to be known in this problem. Suppose we consider estimating $\beta_1, \beta_2$ and $\sigma_w^2$ by least squares, or equivalently, by maximum likelihood if the $w_t$ are assumed to be Gaussian.

(a) Prove, for a fixed $\nu_k$, the minimum squared error is attained by

$$\begin{pmatrix} \widehat{\beta}_1 \\ \widehat{\beta}_2 \end{pmatrix} = 2n^{-1/2} \begin{pmatrix} X_c(\nu_k) \\ X_s(\nu_k) \end{pmatrix},$$

where the cosine and sine transforms (3.41) and (3.42) appear on the right-hand side.

(b) Prove that the error sum of squares can be written as

$$SSE = \sum_{t=1}^{n} x_t^2 - 2I_x(\nu_k)$$

so that the value of $\nu_k$ that minimizes squared error is the same as the value that maximizes the periodogram $I_x(\nu_k)$ estimator (3.43).

(c) Under the Gaussian assumption and fixed $\nu_k$, show the likelihood ratio test of no regression leads to an $F$-statistic that is a monotone function of $I_x(\nu_k)$.

*Section 3.6*

**3.14** Suppose a sample time series with $n = 256$ points is available from the first order autoregressive model. Furthermore, suppose a sample spectrum computed with $L = 3$ yields the estimated value $\widehat{f}_x(1/8) = 2.25$. Is this sample value consistent with $\sigma_w^2 = 1, \phi = .5$? Repeat using $L = 11$ if we just happen to obtain the same sample value.

**3.15** The levels of salt concentration known to have occurred over rows, corresponding to the average temperature levels for the soil science data considered in Figures 1.25 and 1.26, are shown in Figure (3.19).

(a) Identify the dominant frequencies by performing separate spectral analyses on the two series. Include confidence intervals for the dominant frequencies.

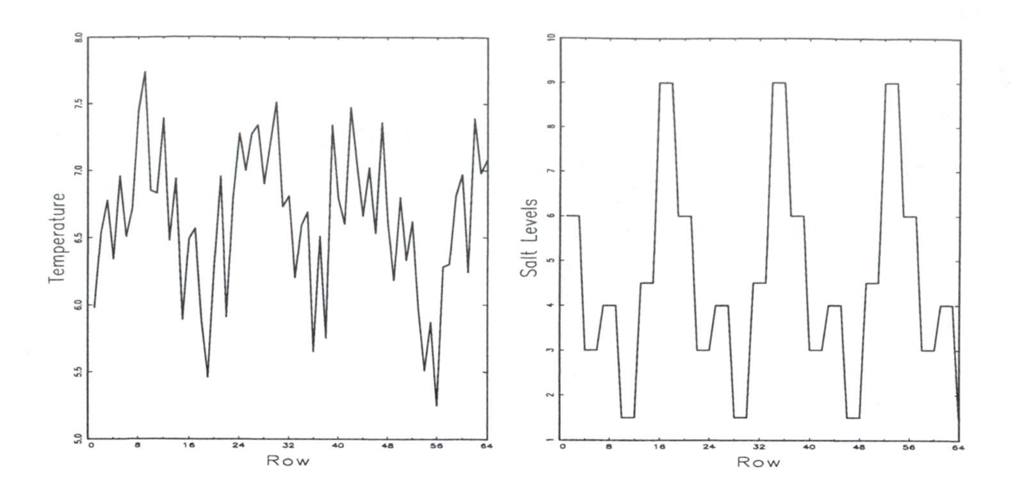


**Figure 3.19:** Temperature and salt profiles over 64 rows at 17-ft spacing

(b) Analyze the coherence function to determine if the dominant frequency is coherent.

**3.16** Consider two time series

$$x_t = w_t - w_{t-1},$$

$$y_t = \frac{1}{2}(w_t + w_{t-1}),$$

formed from the white noise series $w_t$ with variance $\sigma_w^2 = 1$.

(a) Are $x_t$ and $y_t$ jointly stationary?. Recall the cross-covariance function must also be a function only of the lag $h$ and cannot depend on time.

(b) Compute the spectra $f_y(\nu)$ and $f_x(\nu)$, and comment on the difference between the two results.

(c) Suppose sample spectral estimators $\widehat{f}_y(.10)$ are computed for the series using $L = 3$. Find $a$ and $b$ such that

$$P\left\{a \leq \widehat{f}_y(.10) \leq b\right\} = .90.$$

This expression gives two points which will contain 90% of the sample spectral values. Put 5% of the area in each tail.

**3.17** Consider the bivariate time series records containing monthly U.S. production as measured monthly by the Federal Reserve Board Production Index and unemployment as given in Figure 2.26.

(a) Compute the spectrum and the log spectrum for each series, and identify statistically significant peaks. Explain what might be generating the peaks. Compute the coherence, and explain what is meant when a high coherence is observed at a particular frequency.

(b) What would be the effect of applying the filter

$$u_t = x_t - x_{t-1}$$

followed by

$$v_t = u_t - u_{t-12}$$

to the series given above? Plot the predicted frequency responses of the simple difference filter and of the seasonal difference of the first difference.

(c) Apply the filters successively to one of the two series and plot the output. Examine the output after taking a first difference and comment on whether stationarity is a reasonable assumption. Why or why not? Plot after taking the seasonal difference of the first difference. What can be noticed about the output that is consistent with what you have predicted from the frequency response? Verify by computing the spectrum of the output after filtering.

**3.18** To verify the approximation to the expectation of the sample spectral estimator is (3.73) when a taper of the form (3.71) is applied, first show

$$E|Y(\nu_k)|^2 = \int_{-1/2}^{1/2} |H_n(\nu_k - \nu)|^2 f_x(\nu)\, d\nu$$

where $H_n(\nu)$ is defined in (3.75). Then use the result to verify (3.73). In what sense is (3.73) an approximation?

*Section 3.7*

**3.19** Often, the periodicities in the sunspot series are investigated by fitting an autoregressive spectrum of sufficiently high order. Figure 3.20 shows the semi yearly smoothed (12 month moving average) sunspot numbers from June 1749 to December 1978 with $n = 459$ points that were taken twice per year. The main periodicity is often stated to be in the neighborhood of 11 years. Fit an autoregressive spectral estimator using SIC to determine the order. Compare the result with a conventional nonparametric spectral estimator, using the methods of Section 3.6.

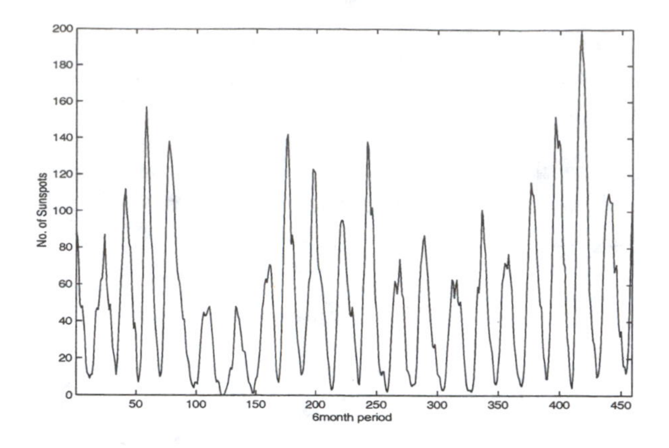


**Figure 3.20:** Smoothed 12-month sunspot numbers sampled twice per year, $n = 459$

**3.20** Suppose we wish to test the noise alone hypothesis $H_0 : x_t = n_t$ against the signal-plus-noise hypothesis $H_1 : x_t = s_t + n_t$, where $s_t$ and $n_t$ are uncorrelated zero-mean stationary processes with spectra $f_s(\nu)$ and $f_n(\nu)$. Suppose that we want the test over a band of frequencies of the form $\nu_k^n + \ell/n, \ell = 0, \pm 1, \pm 2, \ldots, \pm(L-1)/2$ near some fixed frequency $\nu$. Assume that both the signal and noise spectra are approximately constant over the interval.

(a) Prove the approximate likelihood-based test statistic for testing $H_0$ against $H_1$ is proportional to

$$T = \sum_{\ell} |X(\nu_k^n + \ell/n)|^2 \left( \frac{1}{f_n(\nu)} - \frac{1}{f_s(\nu) + f_n(\nu)} \right).$$

(b) Find the approximate distributions of $T$ under $H_0$ and $H_1$.

(c) Define the false alarm and signal detection probabilities as $P_F = P\{T > K|H_0\}$ and $P_d = P\{T > k|H_1\}$, respectively. Express these probabilities in terms of the signal-to-noise ratio $f_s(\nu)/f_n(\nu)$ and appropriate chi-squared integrals.

*Section 3.8*

**3.21** Consider the problem of approximating the filter output

$$y_t = \sum_{k=-\infty}^{\infty} a_k x_{t-k}, \quad \sum_{-\infty}^{\infty} |a_k| < \infty,$$

by

$$y_t^M = \sum_{|k|<M/2} a_k^M x_{t-k}$$

for $t = M/2-1, M/2, \ldots, n-M/2$, where $x_t$ is available for $t = 1, \ldots, n$ and

$$a_t^M = M^{-1} \sum_{k=0}^{M-1} A(\nu_k) \exp\{2\pi i \nu_k t\}$$

with $\nu_k = k/M$. Prove

$$E\{(y_t - y_t^M)^2\} \leq 4\gamma_x(0) \Bigg( \sum_{|k| \geq M/2} |a_k| \Bigg)^2.$$

**3.22** Prove the squared coherence $\rho^2_{y \cdot x}(\nu) = 1$ for all $\nu$ when

$$y_t = \sum_{r=-\infty}^{\infty} a_r x_{t-r},$$

that is, when $x_t$ and $y_t$ can be related exactly by a linear filter.

**3.23** Figure 3.21 contains 454 months of measured values for the climatic variables air temperature, dew point, cloud cover, wind speed, precipitation, and inflow at Shasta Lake in California. We would like to look at possible relations among the weather factors and between the weather factors and the inflow to Shasta Lake.

(a) Argue the strongest determinant of the inflow series is precipitation using the coherence functions. Use transformed inflow $I_t = \log i_t$, where $i_t$ is inflow, and transformed precipitation $P_t = \sqrt{p_t}$, where $p_t$ is precipitation. It should be mentioned here that Chapter 5 discusses methods for determining whether inflow might depend jointly on several input series.

(b) Using the estimated impulse response function, argue for the model

$$I_t = \alpha_0 + \frac{\alpha_1}{1 - \phi B} P_t,$$

where the notation is as discussed in Chapter 2. What would be a reasonable value for $\phi$? Assume the means are taken out of the series before the analysis begins.

*Section 3.9*

**3.24** Consider the *signal plus noise* model

$$y_t = \sum_{r=-\infty}^{\infty} a_r x_{t-r} + v_t,$$

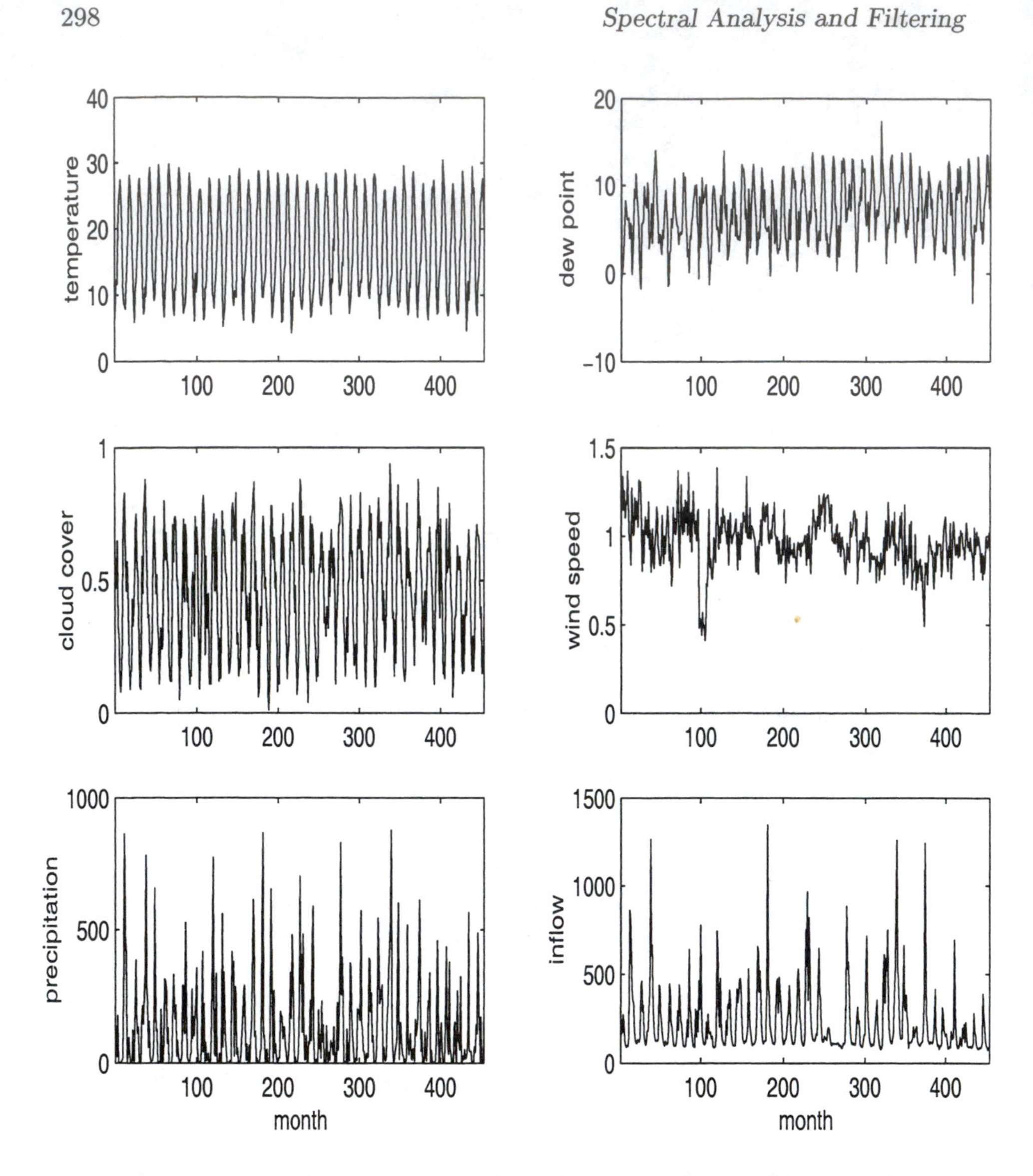


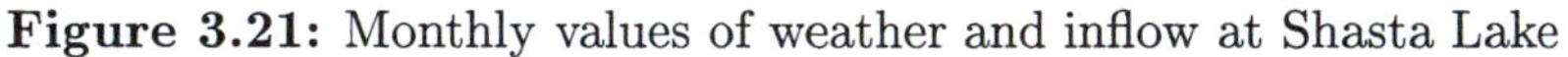

**Figure 3.21:** Monthly values of weather and inflow at Shasta Lake

where the signal and noise series, $x_t$ and $v_t$ are both stationary with spectra $f_x(\nu)$ and $f_v(\nu)$ respectively. Assuming that $x_t$ and $v_t$ are independent of each other for all $t$, verify that (3.115) and (3.116).

**3.25** Consider the model

$$y_t = x_t + v_t,$$

where

$$x_t = \phi_1 x_{t-1} + w_t,$$

with $v_t$ white and independent of $x_t$ with $var\ v_t = \sigma_v^2$, $w_t$ white and independent of $v_t$, and $var\ w_t = \sigma_w^2, |\phi_1| < 1$ and $Ex_0 = 0$. Prove that the spectrum of the observed series $y_t$ is

$$f_y(\nu) = \frac{\sigma^2|1 - \theta_1 e^{-2\pi i\nu}|^2}{|1 - \phi_1 e^{-2\pi i\nu}|^2},$$

where

$$\theta_1 = \frac{c \pm \sqrt{c^2 - 4}}{2},$$

$$\sigma^2 = \frac{\sigma_v^2 \phi_1}{\theta_1},$$

and

$$c = \frac{\sigma_w^2 + \sigma_v^2(1 + \phi_1^2)}{\sigma_v^2 \phi_1}.$$

**3.26** Consider the same model as in the preceding problem.

(a) Prove the optimal smoothed estimator of the form

$$\widehat{x}_t = \sum_{s=-\infty}^{\infty} a_s y_{t-s}$$

has

$$a_s = \frac{\sigma_w^2}{\sigma^2} \frac{\theta_1^{|s|}}{1 - \theta_1^2}.$$

(b) Show the mean square error is given by

$$E\{(x_t - \widehat{x}_t)^2\} = \frac{\sigma_v^2 \sigma_w^2}{\sigma^2(1 - \theta_1^2)}$$

.

(c) Compare mean square error of the estimator in part (b) with that of the optimal finite estimator of the form

$$\widehat{x}_t = a_1 y_{t-1} + a_2 y_{t-2}$$

when $\sigma_v^2 = .053, \sigma_w^2 = .172$, and $\phi_1 = .9$.

*Section 3.10*

**3.27** Consider the two-dimensional linear filter given as the output (3.127).

(a) Express the two-dimensional autocovariance function of the output, say, $\gamma_y(h_1, h_2)$, in terms of an infinite sum involving the autocovariance function of $x_{\boldsymbol{s}}$ and the filter coefficients $a_{s_1,s_2}$.

(b) Use the expression derived in (a), combined with (3.126) and (3.129) to derive the spectrum of the filtered output (3.128).

*Section T3.12*

**3.28** Let $w_t$ be a Gaussian white noise series with variance $\sigma_w^2$. If $W(\nu_k)$ denotes the DFT of the series at frequency $\nu_k$, prove that the results of Theorem 3.3 hold without error.

*Section T3.13*

**3.29** For the zero-mean complex random vector $\boldsymbol{z} = \boldsymbol{x}_c - i\boldsymbol{x}_s$, with $\text{cov}(\boldsymbol{z}) = \Sigma = C - iQ$, with $\Sigma = \Sigma^*$, define

$$w = 2\text{Re}(\boldsymbol{a}^*\boldsymbol{z}),$$

where $\boldsymbol{a} = \boldsymbol{a}_c - i\boldsymbol{a}_s$ is an arbitrary non-zero complex vector. Prove

$$\text{cov}(w) = 2\boldsymbol{a}^*\Sigma\boldsymbol{a}.$$

Recall * denotes the complex conjugate transpose.

# CHAPTER 4

# State-Space and Multivariate ARMAX Models

## 4.1 Introduction

A very general model that seems to subsume a whole class of special cases of interest in much the same way that linear regression does is the ***state-space model*** or the ***dynamic linear model (DLM)***, which was introduced in Kalman (1960) and Kalman and Bucy (1961). Although the model was originally introduced as a method primarily for use in aerospace-related research, it has recently been applied to modeling data from economics (Harrison and Stevens, 1976, Harvey and Pierse, 1984, Harvey and Todd, 1983, Kitagawa and Gersch 1984, Shumway and Stoffer, 1982), medicine (Jones, 1984) and the soil sciences (Shumway, 1985).

To understand the state-space model and its capabilities, we should have a basic knowledge of multivariate time series regression techniques. A useful extension of the basic univariate regression model presented in Section 1.8 is the case in which we have more than one output series, that is, ***multivariate regression analysis***. Suppose, instead of a single output variable $y_t$, a collection of $p$ output variables $y_{t1}, y_{t2}, \ldots, y_{tp}$ exist that are related to the inputs as

$$y_{ti} = \beta_{i1} z_{t1} + \beta_{i2} z_{t2} + \ldots \beta_{iq} z_{tq} + w_{it} \tag{4.1}$$

for each of the $i = 1, 2, \ldots, p$ output variables. We assume the $w_{ti}$ variables are correlated over the variable identifier $i$, but are still uncorrelated over time. Formally, we assume $\text{cov}\{w_{is}, w_{jt}\} = \sigma_{ij}$ for $s = t$ and is zero otherwise. Then, writing (4.1) in matrix notation, with $\boldsymbol{y}_t = (y_{t1}, y_{t2}, \ldots, y_{tp})'$ being the vector of outputs, and $\mathcal{B} = \{\beta_{ij}\}, i = 1, \ldots, p, j = 1, \ldots, q$ being an $p \times q$ matrix containing the regression coefficients, leads to the simple looking form

$$\boldsymbol{y}_t = \mathcal{B}\boldsymbol{z}_t + \boldsymbol{w}_t. \tag{4.2}$$

Here, the $p \times 1$ vector process $\boldsymbol{w}_t$ is assumed to be a collection of independent vectors with common covariance matrix $E\{\boldsymbol{w}_t\boldsymbol{w}_t'\} = \Sigma_w$, the $p \times p$ matrix containing the covariances $\sigma_{ij}$. The maximum likelihood estimator for the regression matrix in this case is

$$\widehat{\mathcal{B}} = Y'Z(Z'Z)^{-1}, \tag{4.3}$$

where $Z' = [\boldsymbol{z}_1, \boldsymbol{z}_2, \ldots, \boldsymbol{z}_n]$ is as before and $Y' = [\boldsymbol{y}_1, \boldsymbol{y}_2, \ldots, \boldsymbol{y}_n]$. The error covariance matrix $\Sigma_w$ is estimated by

$$\widehat{\Sigma}_w = \frac{1}{(n-q)} \sum_{t=1}^{n} (\boldsymbol{y}_t - \widehat{\mathcal{B}}\boldsymbol{z}_t)(\boldsymbol{y}_t - \widehat{\mathcal{B}}\boldsymbol{z}_t)'. \tag{4.4}$$

The uncertainty in the estimators can be evaluated from

$$\text{se}(\widehat{\beta}_{ij}) = \sqrt{\widehat{\sigma}_{jj} c_{ii}}, \tag{4.5}$$

for $i = 1, \ldots, q, j = 1, \ldots, p$, where se denotes standard error, $\widehat{\sigma}_{jj}$ is the $j$-th diagonal element of $\widehat{\Sigma}_w$, and $c_{ii}$ is the $i$-th diagonal element of $\left(\sum_{t=1}^{n} \boldsymbol{z}_t\boldsymbol{z}_t'\right)^{-1}$.

Also, the information theoretic criterion changes to

$$\text{AIC} = \ln|\widehat{\Sigma}_w| + \frac{2}{n}\left(pq + \frac{p(p+1)}{2}\right). \tag{4.6}$$

and SIC just replaces the second term in (4.6) by $K \ln n/n$ where $K = pq + p(p+1)/2$. Bedrick and Tsai (1994) have given a corrected form for AIC in the multivariate case as

$$\text{AICc} = \ln|\widehat{\Sigma}_w| + \frac{p(q+n)}{n-q-p-1}. \tag{4.7}$$

Many data sets involve more than one time series, and we are often interested in the possible dynamics relating all series. In this situation, we are interested in modeling and forecasting $p \times 1$ vector-valued time series $\boldsymbol{x}_t = (x_{t1}, \ldots, x_{tp})'$, $t = 0, \pm 1, \pm 2, \ldots$. Unfortunately, extending univariate ARMA models to the multivariate case is not so simple, and we will discuss this topic further in Section 4.12. The multivariate autoregressive model, however, is a straight-forward extension of the univariate AR model.

For the first-order ***vector autoregressive model***, VAR(1), we take

$$\boldsymbol{x}_t = \boldsymbol{\alpha} + \Phi\boldsymbol{x}_{t-1} + \boldsymbol{w}_t, \tag{4.8}$$

where $\Phi$ is a $p \times p$ ***transition matrix*** that expresses the dependence of $\boldsymbol{x}_t$ on $\boldsymbol{x}_{t-1}$. The ***vector white noise*** process $\boldsymbol{w}_t$ is defined by its covariance matrix

$$E\boldsymbol{w}_t\boldsymbol{w}_t' = \Sigma_w, \tag{4.9}$$

and the vector $\boldsymbol{\alpha} = (\alpha_1, \alpha_2, \ldots, \alpha_p)'$ appears as the constant in the regression setting. If $E(\boldsymbol{x}_t) = \boldsymbol{\mu}$, then $\boldsymbol{\alpha} = (I - \Phi)\boldsymbol{\mu}$.

Note the similarity between the VAR model and the multivariate linear regression model (4.2). The regression formulas carry over, and we can, on observing $\boldsymbol{x}_1, \ldots, \boldsymbol{x}_n$, set up the model (4.8) with $\boldsymbol{y}_t = \boldsymbol{x}_t$, $\mathcal{B} = (\boldsymbol{\alpha}, \Phi)$ and $\boldsymbol{z}_t = (1, \boldsymbol{x}_{t-1}')'$. Then, write the solution as (4.3) with the conditional maximum likelihood estimator for the covariance matrix given by

$$\widehat{\Sigma}_w = (n-1)^{-1} \sum_{t=2}^{n} (\boldsymbol{x}_t - \widehat{\boldsymbol{\alpha}} - \widehat{\Phi}\boldsymbol{x}_{t-1})(\boldsymbol{x}_t - \widehat{\boldsymbol{\alpha}} - \widehat{\Phi}\boldsymbol{x}_{t-1})'. \tag{4.10}$$

**Example 4.1 Pollution, Weather, and Mortality**

For example, for the three-dimensional series composed of detrended cardiovascular mortality $x_{t1}$, temperature $x_{t2}$, and particulate levels $x_{t3}$, introduced in Example 1.27, take $\boldsymbol{x}_t = (x_{t1}, x_{t2}, x_{t3})'$ as a vector of dimension $p = 3$. We might envision dynamic relations among the three series defined as the first order relation,

$$x_{t1} = \alpha_1 + \phi_{11}x_{t-1,1} + \phi_{12}x_{t-1,2} + \phi_{13}x_{t-1,3} + w_{t1},$$

which expresses the current value of mortality as a linear combination of its immediate past value and the past values of temperature and particulate levels. Similarly,

$$x_{t2} = \alpha_2 + \phi_{21}x_{t-1,1} + \phi_{22}x_{t-1,2} + \phi_{23}x_{t-1,3} + w_{t2}$$

and

$$x_{t3} = \alpha_3 + \phi_{31}x_{t-1,1} + \phi_{32}x_{t-1,2} + \phi_{33}x_{t-1,3} + w_{t3}$$

express the dependence of temperature and particulate levels on the other series. Of course, methods for the preliminary identification of these models exist, and we will discuss these methods in Section 4.12.

For this particular case, we obtain $\widehat{\boldsymbol{\alpha}} = (-4.57, 6.09, 19.78)'$ and

$$\widehat{\Phi} = \begin{pmatrix} .47(.04) & -.36(.03) & .10(.02) \\ -.24(.04) & .49(.04) & -.13(.02) \\ -.13(.08) & -.48(.07) & .58(.04) \end{pmatrix},$$

where the standard errors, computed as in (4.5), are given in parentheses. Hence, for the vector $(x_{t1}, x_{t2}, x_{t3}) = (M_t, T_t, P_t)$, with $M_t, T_t$ and $P_t$

denoting mortality, temperature, and particulate level, respectively, we obtain the prediction equation for mortality,

$$\widehat{M_t} = -4.57 + .47M_{t-1} - .36T_{t-1} + .10P_{t-1}.$$

Comparing observed and predicted mortality with this model leads to an $R^2$ of about 0.78, whereas the value in the regression model fitted by the method of Example 1.27 gave an $R^2 = 0.69$.

It is easy to extend the VAR(1) process to higher orders, VAR($p^*$). To do this, we use the notation of (4.2) and write the vector of regressors as

$$z_t = (1, \boldsymbol{x}'_{t-1}, \boldsymbol{x}'_{t-2}, \dots \boldsymbol{x}'_{t-p^*})'$$

and the regression matrix as $\mathcal{B} = (\boldsymbol{\alpha}, \Phi_1, \Phi_2, \dots, \Phi_{p^*})$. Then, this regression model can be written as

$$\boldsymbol{x}_t = \boldsymbol{\alpha} + \sum_{k=1}^{p^*} \Phi_k \boldsymbol{x}_{t-k} + \boldsymbol{w}_t \tag{4.11}$$

for $t = p+1, \dots, n$. The $p \times p$ ***error sum of products matrix*** becomes

$$RSP = \sum_{t=p^*+1}^{n} (\boldsymbol{x}_t - \mathcal{B}\boldsymbol{z}_t)(\boldsymbol{x}_t - \mathcal{B}\boldsymbol{z}_t)', \tag{4.12}$$

so that the conditional maximum likelihood estimator for the ***error covariance matrix*** $\Sigma_w$ is

$$\widehat{\Sigma}_w = RSP/(n - p^*), \tag{4.13}$$

as in the multivariate regression case, except now only $n - p^*$ residuals exist in (4.12). For the multivariate case, we have found that the Schwarz criterion

$$\text{SIC} = \log|\widehat{\Sigma}_w| + p^2 p^* \ln n/n, \tag{4.14}$$

gives more reasonable classifications than either AIC or corrected version AICc. The result is consistent with those reported in simulations by Lütkepohl (1985).

**Example 4.2 Mortality, Pollution and Temperature Data**

A trivariate AR(2) model for the data in Example 4.1 yields

$$\widehat{\Phi}_1 = \begin{pmatrix} .30(.04) & -.20(.04) & .04(.02) \\ -.11(.05) & .26(.05) & -.05(.03) \\ .08(.09) & -.39(.09) & .39(.05) \end{pmatrix},$$

Table 4.1: Summary Statistics for Example 4.2

| Order ($p^*$) | $p^2p^*$ | $\lvert\widehat{\Sigma}_w\rvert$ | SIC | AICc |
|---|---|---|---|---|
| 1 | 505 | 118,520 | 11.79 | 14.71 |
| 2 | 503 | 74,708 | 11.44 | 14.26 |
| 3 | 501 | 70,146 | 11.49 | 14.21 |
| 4 | 499 | 65,268 | 11.53 | 14.15 |
| 5 | 497 | 59,684 | 11.55 | 14.08 |

$$\widehat{\Phi}_2 = \begin{pmatrix} .28(.04) & -.08(.04) & .07(.03) \\ -.04(.05) & .36(.05) & -.09(.03) \\ -.33(.09) & .05(.09) & .38(.05) \end{pmatrix}.$$

In Table 4.1, fitting successively higher order models beyond $p^* = 2$ does not improve the value of SIC, and we would tend to settle on the second-order model. Note that the value of AICc continues to decrease as the model order increases.

A $p \times 1$ vector-valued time series $\boldsymbol{x}_t$, for $t = 0, \pm 1, \pm 2, ...$, is said to be ARMA$(p^*, q^*)$ if $\boldsymbol{x}_t$ is stationary and

$$\boldsymbol{x}_t = \boldsymbol{\alpha} + \Phi_1 \boldsymbol{x}_{t-1} + \cdots + \Phi_{p^*} \boldsymbol{x}_{t-p^*} + \boldsymbol{w}_t + \Theta_1 \boldsymbol{w}_{t-1} + \cdots + \Theta_{q^*} \boldsymbol{w}_{t-q^*}, \quad (4.15)$$

with $\Phi_{p^*} \neq 0$, $\Theta_{q^*} \neq 0$, and $\Sigma_w > 0$ (that is, $\Sigma_w$ is positive definite). The coefficient matrices $\Phi_j$; $j = 1, ..., p^*$ and $\Theta_j$; $j = 1, ..., q^*$ are, of course, $p \times p$ matrices. If $\boldsymbol{x}_t$ has mean $\boldsymbol{\mu}$ then $\boldsymbol{\alpha} = (I - \Phi_1 - \cdots - \Phi_{p^*})\boldsymbol{\mu}$. As in the univariate case, we will have to place a number of conditions on the multivariate ARMA model to ensure the model is unique and has desirable properties such as causality. These conditions will be discussed in Section 4.12.

The special form assumed for the constant component, $\boldsymbol{\alpha}$, of the vector ARMA model in (4.15) can be generalized to include a fixed $r \times 1$ vector of inputs, $\boldsymbol{u}_t$. That is, we could have proposed the ***ARMAX model***,

$$\boldsymbol{x}_t = \Gamma \boldsymbol{u}_t + \sum_{j=1}^{p^*} \Phi_j \boldsymbol{x}_{t-j} + \sum_{k=1}^{q^*} \Theta_k \boldsymbol{w}_{t-k} + \boldsymbol{w}_t, \quad (4.16)$$

where $\Gamma$ is a $p \times r$ parameter matrix. The X in ARMAX refers to the exogenous vector process we have denoted here by $\boldsymbol{u}_t$. The introduction of exogenous variables through replacing $\boldsymbol{\alpha}$ by $\Gamma \boldsymbol{u}_t$ does not present any special problems in making inferences. For example, the case of the ARX model, that is, $q^* = 0$ in (4.16), can be estimated using standard regression results. In this case, the model can be written as a multivariate regression model in which the vector of regressors are

$$z_t = (\boldsymbol{u}_t', \boldsymbol{x}_{t-1}', ..., \boldsymbol{x}_{t-p^*}')' \quad (4.17)$$

and the new regression matrix is

$$\mathcal{B} = [\Gamma, \Phi_1, \Phi_2, ..., \Phi_{p^*}]. \tag{4.18}$$

The general ARMA model, (4.15), is a special case of the ARMAX model, (4.16), with r=1, $\boldsymbol{u}_t = 1$, and $\Gamma = \boldsymbol{\alpha}$.

The ***state-space model*** or ***dynamic linear model (DLM)***, in its basic form, retains a VAR(1) as the ***state equation***,

$$\boldsymbol{x}_t = \Phi \boldsymbol{x}_{t-1} + \boldsymbol{w}_t, \tag{4.19}$$

where the state equation determines the rule for the generation of $x_{ti}$ from the past states $x_{t-1,j}, j = 1, \ldots, p$ for $i = 1, \ldots, p$ and time points $t = 1, \ldots, n$. We assume for completeness the $\boldsymbol{w}_t$ are $p \times 1$ independent and identically distributed, zero-mean normal vectors with covariance matrix $Q$. In the DLM, we assume the process starts with a normal vector $\boldsymbol{x}_0$ that has mean $\boldsymbol{\mu}_0$ and $p \times p$ covariance matrix $\Sigma_0$.

The DLM, however, adds an additional component to the model in assuming we do not observe the state vector $\boldsymbol{x}_t$ directly, but can only observe a linear transformed version of it with noise added, say

$$\boldsymbol{y}_t = A_t \boldsymbol{x}_t + \boldsymbol{v}_t \tag{4.20}$$

where $A_t$ is a $q \times p$ ***measurement*** or ***observation matrix***; equation (4.20) is called the ***observation equation***. The model arose originally in the space tracking setting, where the state equation defines the motion equations for the position or ***state*** of a spacecraft with location $\boldsymbol{x}_t$ and $\boldsymbol{y}_t$ reflects information that can be observed from a tracking device such as velocity and azimuth. The observed data are in the $q \times 1$ vectors $\boldsymbol{y}_t$, which can be larger than or smaller than $p$, the dimension of the underlying series of interest. The additive ***observation noise*** $\boldsymbol{v}_t$ is assumed to be white and Gaussian with $q \times q$ covariance matrix $R$. In addition, we initially assume, for simplicity, $\{\boldsymbol{w}_t\}$ and $\{\boldsymbol{v}_t\}$ are uncorrelated; this assumption is not necessary, but it helps in the explanation of first concepts. The case of correlated errors is discussed in Section 4.6. Of course, we can further modify the basic model, (4.19) and (4.20), to include exogenous variables, and we will also discuss this in Section 4.6.

**Example 4.3 A Biomedical Example**

Suppose we consider the problem of monitoring the level of several biomedical parameters monitored after a cancer patient undergoes a bone marrow transplant. The data in Figure 4.1, used by Jones (1984), are measurements made for 91 days on the three variables, log (white blood count), log (platelet), and hematocrit (HCT), denoted $y_{t1}, y_{t2}$, and $y_{t3}$, respectively. Approximately 40% of the values are missing, with missing values occurring primarily after the 35th day. The main objectives are to model

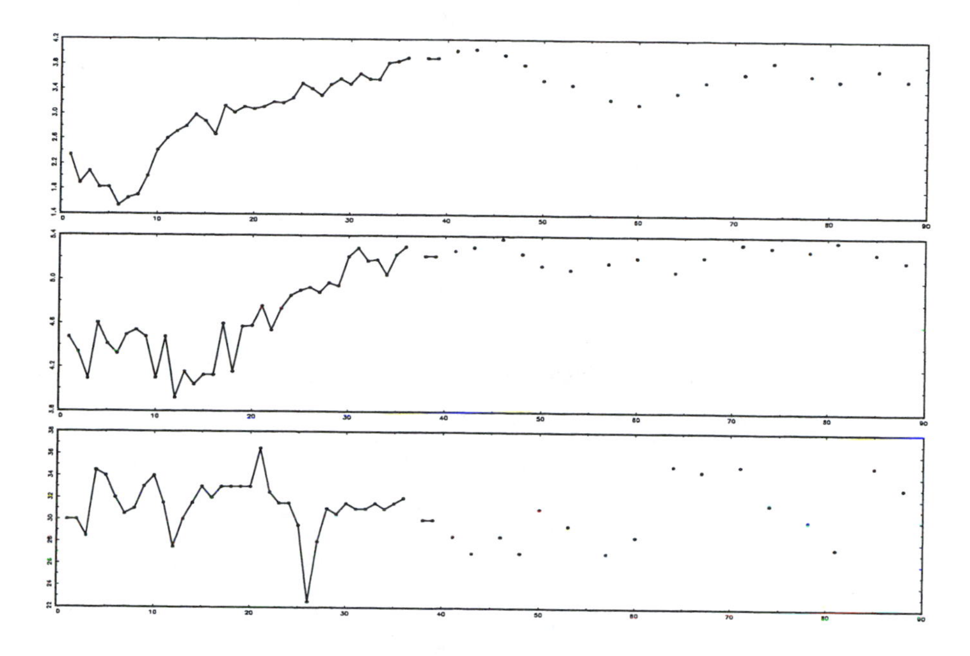

**Figure 4.1:** Longitudinal series of blood parameter levels monitored, log (white blood count) [top], log (platelet) [middle], and hematocrit (HCT) [bottom], after a bone marrow transplant ($n = 91$ days).

the three variables using the state-space approach, and to estimate the missing values. According to Jones, "Platelet count at about 100 days post transplant has previously been shown to be a good indicator of subsequent long term survival." For this particular situation, we model the three variables in terms of the state equation (4.19); that is,

$$\begin{pmatrix} x_{t1} \\ x_{t2} \\ x_{t3} \end{pmatrix} = \begin{pmatrix} \phi_{11} & \phi_{12} & \phi_{13} \\ \phi_{21} & \phi_{22} & \phi_{23} \\ \phi_{31} & \phi_{32} & \phi_{33} \end{pmatrix} \begin{pmatrix} x_{t-1,1} \\ x_{t-1,2} \\ x_{t-1,3} \end{pmatrix} + \begin{pmatrix} w_{t1} \\ w_{t2} \\ w_{t3} \end{pmatrix}. \tag{4.21}$$

The $3 \times 3$ observation matrix, $A_t$, is either the identity matrix, or the identity matrix with all zeros in a row when that variable is missing. The covariance matrices $R$ and $Q$ are $3 \times 3$ matrices with $R = \text{diag}\{r_{11}, r_{22}, r_{33}\}$, a diagonal matrix, required for a simple approach when data are missing.

The model given in (4.19) involving only a single lag is not unduly restrictive. A multivariate model with $p^*$ lags, such as the VAR($p^*$) in (4.11), could be developed by replacing the $p \times 1$ state vector, $\boldsymbol{x}_t$, by the $pp^* \times 1$ state vector

$\boldsymbol{X}_t = (\boldsymbol{x}'_t, \boldsymbol{x}'_{t-1}, \dots, \boldsymbol{x}'_{t-p*+1})'$ and the transition matrix by

$$\Phi = \begin{pmatrix} \Phi_1 & \Phi_2 & \dots & \Phi_{p*-1} & \Phi_{p*} \\ I & 0 & \dots & 0 & 0 \\ 0 & I & \dots & 0 & 0 \\ \vdots & \vdots & \ddots & \vdots & \vdots \\ 0 & 0 & \dots & I & 0 \end{pmatrix}. \tag{4.22}$$

Letting $\boldsymbol{W}_t = (\boldsymbol{w}'_t, \boldsymbol{0}', ..., \boldsymbol{0}')'$ be the new $pp^* \times 1$ state error vector, the new state equation will be

$$\boldsymbol{X}_t = \Phi \boldsymbol{X}_{t-1} + \boldsymbol{W}_t, \tag{4.23}$$

where the new matrix "$Q$" now has the form of a $pp^* \times pp^*$ matrix with $Q$ in the upper right-hand corner and zeros elsewhere. The observation equation can then be written as

$$\boldsymbol{y}_t = \left[A_t \mid 0 \mid \cdots \mid 0\right] \boldsymbol{X}_t + \boldsymbol{v}_t. \tag{4.24}$$

This simple recoding shows one way of handling higher order lags within the context of the single lag structure. Further discussion of this notion is given in Section 4.6.

The real advantages of the state-space formulation, however, do not really come through in the simple example given above. The special forms that can be developed for various versions of the matrix $A$ and for the transition scheme defined by the matrix $\Phi$ allow fitting more parsimonious structures with fewer parameters needed to describe a multivariate time series. We will give some examples of ***structural models*** in Section 4.5, but the simple example shown below is instructive.

**Example 4.4 Global Warming**

Figure 4.2 (see also Figure 1.14) shows two different estimators for the global temperature series from 1880 to 1987, plotted on the same scale. The solid line is considered in the first chapter (see Jones, 1994), which gives average surface air temperature computed from land-based observation stations. The second series (see Parker et al, 1996) gives averages from a number marine-based stations. Conceptually, both series should be measuring the same underlying climatic signal, and we may consider the problem of extracting this underlying signal. We suppose both series are observing the same signal with different noises; that is,

$$y_{t1} = x_t + v_{t1}$$

and

$$y_{t2} = x_t + v_{t2},$$

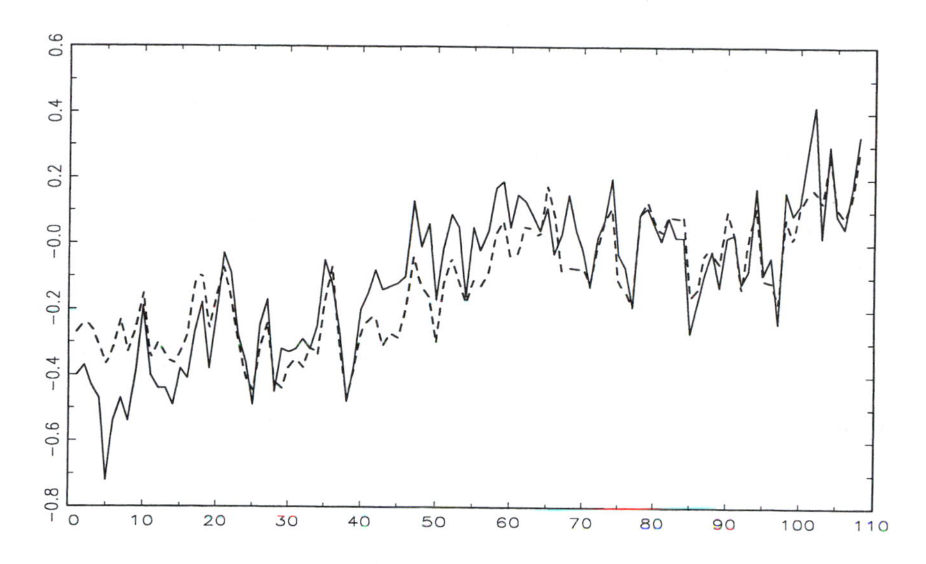


**Figure 4.2:** Two average global temperature deviations for $n = 108$ years in degrees Centigrade (1880-1987). The solid line is the land-based series whereas the dotted line shows the marine-based series.

where $x_t$ is the unknown common signal. Suppose it can be modeled as a random walk of the form

$$x_t = x_{t-1} + w_t, \tag{4.25}$$

which we can argue for by noting the stability of the first difference as has been noted in Chapter 1. Furthermore, the first difference of the observed series will be a first-order moving average under this model, arguing from the fact that the first difference of the land-based series has a peak at lag 1. In this example, $p = 1, q = 2$, and $\phi = 1$ is held at a constant value. The observation equation (4.20) can be written in the form

$$\begin{pmatrix} y_{t1} \\ y_{t2} \end{pmatrix} = \begin{pmatrix} 1 \\ 1 \end{pmatrix} x_t + \begin{pmatrix} v_{t1} \\ v_{t2} \end{pmatrix}, \tag{4.26}$$

and we have the covariance matrices given by $Q = q_{11}$ and

$$R = \begin{pmatrix} r_{11} & r_{12} \\ r_{21} & r_{22} \end{pmatrix}.$$

The introduction of the state-space approach as a tool for modeling data in the social and biological sciences requires model identification and parameter estimation because there is rarely a well-defined differential equation describing the state transition. The questions of general interest for the dynamic linear model (4.19) and (4.20) relate to estimating the unknown parameters $R, Q$, and $\Phi$ that define the particular model, and estimating or forecasting values of the underlying unobserved process $\boldsymbol{x}_t$. The advantages of the state-space formulation are in the ease with which we can treat various missing data configurations and in the incredible array of models that can be generated from (4.19) and (4.20). The analogy between the observation matrix $A_t$ and the design matrix in the usual regresssion and analysis of variance setting is a useful one. We can generate fixed and random effect structures that are either constant or vary over time simply by making appropriate choices for the matrix $A_t$ and the transition structure $\Phi$. We will give only a few examples in this chapter; for further examples, see Harvey (1993) or Shumway (1988).

Before continuing our investigation of the more complex model, it is instructive to consider a simple univariate state-space model.

### Example 4.5 An AR(1) Process with Observational Noise

Figure 4.3 shows $n = 100$ simulated observations from the univariate state-space model,

$$y_t = x_t + v_t, \tag{4.27}$$

where the signal satisfies an AR(1) model

$$x_t = \phi x_{t-1} + w_t, \tag{4.28}$$

for $t = 1, 2, ..., n$. The noise processes are independent and Gaussian, and with $\sigma_w = \sigma_v = 1$. In particular, the state $x_t$ follows a stationary AR(1) model with $\phi = 0.8$, and it is shown as the dark line in that figure. In this model, we do not observe $x_t$ directly, but rather $y_t$, which is the state $x_t$ with added noise $v_t$, as seen by the thin line in Figure 4.3.

In Chapter 2, we investigated the properties of the state, $x_t$, because it is a stationary AR(1) process. For example, we know the autocovariance function of $x_t$ is

$$\gamma_x(h) = \frac{\sigma_w^2}{1 - \phi^2}\, \phi^h, \quad h = 0, 1, 2, \dots . \tag{4.29}$$

But here, we must investigate how the addition of observation noise affects the dynamics. Although it is not a necessary assumption, we have assumed here $x_t$ is stationary. In this case, the observations are also stationary because $y_t$ is the sum of two independent stationary components $x_t$ and $v_t$. We have

$$\gamma_y(0) = \text{var}(y_t) = \text{var}(x_t + v_t) = \frac{\sigma_w^2}{1 - \phi^2} + \sigma_v^2, \tag{4.30}$$

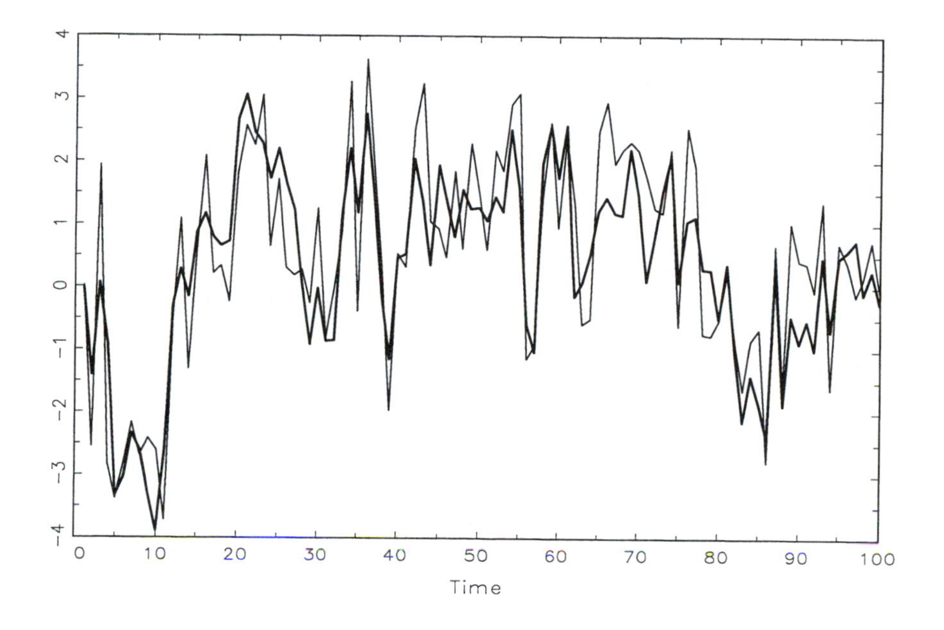


**Figure 4.3:** Simulated data, $n = 100$, from the model (4.27) and (4.28) with $\phi = 0.8$ and $\sigma_w = \sigma_v = 1$. The states, $x_t$, are shown as the dark line, and the observations $y_t$ are shown as the thin line.

and, when $h \geq 1$,

$$\gamma_y(h) = \text{cov}(y_t, y_{t-h}) = \text{cov}(x_t + v_t, x_{t-h} + v_{t-h}) = \gamma_x(h). \tag{4.31}$$

Consequently, for $h \geq 1$, the ACF of the observations is

$$\rho_y(h) = \frac{\gamma_y(h)}{\gamma_y(0)} = \left(1 + \frac{\sigma_v^2}{\sigma_w^2}(1 - \phi^2)\right)^{-1} \phi^h. \tag{4.32}$$

It should be clear from the correlation structure given by (4.32) the observations, $y_t$, are not AR(1) unless $\sigma_v^2 = 0$. In addition, the autocorrelation structure of $y_t$ is identical to the autocorrelation structure of an ARMA(1,1) process, as presented in Example 2.13. Thus, the observations can also be written in an ARMA(1,1) form,

$$y_t = \phi y_{t-1} + \theta u_{t-1} + u_t,$$

where $u_t$ is Gaussian white noise with variance $\sigma_u$, and with $\theta$ and $\sigma_u^2$ suitably chosen (see Example 4.11).

Although an equivalence exists between stationary ARMA models and stationary state-space models (see Section 4.6), it is sometimes easier to work with one form than another. As previously mentioned, in the case of missing data, complex multivariate systems, mixed effects, and certain types of nonstationarity, it is easier to work in the framework of state-space models; in this chapter, we explore some of these situations.

## 4.2 Filtering, Smoothing, and Forecasting

From a practical view, the primary aims of any analysis involving the state-space model as defined by (4.19) and (4.20) would be to produce estimators for the underlying unobserved signal $\boldsymbol{x}_t$, given the data $Y_s = \{\boldsymbol{y}_1, ..., \boldsymbol{y}_s\}$, to time $s$. When $s < t$, the problem is called ***forecasting*** or ***prediction***. When $s = t$, the problem is called ***filtering***, and when $s > t$, the problem is called ***smoothing***. In addition to these estimates, we would also want to measure their precision. The solution to these problems is accomplished via the ***Kalman filter and smoother*** and is the focus of this section.

Throughout this chapter, we will use the following definitions:

$$\boldsymbol{x}_t^s = E(\boldsymbol{x}_t \mid Y_s) \tag{4.33}$$

and

$$P_{t_1,t_2}^s = E\left\{(\boldsymbol{x}_{t_1} - \boldsymbol{x}_{t_1}^s)(\boldsymbol{x}_{t_2} - \boldsymbol{x}_{t_2}^s)'\right\}. \tag{4.34}$$

When $t_1 = t_2$ ($= t$ say) in (4.34), we will write $P_t^s$ for convenience.

In obtaining the filtering and smoothing equations, we will rely heavily on the Gaussian assumption. Even in the non-Gaussian case, the estimators we obtain are the minimum mean-squared error estimators within the class of linear estimators (BLP). That is, we can think of $E$ in (4.33) as the projection operator in the sense of Section T2.16 rather than expectation and $P_t^s$ as the corresponding mean-squared error. When we assume, as in this section, the processes are Gaussian, (4.34) is also the conditional error covariance; that is,

$$P_{t_1,t_2}^s = E\left\{(\boldsymbol{x}_{t_1} - \boldsymbol{x}_{t_1}^s)(\boldsymbol{x}_{t_2} - \boldsymbol{x}_{t_2}^s)' \mid Y_s\right\}.$$

This fact can be seen, for example, by noting the covariance matrix between $(\boldsymbol{x}_t - \boldsymbol{x}_t^s)$ and $Y_s$, for any $t$ and $s$, is zero; we could say they are orthogonal in the sense of Section T2.16. This result implies that $(\boldsymbol{x}_t - \boldsymbol{x}_t^s)$ and $Y_s$ are independent (because of the normality), and hence, the conditional distribution of $(\boldsymbol{x}_t - \boldsymbol{x}_t^s)$ given $Y_s$ is the unconditional distribution of $(\boldsymbol{x}_t - \boldsymbol{x}_t^s)$. Derivations of the filtering and smoothing equations from a Bayesian perspective are given in Meinhold and Singpurwalla (1983); more traditional approaches based on the concept of projection and on multivariate normal distribution theory are given in Jazwinski (1970) and Anderson and Moore (1979).

First, we present the Kalman filter, which gives the filtering and forecasting equations. The name filter comes from the fact that $\boldsymbol{x}_t^t$ is a linear filter of the observations $\boldsymbol{y}_1, ..., \boldsymbol{y}_t$; that is, $\boldsymbol{x}_t^t = \sum_{s=1}^t B_s \boldsymbol{y}_s$ for suitably chosen $p \times q$ matrices $B_s$. The advantage of the Kalman filter is that it specifies how to update the filter from $\boldsymbol{x}_{t-1}^{t-1}$ to $\boldsymbol{x}_t^t$ once a new observation $\boldsymbol{y}_t$ is obtained, without having to reprocess the entire data set $\boldsymbol{y}_1, ..., \boldsymbol{y}_t$.

***Property P4.1: The Kalman Filter***

*For the state-space model specified in (4.19) and (4.20), with initial conditions* $\boldsymbol{x}_0^0 = \boldsymbol{\mu}$ *and* $P_0^0 = \Sigma_0$, *for* $t = 1, ..., n$,

$$\boldsymbol{x}_t^{t-1} = \Phi \boldsymbol{x}_{t-1}^{t-1}, \tag{4.35}$$

$$P_t^{t-1} = \Phi P_{t-1}^{t-1} \Phi' + Q, \tag{4.36}$$

*with*

$$\boldsymbol{x}_t^t = \boldsymbol{x}_t^{t-1} + K_t(\boldsymbol{y}_t - A_t \boldsymbol{x}_t^{t-1}), \tag{4.37}$$

$$P_t^t = [I - K_t A_t] P_t^{t-1}, \tag{4.38}$$

*where*

$$K_t = P_t^{t-1} A_t' [A_t P_t^{t-1} A_t' + R]^{-1} \tag{4.39}$$

*is called the Kalman gain. Prediction for* $t > n$ *is accomplished via (4.35) and (4.36) with initial conditions* $\boldsymbol{x}_n^n$ *and* $P_n^n$.

***Proof.*** The derivations of (4.35) and (4.36) follow from straight forward calculations, because from (4.19) we have

$$\boldsymbol{x}_t^{t-1} = E(\boldsymbol{x}_t \mid Y_{t-1}) = E(\Phi \boldsymbol{x}_{t-1} + \boldsymbol{w}_t \mid Y_{t-1}) = \Phi x_{t-1}^{t-1},$$

and thus

$$\begin{aligned} P_t^{t-1} &= E\left\{(\boldsymbol{x}_t - \boldsymbol{x}_t^{t-1})(\boldsymbol{x}_t - \boldsymbol{x}_t^{t-1})'\right\} \\ &= E\left\{\left[\Phi(\boldsymbol{x}_{t-1} - \boldsymbol{x}_{t-1}^{t-1}) + \boldsymbol{w}_t\right]\left[\Phi(\boldsymbol{x}_{t-1} - \boldsymbol{x}_{t-1}^{t-1}) + \boldsymbol{w}_t\right]'\right\} \\ &= \Phi P_{t-1}^{t-1} \Phi' + Q. \end{aligned}$$

To derive (4.37), we first define the ***innovations*** as

$$\boldsymbol{\epsilon}_t = \boldsymbol{y}_t - E(\boldsymbol{y}_t \mid Y_{t-1}) = \boldsymbol{y}_t - A_t \boldsymbol{x}_t^{t-1}, \tag{4.40}$$

for $t = 1, ..., n$. Note, $E(\boldsymbol{\epsilon}_t) = \boldsymbol{0}$ and

$$\Sigma_t \stackrel{\text{def}}{=} \text{var}(\boldsymbol{\epsilon}_t) = \text{var}[A_t(\boldsymbol{x}_t - \boldsymbol{x}_t^{t-1}) + \boldsymbol{v}_t] = A_t P_t^{t-1} A_t' + R \tag{4.41}$$

In addition, using Theorem 2.2 (iv) of Section T2.16, $E(\boldsymbol{\epsilon}_t \boldsymbol{y}_s') = \boldsymbol{0}$ for $s = 1, ..., t-1$, which in view of the fact the innovation sequence is a Gaussian process, implies that the innovations are independent of the past observations. Furthermore, the conditional covariance between $\boldsymbol{x}_t$ and $\boldsymbol{\epsilon}_t$ given $Y_{t-1}$ is

$$\begin{aligned}
\operatorname{cov}(\boldsymbol{x}_t,\ \boldsymbol{\epsilon}_t \mid Y_{t-1}) &= \operatorname{cov}(\boldsymbol{x}_t,\ \boldsymbol{y}_t - A_t\boldsymbol{x}_t^{t-1} \mid Y_{t-1}) \\
&= \operatorname{cov}(\boldsymbol{x}_t - \boldsymbol{x}_t^{t-1},\ \boldsymbol{y}_t - A_t\boldsymbol{x}_t^{t-1} \mid Y_{t-1}) \\
&= \operatorname{cov}[\boldsymbol{x}_t - \boldsymbol{x}_t^{t-1},\ A_t(\boldsymbol{x}_t - \boldsymbol{x}_t^{t-1}) + \boldsymbol{v}_t] \\
&= P_t^{t-1}A_t'. \qquad (4.42)
\end{aligned}$$

Using these results we have that joint conditional distribution of $\boldsymbol{x}_t$ and $\boldsymbol{\epsilon}_t$ given $Y_{t-1}$ is normal

$$\begin{pmatrix} \boldsymbol{x}_t \\ \boldsymbol{\epsilon}_t \end{pmatrix} \Bigg| Y_{t-1} \sim \mathrm{N}\left( \begin{bmatrix} \boldsymbol{x}_t^{t-1} \\ \mathbf{0} \end{bmatrix}, \begin{bmatrix} P_t^{t-1} & P_t^{t-1}A_t' \\ A_tP_t^{t-1} & \Sigma_t \end{bmatrix} \right).$$

Thus, using (2.234) of Section T2.16, we can write

$$\boldsymbol{x}_t^t = E(\boldsymbol{x}_t|\boldsymbol{y}_1,\dots,\boldsymbol{y}_{t-1},\boldsymbol{y}_t) = E(\boldsymbol{x}_t|Y_{t-1},\boldsymbol{\epsilon}_t) = \boldsymbol{x}_t^{t-1} + K_t\boldsymbol{\epsilon}_t, \qquad (4.43)$$

where

$$K_t = P_t^{t-1}A_t'\Sigma_t^{-1} = P_t^{t-1}A_t'(A_tP_t^{t-1}A_t' + R)^{-1}.$$

The evaluation of $P_t^t$ is obtained by writing

$$\boldsymbol{x}_t - \boldsymbol{x}_t^t = [I - K_tA_t](\boldsymbol{x}_t - \boldsymbol{x}_t^{t-1}) - K_t\boldsymbol{v}_t,$$

and then simplifying the result of the expectation, $E\{(\boldsymbol{x}_t - \boldsymbol{x}_t^t)(\boldsymbol{x}_t - \boldsymbol{x}_t^t)'\}$, to arrive at (4.38). □

Next, we explore the model, prediction, and filtering from a density point of view. First consider the Gaussian DLM as described in (4.19) and (4.20); that is,

$$\boldsymbol{x}_t = \Phi\boldsymbol{x}_{t-1} + \boldsymbol{w}_t \quad \text{and} \quad \boldsymbol{y}_t = A_t\boldsymbol{x}_t + \boldsymbol{v}_t.$$

Recall $\boldsymbol{w}_t$ and $\boldsymbol{v}_t$ are independent, white Gaussian sequences, and the initial state is normal, say, $\boldsymbol{x}_0 \sim \mathrm{N}(\boldsymbol{\mu}_0, \Sigma_0)$. To ease the discussion, we will write $\boldsymbol{\mu}_0 = \boldsymbol{x}_0^0$, $\Sigma_0 = P_0^0$, and we will write the initial state density as $f_0(\boldsymbol{x}_0 - \boldsymbol{x}_0^0)$, where $f_0(\cdot)$ represents the $p$-variate normal density with mean zero and variance-covariance matrix $P_0^0$. Similarly, letting $p_\Theta(\cdot)$ denote a generic density function with parameters represented by $\Theta$, we could describe the state relationship as

$$p_\Theta(\boldsymbol{x}_t|\boldsymbol{x}_{t-1},\boldsymbol{x}_{t-2},\dots,\boldsymbol{x}_0) = p_\Theta(\boldsymbol{x}_t|\boldsymbol{x}_{t-1}) = f_w(\boldsymbol{x}_t - \Phi\boldsymbol{x}_{t-1}), \qquad (4.44)$$

where $f_w(\cdot)$ represents the $p$-variate normal density with mean zero and variance-covariance matrix $Q$. In (4.44), we are stating the process is Markovian, linear, and Gaussian. The relationship of the observations to the state process is written as

$$p_\Theta(\boldsymbol{y}_t|\boldsymbol{x}_t, Y_{t-1}) = p_\Theta(\boldsymbol{y}_t|\boldsymbol{x}_t) = f_v(\boldsymbol{y}_t - A_t\boldsymbol{x}_t), \qquad (4.45)$$

where $f_v(\cdot)$ represents the $q$-variate normal density with mean zero and variance-covariance matrix $R$. In (4.45), we are stating the observations are conditionally independent given the state, and the observations are linear and Gaussian. Note (4.44), (4.45), and the initial density, $f_0(\cdot)$, completely specify the likelihood (or, equivalently, the model),

$$\begin{aligned} L_{X,Y}(\Theta) &= p_\Theta(\boldsymbol{x}_0, \boldsymbol{x}_1, ..., \boldsymbol{x}_n, \boldsymbol{y}_1, ..., \boldsymbol{y}_n) \\ &= f_0(\boldsymbol{x}_0 - \boldsymbol{x}_0^0) \prod_{t=1}^{n} f_w(\boldsymbol{x}_t - \Phi \boldsymbol{x}_{t-1}) f_v(\boldsymbol{y}_t - A_t \boldsymbol{x}_t), \end{aligned} \tag{4.46}$$

where $\Theta = \{\boldsymbol{x}_0^0, P_0^0, \Phi, Q, R\}$.

Given the data, $Y_{t-1} = \{\boldsymbol{y}_1, ..., \boldsymbol{y}_{t-1}\}$, through time $t-1$, and the current filter density, $p_\Theta(\boldsymbol{x}_{t-1} \mid Y_{t-1})$, Property 4.1 tells us, via conditional means and variances, how to recursively generate the Gaussian forecast density, $p_\Theta(\boldsymbol{x}_t \mid Y_{t-1})$, and how to update the density given the current observation, $\boldsymbol{y}_t$, to obtain the Gaussian filter density, $p_\Theta(\boldsymbol{x}_t \mid Y_t)$. In terms of densities, the Kalman filter can be seen as a simple Bayesian updating scheme, where, to determine the forecast and filter densities, we have

$$\begin{aligned} p_\Theta(\boldsymbol{x}_t \mid Y_{t-1}) &= \int_{R^p} p_\Theta(\boldsymbol{x}_t, \boldsymbol{x}_{t-1} \mid Y_{t-1}) \, d\boldsymbol{x}_{t-1} \\ &= \int_{R^p} p_\Theta(\boldsymbol{x}_t \mid \boldsymbol{x}_{t-1}) p_\Theta(\boldsymbol{x}_{t-1} \mid Y_{t-1}) \, d\boldsymbol{x}_{t-1} \\ &= \int_{R^p} f_w(\boldsymbol{x}_t - \Phi \boldsymbol{x}_{t-1}) p_\Theta(\boldsymbol{x}_{t-1} \mid Y_{t-1}) d\boldsymbol{x}_{t-1}, \end{aligned} \tag{4.47}$$

which simplifies to the $p$-variate $\mathrm{N}(\boldsymbol{x}_t^{t-1}, P_t^{t-1})$ density, and

$$\begin{aligned} p_\Theta(\boldsymbol{x}_t \mid Y_t) &= p_\Theta(\boldsymbol{x}_t \mid \boldsymbol{y}_t, Y_{t-1}) \\ &\propto p_\Theta(\boldsymbol{y}_t \mid \boldsymbol{x}_t) \, p_\Theta(\boldsymbol{x}_t \mid Y_{t-1}), \\ &= f_v(\boldsymbol{y}_t - A_t \boldsymbol{x}_t) p_\Theta(\boldsymbol{x}_t \mid Y_{t-1}), \end{aligned} \tag{4.48}$$

from which we can deduce $p_\Theta(\boldsymbol{x}_t \mid Y_t)$ is the $p$-variate $\mathrm{N}(\boldsymbol{x}_t^t, P_t^t)$ density. These statements are true for $t = 1, ..., n$, with initial condition $p_\Theta(\boldsymbol{x}_0 \mid Y_0) = f_0(\boldsymbol{x}_0 - \boldsymbol{x}_0^0)$. The prediction and filter recursions of Property P4.1 could also have been calculated directly from the density relationships (4.47) and (4.48) using multivariate normal distribution theory.

Next, we consider the problem of obtaining estimators for $\boldsymbol{x}_t$ based on the entire data sample $\boldsymbol{y}_1, ..., \boldsymbol{y}_n$, where $t \le n$, namely, $\boldsymbol{x}_t^n$. These estimators are called smoothers because a time plot of the sequence $\{\boldsymbol{x}_t^n;\ t = 1, ..., n\}$ is typically smoother than the forecasts $\{\boldsymbol{x}_t^{t-1};\ t = 1, ..., n\}$ or the filters $\{\boldsymbol{x}_t^t;\ t = 1, ..., n\}$. As is obvious from the above remarks, smoothing implies that each estimated value is a function of the present, future, and past, whereas the filtered estimator depends on the present and past. The forecast depends only on the past, as usual.

***Property P4.2: The Kalman Smoother***
*For the state-space model specified in (4.19) and (4.20), with initial conditions $\boldsymbol{x}_n^n$ and $P_n^n$ obtained via Property P4.1, for $t = n, n-1, ..., 1$,*

$$\boldsymbol{x}_{t-1}^n = \boldsymbol{x}_{t-1}^{t-1} + J_{t-1}\left(\boldsymbol{x}_t^n - \boldsymbol{x}_t^{t-1}\right), \tag{4.49}$$

$$P_{t-1}^n = P_{t-1}^{t-1} + J_{t-1}\left(P_t^n - P_t^{t-1}\right)J_{t-1}', \tag{4.50}$$

*where*

$$J_{t-1} = P_{t-1}^{t-1}\Phi'\left[P_t^{t-1}\right]^{-1}. \tag{4.51}$$

***Proof.*** The smoother can be derived in many ways. Here, we find it instructive to take advantage of Gaussian assumption and use a maximum likelihood technique that was presented in Rauch et al (1965). A derivation based solely on the Projection Theorem of Section T2.15 is discussed in Problem 4.6. Recall $\boldsymbol{x}_n^n$ and $P_n^n$ are available from the Kalman filter. We use the notation $Y_s = \{\boldsymbol{y}_1, ..., \boldsymbol{y}_s\}$.

Consider the problem of obtaining the MLEs of $\boldsymbol{x}_{t-1}$ and $\boldsymbol{x}_t$, for $t \le n$, based on the data $Y_n$. The conditional means $\boldsymbol{x}_{t-1}^n$ and $\boldsymbol{x}_t^n$, are those values of $\boldsymbol{x}_{t-1}$ and $\boldsymbol{x}_t$, respectively, that maximize the joint Gaussian density

$$f(\boldsymbol{x}_{t-1}, \boldsymbol{x}_t | Y_n). \tag{4.52}$$

We write

$$\begin{aligned} f(\boldsymbol{x}_{t-1}, \boldsymbol{x}_t|Y_n) &\propto f(\boldsymbol{x}_{t-1}, \boldsymbol{x}_t, Y_n) = f(\boldsymbol{x}_{t-1}, \boldsymbol{x}_t, Y_{t-1}, \boldsymbol{y}_t, ..., \boldsymbol{y}_n) \\ &= f(Y_{t-1}) f(\boldsymbol{x}_{t-1}, \boldsymbol{x}_t|Y_{t-1}) f(\boldsymbol{y}_t, ..., \boldsymbol{y}_n|\boldsymbol{x}_{t-1}, \boldsymbol{x}_t, Y_{t-1}). \end{aligned}$$

From the model, (4.19) and (4.20), it follows that

$$f(\boldsymbol{x}_{t-1}, \boldsymbol{x}_t|Y_{t-1}) = f(\boldsymbol{x}_{t-1}|Y_{t-1}) f(\boldsymbol{x}_t|\boldsymbol{x}_{t-1}, Y_{t-1}) = f(\boldsymbol{x}_{t-1}|Y_{t-1}) f(\boldsymbol{x}_t|\boldsymbol{x}_{t-1}),$$

and

$$f(\boldsymbol{y}_t, ..., \boldsymbol{y}_n|\boldsymbol{x}_{t-1}, \boldsymbol{x}_t, Y_{t-1}) = f(\boldsymbol{y}_t, ..., \boldsymbol{y}_n|\boldsymbol{x}_t),$$

independent of $\boldsymbol{x}_{t-1}$.

Finally, the conditional joint density, (4.52), has the form

$$f(\boldsymbol{x}_{t-1}, \boldsymbol{x}_t|Y_n) = c(\boldsymbol{x}_t) f(\boldsymbol{x}_{t-1}|Y_{t-1}) f(\boldsymbol{x}_t|\boldsymbol{x}_{t-1}), \tag{4.53}$$

where $c(\boldsymbol{x}_t)$ is independent of $\boldsymbol{x}_{t-1}$. The conditional densities in (4.53) are Gaussian, in particular,

$$\boldsymbol{x}_{t-1}|Y_{t-1} \sim \mathrm{N}(\boldsymbol{x}_{t-1}^{t-1}, P_{t-1}^{t-1}),$$

and

$$\boldsymbol{x}_t|\boldsymbol{x}_{t-1} \sim \mathrm{N}(\Phi\boldsymbol{x}_{t-1}, Q).$$

Then, we wish to minimize

$$\begin{aligned} -2\ln f(\boldsymbol{x}_{t-1}, \boldsymbol{x}_t | Y_n) &\propto \left(\boldsymbol{x}_{t-1} - \boldsymbol{x}_{t-1}^{t-1}\right) \left[P_{t-1}^{t-1}\right]^{-1} \left(\boldsymbol{x}_{t-1} - \boldsymbol{x}_{t-1}^{t-1}\right)' \\ &+ \left(\boldsymbol{x}_t - \Phi \boldsymbol{x}_{t-1}\right) Q^{-1} \left(\boldsymbol{x}_t - \Phi \boldsymbol{x}_{t-1}\right)' + d(\boldsymbol{x}_t), \end{aligned}$$

with respect to $\boldsymbol{x}_{t-1}$ and $\boldsymbol{x}_t$, where $d(\boldsymbol{x}_t)$ is independent of $\boldsymbol{x}_{t-1}$. Suppose we have $\boldsymbol{x}_t^n$ available. Then $\boldsymbol{x}_{t-1}^n$ is found by minimizing the criterion function

$$\begin{aligned} l(\boldsymbol{x}_{t-1}) &= \left(\boldsymbol{x}_{t-1} - \boldsymbol{x}_{t-1}^{t-1}\right) \left[P_{t-1}^{t-1}\right]^{-1} \left(\boldsymbol{x}_{t-1} - \boldsymbol{x}_{t-1}^{t-1}\right)' \\ &+ \left(\boldsymbol{x}_t^n - \Phi \boldsymbol{x}_{t-1}\right) Q^{-1} \left(\boldsymbol{x}_t^n - \Phi \boldsymbol{x}_{t-1}\right)', \end{aligned}$$

with respect to $\boldsymbol{x}_{t-1}$. Differentiating $l(\boldsymbol{x}_{t-1})$ with respect to $\boldsymbol{x}_{t-1}$ and setting the result equal to zero, we obtain

$$\boldsymbol{x}_{t-1}^n = \left\{\left[P_{t-1}^{t-1}\right]^{-1} + \Phi' Q^{-1} \Phi\right\}^{-1} \left\{\left[P_{t-1}^{t-1}\right]^{-1} \boldsymbol{x}_{t-1}^{t-1} + \Phi' Q^{-1} \boldsymbol{x}_t^n\right\}. \tag{4.54}$$

Equation (4.54) gives the desired relationship for obtaining the smoothers recursively, $t = n, n-1, ..., 1$, based on the filtered values $\boldsymbol{x}_{t-1}^{t-1}$ and initial condition $\boldsymbol{x}_n^n$ obtained from Property 4.1. Equation (4.54) can be simplified to (4.49) using the following well-known matrix relationships that we state without proof; details can be found in Rao (1973, Section 1b). Let $A$, $B$, and $C$ be $p \times p$, $q \times q$, and $q \times p$ matrices, respectively, where $A$ and $B$ are positive definite. Then, the following hold:

$$(A^{-1} + C'B^{-1}C)^{-1} = A - AC'(CAC' + B)^{-1}CA, \tag{4.55}$$

$$(A^{-1} + C'B^{-1}C)^{-1}C'B^{-1} = AC'(CAC' + B)^{-1}. \tag{4.56}$$

Using relationships (4.55) and (4.56), with $A = P_{t-1}^{t-1}$, $B = Q$, and $C = \Phi$, in (4.54), we obtain the simplification (Problem 4.5)

$$\boldsymbol{x}_{t-1}^n = \boldsymbol{x}_{t-1}^{t-1} + J_{t-1}\left(\boldsymbol{x}_t^n - \Phi \boldsymbol{x}_{t-1}^{t-1}\right), \tag{4.57}$$

where

$$J_{t-1} = P_{t-1}^{t-1}\Phi'[\Phi P_{t-1}^{t-1}\Phi' + Q]^{-1} = P_{t-1}^{t-1}\Phi'\left[P_t^{t-1}\right]^{-1}.$$

Thus, (4.57) is of the form given in the Kalman smoother.

The recursion for the error covariance, $P_{t-1}^n$, is obtained by straight-forward calculation. Using (4.57) we obtain

$$\boldsymbol{x}_{t-1} - \boldsymbol{x}_{t-1}^n = \boldsymbol{x}_{t-1} - \boldsymbol{x}_{t-1}^{t-1} - J_{t-1}\left(\boldsymbol{x}_t^n - \Phi \boldsymbol{x}_{t-1}^{t-1}\right),$$

or

$$\left(\boldsymbol{x}_{t-1} - \boldsymbol{x}_{t-1}^n\right) + J_{t-1}\boldsymbol{x}_t^n = \left(\boldsymbol{x}_{t-1} - \boldsymbol{x}_{t-1}^{t-1}\right) + J_{t-1}\Phi \boldsymbol{x}_{t-1}^{t-1}. \tag{4.58}$$

Multiplying each side of (4.58) by the transpose of itself and talking expectation, we have

$$P_{t-1}^n + J_{t-1}E(\boldsymbol{x}_t^n \boldsymbol{x}_t^{n'})J_{t-1'} = P_{t-1}^{t-1} + J_{t-1}\Phi E(\boldsymbol{x}_{t-1}^{t-1}\boldsymbol{x}_{t-1}^{t-1'})\Phi' J_{t-1'}, \tag{4.59}$$

using the fact the cross-product terms are zero. But,

$$E(\boldsymbol{x}_t^n \boldsymbol{x}_t^{n'}) = E(\boldsymbol{x}_t \boldsymbol{x}_t') - P_t^n = \Phi E(\boldsymbol{x}_{t-1} \boldsymbol{x}_{t-1}')\Phi' + Q - P_t^n,$$

and

$$E(\boldsymbol{x}_{t-1}^{t-1} \boldsymbol{x}_{t-1}^{t-1'}) = E(\boldsymbol{x}_{t-1} \boldsymbol{x}_{t-1}') - P_{t-1}^{t-1},$$

so (4.59) simplifies to (4.50).

**Example 4.6 Filtering and Smoothing for Example 4.5**

In this example, we consider the simulated data in Example 4.5 and we concentrate on initial state $x_0$ and the first ten values of the state, $x_t$, $t = 1, ..., 10$. We use the known parameters $\phi = 0.8$, $\sigma_w = \sigma_v = 1$ because we discuss estimation in the next section. In this case, the Kalman filter is initialized by $x_0^0 = E(x_0) = 0$ and $P_0^0 = \text{var}(x_0) = \sigma_w^2/(1-\phi^2) = 2.78$, and the results of applying the predictor, the filter, and the smoother to the data are exhibited in Table 4.2. Note immediately from Table 4.2 one-step-ahead prediction is more uncertain than the corresponding filtered value, which, in turn, is more uncertain than the corresponding smoother value (that is $P_t^{t-1} > P_t^t > P_t^n$). Also, in each case, the error variances stabilize quickly.

For example, using Property 4.1, the one-step-ahead forecast of $x_1$ is

$$x_1^0 = 0.8x_0^0 = 0.$$

The error variance is

$$P_1^0 = E(x_1 - x_1^0)^2 = \phi^2 P_0^0 + \sigma_w^2 = 0.8^2(2.78) + 1 = 2.78.$$

The filtered value of $x_1$ is

$$x_1^1 = x_1^0 + K_1 \left(y_1 - x_1^0\right) = 0 + \frac{2.78}{3.78}(0.02 - 0) = 0.01,$$

where the Kalman gain is

$$K_1 = \frac{P_1^0}{P_1^0 + \sigma_v^2} = \frac{2.78}{3.78}.$$

The error variance of the filter estimator is

$$P_1^1 = P_1^0 \left(1 - \frac{P_1^0}{P_1^0 + \sigma_v^2}\right) = 2.78 \left(1 - \frac{2.78}{3.78}\right) = 0.74.$$

The next step is to calculate

$$x_2^1 = 0.8x_1^1 = 0.01 \quad \text{and} \quad P_2^1 = 0.8^2(0.74) + 1 = 1.47,$$

**Table 4.2:** Forecasts, Filters, and Smoothers for Example 4.5 Data

| $t$ | $y_t$ | $x_t$ | $x_t^{t-1}(P_t^{t-1})$ | $x_t^t$ $(P_t^t)$ | $x_t^n$ $(P_t^n)$ |
|---|---|---|---|---|---|
| 0 | — | 1.40 | — (—) | 0.00 (2.78) | -0.37 (1.37) |
| 1 | 0.02 | -0.02 | 0.00 (2.78) | 0.01 (0.74) | -0.46 (0.58) |
| 2 | -2.55 | -1.41 | 0.01 (1.47) | -1.51 (0.60) | -1.17 (0.49) |
| 3 | 1.93 | 0.07 | -1.21 (1.38) | 0.61 (0.58) | -0.21 (0.48) |
| 4 | -2.83 | -0.93 | 0.49 (1.37) | -1.43 (0.58) | -1.94 (0.48) |
| 5 | -3.38 | -3.34 | -1.14 (1.37) | -2.43 (0.58) | -2.65 (0.48) |
| 6 | -2.81 | -3.04 | -1.95 (1.37) | -2.44 (0.58) | -2.58 (0.48) |
| 7 | -2.16 | -2.33 | -1.96 (1.37) | -2.07 (0.58) | -2.34 (0.48) |
| 8 | -2.68 | -2.59 | -1.66 (1.37) | -2.25 (0.58) | -2.45 (0.48) |
| 9 | -2.41 | -3.30 | -1.80 (1.37) | -2.16 (0.58) | -2.41 (0.48) |
| 10 | -2.60 | -3.89 | -1.72 (1.37) | -2.23 (0.58) | -2.45 (0.48) |

for prediction, and, for filtering,

$$x_2^2 = 0.01 + \left(\frac{1.47}{2.47}\right)(-2.55 - 0.01) = -1.51,$$

$$P_2^2 = 1.47\left(1 - \frac{1.47}{2.47}\right) = 0.60.$$

To compute the smoothers, we use Property P4.2, starting with $x_{100}^{100}$ and $P_{100}^{100}$ obtained from the filter, Property P4.1. The recursion goes backward, computing $x_{99}^{100}$ and $P_{99}^{100}$ from $x_{100}^{100}$ and $P_{100}^{100}$, and so on. For example, the values of the smoother and its error variance at $t = 10$ are

$$x_{10}^{100} = -2.45 \quad \text{and} \quad P_{10}^{100} = 0.48.$$

Thus, using the values in Table 4.2,

$$x_9^{100} = x_9^9 + J_9(x_{10}^{100} - x_{10}^9) = -2.16 + 0.34(-2.45 + 1.72) = -2.41,$$

where

$$J_9 = \frac{\phi P_9^9}{P_{10}^9} = \frac{0.8\ 0.58}{1.37} = 0.34.$$

The error variance of this smoothed estimate is

$$P_9^{100} = P_9^9 + J_9^2(P_{10}^{100} - P_{10}^9) = 0.58 + 0.34^2(0.48 - 1.37) = 0.48.$$

In the next section, we will need a set of recursions for obtaining $P_{t,t-1}^n$, as defined in (4.34). We give the necessary recursion in the following property.

***Property P4.3: The Lag-One Covariance Smoother***
*For the state-space model specified in (4.19) and (4.20), with $K_t$, $J_t$ ($t = 1, ..., n$), and $P_n^n$ obtained from Properties P4.1 and P4.2, and with initial condition*

$$P_{n,n-1}^n = (I - K_n A_n)\Phi P_{n-1}^{n-1}, \tag{4.60}$$

*for $t = n, n-1, ..., 2$,*

$$P_{t-1,t-2}^n = P_{t-1}^{t-1} J_{t-2}' + J_{t-1}\left(P_{t,t-1}^n - \Phi P_{t-1}^{t-1}\right) J_{t-2}'. \tag{4.61}$$

***Proof.*** To derive the initial term (4.60), we first define

$$\widetilde{\boldsymbol{x}}_t^s = \boldsymbol{x}_t - \boldsymbol{x}_t^s.$$

Then, using (4.37) and (4.49), we write

$$\begin{aligned} P_{t,t-1}^t &= E\left(\widetilde{\boldsymbol{x}}_t^t \, \widetilde{\boldsymbol{x}}_{t-1}^{t'}\right) \\ &= E\left\{[\widetilde{\boldsymbol{x}}_t^{t-1} - K_t(\boldsymbol{y}_t - A_t \boldsymbol{x}_t^{t-1})][\widetilde{\boldsymbol{x}}_{t-1}^{t-1} - J_t K_t(\boldsymbol{y}_t - A_t \boldsymbol{x}_t^{t-1})]'\right\} \\ &= E\left\{[\widetilde{\boldsymbol{x}}_t^{t-1} - K_t(A_t \widetilde{\boldsymbol{x}}_t^{t-1} + \boldsymbol{v}_t)][\widetilde{\boldsymbol{x}}_{t-1}^{t-1} - J_t K_t(A_t \widetilde{\boldsymbol{x}}_t^{t-1} + \boldsymbol{v}_t)]'\right\}. \end{aligned}$$

Expanding terms and taking expectation, we arrive at

$$P_{t,t-1}^t = P_{t,t-1}^{t-1} - P_t^{t-1} A_t' K_t' J_{t-1}' - K_t A_t P_{t,t-1}^{t-1} + K_t(A_t P_t^{t-1} A_t' + R) K_t' J_{t-1}',$$

noting $E(\widetilde{\boldsymbol{x}}_t^{t-1} \boldsymbol{v}_t') = \boldsymbol{0}$. The final simplification occurs by realizing that $K_t(A_t P_t^{t-1} A_t' + R) = P_t^{t-1} A_t'$, and $P_{t,t-1}^{t-1} = \Phi P_{t-1}^{t-1}$. These relationships hold for any $t = 1, ..., n$, and (4.60) is the case $t = n$.

We give the basic steps in the derivation of (4.61). The first step is to use (4.49) to write

$$\widetilde{\boldsymbol{x}}_{t-1}^n + J_{t-1} \boldsymbol{x}_t^n = \widetilde{\boldsymbol{x}}_{t-1}^{t-1} + J_{t-1} \Phi \boldsymbol{x}_{t-1}^{t-1} \tag{4.62}$$

and

$$\widetilde{\boldsymbol{x}}_{t-2}^n + J_{t-2} \boldsymbol{x}_{t-1}^n = \widetilde{\boldsymbol{x}}_{t-2}^{t-2} + J_{t-2} \Phi \boldsymbol{x}_{t-2}^{t-2}. \tag{4.63}$$

Next, multiply the left-hand-side of (4.62) by the transpose of the left-hand-side of (4.63), and equate that to the corresponding result of the right-hand-sides of (4.62) and (4.63). Then, taking expectation of both sides, the left-hand-side result reduces to

$$P_{t-1,t-2}^n + J_{t-1} E(\boldsymbol{x}_t^n \boldsymbol{x}_{t-1}^{n'}) J_{t-2}' \tag{4.64}$$

and the right-hand-side result reduces to

$$\begin{aligned} P_{t-1,t-2}^{t-2} &- K_{t-1} A_{t-1} P_{t-1,t-2}^{t-2} + J_{t-1} \Phi K_{t-1} A_{t-1} P_{t-1,t-2}^{t-2} \\ &+ J_{t-1} \Phi E(\boldsymbol{x}_{t-1}^{t-1} \boldsymbol{x}_{t-2}^{t-2'}) \Phi' J_{t-2}'. \end{aligned} \tag{4.65}$$

In (4.64), write

$$E(\boldsymbol{x}_t^n \boldsymbol{x}_{t-1}^{n'}) = E(\boldsymbol{x}_t \boldsymbol{x}_{t-1}') - P_{t,t-1}^n = \Phi E(\boldsymbol{x}_{t-1} \boldsymbol{x}_{t-2}')\Phi' + \Phi Q - P_{t,t-1}^n,$$

and in (4.65), write

$$E(\boldsymbol{x}_{t-1}^{t-1} \boldsymbol{x}_{t-2}^{t-2'}) = E(\boldsymbol{x}_{t-1}^{t-2} \boldsymbol{x}_{t-2}^{t-2'}) = E(\boldsymbol{x}_{t-1} \boldsymbol{x}_{t-2}') - P_{t-1,t-2}^{t-2}.$$

Equating (4.64) to (4.65) using these relationships and simplifying the result leads to (4.61). □

Finally, although it would be inconvenient, the lag-one covariance smoothers, $P_{t-1,t-2}^n$, could also be obtained by stacking the state vectors and observation vectors as $\boldsymbol{x}(t) = (\boldsymbol{x}_t', \boldsymbol{x}_{t-1}')'$ and $\boldsymbol{y}(t) = (\boldsymbol{y}_t', \boldsymbol{y}_{t-1}')'$, respectively, and then running the Kalman filter and smoother on these vectors with the parameters matrices appropriately reconfigured. In this case, the smoother variance of the stacked data would have the form

$$P_{(t)}^{(n)} = \begin{pmatrix} P_t^n & P_{t,t-1}^n \\ P_{t,t-1}^{n'} & P_{t-1}^n \end{pmatrix},$$

where subscript $(t)$ and superscript $(n)$ refer to operations on the stacked values.

## 4.3 Maximum Likelihood Estimation

Estimation of the parameters, $\boldsymbol{\mu}_0$, $\Sigma_0$, $\Phi$, $Q$, and $R$, that specify the state-space model, (4.19) and (4.20), is quite involved. We use $\Theta = \{\boldsymbol{\mu}_0, \Sigma_0, \Phi, Q, R\}$ to represent the vector of parameters containing the elements of the initial mean and covariance $\boldsymbol{\mu}_0$ and $\Sigma_0$, the transition matrix $\Phi$, and the state and observation covariance matrices $Q$ and $R$. We use maximum likelihood under the assumption that the initial state is normal, $\boldsymbol{x}_0 \sim \mathrm{N}(\boldsymbol{\mu}_0, \Sigma_0)$, and the errors $\boldsymbol{w}_1, \dots, \boldsymbol{w}_n$ and $\boldsymbol{v}_1, \dots, \boldsymbol{v}_n$ are jointly normal and uncorrelated vector variables. We continue to assume, for simplicity, $\{\boldsymbol{w}_t\}$ and $\{\boldsymbol{v}_t\}$ are uncorrelated.

The likelihood is computed by noting the ***innovations*** $\epsilon_1, \epsilon_2, \dots, \epsilon_n$, defined by (4.40),

$$\epsilon_t = \boldsymbol{y}_t - A_t \boldsymbol{x}_t^{t-1},$$

are a simple one-to-one linear transformation of the data $Y_n = \{\boldsymbol{y}_1, \boldsymbol{y}_2, \dots, \boldsymbol{y}_n\}$. The ***innovations form of the likelihood function*** was given by Schweppe (1965) and proceeds by noting the innovations are independent Gaussian random vectors with zero means and, as shown in (4.41), covariance matrices

$$\Sigma_t = A_t P_t^{t-1} A_t' + R. \tag{4.66}$$

Hence, ignoring a constant, we may write the likelihood, $L_Y(\Theta)$, as

$$-2\ln L_Y(\Theta) = \sum_{t=1}^{n} \log|\Sigma_t(\Theta)| + \sum_{t=1}^{n} \epsilon_t(\Theta)'\Sigma_t(\Theta)^{-1}\epsilon_t(\Theta), \tag{4.67}$$

where we have emphasized the dependence of the innovations on the parameters $\Theta$. Of course, (4.67) is a highly nonlinear and complicated function of the unknown parameters. The usual procedure is to fix $\boldsymbol{x}_0$ and then develop a set of recursions for the log likelihood function and its first two derivatives (for example, Gupta and Mehra, 1974). Then, a Newton–Raphson algorithm (see Example 2.28) can be used successively to update the parameter values until the log likelihood is maximized. This approach is advocated, for example, by Jones (1980), who developed ARMA estimation by putting the ARMA model in state-space form. For the univariate case, (4.67) is identical, in form, to the likelihood for the ARMA model given in (2.137).

The steps involved in performing a Newton–Raphson estimation procedure are as follows.

1. Select initial values for the parameters, say, $\Theta^{(0)}$.
2. Run the Kalman filter, Property 4.1, using the initial parameter values, $\Theta^{(0)}$, to obtain a set of innovations and error covariances, say, $\{\epsilon_t^{(0)};\ t = 1, ..., n\}$ and $\{\Sigma_t^{(0)};\ t = 1, ..., n\}$.
3. Run one iteration of a Newton–Raphson procedure to obtain a new set of estimates, say $\Theta^{(1)}$.
4. At iteration $j$, $(j = 1, 2, ...)$, repeat step 2 using $\Theta^{(j)}$ in place of $\Theta^{(j-1)}$ to obtain a new set of innovation values $\{\epsilon_t^{(j)};\ t = 1, ..., n\}$ and $\{\Sigma_t^{(j)};\ t = 1, ..., n\}$. Then repeat step 3 to obtain a new estimate $\Theta^{(j+1)}$. Stop when the estimates or the likelihood stabilize; for example, stop when the values of $\Theta^{(j+1)}$ differ from $\Theta^{(j)}$, or when $L_Y(\Theta^{(j+1)})$ differs from $L_Y(\Theta^{(j)})$, by some predetermined, but small amount.

**Example 4.7 Newton–Raphson for Example 4.5**

In this example, we generated data, $y_1, ..., y_{100}$, using the model in Example 4.5, to perform a Newton–Raphson estimation of the parameters $\phi$, $\sigma_w^2$, and $\sigma_v^2$. In the notation of Section 4.2, we put $Q = \sigma_w^2$ and $R = \sigma_v^2$.

In the simple case of an AR(1) with observational noise, initial estimation can be accomplished using the results of Example 4.5. For example, using (4.32), $\rho_y(2)/\rho_y(1) = \phi$. From this data set, we obtained $\widehat{\rho}_y(1) = 0.548$, $\widehat{\rho}_y(2) = 0.427$, so initially, we set $\phi^{(0)} = 0.427/0.548 = 0.779$. Similarly, from (4.31), $\gamma_x(1) = \gamma_y(1) = \phi\sigma_w^2/(1 - \phi^2)$, so that, with $\widehat{\gamma}_y(1) = 1.955$, initially, we set $Q^{(0)} = (1 - 0.779^2)\ 1.955/0.779 = 0.987$. Finally, from

**Table 4.3:** Newton–Raphson Estimation Results for Example 4.5 Data

| iteration($j$) | $\phi^{(j)}$ | $Q^{(j)}$ | $R^{(j)}$ | $-2\ln L_Y$ |
|---|---|---|---|---|
| 0 | 0.779 | 0.987 | 1.064 | 191.5546 |
| 1 | 0.817 | 0.991 | 1.064 | 191.1706 |
| 2 | 0.818 | 0.996 | 1.061 | 191.1646 |
| 3 | 0.812 | 1.077 | 1.007 | 191.1015 |
| 4 | 0.805 | 1.117 | 0.977 | 191.0864 |
| 5 | 0.801 | 1.132 | 0.965 | 191.0833 |
| 6 | 0.800 | 1.133 | 0.962 | 191.0828 |
| 7 | 0.800 | 1.130 | 0.962 | 191.0826 |
| 8 | 0.800 | 1.129 | 0.961 | 191.0825 |

this data, we obtained $\widehat{\gamma}_y(0) = 3.574$, so, using (4.30) and the initial values $\phi^{(0)}$ and $Q^{(0)}$, we obtain an initial estimate of $\sigma_v^2$, namely, $R^{(0)} = 3.574 - [0.987/(1 - 0.779^2)] = 1.064$.

Newton–Raphson estimation was accomplished using the Gauss program `optmum`. In that program, we must provide an evaluation of the function to be minimized, namely, $-\ln L_Y(\Theta)$. In this case, the "function call" combines steps 2 and 3, using the current values of the parameters, $\Theta^{(j-1)}$, to obtain first the filtered values, then the innovation values, and then calculating the criterion function, $-\ln L_Y(\Theta^{(j-1)})$, to be minimized. We can also provide analytic forms of the ***gradient vector***, $-\partial \ln L_Y(\Theta)/\partial\Theta$, and the ***Hessian matrix***, $-\partial^2 \ln L_Y(\Theta)/\partial\Theta\ \partial\Theta'$, in the optimization routine, or allow the program to calculate these values numerically. In this example, we let the program proceed numerically and we note the need to be cautious when calculating gradients numerically. For better stability, e can also provide an iterative solution for obtaining analytic gradients and Hessians of the log likelihood function; for details, see Problems 4.11 and 4.12; also, see Gupta and Mehra (1974). Table 4.3 lists the outcome of the iterations.

The final estimates, along with their standard errors (in parentheses), were

$$\widehat{\phi} = 0.800\ (0.087), \quad \widehat{\sigma}_w^2 = 1.129\ (0.472), \quad \widehat{\sigma}_v^2 = 0.961\ (0.362).$$

The standard errors are a byproduct of the estimation procedure, and we will discuss their evaluation later in this section, after Property P4.4.

In addition to Newton–Raphson, Shumway and Stoffer (1982) presented a conceptually simpler estimation procedure based on the EM (***expectation-maximization***) algorithm (Dempster et al 1977). The basic idea is that if we could observe the states, $X_n = \{\boldsymbol{x}_0, \boldsymbol{x}_1, ..., \boldsymbol{x}_n\}$, in addition to the observations $Y_n = \{\boldsymbol{y}_1, ..., \boldsymbol{y}_n\}$, then we would consider $\{X_n, Y_n\}$ as the ***complete data***, with the joint density

$$f_\Theta(X_n, Y_n) = f_{\mu_0,\Sigma_0}(\boldsymbol{x}_0) \prod_{t=1}^n f_{\Phi,Q}(\boldsymbol{x}_t|\boldsymbol{x}_{t-1}) \prod_{t=1}^n f_R(\boldsymbol{y}_t|\boldsymbol{x}_t). \tag{4.68}$$

Under the Gaussian assumption and ignoring constants, the complete data likelihood, (4.68), can be written as

$$\begin{aligned} -2\ln L_{X,Y}(\Theta) &= \ln|\Sigma_0| + (\boldsymbol{x}_0 - \boldsymbol{\mu}_0)'\Sigma_0^{-1}(\boldsymbol{x}_0 - \boldsymbol{\mu}_0) \\ &+ \ln|Q| + \sum_{t=1}^n (\boldsymbol{x}_t - \Phi\boldsymbol{x}_{t-1})'Q^{-1}(\boldsymbol{x}_t - \Phi\boldsymbol{x}_{t-1}) \\ &+ \ln|R| + \sum_{t=1}^n (\boldsymbol{y}_t - A_t\boldsymbol{x}_t)'R^{-1}(\boldsymbol{y}_t - A_t\boldsymbol{x}_t). \end{aligned} \tag{4.69}$$

Thus, in view of (4.69), if we did have the complete data, we could then use the results from multivariate normal theory to easily obtain the MLEs of $\Theta$. We do not have the complete data; however, the EM algorithm gives us an iterative method for finding the MLEs of $\Theta$ based on the ***incomplete data***, $Y_n$, by successively maximizing the conditional expectation of the complete data likelihood. To implement the EM algorithm, we write, at iteration $j$, $(j = 1, 2, ...)$,

$$Q\left(\Theta \mid \Theta^{(j-1)}\right) = E\left\{-2\ln L_{X,Y}(\Theta) \mid Y_n, \Theta^{(j-1)}\right\}. \tag{4.70}$$

Calculation of (4.70) is the ***expectation step***. Of course, given the current value of the parameters, $\Theta^{(j-1)}$, we can use Property P4.2 to obtain the desired conditional expectations as smoothers. This property yields

$$\begin{aligned} Q\left(\Theta \mid \Theta^{(j-1)}\right) &= \ln|\Sigma_0| + \operatorname{tr}\left\{\Sigma_0^{-1}[P_0^n + (\boldsymbol{x}_0^n - \boldsymbol{\mu}_0)(\boldsymbol{x}_0^n - \boldsymbol{\mu}_0)']\right\} \\ &+ \ln|Q| + \operatorname{tr}\left\{Q^{-1}[S_{11} - S_{10}\Phi' - \Phi S_{10}' + \Phi S_{00}\Phi']\right\} \\ &+ \ln|R| \\ &+ \operatorname{tr}\left\{R^{-1}\sum_{t=1}^n [(\boldsymbol{y}_t - A_t\boldsymbol{x}_t^n)(\boldsymbol{y}_t - A_t\boldsymbol{x}_t^n)' + A_t P_t^n A_t']\right\}, \end{aligned} \tag{4.71}$$

where

$$S_{11} = \sum_{t=1}^n (\boldsymbol{x}_t^n \boldsymbol{x}_t^{n\prime} + P_t^n), \tag{4.72}$$

$$S_{10} = \sum_{t=1}^n (\boldsymbol{x}_t^n \boldsymbol{x}_{t-1}^n{}' + P_{t,t-1}^n), \tag{4.73}$$

and

$$S_{00} = \sum_{t=1}^{n} (\boldsymbol{x}_{t-1}^n \boldsymbol{x}_{t-1}^{n}{}' + P_{t-1}^n). \tag{4.74}$$

In (4.71)-(4.74), the smoothers are calculated under the present value of the parameters $\Theta^{(j-1)}$; for simplicity, we have not explicitly displayed this fact.

Minimizing (4.71) with respect to the parameters, at iteration $j$, constitutes the ***maximization step***, and is analogous to the usual multivariate regression approach, which yields the updated estimates

$$\Phi^{(j)} = S_{10} S_{00}^{-1}, \tag{4.75}$$

$$Q^{(j)} = n^{-1} \left( S_{11} - S_{10} S_{00}^{-1} S_{10}' \right), \tag{4.76}$$

and

$$R^{(j)} = n^{-1} \sum_{t=1}^{n} [(\boldsymbol{y}_t - A_t \boldsymbol{x}_t^n)(\boldsymbol{y}_t - A_t \boldsymbol{x}_t^n)' + A_t P_t^n A_t']. \tag{4.77}$$

The initial mean and covariance cannot be estimated simultaneously, so it is conventional to fix both or to fix the covariance matrix and use the estimator

$$\boldsymbol{\mu}_0{}^{(j)} = \boldsymbol{x}_0^n \tag{4.78}$$

obtained from minimizing (4.71) under that assumption.

The overall procedure can be regarded as simply alternating between the Kalman filtering and smoothing recursions and the multivariate normal maximum likelihood estimators, as given by (4.75)-(4.78). Convergence results for the EM algorithm under general conditions can be found in Wu (1983). We summarize the iterative procedure as follows.

1. Initialize the procedure by selecting starting values for the parameters $\Theta^{(0)} = \{\boldsymbol{\mu}_0, \Phi, Q, R\}$, and fix $\Sigma_0$.

   On iteration $j$, ($j = 1, 2, ...$):

2. Compute the incomplete-data likelihood, $-2 \ln L_Y(\Theta^{(j-1)})$; see equation (4.67).

3. Perform the E-Step. Use Properties 4.1, 4.2, and 4.3 to obtain the smoothed values $\boldsymbol{x}_t^n, P_t^n$ and $P_{t,t-1}^n$, for $t = 1, ..., n$, using the parameters $\Theta^{(j-1)}$. Use the smoothed values to calculate $S_{11}, S_{10}, S_{00}$ given in (4.72)-(4.74).

4. Perform the M-Step. Update the estimates, $\boldsymbol{\mu}_0, \Phi, Q$, and $R$ using (4.75)-(4.78), to obtain $\Theta^{(j)}$.

5. Repeat Steps 2 – 4 to convergence.

**Example 4.8 EM Algorithm for Example 4.5**

Using the same data generated in Example 4.7, we performed an EM algorithm estimation of the parameters $\phi$, $\sigma_w^2$ and $\sigma_v^2$. The initial values are the same as in Example 4.7 and Table 4.4 shows the results of the estimation procedure. The convergence rate of the EM algorithm compared with the Newton–Raphson procedure is slow.

The final estimates, along with their standard errors (in parentheses), were

$$\widehat{\phi} = 0.797\ (0.094), \quad \widehat{\sigma}_w^2 = 1.134\ (0.510), \quad \widehat{\sigma}_v^2 = 0.961\ (0.394).$$

We will discuss the evaluation of the estimated standard errors later in this section, after Property P4.4.

**Table 4.4:** EM Algorithm Estimation Results for Example 4.5 Data

| iteration($j$) | $\phi^{(j)}$ | $Q^{(j)}$ | $R^{(j)}$ | $-2\ln L_Y$ |
|---|---|---|---|---|
| 0 | 0.779 | 0.987 | 1.064 | 191.5546 |
| 1 | 0.808 | 1.016 | 1.057 | 191.1595 |
| 2 | 0.811 | 1.026 | 1.047 | 191.1377 |
| 3 | 0.811 | 1.033 | 1.039 | 191.1285 |
| 4 | 0.810 | 1.040 | 1.032 | 191.1214 |
| 5 | 0.809 | 1.046 | 1.026 | 191.1156 |
| 6 | 0.808 | 1.053 | 1.021 | 191.1107 |
| 7 | 0.807 | 1.059 | 1.016 | 191.1066 |
| 8 | 0.806 | 1.065 | 1.012 | 191.1030 |
| 9 | 0.806 | 1.070 | 1.007 | 191.0999 |
| 10 | 0.805 | 1.075 | 1.004 | 191.0974 |
| 20 | 0.800 | 1.112 | 0.976 | 191.0858 |
| 30 | 0.797 | 1.134 | 0.961 | 191.0846 |

### Asymptotic Distribution of the MLEs

The asymptotic distribution of estimators of the model parameters, say, $\widehat{\Theta}_n$, is studied extensively in Caines (1988, Chapters 7 and 8), and in Hannan and Deistler (1988, Chapter 4). In both of these references, the consistency and asymptotic normality of the estimators is established under general conditions. Although we will only state the basic result, some crucial elements are needed to establish large sample properties of the estimators. These conditions, observability, controllability, and the stability of the filter, assure that, for large $t$, the innovations $\epsilon_t$ are basically copies of each other (that is, independent and identically distributed) with a stable covariance matrix $\Sigma$ that does not depend on $t$ and that, asymptotically, the innovations contain all of the information about the unknown parameters. Although it is not necessary, for simplicity, we shall assume here $A_t \equiv A$ for all $t$. Details on departures from this assumption can be found in Jazwinski (1970, Sections 7.6 and 7.8).

For ***stability of the filter***, we assume ***the eigenvalues of $\Phi$ are less than one in absolute value***; this assumption can be weakened (for example, see Harvey, 1991, Section 4.3), but we retain it for simplicity. This assumption is enough to ensure the stability of the filter in that, as $t \to \infty$, the filter error covariance matrix $P_t^t$ converges to $P$, the steady-state error covariance matrix, the gain matrix $K_t$ converges to $K$, the steady-state gain matrix, from which it follows that the innovation variance–covariance matrix $\Sigma_t$ converges to $\Sigma$, the steady-state variance–covariance matrix of the stable innovations; details can be found in Jazwinski (1970, Sections 7.6 and 7.8) and Anderson and Moore (1979, Section 4.4). In particular, the steady-state filter error covariance matrix, $P$, satisfies the Riccati equation:

$$= \Phi[P - PA'(APA' + R)^{-1}AP]\Phi' + Q;$$

the steady-state gain matrix satisfies $K = PA'[APA' + R]^{-1}$. In Example 4.6, for all practical purposes, stability was reached by the fourth observation.

When the process is in steady-state, we may consider $\boldsymbol{x}_{t+1}^t$ as the steady-state predictor and interpret it as $\boldsymbol{x}_{t+1}^t = E(\boldsymbol{x}_{t+1} \mid \boldsymbol{y}_t, \boldsymbol{y}_{t-1}, ...)$. As can be seen from (4.35) and (4.37), the steady-state predictor can be written as

$$\begin{aligned} \boldsymbol{x}_{t+1}^t &= \Phi[I - KA]\boldsymbol{x}_t^{t-1} + Ky_t \\ &= \Phi\boldsymbol{x}_t^{t-1} + K\epsilon_t, \end{aligned} \tag{4.79}$$

where $\boldsymbol{\epsilon}_t$ is the ***steady-state innovation*** process given by

$$\epsilon_t = y_t - E(\boldsymbol{y}_t \mid \boldsymbol{y}_{t-1}, \boldsymbol{y}_{t-2}, ...).$$

In this case, $\boldsymbol{\epsilon}_t \sim \text{iid N}(\mathbf{0}, \Sigma)$, where $\Sigma = APA' + R$. In steady-state, the observations can be written as

$$\boldsymbol{y}_t = A\boldsymbol{x}_t^{t-1} + \boldsymbol{\epsilon}_t. \tag{4.80}$$

Together, (4.79) and (4.80) make up the ***steady-state innovations form*** of the dynamic linear model.

***Observability*** focuses on the question of how much information can be gained about the $p$-dimensional state vector $\boldsymbol{x}_t$ from $p$ future observations $\{\boldsymbol{y}_t, \boldsymbol{y}_{t+1}, ..., \boldsymbol{y}_{t+p-1}\}$. Consider the state without any noise term,

$$\boldsymbol{x}_{t+p} = \Phi\boldsymbol{x}_{t+p-1} = \cdots = \Phi^p\boldsymbol{x}_t.$$

Then, the data (without observational noise) satisfy

$$\boldsymbol{y}_{t+j} = A\boldsymbol{x}_{t+j} = A\Phi^j\boldsymbol{x}_t, \quad j = 0, ..., p-1,$$

or

$$(\boldsymbol{y}'_t, ..., \boldsymbol{y}'_{t+p-1}) = \boldsymbol{x}'_t[A', \Phi' A', ..., \Phi'^{p-1} A'].$$

Hence, if the ***observability matrix*** $\mathcal{O}' = [A', \Phi' A', ..., \Phi'^{p-1} A']$ has full rank $p$, we may explicitly solve for $\boldsymbol{x}_t$ in terms of $\boldsymbol{y}_{t:p} = (\boldsymbol{y}'_t, ..., \boldsymbol{y}'_{t+p-1})'$, namely,

$$\boldsymbol{x}_t = (\mathcal{O}'\mathcal{O})^{-1}\mathcal{O}'\boldsymbol{y}_{t:p},$$

and the system is said to be observable.

In a similar manner, to define ***controllability***, we assume the matrix $\mathcal{C} = [I, \Phi, \Phi^2, ..., \Phi^{p-1}]$ has full rank $p$. Controllability has to do with the fact that the state equation, (4.19), satisfies

$$\boldsymbol{x}_{t+p} = \sum_{j=0}^{p-1} \Phi^j \boldsymbol{w}_{t+p-j} + \Phi^p \boldsymbol{x}_t = \mathcal{C}\boldsymbol{w}_{p:t} + \Phi^p \boldsymbol{x}_t,$$

where $\boldsymbol{w}_{p:t} = (\boldsymbol{w}'_{t+p}, ..., \boldsymbol{w}'_{t+1})'$. If we think of the variables $\{\boldsymbol{w}_{t+p}, ..., \boldsymbol{w}_{t+1}\}$ as "controlling" the state output $\boldsymbol{x}_t$, and we act as if we are free to choose the $\boldsymbol{w}_t$ at will, the fact that $\mathcal{C} = [I, \Phi, \Phi^2, ..., \Phi^{p-1}]$ is full rank means any desired value of $\boldsymbol{x}_{t+p}$ can be obtained from any initial state $\boldsymbol{x}_t$ by control of $\boldsymbol{w}_{p:t}$. In particular, we can put $\boldsymbol{w}_{p:t} = \mathcal{C}'(\mathcal{C}'\mathcal{C})^{-1}(\boldsymbol{x}_{t+p} - \Phi^p \boldsymbol{x}_t)$.

The key point about controllability and observability is that these conditions are necessary and sufficient to ensure the state-space model has the smallest possible dimension; details can be found in Hannan and Diestler (1988, Section 2.3). As a simple example, suppose the state system is bivariate with $\boldsymbol{x}_t = (x_{t1}, x_{t2})'$ and $\Phi = \text{diag}\{\phi_1, \phi_2\}$, and $y_t = [1, 0]\boldsymbol{x}_t + v_t$; that is, $y_t = x_{t1} + v_t$. Clearly we could not hope to reasonably estimate $\phi_2$. This system is not observable because $\mathcal{O}$ has rank one. Additional details on this point can be found in Jazwinski (1970, Section 7.5).

In the following property, we assume the Gaussian state-space model (4.19) and (4.20), with $A_t \equiv A$, is observable and controllable, and the eigenvalues of $\Phi$ are within the unit circle. We denote the true parameters by $\Theta_0$, and we assume the dimension of $\Theta_0$ is the dimension of the parameter space. Although it is not necessary to assume $\boldsymbol{w}_t$ and $\boldsymbol{v}_t$ are Gaussian, certain additional conditions would have to apply and adjustments to the asymptotic covariance matrix would have to be made (see Caines, 1988, Chapter 8).

***Property P4.4: Asymptotic Distribution of the Estimators***
*Under general conditions, let $\widehat{\Theta}_n$ be the estimator of $\Theta_0$ obtained by maximizing the innovations likelihood, $L_Y(\Theta)$, as given in (4.67). Then, as $n \to \infty$,*

$$\sqrt{n}\left(\widehat{\Theta}_n - \Theta_0\right) \xrightarrow{d} \mathrm{N}\left[0,\ \mathcal{I}(\Theta_0)^{-1}\right],$$

*where $\mathcal{I}(\Theta)$ is the asymptotic information matrix given by*

$$\mathcal{I}(\Theta) = \lim_{n\to\infty} n^{-1} E\left[-\partial^2 \ln L_Y(\Theta)/\partial\Theta\, \partial\Theta'\right].$$

Precise details and the proof of Property P4.4 are given in Caines (1988, Chapter 7) and in Hannan and Deistler (1988, Chapter 4). For a Newton procedure, the Hessian matrix (as described in Example 4.7) at the time of convergence can be used as an estimate of $n\mathcal{I}(\Theta_0)$ to obtain estimates of the standard errors. In the case of the EM algorithm, no derivatives are calculated, but we may include a numerical evaluation of the Hessian matrix at the time of convergence to obtain estimated standard errors. Also, extensions of the EM algorithm exist, such as the SEM algorithm (Meng and Rubin, 1991), that include a procedure for the estimation of standard errors.

In Example 4.7, the estimated standard errors were obtained numerically from the Gauss procedure `optmum` used to maximize the likelihood. In Example 4.8, we used the Gauss procedure `hessp` to compute the numerical Hessian matrix of $-\ln L_Y(\widehat{\Theta})$, where $\widehat{\Theta}$ is the vector of parameters estimates at the time of convergence.

## 4.4 Missing Data Modifications

An attractive feature available within the state-space framework is its ability to treat time series that have been observed irregularly over time. For example, Palma and Chan (1997) used the state-space model for estimation and forecasting of long memory (specifically, fractionally integrated ARMA, or ARFIMA, processes) time series with missing observations. The EM algorithm allows parts of the observation vector $\boldsymbol{y}_t$ to be missing at a number of observation times. Shumway and Stoffer (1982) described the modifications necessary for the special case in which the subvectors of $\boldsymbol{v}_t$ corresponding to the observed and unobserved parts of $\boldsymbol{y}_t$ happen to be uncorrelated. Here, we will also discuss the general case.

Suppose, at a given time $t$, we define the partition of the $q \times 1$ observation vector $\boldsymbol{y}_t = (\boldsymbol{y}_t^{(1)'}, \boldsymbol{y}_t^{(2)'})'$, where the first $q_{1t} \times 1$ component is observed and the second $q_{2t} \times 1$ component is unobserved, $q_{1t} + q_{2t} = q$. Then, write the partitioned observation equation

$$\begin{pmatrix} \boldsymbol{y}_t^{(1)} \\ \boldsymbol{y}_t^{(2)} \end{pmatrix} = \begin{bmatrix} A_t^{(1)} \\ A_t^{(2)} \end{bmatrix} \boldsymbol{x}_t + \begin{pmatrix} \boldsymbol{v}_t^{(1)} \\ \boldsymbol{v}_t^{(2)} \end{pmatrix}, \tag{4.81}$$

where $A_t^{(1)}$ and $A_t^{(2)}$ are, respectively, the $q_{1t} \times p$ and $q_{2t} \times p$ partitioned observation matrices, and

$$\text{cov}\begin{pmatrix} \boldsymbol{v}_t^{(1)} \\ \boldsymbol{v}_t^{(2)} \end{pmatrix} = \begin{bmatrix} R_{11t} & R_{12t} \\ R_{21t} & R_{22t} \end{bmatrix} \tag{4.82}$$

denotes the covariance matrix of the measurement errors between the observed and unobserved parts. Stoffer (1982) established the filtering equations, Properties 4.1, hold for the missing data case if, at update $t$, we make the replacements

$$\boldsymbol{y}_{(t)} = \begin{pmatrix} \boldsymbol{y}_t^{(1)} \\ \boldsymbol{0} \end{pmatrix}, \quad A_{(t)} = \begin{bmatrix} A_t^{(1)} \\ 0 \end{bmatrix}, \quad R_{(t)} = \begin{bmatrix} R_{11t} & 0 \\ 0 & R_{22t} \end{bmatrix}, \tag{4.83}$$

for $\boldsymbol{y}_t$, $A_t$, and $R$, respectively, in (4.37)-(4.39).

Once the "missing data" filtered values have been obtained, Stoffer (1982) also established the smoother values can be processed using Properties P4.2 and P4.3 with the values obtained from the missing data-filtered values. *The implication of these results is that, if $\boldsymbol{y}_t$ is incomplete, the filtered and smoothed estimators can be calculated from the usual equations by entering zeros in the observation vector when data are missing, by zeroing out the corresponding rows of the design matrix $A_t$, and by entering zeros in the off-diagonal elements of $R$ that correspond to $R_{12t}$ and $R_{21t}$ at update $t$ in the filter equation (4.39).* In doing this procedure, the state estimators are

$$\boldsymbol{x}_t^{(s)} = E(\boldsymbol{x}_t \mid \boldsymbol{y}_1^{(1)}, ..., \boldsymbol{y}_s^{(1)}), \tag{4.84}$$

with error variance–covariance matrix

$$P_t^{(s)} = E\left\{(\boldsymbol{x}_t - \boldsymbol{x}_t^{(s)})(\boldsymbol{x}_t - \boldsymbol{x}_t^{(s)})'\right\}. \tag{4.85}$$

The missing data lag-one smoother covariances will be denoted by $P_{t,t-1}^{(n)}$.

The maximum likelihood estimators, as computed in the EM procedure, must also be modified in the missing data case. Now, we consider

$$Y_n^{(1)} = \{\boldsymbol{y}_1^{(1)}, ..., \boldsymbol{y}_n^{(1)}\} \tag{4.86}$$

as the incomplete data, and $X_n, Y_n$, as defined in (4.68), as the complete data. In this case, the complete data likelihood, (4.68), or equivalently (4.69), is the same, but to implement the E-step, at iteration $j$, we must calculate

$$\begin{aligned} Q\left(\Theta \mid \Theta^{(j-1)}\right) &= E\left\{-2\ln L_{X,Y}(\Theta) \mid Y_n^{(1)}, \Theta^{(j-1)}\right\} \\ &= E_*\left\{\ln|\Sigma_0| + \text{tr }\Sigma_0^{-1}(\boldsymbol{x}_0 - \boldsymbol{\mu}_0)(\boldsymbol{x}_0 - \boldsymbol{\mu}_0)' \mid Y_n^{(1)}\right\} \\ &+ E_*\left\{\ln|Q| + \sum_{t=1}^n \text{tr }Q^{-1}(\boldsymbol{x}_t - \Phi\boldsymbol{x}_{t-1})(\boldsymbol{x}_t - \Phi\boldsymbol{x}_{t-1})' \mid Y_n^{(1)}\right\} \\ &+ E_*\left\{\ln|R| + \sum_{t=1}^n \text{tr }R^{-1}(\boldsymbol{y}_t - A_t\boldsymbol{x}_t)(\boldsymbol{y}_t - A_t\boldsymbol{x}_t)' \mid Y_n^{(1)}\right\}, \end{aligned} \tag{4.87}$$

where $E_*$ denotes the conditional expectation under $\Theta^{(j-1)}$ and *tr* denotes trace. The first two terms in (4.87) will be like the first two terms of (4.71) with the smoothers $\boldsymbol{x}_t^n$, $P_t^n$, and $P_{t,t-1}^n$ replaced by their missing data counterparts,

$\boldsymbol{x}_t^{(n)}$, $P_t^{(n)}$, and $P_{t,t-1}^{(n)}$. What changes in the missing data case is the third term of (4.87), where we must evaluate $E_*(\boldsymbol{y}_t^{(2)} \mid Y_n^{(1)})$ and $E_*(\boldsymbol{y}_t^{(2)}\boldsymbol{y}_t^{(2)\prime} \mid Y_n^{(1)})$. In Stoffer (1982), it is shown that

$$E_*\left\{(\boldsymbol{y}_t - A_t\boldsymbol{x}_t)(\boldsymbol{y}_t - A_t\boldsymbol{x}_t)' \mid Y_n^{(1)}\right\}$$

$$= \begin{pmatrix} \boldsymbol{y}_t^{(1)} - A_t^{(1)}\boldsymbol{x}_t^{(n)} \\ R_{*21t}R_{*11t}^{-1}(\boldsymbol{y}_t^{(1)} - A_t^{(1)}\boldsymbol{x}_t^{(n)}) \end{pmatrix} \begin{pmatrix} \boldsymbol{y}_t^{(1)} - A_t^{(1)}\boldsymbol{x}_t^{(n)} \\ R_{*21t}R_{*11t}^{-1}(\boldsymbol{y}_t^{(1)} - A_t^{(1)}\boldsymbol{x}_t^{(n)}) \end{pmatrix}'$$

$$+ \begin{pmatrix} A_t^{(1)} \\ R_{*21t}R_{*11t}^{-1}A_t^{(1)} \end{pmatrix} P_t^{(n)} \begin{pmatrix} A_t^{(1)} \\ R_{*21t}R_{*11t}^{-1}A_t^{(1)} \end{pmatrix}'$$

$$+ \begin{pmatrix} 0 & 0 \\ 0 & R_{*22t} - R_{*21t}R_{*11t}^{-1}R_{*12t} \end{pmatrix}. \tag{4.88}$$

In (4.88), the values of $R_{*ikt}$, for $i, k = 1, 2$, are the current values specified by $\Theta^{(j-1)}$. In addition, $\boldsymbol{x}_t^{(n)}$ and $P_t^{(n)}$ are the values obtained by running the smoother under the current parameter estimates specified by $\Theta^{(j-1)}$.

In the case in which observed and unobserved components have uncorrelated errors, that is, $R_{*12t}$ is the zero matrix, (4.88) can be simplified to

$$E_*\left\{(\boldsymbol{y}_t - A_t\boldsymbol{x}_t)(\boldsymbol{y}_t - A_t\boldsymbol{x}_t)' \mid Y_n^{(1)}\right\}$$

$$= \left(\boldsymbol{y}_{(t)} - A_{(t)}\boldsymbol{x}_t^{(n)}\right)\left(\boldsymbol{y}_{(t)} - A_{(t)}\boldsymbol{x}_t^{(n)}\right)' + A_{(t)}P_t^{(n)}A_{(t)}'$$

$$+ \begin{pmatrix} 0 & 0 \\ 0 & R_{*22t} \end{pmatrix}, \tag{4.89}$$

where $\boldsymbol{y}_{(t)}$ and $A_{(t)}$ are defined in (4.83).

In this simplified case, the "missing data" M-step looks like the M-step given in (4.72)-(4.78). That is, with

$$S_{(11)} = \sum_{t=1}^{n}(\boldsymbol{x}_t^{(n)}\boldsymbol{x}_t^{(n)\prime} + P_t^{(n)}), \tag{4.90}$$

$$S_{(10)} = \sum_{t=1}^{n}(\boldsymbol{x}_t^{(n)}\boldsymbol{x}_{t-1}^{(n)\prime} + P_{t,t-1}^{(n)}), \tag{4.91}$$

and

$$S_{(00)} = \sum_{t=1}^{n}(\boldsymbol{x}_{t-1}^{(n)}\boldsymbol{x}_{t-1}^{(n)\prime} + P_{t-1}^{(n)}), \tag{4.92}$$

where the smoothers are calculated under the present value of the parameters $\Theta^{(j-1)}$ using the missing data modifications, at iteration $j$, the *maximization step* is

$$\Phi^{(j)} = S_{(10)}S_{(00)}^{-1}, \tag{4.93}$$

$$Q^{(j)} = n^{-1}\left(S_{(11)} - S_{(10)}S_{(00)}^{-1}S_{(10)}'\right), \tag{4.94}$$

and

$$\begin{aligned} R^{(j)} &= n^{-1}\sum_{t=1}^{n} D_t\left\{\left(\boldsymbol{y}_{(t)} - A_{(t)}\boldsymbol{x}_t^{(n)}\right)\left(\boldsymbol{y}_{(t)} - A_{(t)}\boldsymbol{x}_t^{(n)}\right)' + A_{(t)}P_t^{(n)}A_{(t)}' \right. \\ &+ \left.\begin{pmatrix} 0 & 0 \\ 0 & R_{22t}^{(j-1)} \end{pmatrix}\right\} D_t', \end{aligned} \tag{4.95}$$

where $D_t$ is a permutation matrix that reorders the variables at time $t$ in their original order and $\boldsymbol{y}_{(t)}$ and $A_{(t)}$ are defined in (4.83). For example, suppose $q = 3$ and at time $t$, $y_{t2}$ is missing. Then,

$$\boldsymbol{y}_{(t)} = \begin{pmatrix} y_{t1} \\ y_{t3} \\ 0 \end{pmatrix}, \quad A_{(t)} = \begin{bmatrix} A_{t1} \\ A_{t3} \\ \mathbf{0}' \end{bmatrix}, \quad \text{and} \quad D_t = \begin{bmatrix} 1 & 0 & 0 \\ 0 & 0 & 1 \\ 0 & 1 & 0 \end{bmatrix},$$

where $A_{ti}$ is the $i$th row of $A_t$ and $\mathbf{0}'$ is a $1 \times p$ vector of zeros. In (4.95), only $R_{11t}$ gets updated, and $R_{22t}$ at iteration $j$ is simply set to its value from the previous iteration, $j-1$. Of course, if we cannot assume $R_{12t} = 0$, (4.95) must be changed accordingly using (4.88), but (4.93) and (4.94) remain the same. As before, the initial covariance matrix $\Sigma_0$ is held fixed and

$$\boldsymbol{\mu}_0{}^{(j)} = \boldsymbol{x}_0^{(n)}. \tag{4.96}$$

**Example 4.9 Longitudinal Biomedical Data**

We consider the biomedical data in Example 4.3 which has portions of the three-dimensional vector missing after the 40th day. The maximum likelihood procedure yielded the estimators

$$\widehat{\Phi} = \begin{pmatrix} 1.00 & -.06 & .01 \\ .07 & .91 & .01 \\ -.73 & 1.12 & .90 \end{pmatrix}, \quad \widehat{Q} = \begin{pmatrix} .013 & -.002 & -.009 \\ -.002 & .004 & .020 \\ -.009 & .020 & 1.786 \end{pmatrix},$$

and $\widehat{R} = \text{diag}\{.013, .025, 2.41\}$ for the transition, state error covariance and observation error covariance matrices, respectively. The coupling between the first and second series is relatively weak, whereas the third series HCT is strongly related to the first two; that is,

$$\widehat{x}_{t3} = -.73x_{t-1,1} + 1.12x_{t-1,2} + .90x_{t-1,3}.$$

Hence, the HCT is negatively correlated with white blood count and positively correlated with platelet count. Byproducts of the procedure are estimated trajectories for all three longitudinal series and their respective prediction intervals. In particular, we obtain the smoothed values $x_t^n$ for critical post-transplant platelet count.

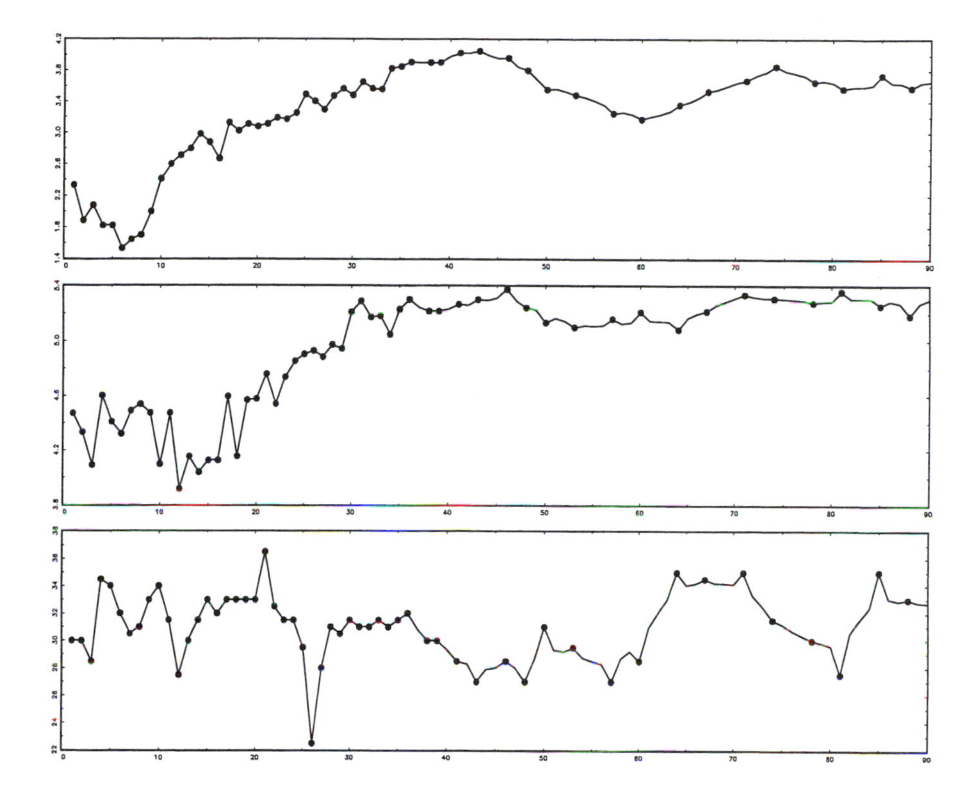

**Figure 4.4:** Smoothed values for various components in the blood parameter tracking problem, log (white blood count) [top], log (platelet) [middle], and hematocrit (HCT) [bottom]. The actual data are shown as points, and the smoothed values are shown as lines.

## 4.5 Structural Models: Signal Extraction and Forecasting

In order to develop computing techniques for handling a versatile cross section of possible models, it is necessary to restrict the state-space model somewhat, and we consider one possible class of specializations in this section. The components of the model are taken as linear processes that can be adapted to represent fixed and disturbed trends and periodicities as well as classical autoregressions. The observed series is regarded as being a sum of component signal series. To illustrate the possibilities, consider the economic example

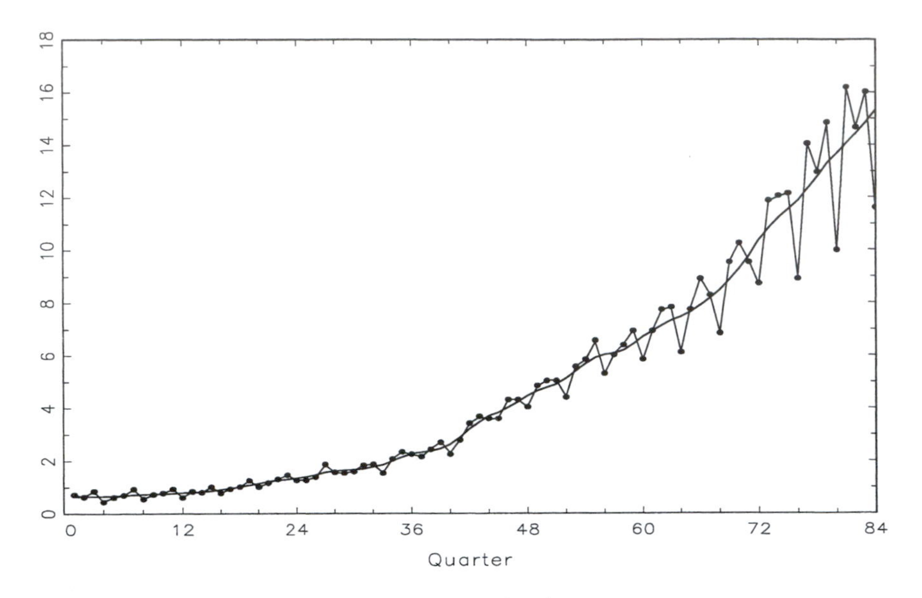


**Figure 4.5:** Estimated trend component ($T_t^n$) and estimated trend plus seasonal component ($T_t^n + S_t^n$) for the Johnson and Johnson quarterly earnings series. The actual data are shown as points, and the smoothers are shown as lines.

given below that shows how to fit a sum of trend, seasonal, and irregular components the quarterly earnings data that we have considered before.

**Example 4.10 Johnson & Johnson Quarterly Earnings**

Consider the quarterly earnings series from the U.S. company Johnson & Johnson as given in Figure 1.1. The series is highly nonstationary, and there is both a trend signal that is gradually increasing over time and a seasonal component that cycles every four quarters or once per year. The seasonal component is getting larger over time as well. Transforming into logarithms or even taking the $n$th root does not seem to make the series stationary, as there is a slight bend to the transformed curve. Suppose, however, we consider the series to be the sum of a trend component, a seasonal component, and a white noise. That is, let the observed series be expressed as

$$y_t = T_t + S_t + v_t, \tag{4.97}$$

where $T_t$ is trend and $S_t$ is the seasonal component. Suppose we allow trend to increase exponentially; that is,

$$T_t = \phi T_{t-1} + w_{t1}, \tag{4.98}$$

where the coefficient $\phi > 1$ characterizes the increase. Let the seasonal component be modeled as

$$S_t + S_{t-1} + S_{t-2} + S_{t-3} = w_{t2}, \tag{4.99}$$

which corresponds to assuming the seasonal component is expected to sum to zero over a complete period or four quarters. To express this model in state-space form, let $\boldsymbol{x}_t' = (T_t, S_t, S_{t-1}, S_{t-2})$ be the state vector so the observation equation (4.20) can be written as

$$y_t = \begin{pmatrix} 1 & 1 & 0 & 0 \end{pmatrix} \begin{pmatrix} T_t \\ S_t \\ S_{t-1} \\ S_{t-2} \end{pmatrix} + v_t,$$

with the state equation written as

$$\begin{pmatrix} T_t \\ S_t \\ S_{t-1} \\ S_{t-2} \end{pmatrix} = \begin{pmatrix} \phi & 0 & 0 & 0 \\ 0 & -1 & -1 & -1 \\ 0 & 1 & 0 & 0 \\ 0 & 0 & 1 & 0 \end{pmatrix} \begin{pmatrix} T_{t-1} \\ S_{t-1} \\ S_{t-2} \\ S_{t-3} \end{pmatrix} + \begin{pmatrix} w_{t1} \\ w_{t2} \\ 0 \\ 0 \end{pmatrix},$$

where $R = r_{11}$ and

$$Q = \begin{pmatrix} q_{11} & 0 & 0 & 0 \\ 0 & q_{22} & 0 & 0 \\ 0 & 0 & 0 & 0 \\ 0 & 0 & 0 & 0 \end{pmatrix}.$$

The model reduces to state-space form, (4.19) and (4.20), with $p = 4$ and $q = 1$. The parameters to be estimated are $r_{11}$, the noise variance in the measurement equations, $q_{11}$ and $q_{22}$, the model variances corresponding to the trend and seasonal components and $\phi$, the transition parameter that models the growth rate. Growth is about 3% per year, and we began with $\phi = 1.03$. The initial mean was fixed at $\boldsymbol{\mu}_0 = (.5, .3, .2, .1)'$, with uncertainty modeled by the diagonal covariance matrix with $\Sigma_{0ii} = .01, i = 1, \ldots, 4$. Initial state covariance values were taken as $q_{11} = .01, q_{22} = .10$, corresponding to relatively low uncertainty in the trend model compared with that in the seasonal model. The measurement error covariance was started at $r_{11} = .04$. After 70 iterations of the EM algorithm, we obtained an initial mean of $\widehat{\boldsymbol{\mu}_0} = (.55, .21, .15, .06)'$, and the transition parameter stabilized at $\widehat{\phi} = 1.035$, corresponding to exponential growth with inflation at about 3.5% per year. The measurement uncertainty was small at $\widehat{r}_{11} = .0086$, compared with the model uncertainties $\widehat{q}_{11} = .0169$ and $\widehat{q}_{22} = .0497$. From initial guesses, the trend uncertainty increased and the seasonal uncertainty decreased. Figure 4.5 shows the smoothed trend estimate and the exponentially increasing seasonal components. We may also consider forecasting the Johnson

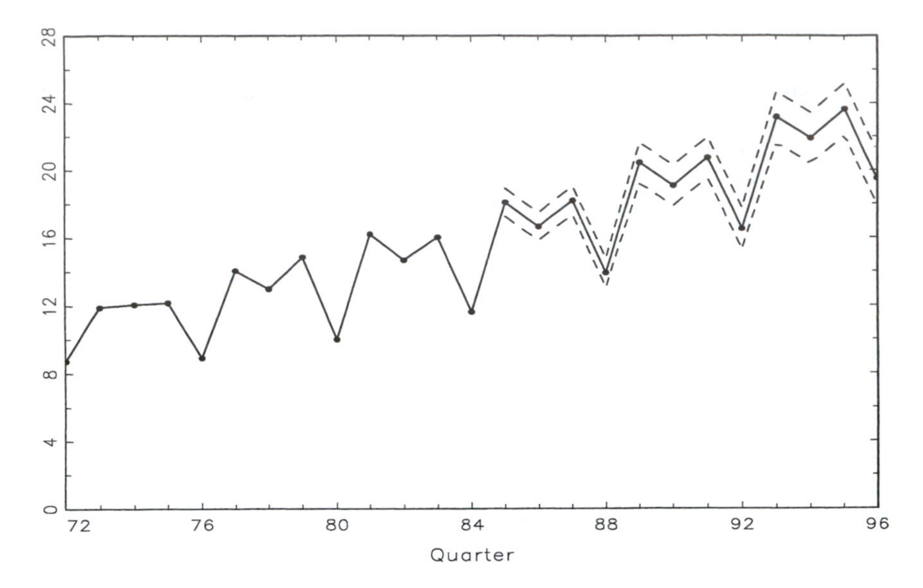


**Figure 4.6:** A 12-quarter forecast for the Johnson & Johnson quarterly earnings series. The last three years of data (quarters 72-84), are shown as points connected by a solid line. The forecasts are shown as points connected by a solid line (quarters 85-96) and dotted lines are upper and lower 95% prediction intervals.

& Johnson series, and the result of a 12-quarter forecast is shown in Figure 4.6 as basically an extension of the latter part of the observed data.

## 4.6 ARMAX Models in State-Space Form

We may add exogenous variables, $\boldsymbol{u}_t$, an $r \times 1$ vector of fixed inputs, to the state-space system, (4.19) and (4.20), as was done with ARMA models in (4.16) of Section 4.1. In the case of state-space models, exogenous inputs can enter in the state equation, the observation equation, or both.

Sometimes, it is advantageous to write the state-space model in a slightly different way, as is done by numerous authors; for example, Anderson and Moore (1970) and Hannan and Deistler (1988). Here, we write the state-space model as

$$\boldsymbol{x}_{t+1} = \Phi \boldsymbol{x}_t + \Upsilon \boldsymbol{u}_t + \boldsymbol{w}_t \qquad t = 0, 1, ..., n \tag{4.100}$$

$$y_t = A_t x_t + \Gamma u_t + v_t \qquad t = 1, ..., n \tag{4.101}$$

where, in the state equation, $x_0 \sim N(\mu_0, \Sigma_0)$, $\Phi$ is $p \times p$, and $\Upsilon$ is $p \times r$. In the observation equation, $A_t$ is $q \times p$ and $\Gamma$ is $q \times r$. Here, $w_t$ and $v_t$ are still white noise series (both independent of $x_0$), with $\text{var}(w_t) = Q$, $\text{var}(v_t) = R$, but we also allow the state noise and observation noise to be correlated at time $t$; that is,

$$\text{cov}(w_t, v_t) = E(w_t v_t') = S \tag{4.102}$$

and zero otherwise; note, $S$ is a $p \times q$ matrix. To obtain the innovations, $\epsilon_t = y_t - A_t x_t^{t-1} - \Gamma u_t$, and the innovation variance $\Sigma_t = A_t P_t^{t-1} A_t' + R$, in this case, we need the one-step-ahead state predictions. Of course, the filtered estimates will also be of interest, and they will be needed for smoothing. Property P4.2 (the smoother) as displayed in Section 4.2 still holds. The following property generates the predictor $x_{t+1}^t$ from the past predictor $x_t^{t-1}$ when the noise terms are correlated and exhibits the filter update.

***Property P4.5: The Kalman Filter with Correlated State and Measurement Noise***

*For the state-space model specified in (4.100) and (4.101), with initial conditions $x_1^0$ and $P_1^0$, for $t = 1, ..., n$,*

$$x_{t+1}^t = \Phi x_t^{t-1} + \Upsilon u_t + K_t^*(y_t - A_t x_t^{t-1} - \Gamma u_t), \tag{4.103}$$

$$P_{t+1}^t = [\Phi - K_t^* A_t] P_t^{t-1} [\Phi - K_t^* A_t]' + Q + K_t^* R K_t^{*'} - S K_t^{*'} - K_t^* S', \tag{4.104}$$

*where the new gain matrix is given by*

$$K_t^* = [\Phi P_t^{t-1} A_t' + S][[A_t P_t^{t-1} A_t' + R]^{-1}. \tag{4.105}$$

*The filter update, given a new observation $y_{t+1}$ and input $u_{t+1}$ is given by*

$$x_{t+1}^{t+1} = x_{t+1}^t + P_{t+1}^t A_{t+1}' \left[A_{t+1} P_{t+1}^t A_{t+1}' + R\right]^{-1} \epsilon_{t+1}, \tag{4.106}$$

$$P_{t+1}^{t+1} = P_{t+1}^t - P_{t+1}^t A_{t+1}' \left[A_{t+1} P_{t+1}^t A_{t+1}' + R\right]^{-1} A_{t+1} P_{t+1}^t. \tag{4.107}$$

The derivation of Property P4.5 is similar to the derivation of the Kalman filter in Property P4.1 (Problem 4.17). Note, (4.106) and (4.107) are identical to (4.35) and (4.36).

Consider a $p$-dimensional ARMAX model given by,

$$y_t = \Gamma u_t + \sum_{j=1}^{p*} \Phi_j y_{t-j} + \sum_{k=1}^{q*} \Theta_k v_{t-k} + v_t. \tag{4.108}$$

The $\Phi$s and $\Theta$s are $p \times p$ matrices, $\Gamma$ is $p \times r$, and $v_t$ is a $p \times 1$ white noise process; in fact, (4.108) and (4.16) are identical models, but here, we have written the observations as $y_t$. We now have the following property.

***Property P4.6: A State-Space Form of ARMAX***
*For $p^* \geq q^*$, the state-space model given by*

$$\boldsymbol{x}_{t+1} = \begin{bmatrix} \Phi_1 & I & 0 & \cdots & 0 \\ \Phi_2 & 0 & I & \cdots & 0 \\ \vdots & \vdots & \vdots & \ddots & \vdots \\ \Phi_{p*-1} & 0 & 0 & \cdots & I \\ \Phi_{p*} & 0 & 0 & \cdots & 0 \end{bmatrix} \boldsymbol{x}_t + \begin{bmatrix} \Theta_1 + \Phi_1 \\ \vdots \\ \Theta_{q*} + \Phi_{q*} \\ \Phi_{q*+1} \\ \vdots \\ \Phi_{p*} \end{bmatrix} \boldsymbol{v}_t, \tag{4.109}$$

$$\boldsymbol{y}_t = [I, 0, \cdots, 0]\boldsymbol{x}_t + \Gamma \boldsymbol{u}_t + \boldsymbol{v}_t, \tag{4.110}$$

*implies the ARMAX model (4.108). The state process, $\boldsymbol{x}_t$, is $pp^* \times 1$, and the observations process $\boldsymbol{y}_t$ is $p \times 1$. If $p^* < q^*$, set $\Phi_{p*+1} = \cdots = \Phi_{q*} = 0$, in which case $p^* = q^*$ and (4.109)-(4.110) still apply.*

This form of the model is somewhat different than the form suggested in Section 4.1, equations (4.22)-(4.24). For example, in (4.24), by setting $A_t$ equal to the $p \times p$ identity matrix (for all $t$) and setting $R = 0$ implies the data $y_t$ in (4.24) follow a VAR($p^*$) process. In doing so, however, we do not make use of the ability to allow for correlated state and observation error, so a nonsingularity is introduced into the system in the form of $R = 0$. The method in Property P4.6 avoids that problem, and points out the fact that the same model can take many forms. We do not prove Property P4.6 directly, but the following example should suggest how to establish the general result.

**Example 4.11 Univariate ARMA(1,1) in State-Space Form**

Consider the univariate ARMA(1,1) model $y_t = \phi y_{t-1} + \theta v_{t-1} + v_t$. Using Property P4.6, we can write the model as

$$x_{t+1} = \phi x_t + w_t, \qquad \text{(state eqn)}, \tag{4.111}$$

where $w_t = (\theta + \phi)v_t$ and

$$y_t = x_t + v_t, \qquad \text{(obs eqn)}. \tag{4.112}$$

In this case, $\text{cov}(w_t, v_t) = (\theta+\phi)^2\text{var}(v_t) = (\theta+\phi)^2 R$, and $\text{cov}(w_t, v_s) = 0$ when $s \neq t$, so Property P4.5 would apply. To verify (4.111) and (4.112) specify an ARMA(1,1) model, we have

$$\begin{aligned} y_t &= x_t + v_t && \text{from (4.112)} \\ &= \phi x_{t-1} + (\theta + \phi)v_{t-1} + v_t && \text{from (4.111)} \\ &= \phi(x_{t-1} + v_{t-1}) + \theta v_{t-1} + v_t && \\ &= \phi y_{t-1} + \theta v_{t-1} + v_t, && \text{from (4.112)}. \end{aligned}$$

Properties P4.5 and P4.6, together, can be used to accomplish maximum likelihood estimation for ARMAX models. In this case, the likelihood would be in the innovations form given in Chapter 2, equation (2.135), or equivalently (4.67), and estimation could be accomplished using Newton–Raphson or the EM algorithm as described in Section 4.3.

## 4.7 Bootstrapping State-Space Models

Although, in Section 4.3, we discussed the fact that, under general conditions (which we assume to hold in this section), the MLEs of the parameters of a DLM are consistent and asymptotically normal, time series data are often of short or moderate length. Several researchers have found evidence that samples must be fairly large before asymptotic results are applicable (Dent and Min, 1978; Ansley and Newbold, 1980). Moreover, as we discussed in Section 2.7, Example 2.32, problems occur if the parameters are near the boundary of the parameter space. In this section, we discuss an algorithm for bootstrapping state-space models; this algorithm and its justification, including the non-Gaussian case, along with numerous examples, can be found in Stoffer and Wall (1991). In view of Section 4.6, anything we do or say here about DLMs applies equally to ARMAX models.

Using the DLM given by (4.100)–(4.102) and Property P4.5, we write the ***innovations form of the filter*** as

$$\begin{aligned}
\boldsymbol{\epsilon}_t &= \boldsymbol{y}_t - A\boldsymbol{x}_t^{t-1} - \Gamma\boldsymbol{u}_t, &(4.113)\\
\Sigma_t &= AP_t^{t-1}A' + R, &(4.114)\\
\boldsymbol{x}_{t+1}^t &= \Phi\boldsymbol{x}_t^{t-1} + \Upsilon\boldsymbol{u}_t + K_t\boldsymbol{\epsilon}_t, &(4.115)\\
K_t &= [\Phi P_t^{t-1}A' + S]\Sigma_t^{-1}, &(4.116)\\
P_{t+1}^t &= \Phi P_t^{t-1}\Phi' + Q + K_t\Sigma_t K_t'. &(4.117)
\end{aligned}$$

This form of the filter is just a rearrangement of the filter given in Property 4.5; we have dropped the * in the new form of the gain matrix. For ease, we address the case in which the measurement matrix is constant for all $t$, i.e., $A_t = A$.

In addition, we can rewrite the model to obtain the ***innovations form of the model***,

$$\begin{aligned}
\boldsymbol{x}_{t+1}^t &= \Phi\boldsymbol{x}_t^{t-1} + \Upsilon\boldsymbol{u}_t + K_t\boldsymbol{\epsilon}_t, &(4.118)\\
\boldsymbol{y}_t &= A\boldsymbol{x}_t^{t-1} + \Gamma\boldsymbol{u}_t + \boldsymbol{\epsilon}_t. &(4.119)
\end{aligned}$$

This form of the model is a rewriting of (4.113) and (4.115), and it accommodates the bootstrapping algorithm.

As discussed in Example 2.32 and Example 4.6, although the innovations $\boldsymbol{\epsilon}_t$ are uncorrelated, initially, $\Sigma_t$ can be different for different time points $t$. Thus, in a resampling procedure, we can either ignore the first few values of $\boldsymbol{\epsilon}_t$ until

$\Sigma_t$ stabilizes or we can work with the ***standardized innovations***

$$e_t = \Sigma_t^{-1/2} \epsilon_t, \tag{4.120}$$

so we are guaranteed these innovations have, at least, the same first two moments. In (4.120), $\Sigma_t^{1/2}$ denotes the unique square root matrix of $\Sigma_t$ defined by $\Sigma_t^{1/2}\Sigma_t^{1/2} = \Sigma_t$. In what follows, we base the bootstrap procedure on the standardized innovations, but we stress the fact that, even in this case, ignoring startup values might be necessary, as noted by Stoffer and Wall (1991).

The model coefficients and the correlation structure of the model are uniquely parameterized by a $k \times 1$ parameter vector $\Theta_0$; that is, $\Phi = \Phi(\Theta_0)$, $\Upsilon = \Upsilon(\Theta_0)$, $Q = Q(\Theta_0)$, $A = A(\Theta_0)$, $\Gamma = \Gamma(\Theta_0)$, and $R = R(\Theta_0)$. Recall the innovations form of the Gaussian likelihood (ignoring a constant) is

$$\begin{aligned} -2\ln L_Y(\Theta) &= \sum_{t=1}^{n} \ln|\Sigma_t(\Theta)| + \epsilon_t(\Theta)'\Sigma_t(\Theta)^{-1}\epsilon_t(\Theta) \\ &= \sum_{t=1}^{n} \ln|\Sigma_t(\Theta)| + e_t(\Theta)'e_t(\Theta). \end{aligned} \tag{4.121}$$

We stress the fact that it is not necessary for the model to be Gaussian to consider (4.121) as the criterion function to be used for parameter estimation. Furthermore, under general conditions, the Gaussian MLE of $\Theta$, even when the process is non-Guassian, is asymptotically optimal; details can be found in Caines (1988, Chapter 8).

Let $\widehat{\Theta}$ denote the MLE of $\Theta_0$, that is, $\widehat{\Theta} = \operatorname{argmax}_\Theta L_Y(\Theta)$, obtained by the methods discussed in Section 4.3. Let $\epsilon_t(\widehat{\Theta})$ and $\Sigma_t(\widehat{\Theta})$ be the innovation values obtained by running the filter, (4.113)-(4.117), under $\widehat{\Theta}$. Once this has been done, the bootstrap procedure is accomplished by the following steps.

1. Construct the standardized innovations

$$e_t(\widehat{\Theta}) = \Sigma_t^{-1/2}(\widehat{\Theta})\epsilon_t(\widehat{\Theta}).$$

2. Sample, with replacement, $n$ times from the set $\{e_1(\widehat{\Theta}), ..., e_n(\widehat{\Theta})\}$ to obtain $\{e_1^*(\widehat{\Theta}), ..., e_n^*(\widehat{\Theta})\}$, a bootstrap sample of standardized innovations.

3. Construct a bootstrap data set $\{y_1^*, ..., y_n^*\}$ as follows. Define the $(p+q) \times 1$ vector $\xi_t = (x_{t+1}^{t'}, y_t')'$. Stacking (4.118) and (4.119) results in a vector first-order equation for $\xi_t$ given by

$$\xi_t = F\xi_{t-1} + Gu_t + H_t e_t, \tag{4.122}$$

where

$$F = \begin{bmatrix} \Phi & 0 \\ A & 0 \end{bmatrix}, \quad G = \begin{bmatrix} \Upsilon \\ \Gamma \end{bmatrix}, \quad H_t = \begin{bmatrix} K_t\Sigma_t^{-1/2} \\ \Sigma_t^{-1/2} \end{bmatrix}.$$

Thus, to construct the bootstrap data set, solve (4.122) using $\boldsymbol{e}_t^*(\widehat{\Theta})$ in place of $\boldsymbol{e}_t$. The exogenous variables $\boldsymbol{u}_t$ and the initial conditions of the Kalman filter remain fixed at their given values, and the parameter vector is held fixed at $\widehat{\Theta}$.

4. Using the bootstrap data set $\{\boldsymbol{y}_t^*; t = 1, ..., n\}$, construct a likelihood, $L_{Y^*}(\Theta)$, and obtain the MLE of $\Theta$, say, $\widehat{\Theta}^*$.

5. Repeat steps 2 through 4, a large number, $B$, of times, obtaining a bootstrapped set of parameter estimates $\{\widehat{\Theta}_b^*;\ b = 1, ..., B\}$. The finite sample distribution of $\widehat{\Theta} - \Theta_0$ may be approximated by the distribution of $\widehat{\Theta}_b^* - \widehat{\Theta}$, $b = 1, ..., B$.

In the next example, we discuss the case of a linear regression model, but where the regression coefficients are stochastic and allowed to vary with time. The state-space model provides a convenient setting for the analysis of such models.

**Example 4.12 Stochastic Regression**

Figure 4.7 shows the interest rate recorded for three-month treasury bills (line–squares), $y_t$, and the quarterly inflation rate (dotted line–circles) in the Consumer Price Index, $z_t$, from the first quarter of 1953 through the second quarter of 1965, $n = 50$ observations. These data were analyzed by Newbold and Bos (1985, pp. 61-73).

In this analysis, the treasury bill interest rate is modeled as being linearly related to quarterly inflation as

$$y_t = \alpha + \beta_t z_t + v_t,$$

where $\alpha$ is a fixed constant, $\beta_t$ is a stochastic regression coefficient, and $v_t$ is white noise with variance $\sigma_v^2$. The stochastic regression term, which comprises the state variable, is specified by a first-order autoregression,

$$(\beta_t - b) = \phi(\beta_{t-1} - b) + w_t,$$

where $b$ is a constant, and $w_t$ is white noise with variance $\sigma_w^2$. The noise processes, $v_t$ and $w_t$, are assumed to be uncorrelated.

Using the notation of the state-space model (4.100) and (4.101), we have in the state equation, $\boldsymbol{x}_t = \beta_t$, $\Phi = \phi$, $\boldsymbol{u}_t \equiv 1$, $\Upsilon = (1 - \phi)b$, $Q = \sigma_w^2$, and in the observation equation, $A_t = z_t$, $\Gamma = \alpha$, $R = \sigma_v^2$, and $S = 0$. The parameter vector is $\Theta = (\phi, \alpha, b, \sigma_w, \sigma_v)'$. The results of the Newton–Raphson estimation procedure are listed in Table 4.5. Also shown in the Table 4.5 are the corresponding standard errors obtained from $B = 500$ runs of the bootstrap. These standard errors are simply the standard deviations of the bootstrapped estimates, that is, the square

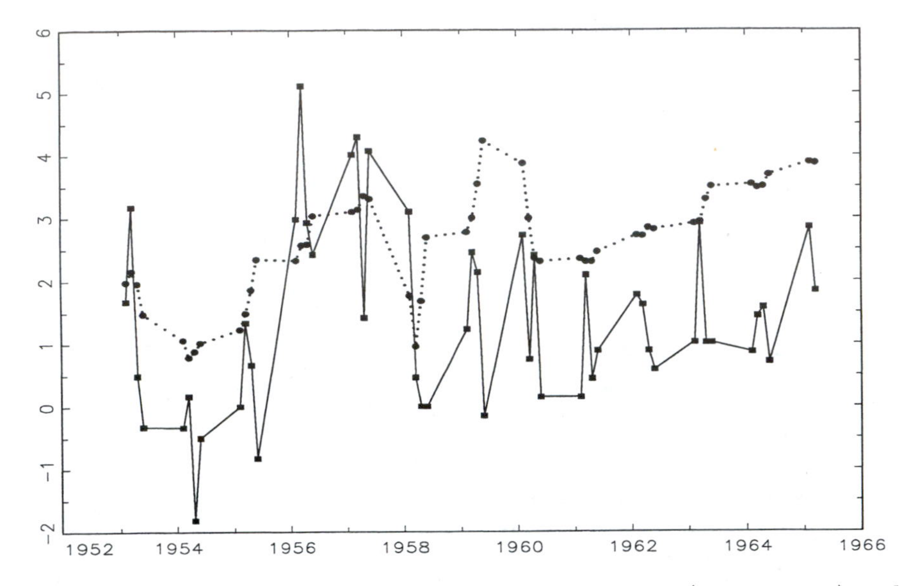


**Figure 4.7:** Interest rate for three-month treasury bills (line–squares) and quarterly inflation rate (dotted line–circles) in the Consumer Price Index, 1953:1 to 1965:2.

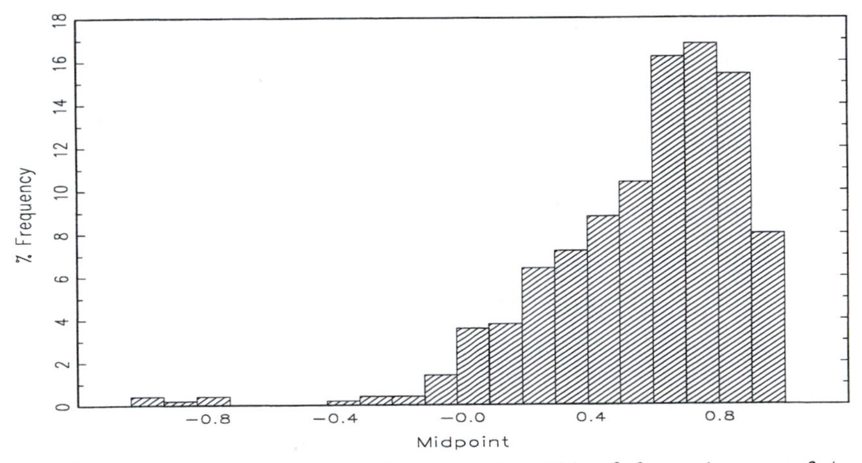


**Figure 4.8:** Bootstrap distribution, $B = 500$, of the estimator of $\phi$.

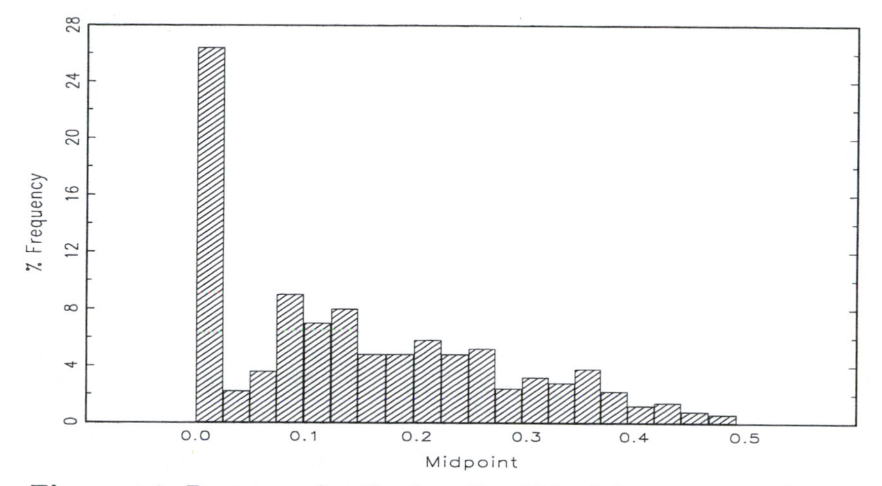


**Figure 4.9:** Bootstrap distribution, $B = 500$, of the estimator of $\sigma_w$.

**Table 4.5:** Comparison of Asymptotic Standard Errors and Bootstrapped Standard Errors ($B = 500$)

| Parameter | MLE | Asymptotic Standard Error | Bootstrap Standard Error |
|---|---|---|---|
| $\phi$ | 0.841 | 0.200 | 0.304 |
| $\alpha$ | -0.771 | 0.645 | 0.645 |
| $b$ | 0.855 | 0.278 | 0.277 |
| $\sigma_w$ | 0.127 | 0.092 | 0.182 |
| $\sigma_v$ | 1.131 | 0.142 | 0.217 |

root of $\sum_{b=1}^{B}(\Theta_{ib}^* - \bar{\Theta}_i^*)^2/(B-1)$, where $\Theta_i$, represents the $i$th parameter, $i = 1, ..., 5$, and $\bar{\Theta}_i^* = \sum_{b=1}^{B} \Theta_{ib}^*/B$.

The asymptotic standard errors listed in Table 4.5 are typically smaller than those obtained from the bootstrap. This result is the most pronounced in the estimates of $\phi$, $\sigma_w$, and $\sigma_v$, where the bootstrapped standard errors are about 50% larger than the corresponding asymptotic value. Also, asymptotic theory prescribes the use of normal theory when dealing with the parameter estimates. The bootstrap, however, allows us to investigate the small sample distribution of the estimators and, hence, provides more insight into the data analysis.

For example, Figure 4.8 shows the bootstrap distribution of the estimator of $\phi$. This distribution is highly skewed with values concentrated around 0.8, but with a long tail to the left. Some quantiles of the bootstrapped distribution of $\phi$ are -0.09 (2.5%), 0.03 (5%), 0.16 (10%), 0.87 (90%), 0.92

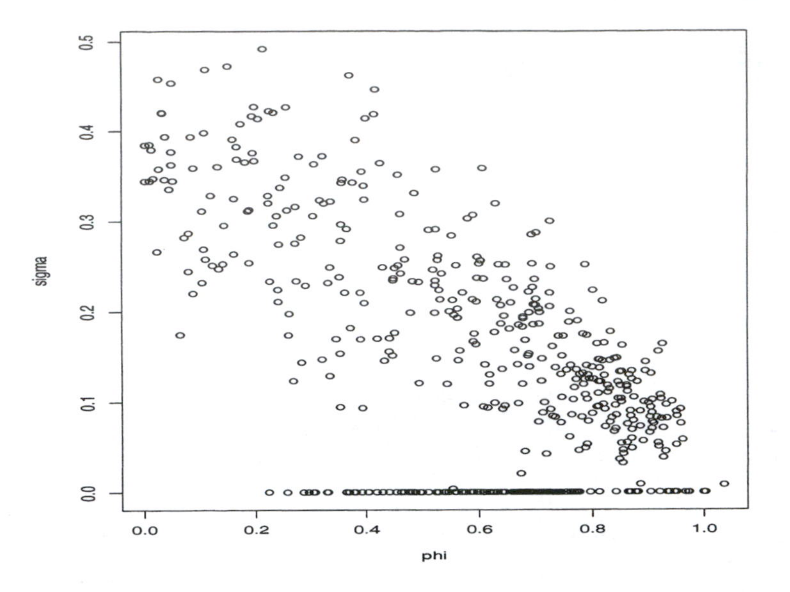


**Figure 4.10:** Joint bootstrap distribution, $B = 500$, of the estimators of $\phi$ and $\sigma_w$. Only the values corresponding to $\widehat{\phi}^* \geq 0$ are shown.

(95%), 0.94 (97.5%), and they can be used to obtain confidence intervals. For example, a 90% confidence interval for $\phi$ would be approximated by (0.03, 0.92). This interval is rather wide, and we will interpret this after we discuss the results of the estimation of $\sigma_w$.

Figure 4.9 shows the bootstrap distribution of $\widehat{\sigma}_w$. The distribution is concentrated at two locations, one at approximately $\widehat{\sigma}_w = 0.15$ and the other at $\widehat{\sigma}_w = 0$. The cases in which $\widehat{\sigma}_w \approx 0$ correspond to deterministic state dynamics. When $\sigma_w = 0$ and $|\phi| < 1$, then $\beta_t \approx b$ for large $t$, so the approximately 25% of the cases in which $\widehat{\sigma}_w \approx 0$ suggest a fixed state, or constant coefficient model. The cases in which $\widehat{\sigma}_w$ is away from zero would suggest a truly stochastic regression parameter. To investigate this matter further, Figure 4.10 shows the joint bootstrapped estimates, $(\widehat{\phi}, \widehat{\sigma}_w)$, for positive values of $\widehat{\phi}$. The joint distribution suggests $\widehat{\sigma}_w > 0$ corresponds to $\widehat{\phi} \approx 0$. When $\phi = 0$, the state dynamics are given by $\beta_t = b + w_t$. If, in addition, $\sigma_w$ is small relative to $b$, the system is nearly deterministic; that is, $\beta_t \approx b$. Considering these results, the bootstrap analysis leads us to conclude the dynamics of the data are best described in terms of a fixed regression effect.

## 4.8 Dynamic Linear Models with Switching

The problem of modeling changes in regimes for vector-valued times series has been of interest in many different fields. In Section 2.13, we explored the idea that the dynamics of the system of interest might change over the course of time. In Example 2.51, we saw that pneumonia and influenza mortality rates behave differently when a flu epidemic occurs than when no epidemic occurs. As another example, some authors (for example, Hamilton, 1989, or McCulloch and Tsay, 1993) have explored the possibility the dynamics of the quarterly U.S. GNP series (say, $y_t$) analyzed in Example 2.34 might be different during expansion ($\nabla \log y_t > 0$) than during contraction ($\nabla \log y_t < 0$). In this section, we will concentrate on the method presented in Shumway and Stoffer (1991). One way of modeling change in an evolving time series is by assuming the dynamics of some underlying model changes discontinuously at certain undetermined points in time. Our starting point is the DLM given in Section 4.1, namely,

$$\boldsymbol{x}_t = \Phi \boldsymbol{x}_{t-1} + \boldsymbol{w}_t, \tag{4.123}$$

to describe the $p \times 1$ state dynamics, and

$$\boldsymbol{y}_t = A_t \boldsymbol{x}_t + \boldsymbol{v}_t \tag{4.124}$$

to describe the $q \times 1$ observation dynamics. Recall $\boldsymbol{w}_t$ and $\boldsymbol{v}_t$ are Gaussian white noise sequences with $\text{var}(\boldsymbol{w}_t) = Q$, $\text{var}(\boldsymbol{v}_t) = R$, and $\text{cov}(\boldsymbol{w}_t, \boldsymbol{v}_s) = 0$ for all $s$ and $t$.

Generalizations of (4.123) and (4.124) to include the possibility of changes occurring over time have been approached by allowing changes in the error covariances (Harrison and Stevens, 1976, Gordon and Smith, 1988, 1990) or by assigning mixture distributions to the observation errors $\boldsymbol{v}_t$ (Peña and Guttman, 1988). Approximations to filtering were derived in all of the aforementioned articles. An application to monitoring renal transplants was described in Smith and West (1983) and in Gordon and Smith (1990). Changes can also be modeled in the classical regression case by allowing switches in the design matrix, as in Quandt (1972).

Switching via a stationary Markov chain with independent observations has been developed by Lindgren (1978) and Goldfeld and Quandt (1973). In the Markov chain approach, we declare the dynamics of the system at time $t$ is generated by one of $m$ possible regimes evolving according to a Markov chain over time. As a simple example, suppose the dynamics of a univariate time series, $y_t$, is generated by either the model (1) $y_t = \beta_1 y_{t-1} + w_t$ or the model (2) $y_t = \beta_2 y_{t-1} + w_t$. We will write the model as $y_t = \phi_t y_{t-1} + w_t$ such that $\Pr(\phi_t = \beta_j) = \pi_j$, $j = 1, 2$, $\pi_1 + \pi_2 = 1$, and with the Markov property

$$\Pr(\phi_t = \beta_j \mid \phi_{t-1} = \beta_i, \phi_{t-2} = \beta_{i_2}, \ldots) = \Pr(\phi_t = \beta_j \mid \phi_{t-1} = \beta_i) = \pi_{ij},$$

for $i, j = 1, 2$ (and $i_2, \ldots = 1, 2$). As previously mentioned, Markov switching for dependent data has been applied by Hamilton (1989) to detect changes between positive and and negative growth periods in the economy. Applications to speech recognition have been considered by Juang and Rabiner (1985). The case in which the particular regime is unknown to the observer comes under the heading of ***hidden Markov models***, and the techniques related to analyzing these models are summarized in Rabiner and Juang (1986). An application of the idea of switching to the tracking of multiple targets has been considered in Bar-Shalom (1978), who obtained approximations to Kalman filtering in terms of weighted averages of the innovations.

**Example 4.13 Tracking Multiple Targets**

The approach of Shumway and Stoffer (1991) was motivated primarily by the problem of tracking a large number of moving targets using a vector $\boldsymbol{y}_t$ of sensors. In this problem, we do not know at any given point in time which target any given sensor has detected. Hence, it is the structure of the measurement matrix $A_t$ in (4.124) that is changing, and not the dynamics of the signal $\boldsymbol{x}_t$ or the noises, $\boldsymbol{w}_t$ or $\boldsymbol{v}_t$. As an example, consider a $3 \times 1$ vector of satellite measurements $\boldsymbol{y}_t = (y_{t1}, y_{t2}, y_{t3})'$ that are observations on some combination of a $3 \times 1$ vector of targets or signals, $\boldsymbol{x}_t = (x_{t1}, x_{t2}, x_{t3})'$. For the measurement matrix

$$A_t = \begin{bmatrix} 1 & 0 & 0 \\ 1 & 0 & 0 \\ 1 & 0 & 0 \end{bmatrix}$$

in the model (4.124), all sensors are observing the first target, $x_{t1}$, whereas for the measurement matrix

$$A_t = \begin{bmatrix} 0 & 1 & 0 \\ 1 & 0 & 0 \\ 0 & 0 & 1 \end{bmatrix}$$

the first sensor, $y_{t1}$, observes the second target, $x_{t2}$; the second sensor, $y_{t2}$, observes the first target, $x_{t1}$; and the third sensor, $y_{t3}$, observes the third target, $x_{t3}$. All possible detection configurations will define a set of possible values for $A_t$, say, $\{M_1, M_2, ..., M_m\}$, as a collection of plausible measurement matrices.

**Example 4.14 Modeling Economic Change**

As another example of the switching model presented in this section, consider the case in which the dynamics of the linear model changes suddenly over the history of a given realization. For example, Lam (1990) has given the following generalization of Hamilton's (1989) model for detecting positive and negative growth periods in the economy. Suppose the data are generated by

$$y_t = z_t + n_t, \tag{4.125}$$

where $z_t$ is an autoregressive series and $n_t$ is a random walk with a drift that switches between two values $\alpha_0$ and $\alpha_0 + \alpha_1$. That is,

$$n_t = n_{t-1} + \alpha_0 + \alpha_1 S_t, \tag{4.126}$$

with $S_t = 0$ or 1, depending on whether the system is in state 1 or state 2. For the purpose of illustration, suppose

$$z_t = \phi_1 z_{t-1} + \phi_2 z_{t-2} + w_t \tag{4.127}$$

is an AR(2) series with $\text{var}(w_t) = \sigma_w^2$. Lam (1990) wrote (4.125) in a differenced form

$$\nabla y_t = z_t - z_{t-1} + \alpha_0 + \alpha_1 S_t, \tag{4.128}$$

which we may take as the observation equation (4.124) with state vector

$$\boldsymbol{x}_t = (z_t, z_{t-1}, \alpha_0, \alpha_1)' \tag{4.129}$$

and

$$M_1 = [1, -1, 1, 0] \quad \text{and} \quad M_2 = [1, -1, 1, 1] \tag{4.130}$$

determining the two possible economic conditions. The state equation, (4.123), is of the form

$$\begin{pmatrix} z_t \\ z_{t-1} \\ \alpha_0 \\ \alpha_1 \end{pmatrix} = \begin{bmatrix} \phi_1 & \phi_2 & 0 & 0 \\ 1 & 0 & 0 & 0 \\ 0 & 0 & 1 & 0 \\ 0 & 0 & 0 & 1 \end{bmatrix} \begin{pmatrix} z_{t-1} \\ z_{t-2} \\ \alpha_0 \\ \alpha_1 \end{pmatrix} + \begin{pmatrix} w_t \\ 0 \\ 0 \\ 0 \end{pmatrix}. \tag{4.131}$$

The observation equation, (4.124), in this case is

$$\nabla y_t = A_t \boldsymbol{x}_t + v_t, \tag{4.132}$$

where $\Pr(A_t = M_1) = 1 - \Pr(A_t = M_2)$, with $M_1$ and $M_2$ given in (4.130).

To incorporate a reasonable switching structure for the measurement matrix into the DLM that is compatible with both practical situations previously described, we assume that the $m$ possible configurations are states in a nonstationary, independent process defined by the time-varying probabilities

$$\pi_j(t) = \Pr(A_t = M_j), \tag{4.133}$$

for $j = 1, ..., m$ and $t = 1, 2, ..., n$. Important information about the current state of the measurement process is given by the filtered probabilities of being in state $j$, defined as the conditional probabilities

$$\pi_j(t|t) = \Pr(A_t = M_j | Y_t), \tag{4.134}$$

which also vary as a function of time. In (4.134), we have used the notation $Y_s = \{\boldsymbol{y}_1, ..., \boldsymbol{y}_s\}$. The filtered probabilities (4.134) give the time-varying estimates of the probability of being in state $j$ given the data to time $t$.

It will be important for us to obtain estimators of the configuration probabilities, $\pi_j(t|t)$, the predicted and filtered state estimators, $\boldsymbol{x}_t^{t-1}$ and $\boldsymbol{x}_t^t$, and the corresponding error covariance matrices $P_t^{t-1}$ and $P_t^t$. Of course, the predictor and filter estimators will depend on the parameters, $\Theta$, of the DLM. In many situations, the parameters will be unknown and we will have to estimate them. Our focus will be on maximum likelihood estimation, but other authors have taken a Bayesian approach that assigns priors to the parameters, and then seeks posterior distributions of the model parameters; see, for example, Gordon and Smith (1990), Peña and Guttman (1988), or McCulloch and Tsay (1993).

We now establish the recursions for the filters associated with the state $\boldsymbol{x}_t$ and the switching process, $A_t$. As discussed in Section 4.3, the filters are also an essential part of the maximum likelihood procedure. The predictors, $\boldsymbol{x}_t^{t-1} = E(\boldsymbol{x}_t|Y_{t-1})$, and filters, $\boldsymbol{x}_t^t = E(\boldsymbol{x}_t|Y_t)$, and their associated error variance–covariance matrices, $P_t^{t-1}$ and $P_t^t$, are given by

$$\boldsymbol{x}_t^{t-1} = \Phi \boldsymbol{x}_{t-1}^{t-1}, \tag{4.135}$$

$$P_t^{t-1} = \Phi P_{t-1}^{t-1} \Phi' + Q, \tag{4.136}$$

$$\boldsymbol{x}_t^t = \boldsymbol{x}_t^{t-1} + \sum_{j=1}^m \pi_j(t|t) K_{tj} \boldsymbol{\epsilon}_{tj}, \tag{4.137}$$

$$P_t^t = \sum_{j=1}^m \pi_j(t|t)(I - K_{tj} M_j) P_t^{t-1}, \tag{4.138}$$

$$K_{tj} = P_t^{t-1} M_j' \Sigma_{tj}^{-1}, \tag{4.139}$$

where the innovation values in (4.137) and (4.139) are

$$\boldsymbol{\epsilon}_{tj} = \boldsymbol{y}_t - M_j \boldsymbol{x}_t^{t-1}, \tag{4.140}$$

$$\Sigma_{tj} = M_j P_t^{t-1} M_j' + R, \tag{4.141}$$

for $j = 1, ..., m$. Equations (4.135)-(4.139) exhibit the filter values as weighted linear combinations of the $m$ innovation values, (4.140)-(4.141), corresponding to each of the possible measurement matrices. The equations are similar to the approximations introduced by Bar-Shalom and Tse (1975), by Gordon and Smith (1990), and Peña and Guttman (1988).

To verify (4.137), let the indicator $I(A_t = M_j) = 1$ when $A_t = M_j$, and zero otherwise. Then, using (4.37) and Theorem 2.2 (iv) of Section T2.16,

$$\boldsymbol{x}_t^t \;=\; E(\boldsymbol{x}_t|Y_t) = E[E(\boldsymbol{x}_t|Y_t, A_t) \mid Y_t]$$

$$
\begin{aligned}
&= E\left\{\sum_{j=1}^{m} E(\boldsymbol{x}_t|Y_t, A_t = M_j)I(A_t = M_j) \mid Y_t\right\} \\
&= E\left\{\sum_{j=1}^{m} [\boldsymbol{x}_t^{t-1} + K_{tj}(\boldsymbol{y}_t - M_j\boldsymbol{x}_t^{t-1})]I(A_t = M_j) \mid Y_t\right\} \\
&= \sum_{j=1}^{m} \pi_j(t|t)[\boldsymbol{x}_t^{t-1} + K_{tj}(\boldsymbol{y}_t - M_j\boldsymbol{x}_t^{t-1})],
\end{aligned}
$$

where $K_{tj}$ is given by (4.139). Equation (4.138) is derived in a similar fashion; the other relationships, (4.135), (4.136), and (4.139), follow from straightforward applications of the Kalman filter results given in Property P4.1.

Next, we derive the filters $\pi_j(t|t)$. Let $f_j(t|t-1)$ denote the conditional density of $\boldsymbol{y}_t$ given the past $\boldsymbol{y}_1, ..., \boldsymbol{y}_{t-1}$, and $A_t = M_j$, for $j = 1, ..., n$. Then,

$$
\pi_j(t|t) = \frac{\pi_j(t) f_j(t|t-1)}{\sum_{k=1}^{m} \pi_k(t) f_k(t|t-1)}, \tag{4.142}
$$

where we assume the distribution $\pi_j(t)$, for $j = 1, ..., m$ has been specified before observing $\boldsymbol{y}_1, ..., \boldsymbol{y}_t$ (details follow as in Example 4.15 below). If the investigator has no reason to prefer one state over another at time $t$, the choice of uniform priors, $\pi_j(t) = m^{-1}$, for $j = 1, ..., m$, will suffice. Smoothness can be introduced by letting

$$
\pi_j(t) = \sum_{i=1}^{m} \pi_i(t-1|t-1)\pi_{ij}, \tag{4.143}
$$

where the nonnegative weights $\pi_{ij}$ are chosen so $\sum_{i=1}^{m} \pi_{ij} = 1$. If the $A_t$ process was Markov with transition probabilities $\pi_{ij}$, then (4.143) would be the update for the filter probability, as shown in the next example.

### Example 4.15 Hidden Markov Chain Model

If $\{A_t\}$ is a hidden Markov chain with stationary transition probabilities $\pi_{ij} = \Pr(A_t = M_j|A_{t-1} = M_i)$, for $i, j = 1, ..., m$, letting $p(\cdot)$ denote a generic probability function, we have

$$
\begin{aligned}
\pi_j(t|t) &= \frac{p(A_t = M_j, \boldsymbol{y}_t, Y_{t-1})}{p(\boldsymbol{y}_t, Y_{t-1})} \\
&= \frac{p(Y_{t-1})p(A_t = M_j \mid Y_{t-1})p(\boldsymbol{y}_t \mid A_t = M_j, Y_{t-1})}{p(Y_{t-1})p(\boldsymbol{y}_t \mid Y_{t-1})} \\
&= \frac{\pi_j(t|t-1)f_j(t|t-1)}{\sum_{k=1}^{m} \pi_k(t|t-1)f_k(t|t-1)}.
\end{aligned} \tag{4.144}
$$

In the Markov case, the conditional probabilities

$$\pi_j(t|t-1) = \Pr(A_t = M_j \big| Y_{t-1})$$

in (4.144) replace the unconditional probabilities, $\pi_j(t) = \Pr(A_t = M_j)$, in (4.142).

To evaluate (4.144), we must be able to calculate $\pi_j(t|t-1)$ and $f_j(t|t-1)$. We will discuss the calculation of $f_j(t|t-1)$ after this example. To derive $\pi_j(t|t-1)$, note,

$$\begin{aligned} \pi_j(t|t-1) &= \Pr(A_t = M_j \big| Y_{t-1}) \\ &= \sum_{i=1}^{m} \Pr(A_t = M_j, A_{t-1} = M_i \big| Y_{t-1}) \\ &= \sum_{i=1}^{m} \Pr(A_t = M_j \big| A_{t-1} = M_i) \Pr(A_{t-1} = M_i \big| Y_{t-1}) \\ &= \sum_{i=1}^{m} \pi_{ij} \pi_i(t-1|t-1). \end{aligned} \tag{4.145}$$

Expression (4.143) comes from equation (4.145), where, as previously noted, we replace $\pi_j(t|t-1)$ by $\pi_j(t)$.

The difficulty in extending the approach here to the Markov case is the dependence among the $\boldsymbol{y}_t$, which makes it necessary to enumerate over all possible histories to derive the filtering equations. This problem will be evident when we derive the conditional density $f_j(t|t-1)$. Equation (4.143) has $\pi_j(t)$ as a function of the past observations, $Y_{t-1}$, which is inconsistent with our model assumption. Nevertheless, this seems to be a reasonable compromise that allows the data to modify the probabilities $\pi_j(t)$, without having to develop a highly computer-intensive technique.

As previously suggested, the computation of $f_j(t|t-1)$, without some approximations, is highly computer-intensive. To evaluate $f_j(t|t-1)$, consider the event

$$A_1 = M_{j_1}, \; \dots \; , A_{t-1} = M_{j_{t-1}}, \tag{4.146}$$

for $j_i = 1, ..., m$, and $i = 1, ..., t-1$, which specifies a specific set of measurement matrices through the past; we will write this event as $A_{(t-1)} = M_{(\ell)}$. Because $m^{t-1}$ possible outcomes exist for $A_1, ..., A_{t-1}$, the index $\ell$ runs through $\ell = 1, ..., m^{t-1}$. Using this notation, we may write

$$\begin{aligned} & f_j(t|t-1) \\ &\quad = \sum_{\ell=1}^{m^{t-1}} \Pr\{A_{(t-1)} = M_{(\ell)} \mid Y_{t-1}\} f(\boldsymbol{y}_t \mid Y_{t-1}, A_t = M_j, A_{(t-1)} = M_{(\ell)}) \\ &\quad \equiv \sum_{\ell=1}^{m^{t-1}} \alpha(\ell) \, \mathrm{N}\left(\boldsymbol{y}_t \;\middle|\; \boldsymbol{\mu}_{tj}(\ell), \Sigma_{tj}(\ell)\right), \quad j = 1, ..., m, \end{aligned} \tag{4.147}$$

where the notation $\mathrm{N}(\cdot \mid \boldsymbol{b}, B)$ represents the normal density with mean vector $\boldsymbol{b}$ and variance–covariance matrix $B$. That is, $f_j(t|t-1)$ is a mixture of normals with nonnegative weights $\alpha(\ell) = \Pr\{A_{(t-1)} = M_{(\ell)} \mid Y_{t-1}\}$ such that $\sum_\ell \alpha(\ell) = 1$, and with each normal distribution having mean vector

$$\boldsymbol{\mu}_{tj}(\ell) = M_j \boldsymbol{x}_t^{t-1}(\ell) = M_j E[\boldsymbol{x}_t \mid Y_{t-1}, A_{(t-1)} = M_{(\ell)}] \tag{4.148}$$

and covariance matrix

$$\Sigma_{tj}(\ell) = M_j P_t^{t-1}(\ell) M_j' + R. \tag{4.149}$$

This result follows because the conditional distribution of $\boldsymbol{y}_t$ in (4.147) is identical to the fixed measurement matrix case presented in Section 4.2. The values in (4.148) and (4.149), and hence the densities, $f_j(t|t-1)$, for $j = 1, ..., m$, can be obtained directly from the Kalman filter, Property P4.1, with the measurement matrices $A_{(t-1)}$ fixed at $M_{(\ell)}$.

Although $f_j(t|t-1)$ is given explicitly in (4.147), its evaluation is highly computer intensive. For example, with $m = 2$ states and $n = 20$ observations, we have to filter over $2 + 2^2 + \cdots + 2^{20}$ possible sample paths; note, $2^{20} = 1{,}048{,}576$. One remedy is to trim (remove), at each $t$, highly improbable sample paths; that is, remove events in (4.146) with extremely small probability of occurring, and then evaluate $f_j(t|t-1)$ as if the trimmed sample paths could not have occurred. Another alternative, as suggested by Gordon and Smith (1990) and Shumway and Stoffer (1991), is to approximate $f_j(t|t-1)$ using the closest (in the sense of Kulback–Leibler distance) normal distribution. In this case, the approximation leads to choosing normal distribution with the same mean and variance associated with $f_j(t|t-1)$; that is, we approximate $f_j(t|t-1)$ by a normal with mean $M_j \boldsymbol{x}_t^{t-1}$ and variance $\Sigma_{tj}$ given in (4.141).

To develop a procedure for maximum likelihood estimation, the joint density of the data is

$$\begin{aligned} f(\boldsymbol{y}_1, ..., \boldsymbol{y}_n) &= \prod_{t=1}^n f(\boldsymbol{y}_t | Y_{t-1}) \\ &= \prod_{t=1}^n \sum_{j=1}^m \Pr(A_t = M_j | Y_{t-1}) f(\boldsymbol{y}_t | A_t = M_j, Y_{t-1}), \end{aligned}$$

and hence, the likelihood can be written as

$$\ln L_Y(\Theta) = \sum_{t=1}^n \ln \left( \sum_{j=1}^m \pi_j(t) f_j(t|t-1) \right). \tag{4.150}$$

For the hidden Markov model, $\pi_j(t)$ would be replaced by $\pi_j(t|t-1)$. In (4.150), we will use the normal approximation to $f_j(t|t-1)$. That is, henceforth, we will consider $f_j(t|t-1)$ as the normal, $\mathrm{N}(M_j \boldsymbol{x}_t^{t-1}, \Sigma_{tj})$, density, where $\boldsymbol{x}_t^{t-1}$ is given in (4.135) and $\Sigma_{tj}$ is given in (4.141). We may consider maximizing (4.150) directly as a function of the parameters $\Theta = \{\boldsymbol{\mu}_0, \Phi, Q, R\}$ using a Newton method, or we may consider applying the EM algorithm to the complete data likelihood.

To apply the EM algorithm as in Section 4.3, we call $\boldsymbol{x}_0, \boldsymbol{x}_1, ..., \boldsymbol{x}_n, A_1, ..., A_n$, and $\boldsymbol{y}_1, ..., \boldsymbol{y}_n$, the complete data, with likelihood given by

$$\begin{aligned} -2\ln L_{X,A,Y}(\Theta) &= \ln|\Sigma_0| + (\boldsymbol{x}_0 - \boldsymbol{\mu}_0)'\Sigma_0^{-1}(\boldsymbol{x}_0 - \boldsymbol{\mu}_0) \\ &+ \ln|Q| + \sum_{t=1}^{n}(\boldsymbol{x}_t - \Phi\boldsymbol{x}_{t-1})'Q^{-1}(\boldsymbol{x}_t - \Phi\boldsymbol{x}_{t-1}) \\ &- 2\sum_{t=1}^{n}\sum_{j=1}^{m} I(A_t = M_j)\ln\pi_j(t) \\ &+ \ln|R| + \sum_{t=1}^{n}(\boldsymbol{y}_t - A_t\boldsymbol{x}_t)'R^{-1}(\boldsymbol{y}_t - A_t\boldsymbol{x}_t). \end{aligned} \tag{4.151}$$

As discussed in Section 4.3, we require the maximization of the conditional expectation

$$Q\left(\Theta \mid \Theta^{(k-1)}\right) = E\left\{-2\ln L_{X,A,Y}(\Theta) \,\middle|\, Y_n, \Theta^{(k-1)}\right\}, \tag{4.152}$$

with respect to $\Theta$ at each iteration, $k = 1, 2, ...$ . The calculation and maximization of (4.152) is similar to the case of (4.70) in Section 4.3. In particular, with

$$\pi_j(t|n) = E[I(A_t = M_j) \mid Y_n], \tag{4.153}$$

we obtain on iteration $k$,

$$\pi_j^{(k)}(t) = \pi_j(t|n), \tag{4.154}$$

$$\boldsymbol{\mu}_0^{(k)} = \boldsymbol{x}_0^n, \tag{4.155}$$

$$\Phi^{(k)} = S_{10}S_{00}^{-1}, \tag{4.156}$$

$$Q^{(k)} = n^{-1}\left(S_{11} - S_{10}S_{00}^{-1}S_{10}'\right), \tag{4.157}$$

and

$$R^{(k)} = n^{-1}\sum_{t=1}^{n}\sum_{j=1}^{m}\pi_j(t|n)\left[(\boldsymbol{y}_t - M_j\boldsymbol{x}_t^n)(\boldsymbol{y}_t - M_j\boldsymbol{x}_t^n)' + M_jP_t^nM_j'\right]. \tag{4.158}$$

where $S_{11}, S_{10}, S_{00}$ are given in (4.72)-(4.74). As before, at iteration $k$, the filters and the smoothers are calculated using the current values of the parameters, $\Theta^{(k-1)}$, and $\Sigma_0$ is held fixed. Filtering is accomplished by using (4.135)-(4.139). Smoothing is derived in a similar manner to the derivation of the filter, and one is lead to the smoother given in Property P4.2 and P4.3, with one exception, the initial smoother covariance, (4.60), is now

$$P^n_{n,n-1} = \sum_{j=1}^{m} \pi_j(n|n)(I - K_{tj}M_j)\Phi P^{n-1}_{n-1}. \tag{4.159}$$

Unfortunately, the computation of $\pi_j(t|n)$ is excessively complicated, and requires integrating over mixtures of normal distributions. Shumway and Stoffer (1991) suggest approximating the smoother $\pi_j(t|n)$ by the filter $\pi_j(t|t)$, and find the approximation works well.

**Example 4.16 Analysis of Influenza Data**

We use the results of this section to analyze the U.S. monthly pneumonia and influenza mortality data (1968-1978) presented in Section 2.12, Figure 2.33. Letting $y_t$ denote the mortality caused by pneumonia and influenza at month $t$, we model $y_t$ in terms of a structural component model coupled with a hidden Markov process that determines whether a flu epidemic exists.

The model consists of three structural components. The first component, $x_{t1}$, is an AR(2) process chosen to represent the periodic (seasonal) component of the data,

$$x_{t1} = \alpha_1 x_{t-1,1} + \alpha_2 x_{t-2,1} + w_{t1}, \tag{4.160}$$

where $w_{t1}$ is white noise, with $\text{var}(w_{t1}) = \sigma_1^2$. The second component, $x_{t2}$, is an AR(1) process with a nonzero constant term, which is chosen to represent the sharp rise in the data during an epidemic,

$$x_{t2} = \beta_0 + \beta_1 x_{t-1,2} + w_{t2}, \tag{4.161}$$

where $w_{t2}$ is white noise, with $\text{var}(w_{t2}) = \sigma_2^2$. The third component, $x_{t3}$, is a fixed trend component given by,

$$x_{t3} = x_{t-1,3} + w_{t3}, \tag{4.162}$$

where $\text{var}(w_{t3}) = 0$. The case in which $\text{var}(w_{t3}) > 0$, which corresponds to a stochastic trend (random walk), was tried here, but the estimation became unstable, and lead to us fitting a fixed, rather than stochastic, trend. Thus, in the final model, the trend component satisfies $\nabla x_{t3} = 0$; recall in Example 2.51 the data were also differenced once before fitting the model.

Throughout the years, periods of normal influenza mortality (state 1) are modeled as

$$y_t = x_{t1} + x_{t3} + v_t, \tag{4.163}$$

**Table 4.6:** Estimation Results for Influenza Data

| Parameter | Initial Estimate | Final Estimate |
|---|---|---|
| $\alpha_1$ | 1.401 (0.079) | 1.379 (0.073) |
| $\alpha_2$ | -0.618 (0.091) | -0.575 (0.075) |
| $\beta_0$ | 0.162 (0.042) | 0.201 (0.028) |
| $\beta_1$ | 0.156 (0.142) | — |
| $\sigma_1$ | 0.023 (0.001) | 0.023 (0.001) |
| $\sigma_2$ | 0.105 (0.015) | 0.108 (0.016) |
| $\sigma_v$ | 0.000 (0.032) | — |

Estimated standard errors are shown in parentheses.

where the measurement error, $v_t$, is white noise with $\text{var}(v_t) = \sigma_v^2$. When an epidemic occurs (state 2), mortality is modeled as

$$y_t = x_{t1} + x_{t2} + x_{t3} + v_t. \tag{4.164}$$

The model specified in (4.160)-(4.164) can be written in the general state-space form. The state equation is

$$\begin{pmatrix} x_{t1} \\ x_{t-1,1} \\ x_{t2} \\ x_{t3} \end{pmatrix} = \begin{bmatrix} \alpha_1 & \alpha_2 & 0 & 0 \\ 1 & 0 & 0 & 0 \\ 0 & 0 & \beta_1 & 0 \\ 0 & 0 & 0 & 1 \end{bmatrix} \begin{pmatrix} x_{t-1,1} \\ x_{t-2,1} \\ x_{t-1,2} \\ x_{t-1,3} \end{pmatrix} + \begin{pmatrix} 0 \\ 0 \\ \beta_0 \\ 0 \end{pmatrix} + \begin{pmatrix} w_{t1} \\ 0 \\ w_{t2} \\ 0 \end{pmatrix}. \tag{4.165}$$

Of course, (4.165) can be written in the standard state-equation form as

$$\boldsymbol{x}_t = \Phi \boldsymbol{x}_{t-1} + \boldsymbol{\alpha} + \boldsymbol{w}_t, \tag{4.166}$$

where $\boldsymbol{x}_t = (x_{t1}, x_{t-1,1}, x_{t2}, x_{t3})'$, $\boldsymbol{\alpha} = (0, 0, \beta_0, 0)'$, and $Q$ is a $4 \times 4$ matrix with $\sigma_1^2$ as the (1,1)-element, $\sigma_2^2$ as the (3,3)-element, and the remaining elements set equal to zero. With this model, the filter equation (4.135) will be $\boldsymbol{x}_t^{t-1} = \Phi \boldsymbol{x}_{t-1}^{t-1} + \boldsymbol{\alpha}$. The observation equation is

$$y_t = A_t \boldsymbol{x}_t + v_t, \tag{4.167}$$

where $A_t$ is $1 \times 4$, and $v_t$ is white noise with $\text{var}(v_t) = R = \sigma_v^2$. We assume all components of variance $w_{t1}$, $w_{t2}$, and $v_t$ are uncorrelated.

As discussed in (4.163) and (4.164), $A_t$ can take one of two possible forms

$$\begin{aligned} A_t &= M_1 = [1, 0, 0, 1] \quad \text{no epidemic,} \\ A_t &= M_2 = [1, 0, 1, 1] \quad \text{epidemic,} \end{aligned}$$

corresponding to the two possible states of (1) no flu epidemic and (2) flu epidemic, such that $\Pr(A_t = M_1) = 1 - \Pr(A_t = M_2)$. In this

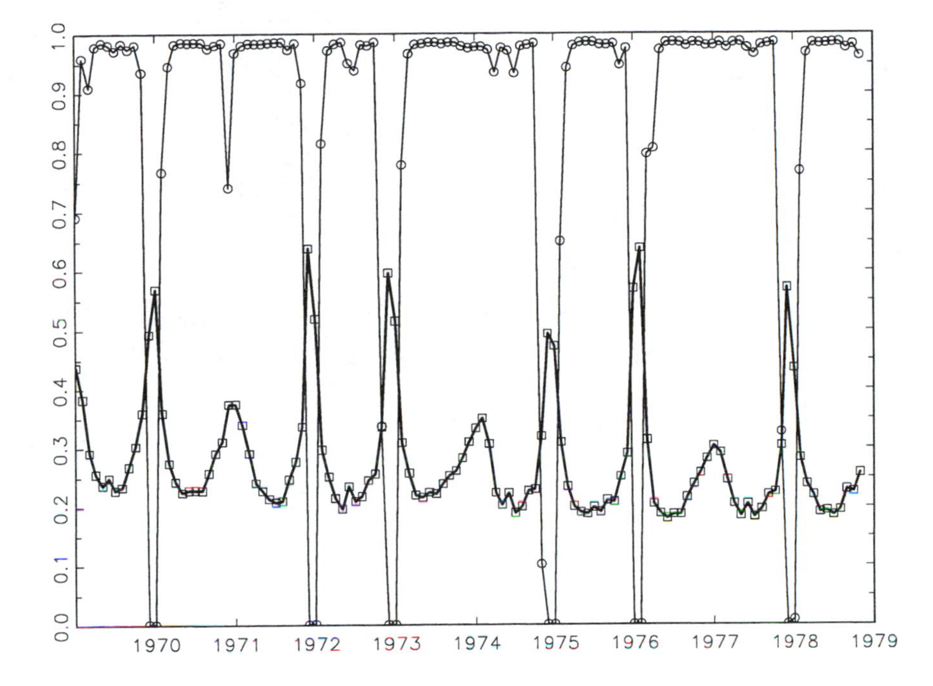


**Figure 4.11:** Influenza data, $y_t$, (dark line-squares) and the predicted probability that no epidemic occurs in month $t$ given the past, $\widehat{\pi}_1(t|t-1)$ (line-circles) for the ten-year period 1969-1978; 1968 is not shown.

example, we will assume $A_t$ is a hidden Markov chain, and hence we use the updating equations given in Example 4.15, (4.144) and (4.145), with transition probabilities $\pi_{11} = \pi_{22} = .75$ (and, thus, $\pi_{12} = \pi_{21} = .25$).

Parameter estimation was accomplished using a quasi-Newton–Raphson procedure to maximize the approximate log likelihood given in (4.150), with initial values of $\pi_1(1|0) = \pi_2(1|0) = 0.5$. Table 4.6 shows the results of the estimation procedure. On the initial fit, two estimates are not significant, namely, $\widehat{\beta}_1$ and $\widehat{\sigma}_v$. When $\sigma_v^2 = 0$, there is no measurement error, and the variability in data is explained solely by the variance components of the state system, namely, $\sigma_1^2$ and $\sigma_2^2$. The case in which $\beta_1 = 0$ corresponds to a simple level shift during a flu epidemic. In the final model, with $\beta_1$ and $\sigma_v^2$ removed, the estimated level shift ($\widehat{\beta}_0$) corresponds to an increase in mortality by about .2 per 1000 during a flu epidemic. The estimates for the final model are also listed in Table 4.6.

Figure 4.11 shows a plot of the data, $y_t$, for the ten-year period of

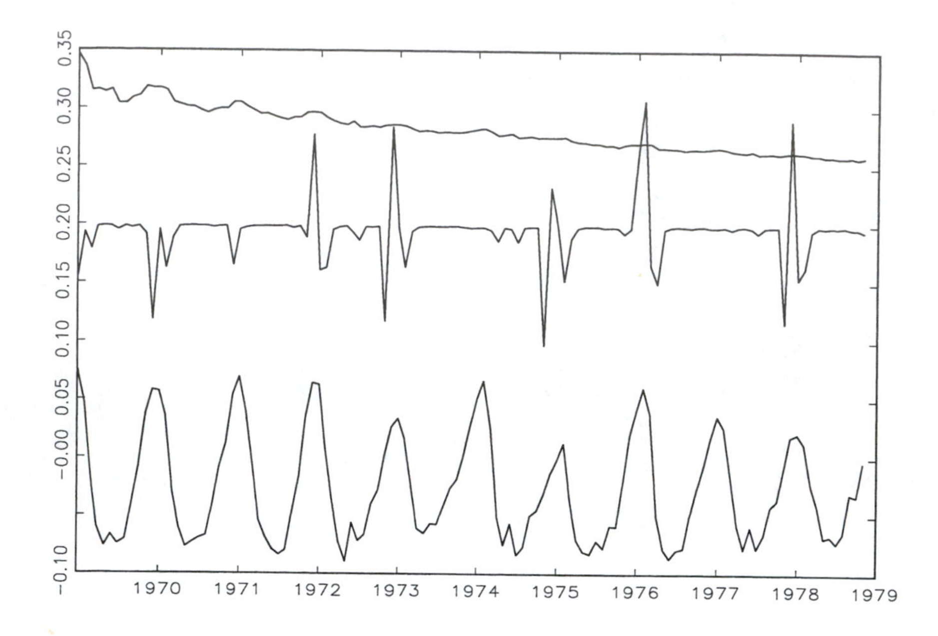


**Figure 4.12:** The three filtered structural components of influenza mortality: $\widehat{x}_{t1}^t$ (*cyclic trace*), $\widehat{x}_{t2}^t$ (*spiked trace*), and $\widehat{x}_{t3}^t$ (*negative linear trace*) for the ten-year period of 1969-1978.

1969-1978 as well as the estimated approximate conditional probabilities $\widehat{\pi}_1(t|t-1)$, that is, the predicted probability no epidemic occurs in month $t$ given the past, $y_1, ..., y_{t-1}$. The results for the first year of the data, 1968, are not included in the figure because of initial instabilities of the filter. Of course, the estimated predicted probability a flu epidemic will occur next month is $\widehat{\pi}_2(t|t-1) = 1 - \widehat{\pi}_1(t|t-1)$. Thus, a good estimator would have small values of $\widehat{\pi}_1(t|t-1)$ corresponding to peaks in $y_t$. Except for initial values where instability exists, the estimated prediction probabilities are right on the mark. That is, the predicted probability of a flu epidemic exceeds the probability of no epidemic when indeed a flu epidemic occurred the next month.

Figure 4.12 shows the estimated filtered values (that is, filtering is done using the parameter estimates) of the three components of the model, $x_{t1}^t$, $x_{t2}^t$, and $x_{t3}^t$. Except for initial instability (which is not shown), $\widehat{x}_{t1}^t$ represents the seasonal (cyclic) aspect of the data, $\widehat{x}_{t2}^t$ represents the spikes during a flu epidemic, and $\widehat{x}_{t3}^t$ represents the slow decline in flu mortality over the ten-year period of 1969-1978.

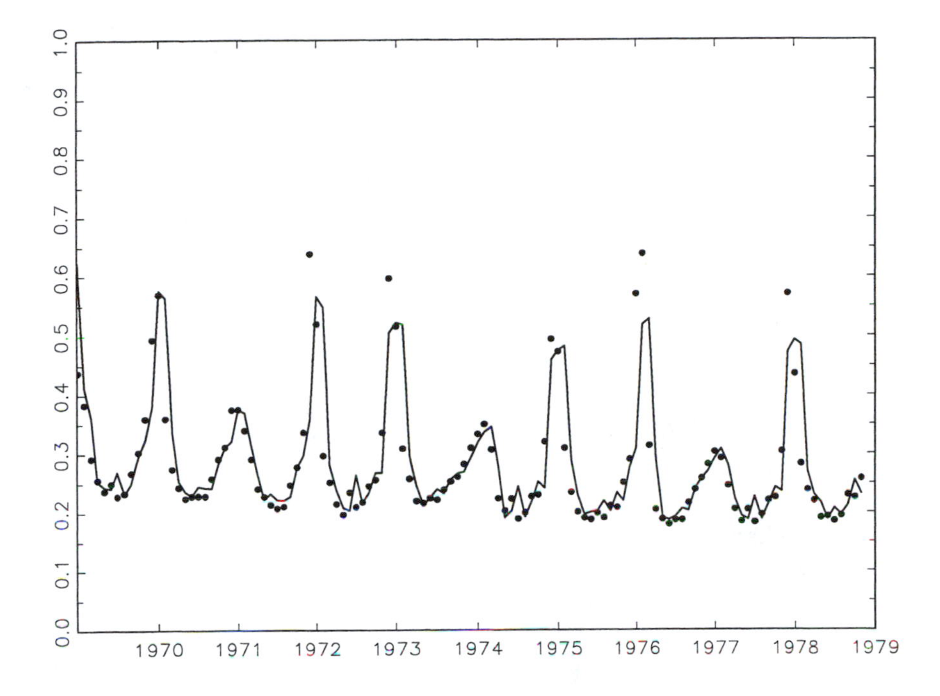


**Figure 4.13:** One-month-ahead prediction, $\widehat{y}_t^{t-1}$ (line), of the number of deaths caused by pneumonia and influenza, $y_t$ (points) for 1969-1978. The standard error of the prediction is 0.02 when a flu epidemic is not predicted, and 0.11 when a flu epidemic is predicted.

One-month-ahead prediction, say, $\widehat{y}_t^{t-1}$, is obtained as follows,

$$\widehat{y}_t^{t-1} = M_1 \widehat{\boldsymbol{x}}_t^{t-1} \quad \text{if} \quad \widehat{\pi}_1(t|t-1) > \widehat{\pi}_2(t|t-1),$$

$$\widehat{y}_t^{t-1} = M_2 \widehat{\boldsymbol{x}}_t^{t-1} \quad \text{if} \quad \widehat{\pi}_1(t|t-1) \le \widehat{\pi}_2(t|t-1).$$

Of course, $\widehat{\boldsymbol{x}}_t^{t-1}$ is the estimated state prediction, obtained via the filter presented in (4.135)-(4.139) (with the addition of the constant term in the model) using the estimated parameters. The results are shown in Figure 4.13. The precision of the forecasts can be measured by the innovation variances, $\Sigma_{t1}$ when no epidemic is predicted, and $\Sigma_{t2}$ when an epidemic is predicted. These values become stable quickly, and when no epidemic is predicted, the estimated standard error of the prediction is approximately 0.02 (this is the square root of $\Sigma_{t1}$ for $t$ large); when a flu epidemic is predicted, the estimated standard error of the prediction is approximately 0.11.

The results of this analysis are impressive given the small number of parameters and the degree of approximation that was made to obtain a computationally simple method for fitting a complex model. In particular, as seen in Figure 4.11, the model is never fooled as to when a flu epidemic will occur. This result is particularly impressive, given that, for example, in the third year, around $t = 36$, it appeared as though an epidemic was about to begin, but it never was realized, and the model predicted no flu epidemic that year. As seen in Figure 4.13, the predicted mortality tends to be underestimated during the peaks, but the true values are typically within one standard error of the predicted value. Further evidence of the strength of this technique can be found in the example given in Shumway and Stoffer (1991).

## 4.9 Nonlinear and Nonnormal State-Space Models Using Monte Carlo Methods

Most of this chapter has focused on linear dynamic models assumed to be Gaussian processes. Historically, these models were convenient because analyzing the data was a relatively simple matter. These assumptions cannot cover every situation, and it is advantageous to explore departures from these assumptions. As seen in Section 4.8, the solution to the nonlinear and non-Gaussian case will require computer-intensive techniques currently in vogue because of the availability of cheap and fast computers. In this section, we take a Bayesian approach to forecasting as our main objective; see West and Harrison (1997) for a detailed account of Bayesian forecasting with dynamic models. Prior to the mid-1980's, a number of approximation methods were developed to filter nonnormal or nonlinear processes in an attempt to circumvent the computational complexity of the analysis of such models. For example, the extended Kalman filter and the Gaussian sum filter (Alspach and Sorensen, 1972) are two such methods described in detail in Anderson and Moore (1979). As in the previous section, these techniques typically rely on approximating the nonnormal distribution by one or several Gaussian distributions or by some other parametric function.

With the advent of cheap and fast computing, a number of authors developed computer-intensive methods based on numerical integration. For example, Kitagawa (1987) proposed a numerical method based on piecewise linear approximations to the density functions for prediction, filtering, and smoothing for non-Gaussian and nonstationary state-space models. Pole and West (1988) used Gaussian quadrature techniques in a Bayesian analysis of nonlinear dynamic models; West and Harrison (1997, Chapter 13) provide a detailed explanation of these and similar methods. ***Markov chain Monte Carlo (MCMC)*** methods refer to Monte Carlo integration methods that use a Markovian updating scheme. We will describe the method in more detail later. The most common MCMC method is the Gibbs sampler, which is essentially a modification of the Metropolis algorithm (Metropolis et al, 1953) developed by Hastings (1970) in the statistical setting and by Geman and Geman (1984) in the context of image restoration. Later, Tanner and Wong (1987) used the ideas in their substitution sampling approach, and Gelfand and Smith (1990) developed the Gibbs sampler for a wide class of parametric models. This technique was first used by Carlin et al (1992) in the context of general nonlinear and non-Gaussian state-space models. Frühwirth-Schnatter (1994) and Carter and Kohn (1994) built on these ideas to develop efficient Gibbs sampling schemes for more restrictive models.

If the model is linear, that is, (4.19) and (4.20) hold, but the distributions are not Gaussian, a non-Gaussian likelihood can be defined by (4.46) in Section 4.2, but where $f_0(\cdot)$, $f_w(\cdot)$ and $f_v(\cdot)$ are not normal densities. In this case, prediction and filtering can be accomplished using numerical integration techniques (e.g., Kitagawa, 1987, Pole and West, 1988) or Monte Carlo techniques (e.g. Frühwirth-Schnatter, 1994, Carter and Kohn, 1994) to evaluate (4.47) and (4.48). Of course, the prediction and filter densities $p_\Theta(\boldsymbol{x}_t \mid Y_{t-1})$ and $p_\Theta(\boldsymbol{x}_t \mid Y_t)$ will no longer be Gaussian and will not generally be of the location-scale form as in the Gaussian case. A rich class of nonnormal densities is given in (4.178).

In general, the state-space model can be given by the following equations:

$$\boldsymbol{x}_t = F_t(\boldsymbol{x}_{t-1}, \boldsymbol{w}_t) \quad \text{and} \quad \boldsymbol{y}_t = H_t(\boldsymbol{x}_t, \boldsymbol{v}_t), \tag{4.168}$$

where $F_t$ and $H_t$ are known functions that may depend on parameters $\Theta$ and $\boldsymbol{w}_t$ and $\boldsymbol{v}_t$ are white noise processes. The main component of the model retained by (4.168) is that the states are Markov, and the observations are conditionally independent, but we do not necessarily assume $F_t$ and $H_t$ are linear, or $\boldsymbol{w}_t$ and $\boldsymbol{v}_t$ are Gaussian. Of course, if $F_t(\boldsymbol{x}_{t-1}, \boldsymbol{w}_t) = \Phi_t \boldsymbol{x}_{t-1} + \boldsymbol{w}_t$ and $H_t(\boldsymbol{x}_t, \boldsymbol{v}_t) = A_t \boldsymbol{x}_t + \boldsymbol{v}_t$ and $\boldsymbol{w}_t$ and $\boldsymbol{v}_t$ are Gaussian, we have the standard DLM (exogenous variables can be added to the model in the usual way). In the general model, (4.168), the likelihood is given by

$$L_{X,Y}(\Theta) = p_\Theta(\boldsymbol{x}_0) \prod_{t=1}^{n} p_\Theta(\boldsymbol{x}_t \mid \boldsymbol{x}_{t-1}) p_\Theta(\boldsymbol{y}_t \mid \boldsymbol{x}_t), \tag{4.169}$$

and the prediction and filter densities, as given by (4.47) and (4.48) in Section 4.2, still hold.

Because our focus is on simulation using MCMC methods, we first describe the technique in a general context.

**Example 4.17 MCMC Techniques and the Gibbs Sampler**

The goal of a Monte Carlo technique, of course, is to simulate a pseudorandom sample of vectors from a desired density function $p_\Theta(\boldsymbol{z})$. In

Markov chain Monte Carlo, we simulate an ordered sequence of pseudo-random vectors, $z_0 \mapsto z_1 \mapsto z_2 \mapsto \cdots$ by specifying a starting value, $z_0$ and then sampling successive values from a transition density $\pi(z_t|z_{t-1})$, for $t = 1, 2, ....$ In this way, conditional on $z_{t-1}$, the $t$-th pseudo-random vector, $z_t$, is simulated independent of its predecessors. This technique alone does not yield a pseudo-random sample because contiguous draws are dependent on each other (that is, we obtain a first-order dependent sequence of pseudo-random vectors). If done appropriately, the dependence between the pseudo-variates $z_t$ and $z_{t+m}$ decays exponentially in $m$, and we may regard the collection $\{z_{t+\ell m}; \ell = 1, 2, ...\}$ for $t$ and $m$ suitably large, as a pseudo-random sample. Alternately, one may repeat the process in parallel, retaining the $m$-th value, on run $g = 1, 2, ...,$ say, $z_m^{(g)}$, for large $m$. Under general conditions, the Markov chain converges in the sense that, eventually, the sequence of pseudo-variates appear stationary and the individual $z_t$ are marginally distributed according to the stationary "target" density $p_\Theta(z)$. Technical details may be found in Tierney (1994).

For Gibbs sampling, suppose we have a collection $\{z_1, ..., z_k\}$ of random vectors with complete conditional densities denoted generically by

$$p_\Theta(z_j \mid z_i, i \neq j) \equiv p_\Theta(z_j \mid z_1, ..., z_{j-1}, z_{j+1}, ..., z_k),$$

for $j = 1, ..., k$, available for sampling. Here, available means pseudo-samples may be generated by some method given the values of the appropriate conditioning random vectors. Under mild conditions, these complete conditionals uniquely determine the full joint density $p_\Theta(z_1, ..., z_k)$ and, consequently, all marginals, $p_\Theta(z_j)$ for $j = 1, ..., k$; details may be found in Besag (1974). The Gibbs sampler generates pseudo-samples from the joint distribution as follows. Start with an arbitrary set of starting values, say, $\{z_{1[0]}, ..., z_{k[0]}\}$. Draw $z_{1[1]}$ from $p_\Theta(z_1|z_{2[0]}, ..., z_{k[0]})$, then draw $z_{2[1]}$ from $p_\Theta(z_2|z_{1[1]}, z_{3[0]}, ..., z_{k[0]})$, and so on up to $z_{k[1]}$ from $p_\Theta(z_k|z_{1[1]}, ..., z_{k-1[1]})$, to complete one iteration. After $\ell$ such iterations, we have the collection $\{z_{1[\ell]}, ..., z_{k[\ell]}\}$. Geman and Geman (1984) showed that under mild conditions, $\{z_{1[\ell]}, ..., z_{k[\ell]}\}$ converges ($\ell \to \infty$) in distribution to a random observation from $p_\Theta(z_1, ..., z_k)$. For this reason, we typically drop the subscript $[\ell]$ from the notation, assuming $\ell$ is sufficiently large for the generated sample to be thought of as a realization from the joint density; hence, we denote this first realization as $\{z_{1[\ell]}^{(1)}, ..., z_{k[\ell]}^{(1)}\} \equiv \{z_1^{(1)}, ..., z_k^{(1)}\}$. This entire process is replicated in parallel, a large number, $G$, of times providing pseudo-random iid collections $\{z_1^{(g)}, ..., z_k^{(g)}\}$, for $g = 1, ..., G$ from the joint distribution. These simulated values can the be used to estimate the marginal densities. In particular, if $p_\Theta(z_j|z_i, i \neq j)$ is available in closed form, then [1]

$$\widehat{p}_\Theta(z_j) = G^{-1} \sum_{g=1}^{G} p_\Theta(z_j \mid z_i^{(g)}, i \neq j). \tag{4.170}$$

Because of the relatively recent appearance of Gibbs sampling methodology, several important theoretical and practical issues are under investigation. These issues include the diagnosis of convergence, modification of the sampling order, efficient estimation, and sequential sampling schemes (as opposed to the parallel processing described above) to mention a few. At this time, the best advice can be obtained from the texts by Gelman et al (1995) and Gilks et al (1996), and we are certain that many more will follow.

Finally, it may be necessary to nest ***rejection sampling*** within the Gibbs sampling procedure. The need for rejection sampling arises when we want to sample from a density, say, $f(z)$, but $f(z)$ is known only up to a proportionality constant, say, $p(z) \propto f(z)$. If a density $g(z)$ is available, and there is a constant $c$ for which $p(z) \leq cg(z)$ for all $z$, the rejection algorithm generates pseudo-variates from $f(z)$ by generating a value, $z^*$ from $g(z)$ and accepting it as a value from $f(z)$ with probability $\pi(z^*) = p(z^*)/[cg(z^*)]$. This algorithm can be quite inefficient if $\pi(\cdot)$ is close to zero; in such cases, more sophisticated envelope functions may be needed. Further discussion of these matters in the case of nonlinear state-space models can be found in Carlin et al (1992, Examples 1.2 and 3.2).

In Example 4.17, the generic random vectors $\boldsymbol{z}_j$ can represent parameter values, such as components of $\Theta$, state values $\boldsymbol{x}_t$, or future observations $\boldsymbol{y}_{n+m}$, for $m \geq 1$. This will become evident in the following examples. Before discussing the general case of nonlinear and nonnormal state-space models, we briefly introduce MCMC methods for the Gaussian DLM, as presented in Frühwirth-Schnatter (1994) and Carter and Kohn (1994).

**Example 4.18 Assessing Model Parameters for the Gaussian DLM**

Consider the Gaussian DLM given by

$$\boldsymbol{x}_t = \Phi_t \boldsymbol{x}_{t-1} + \boldsymbol{w}_t \quad \text{and} \quad y_t = \boldsymbol{a}_t' \boldsymbol{x}_t + v_t. \tag{4.171}$$

The observations are univariate, and the state process is $p$-dimensional; this DLM includes the structural models presented in Section 4.5. The

[1] Approximation (4.170) is based on the fact that, for random variables $x$ and $y$ with joint density $p(x, y)$, the marginal density of $x$ is obtained as follows: $p(x) = \int p(x, y)dy = \int p(x|y)p(y)dy$.

prior on the initial state is $\boldsymbol{x}_0 \sim \mathrm{N}(\boldsymbol{\mu}_0, \Sigma_0)$, and we assume that $\boldsymbol{w}_t \sim$ iid $\mathrm{N}(\mathbf{0}, Q_t)$, independent of $v_t \sim$ iid $\mathrm{N}(0, r_t)$. The collection of unknown model parameters will be denoted by $\Theta$.

To explore how we would assess the values of $\Theta$ using an MCMC technique, we focus on the problem obtaining the posterior distribution, $p(\Theta \mid Y_n)$, of the parameters given the data, $Y_n = \{y_1, ..., y_n\}$ and a prior $\pi(\Theta)$. Of course, these distributions depend on "hyperparameters" that are assumed to be known. (Some authors consider the states $\boldsymbol{x}_t$ as the first level of parameters because they are unobserved. In this case, the values in $\Theta$ are regarded as the hyperparameters, and the parameters of their distributions are regarded as hyper-hyperparameters.) Denoting the entire set of state vectors as $X_n = \{\boldsymbol{x}_0, \boldsymbol{x}_1, ..., \boldsymbol{x}_n\}$, the posterior can be written as

$$p(\Theta \mid Y_n) = \int p(\Theta \mid X_n, Y_n)\; p(X_n, \Theta^* \mid Y_n)\; dX_n\; d\Theta^*. \tag{4.172}$$

Although the posterior, $p(\Theta \mid Y_n)$, may be intractable, conditioning on the states can make the problem manageable in that

$$p(\Theta \mid X_n, Y_n) \propto \pi(\Theta)\; p(x_0 \mid \Theta) \prod_{t=1}^{n} p(\boldsymbol{x}_t \mid \boldsymbol{x}_{t-1}, \Theta)\; p(y_t \mid \boldsymbol{x}_t, \Theta) \tag{4.173}$$

can be easier to work with (either as members of conjugate families or using some rejection scheme); we will discuss this in more detail when we present the nonlinear, non-Gaussian case, but we will assume for the present $p(\Theta \mid X_n, Y_n)$ is in closed form.

Suppose we can obtain $G$ pseudo-random draws, $X_n^{(g)} \equiv (X_n, \Theta^*)^{(g)}$, for $g = 1, ..., G$, from the joint posterior density $p(X_n, \Theta^* \mid Y_n)$. Then (4.172) can be approximated by

$$\widehat{p}(\Theta \mid Y_n) = G^{-1} \sum_{g=1}^{G} p(\Theta \mid X_n^{(g)}, Y_n).$$

A sample from $p(X_n, \Theta^* \mid Y_n)$ is obtained using two different MCMC methods. First, the Gibbs sampler is used, for each $g$, as follows: sample $X_{n[\ell]}$ given $\Theta^*_{[\ell-1]}$ from $p(X_n \mid \Theta^*_{[\ell-1]}, Y_n)$, and then a sample $\Theta^*_{[\ell]}$ from $p(\Theta \mid X_{n[\ell]}, Y_n)$ as given by (4.173), for $\ell = 1, 2, ....$ Stop when $\ell$ is sufficiently large, and retain the final values as $X_n^{(g)}$. This process is repeated $G$ times.

The first step of this method requires simultaneous generation of the state vectors. Because we are dealing with a Gaussian linear model, we can rely on the existing theory of the Kalman filter to accomplish this step. This step is conditional on $\Theta$, and we assume at this point that $\Theta$ is fixed and known. In other words, our goal is to sample the entire set of state vectors, $X_n = \{\boldsymbol{x}_0, \boldsymbol{x}_1, ..., \boldsymbol{x}_n\}$, from the multivariate normal posterior density $p_\Theta(X_n \mid Y_n)$, where $Y_n = \{y_1, ..., y_n\}$ represents the observations. Because of the Markov structure, we can write,

$$p_\Theta(X_n \mid Y_n) = p_\Theta(\boldsymbol{x}_n \mid Y_n) p_\Theta(\boldsymbol{x}_{n-1} \mid \boldsymbol{x}_n, Y_{n-1}) \cdots p_\Theta(\boldsymbol{x}_0 \mid \boldsymbol{x}_1). \quad (4.174)$$

In view of (4.174), it is possible to sample the entire set of state vectors, $X_n$, by sequentially simulating the individual states backward. This process yields a simulation method that Frühwirth–Schnatter (1994) called the forward-filtering, backward-sampling algorithm. In particular, because the processes are Gaussian, we need only obtain the conditional means and variances, say, $\boldsymbol{m}_t = E_\Theta(\boldsymbol{x}_t \mid Y_t, \boldsymbol{x}_{t+1})$, and $V_t = \text{var}_\Theta(\boldsymbol{x}_t \mid Y_t, \boldsymbol{x}_{t+1})$. This conditioning argument is akin to having $\boldsymbol{x}_{t+1}$ as an additional observation on state $\boldsymbol{x}_t$. In particular, using standard multivariate normal distribution theory,

$$\begin{aligned} \boldsymbol{m}_t &= \boldsymbol{x}_t^t + J_t(\boldsymbol{x}_{t+1} - \boldsymbol{x}_{t+1}^t), \\ V_t &= P_t^t - J_t P_{t+1}^t J_t', \end{aligned} \quad (4.175)$$

for $t = n-1, n-2, ..., 0$, where $J_t$ is defined in (4.51). To verify (4.175), the essential part of the Gaussian density (that is, the exponent) of $\boldsymbol{x}_t \mid Y_t, \boldsymbol{x}_{t+1}$ is

$$(\boldsymbol{x}_{t+1} - \Phi_{t+1}\boldsymbol{x}_t)'[Q_{t+1}]^{-1}(\boldsymbol{x}_{t+1} - \Phi_{t+1}\boldsymbol{x}_t) + (\boldsymbol{x}_t - \boldsymbol{x}_t^t)'[P_t^t]^{-1}(\boldsymbol{x}_t - \boldsymbol{x}_t^t),$$

and we simply complete the square; see Frühwirth–Schnatter (1994) or West and Harrison (1997, Section 4.7). Hence, the algorithm is to first sample $\boldsymbol{x}_n$ from a $\text{N}(\boldsymbol{x}_n^n, P_n^n)$, where $\boldsymbol{x}_n^n$ and $P_n^n$ are obtained from the Kalman filter, Property P4.1, and then sample $\boldsymbol{x}_t$ from a $\text{N}(\boldsymbol{m}_t, V_t)$, for $t = n-1, n-2, ..., 0$, where the conditioning value of $\boldsymbol{x}_{t+1}$ is the value previously sampled; $\boldsymbol{m}_t$ and $V_t$ are given in (4.175).

Next, we address an MCMC approach to nonlinear and non-Gaussian state-space modeling that was first presented in Carlin et al (1992). We consider the general model given in (4.168), but with additive errors:

$$\boldsymbol{x}_t = F_t(\boldsymbol{x}_{t-1}) + \boldsymbol{w}_t \quad \text{and} \quad \boldsymbol{y}_t = H_t(\boldsymbol{x}_t) + \boldsymbol{v}_t, \quad (4.176)$$

where $F_t$ and $H_t$ are given, but may also depend on unknown parameters, say, $\Phi_t$ and $A_t$, respectively, the collection of which will be denoted by $\Theta$. The errors are independent white noise sequences with $\text{var}(\boldsymbol{w}_t) = Q_t$ and $\text{var}(\boldsymbol{v}_t) = R_t$. Although time-varying variance–covariance matrices are easily incorporated in this framework, to ease the discussion we focus on the case $Q_t \equiv Q$ and $R_t \equiv R$. Also, although it is not necessary, we assume the initial state condition $\boldsymbol{x}_0$ is fixed and known; this is merely for notational convenience, so we do not have to carry along the additional terms involving $\boldsymbol{x}_0$ throughout the discussion.

In general, the likelihood specification for the model is given by

$$L_{X,Y}(\Theta, Q, R) = \prod_{t=1}^{n} f_1(\boldsymbol{x}_t \mid \boldsymbol{x}_{t-1}, \Theta, Q)\; f_2(\boldsymbol{y}_t \mid \boldsymbol{x}_t, \Theta, R), \tag{4.177}$$

where it is assumed the densities $f_1(\cdot)$ and $f_2(\cdot)$ are scale mixtures of normals. Specifically, for $t = 1, ..., n$,

$$\begin{aligned} f_1(\boldsymbol{x}_t \mid \boldsymbol{x}_{t-1}, \Theta, Q) &= \int f(\boldsymbol{x}_t \mid \boldsymbol{x}_{t-1}, \Theta, Q, \lambda_t)\; p_1(\lambda_t)\; d\lambda_t, \\ f_2(\boldsymbol{y}_t \mid \boldsymbol{x}_t, \Theta, R) &= \int f(\boldsymbol{y}_t \mid \boldsymbol{x}_t, \Theta, R, \omega_t)\; p_2(\omega_t)\; d\omega_t, \end{aligned} \tag{4.178}$$

where conditional on the independent sequences of nuisance parameters $\boldsymbol{\lambda} = (\lambda_t; t = 1, ..., n)$ and $\boldsymbol{\omega} = (\omega_t; t = 1, ..., n)$,

$$\begin{aligned} \boldsymbol{x}_t \mid \boldsymbol{x}_{t-1}, \Theta, Q, \lambda_t &\sim \mathrm{N}\Big(F_t(\boldsymbol{x}_{t-1}; \Theta),\; \lambda_t Q\Big), \\ \boldsymbol{y}_t \mid \boldsymbol{x}_t, \Theta, R, \omega_t &\sim \mathrm{N}\Big(H_t(\boldsymbol{x}_t; \Theta),\; \omega_t R\Big). \end{aligned} \tag{4.179}$$

By varying $p_1(\lambda_t)$ and $p_2(\omega_t)$, we can have a wide variety of non-Gaussian error densities. These densities include, for example, double exponential, logistic, and $t$ distributions in the univariate case and a rich class of multivariate distributions; this is discussed further in Carlin et al (1992). The key to the approach is the introduction of the nuisance parameters $\boldsymbol{\lambda}$ and $\boldsymbol{\omega}$ and the structure (4.179), which lends itself naturally to the Gibbs sampler and allows for the analysis of this general nonlinear and non-Gaussian problem.

According to Example 4.17, to implement the Gibbs sampler, we must be able to sample from the following complete conditional distributions:

(i) $\boldsymbol{x}_t \mid \boldsymbol{x}_{s \neq t}, \boldsymbol{\lambda}, \boldsymbol{\omega}, \Theta, Q, R, Y_n \quad t = 1, ..., n,$

(ii) $\lambda_t \mid \lambda_{s \neq t}, \boldsymbol{\omega}, \Theta, Q, R, Y_n, X_n \sim \lambda_t \mid \Theta, Q, \boldsymbol{x}_t, \boldsymbol{x}_{t-1} \quad t = 1, ..., n,$

(iii) $\omega_t \mid \omega_{s \neq t}, \boldsymbol{\lambda}, \Theta, Q, R, Y_n, X_n \sim \omega_t \mid \Theta, R, \boldsymbol{y}_t, \boldsymbol{x}_t \quad t = 1, ..., n,$

(iv) $Q \mid \boldsymbol{\lambda}, \boldsymbol{\omega}, \Theta, R, Y_n, X_n \sim Q \mid \boldsymbol{\lambda}, Y_n, X_n,$

(v) $R \mid \boldsymbol{\lambda}, \boldsymbol{\omega}, \Theta, Q, Y_n, X_n \sim R \mid \boldsymbol{\omega}, Y_n, X_n,$

(vi) $\Theta \mid \boldsymbol{\lambda}, \boldsymbol{\omega}, Q, R, Y_n, X_n \sim \Theta \mid Y_n, X_n,$

where $X_n = \{\boldsymbol{x}_1, ..., \boldsymbol{x}_n\}$ and $Y_n = \{\boldsymbol{y}_1, ..., \boldsymbol{y}_n\}$. The main difference between this method and the linear Gaussian case is that, because of the generality, we sample the states one-at-a-time rather than simultaneously generating all of them. As discussed in Carter and Kohn (1994), if possible, it is more efficient to generate the states simultaneously as in Example 4.18.

We will discuss items (i) and (ii) above. The third item follows in a similar manner to the second, and items (iv)-(vi) will follow from standard multivariate normal distribution theory and from Wishart distribution theory because of the conditioning on $\boldsymbol{\lambda}$ and $\boldsymbol{\omega}$. We will discuss this matter further in the next example. First, consider the linear model, $F_t(\boldsymbol{x}_{t-1}) = \Phi_t \boldsymbol{x}_{t-1}$, and $H_t(\boldsymbol{x}_t) = A_t \boldsymbol{x}_t$ in (4.176). In this case, for $t = 1, ..., n$, $\boldsymbol{x}_t \bigm| \boldsymbol{x}_{s \neq t}, \boldsymbol{\lambda}, \boldsymbol{\omega}, \Theta, Q, R, Y_n$ has a $p$-dimensional $\mathrm{N}_p(B_t \boldsymbol{b}_t, B_t)$ distribution, with

$$\begin{aligned} B_t^{-1} &= \frac{Q^{-1}}{\lambda_t} + \frac{A_t' R^{-1} A_t}{\omega_t} + \frac{\Phi_{t+1}' Q^{-1} \Phi_{t+1}}{\lambda_{t+1}}, \\ \boldsymbol{b}_t &= \frac{\boldsymbol{x}_{t-1} \Phi_t' Q^{-1}}{\lambda_t} + \frac{\boldsymbol{y}_t R^{-1} A_t}{\omega_t} + \frac{\boldsymbol{x}_{t+1} Q^{-1} \Phi_{t+1}}{\lambda_{t+1}}, \end{aligned} \tag{4.180}$$

where, when $t = n$ in (4.180), terms in the sum with elements having a subscript of $n+1$ are dropped (this is assumed to be the case in what follows, although we do not explicitly state it). This result follows by noting the essential part of the multivariate normal distribution (that is, the exponent) of $\boldsymbol{x}_t \bigm| \boldsymbol{x}_{s \neq t}, \boldsymbol{\lambda}, \boldsymbol{\omega}, \Theta, Q, R, Y_n$ is

$$\begin{aligned} &(\boldsymbol{x}_t - \Phi_t \boldsymbol{x}_{t-1})'(\lambda_t Q)^{-1}(\boldsymbol{x}_t - \Phi_t \boldsymbol{x}_{t-1}) + (\boldsymbol{y}_t - A_t \boldsymbol{x}_t)'(\omega_t R)^{-1}(\boldsymbol{y}_t - A_t \boldsymbol{x}_t) \\ &\quad + (\boldsymbol{x}_{t+1} - \Phi_{t+1} \boldsymbol{x}_t)'(\lambda_{t+1} Q)^{-1}(\boldsymbol{x}_{t+1} - \Phi_{t+1} \boldsymbol{x}_t), \end{aligned} \tag{4.181}$$

which upon manipulation yields (4.180).

### Example 4.19 Nonlinear Models

In the case of nonlinear models, we can use (4.180) with slight modifications. For example, consider the case in which $F_t$ is nonlinear, but $H_t$ is linear, so the observations are $\boldsymbol{y}_t = A_t \boldsymbol{x}_t + \boldsymbol{v}_t$. Then,

$$\boldsymbol{x}_t \bigm| \boldsymbol{x}_{s \neq t}, \boldsymbol{\lambda}, \boldsymbol{\omega}, \Theta, Q, R, Y_n \propto \eta_1(\boldsymbol{x}_t) \mathrm{N}_p(B_{1t} \boldsymbol{b}_{1t}, B_{1t}), \tag{4.182}$$

where

$$\begin{aligned} B_{1t}^{-1} &= \frac{Q^{-1}}{\lambda_t} + \frac{A_t' R^{-1} A_t}{\omega_t}, \\ \boldsymbol{b}_{1t} &= \frac{F_t'(\boldsymbol{x}_{t-1}) Q^{-1}}{\lambda_t} + \frac{\boldsymbol{y}_t R^{-1} A_t}{\omega_t}, \end{aligned}$$

and

$$\eta_1(\boldsymbol{x}_t) = \exp\left\{ -\frac{1}{2\lambda_{t+1}} \Big( \boldsymbol{x}_{t+1} - F_{t+1}(\boldsymbol{x}_t) \Big)' Q^{-1} \Big( \boldsymbol{x}_{t+1} - F_{t+1}(\boldsymbol{x}_t) \Big) \right\}.$$

Because $0 \le \eta_1(\boldsymbol{x}_t) \le 1$, for all $\boldsymbol{x}_t$, the distribution we want to sample from is dominated by the $\mathrm{N}_p(B_{1t}\boldsymbol{b}_{1t}, B_{1t})$ density. Hence, we may use rejection sampling as discussed in Example 4.17 to obtain an observation from the required density. That is, we generate a pseudo-variate from the $\mathrm{N}_p(B_{1t}\boldsymbol{b}_{1t}, B_{1t})$ density and accept it with probability $\eta_1(\boldsymbol{x}_t)$.

We proceed analogously in the case in which $F_t(\boldsymbol{x}_{t-1}) = \Phi_t \boldsymbol{x}_{t-1}$ is linear and $H_t(\boldsymbol{x}_t)$ is nonlinear. In this case,

$$\boldsymbol{x}_t \bigm| \boldsymbol{x}_{s\neq t}, \boldsymbol{\lambda}, \boldsymbol{\omega}, \Theta, Q, R, Y_n \propto \eta_2(\boldsymbol{x}_t)\mathrm{N}_p(B_{2t}\boldsymbol{b}_{2t}, B_{2t}), \tag{4.183}$$

where

$$\begin{aligned} B_{2t}^{-1} &= \frac{Q^{-1}}{\lambda_t} + \frac{\Phi'_{t+1}Q^{-1}\Phi_{t+1}}{\lambda_{t+1}}, \\ \boldsymbol{b}_{2t} &= \frac{\boldsymbol{x}_{t-1}\Phi'_t Q^{-1}}{\lambda_t} + \frac{\boldsymbol{x}_{t+1}Q^{-1}\Phi_{t+1}}{\lambda_{t+1}}, \end{aligned}$$

and

$$\eta_2(\boldsymbol{x}_t) = \exp\left\{-\frac{1}{2\omega_t}\Big(\boldsymbol{y}_t - H_t(\boldsymbol{x}_t)\Big)' R^{-1}\Big(\boldsymbol{y}_t - H_t(\boldsymbol{x}_t)\Big)\right\}.$$

Here, we generate a pseudo-variate from the $\mathrm{N}_p(B_{2t}\boldsymbol{b}_{2t}, B_{2t})$ density and accept it with probability $\eta_2(\boldsymbol{x}_t)$.

Finally, in the case in which both $F_t$ and $H_t$ are nonlinear, we have

$$\boldsymbol{x}_t \bigm| \boldsymbol{x}_{s\neq t}, \boldsymbol{\lambda}, \boldsymbol{\omega}, \Theta, Q, R, Y_n \propto \eta_1(\boldsymbol{x}_t)\eta_2(\boldsymbol{x}_t)\mathrm{N}_p(F_t(\boldsymbol{x}_{t-1}), \lambda_t Q), \tag{4.184}$$

so we sample from a $\mathrm{N}_p(F_t(\boldsymbol{x}_{t-1}), \lambda_t Q)$ density and accept it with probability $\eta_1(\boldsymbol{x}_t)\eta_2(\boldsymbol{x}_t)$.

Determination of (ii), $\lambda_t \bigm| \Theta, Q, \boldsymbol{x}_t, \boldsymbol{x}_{t-1}$ follows directly from Bayes theorem; that is, $p(\lambda_t \bigm| \Theta, Q, \boldsymbol{x}_t, \boldsymbol{x}_{t-1}) \propto p_1(\lambda_t)p(\boldsymbol{x}_t \bigm| \lambda_t, \boldsymbol{x}_{t-1}, \Theta, Q)$. By (4.178), however, we know the normalization constant is given by $f_1(\boldsymbol{x}_t \bigm| \boldsymbol{x}_{t-1}, \Theta, Q)$, and thus the complete conditional density for $\lambda_t$ is of a known functional form.

Many examples of these techniques are given in Carlin et al (1992), including the problem of model choice. In the next example, we consider a univariate nonlinear model in which the state noise process has a $t$-distribution. As noted in Meinhold and Singpurwalla (1989), using $t$-distributions for the error processes is a way of robustifying the Kalman filter against outliers. In this example we present a brief discussion of a detailed analysis presented in Carlin et al (1992, Example 4.2); readers interested in more detail may find it in that article.

**Example 4.20 Analysis of a Nonlinear, Non-Gaussian State-Space Model**

Kitagawa (1987) considered the analysis of data generated from the following univariate nonlinear model:

$$x_t = F_t(x_{t-1}) + w_t \quad \text{and} \quad y_t = H_t(x_t) + v_t \quad t = 1, ..., 100, \tag{4.185}$$

with

$$\begin{aligned} F_t(x_{t-1}) &= \alpha x_{t-1} + \beta x_{t-1}/(1 + x_{t-1}^2) + \gamma \cos[1.2(t-1)], \\ H_t(x_t) &= x_t^2/20, \end{aligned} \tag{4.186}$$

where $x_0 = 0$, $w_t$ are independent random variables having a central $t$-distribution with $\nu = 10$ degrees and scaled so $\text{var}(w_t) = \sigma_w^2 = 10$ [we denote this generically by $t(0, \sigma, \nu)$], and $v_t$ is white standard Gaussian noise, $\text{var}(v_t) = \sigma_v^2 = 1$. The state noise and observation noise are mutually independent. Kitagawa (1987) discussed the analysis of data generated from this model with $\alpha = 0.5$, $\beta = 25$, and $\gamma = 8$ assumed known. We will use these values of the parameters in this example, but we will assume they are unknown. Figure 4.14 shows a typical data sequence $y_t$ and the corresponding state process $x_t$.

Our goal here will be to obtain an estimate of the prediction density $p(x_{101} \mid Y_{100})$. To accomplish this, we use $n = 101$ and consider $y_{101}$ as a latent variable (we will discuss this in more detail shortly). The priors on the variance components are chosen from a conjugate family, that is, $\sigma_w^2 \sim \text{IG}(a_0, b_0)$ independent of $\sigma_v^2 \sim \text{IG}(c_0, d_0)$, where IG denotes the inverse (reciprocal) gamma distribution [$z$ has an inverse gamma distribution if $1/z$ has a gamma distribution; general properties can be found, for example, in Box and Tiao (1973, Section 8.5)]. Then,

$$\begin{aligned} &\sigma_w^2 \mid \boldsymbol{\lambda}, Y_n, X_n \sim \\ &\qquad \text{IG}\left(a_0 + \frac{n}{2}, \left\{\frac{1}{b_0} + \frac{1}{2}\sum_{t=1}^{n}[x_t - F(x_{t-1})]^2/\lambda_t\right\}^{-1}\right), \\ &\sigma_v^2 \mid \boldsymbol{\omega}, Y_n, X_n \sim \\ &\qquad \text{IG}\left(c_0 + \frac{n}{2}, \left\{\frac{1}{d_0} + \frac{1}{2}\sum_{t=1}^{n}[y_t - H(x_t)]^2/\omega_t\right\}^{-1}\right). \end{aligned} \tag{4.187}$$

Next, letting $\nu/\lambda_t \sim \chi_\nu^2$, we get that, marginally, $w_t \mid \sigma_w \sim t(0, \sigma_w, \nu)$, as required, leading to the complete conditional $\lambda_t \mid \sigma_w, \alpha, \beta, \gamma, Y_n, X_n$, for $t = 1, ..., n$, being distributed as

$$\text{IG}\left(\frac{\nu+1}{2}, 2\left\{\frac{[x_t - F(x_{t-1})]^2}{\sigma_w^2} + \nu\right\}^{-1}\right). \tag{4.188}$$

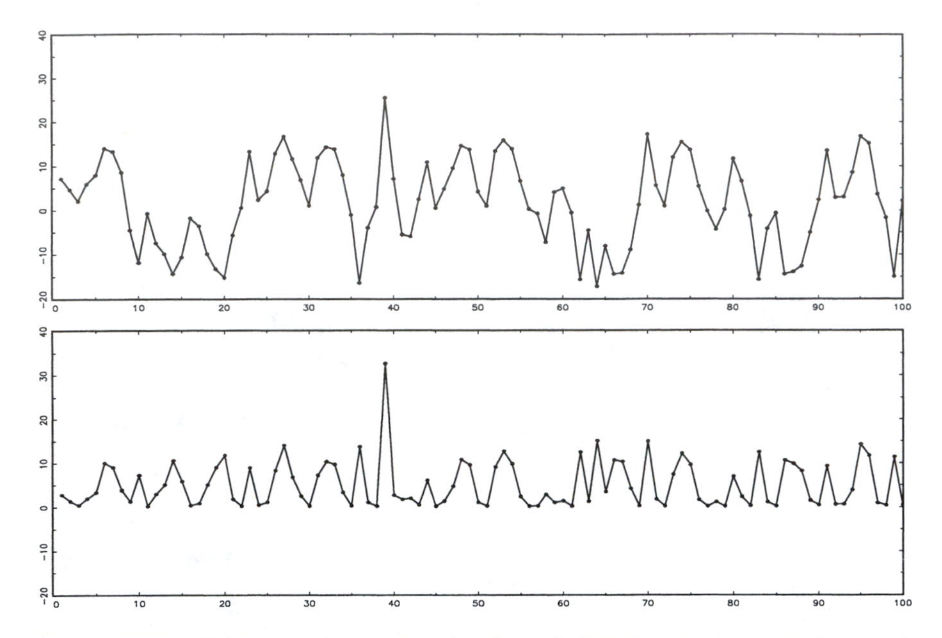


**Figure 4.14:** The state process, $x_t$ (top), and the observations, $y_t$ (bottom), for $t = 1, ..., 100$ generated from the model (4.185).

We take $\omega_t \equiv 1$ for $t = 1, ..., n$, because the observation noise is Gaussian.

For the states, $x_t$, we take a normal prior on the initial state, $x_0 \sim \mathrm{N}(\mu_0, \sigma_0^2)$, and then we use rejection sampling to conditionally generate a state value $x_t$, for $t = 1, ..., n$, as described in Example 4.19, equation (4.184). In this case, $\eta_1(x_t)$ and $\eta_2(x_t)$ are given in (4.182) and (4.183), respectively, with $F_t$ and $H_t$ given by (4.186), $\Theta = (\alpha, \beta, \gamma)'$, $Q = \sigma_w^2$ and $R = \sigma_v^2$. Endpoints take some special consideration; we generate $x_0$ from a $\mathrm{N}(\mu_0, \sigma_0^2)$ and accept it with probability $\eta_1(x_0)$, and we generate $x_{101}$ as usual and accept it with probability $\eta_2(x_{101})$. The last complete conditional depends on $y_{101}$, a latent data value not observed but instead generated according to its complete conditional, which is $\mathrm{N}(x_{101}^2/20, \sigma_v^2)$, because $\omega_{101} = 1$.

The prior on $\Theta = (\alpha, \beta, \gamma)'$ is taken to be trivariate normal with mean $(\mu_\alpha, \mu_\beta, \mu_\gamma)'$ and diagonal variance–covariance matrix $\mathrm{diag}\{\sigma_\alpha^2, \sigma_\beta^2, \sigma_\gamma^2\}$. The necessary conditionals can be found using standard normal theory, as done in (4.180). For example, the complete conditional distribution of $\alpha$ is of the form $\mathrm{N}(Bb, B)$, where

$$B^{-1} = \frac{1}{\sigma_\alpha^2} + \frac{1}{\sigma_w^2} \sum_{t=1}^{n} \frac{x_{t-1}^2}{\lambda_t}$$

and

$$b = \frac{\mu_\alpha}{\sigma_\alpha^2} + \frac{1}{\sigma_w^2} \sum_{t=1}^{n} \frac{x_{t-1}}{\lambda_t} \left( x_t - \beta \frac{x_{t-1}}{1 + x_{t-1}^2} - \gamma \cos[1.2(t-1)] \right).$$

The complete conditional for $\beta$ has the same form, with

$$B^{-1} = \frac{1}{\sigma_\beta^2} + \frac{1}{\sigma_w^2} \sum_{t=1}^{n} \frac{x_{t-1}^2}{\lambda_t (1 + x_{t-1}^2)^2}$$

and

$$b = \frac{\mu_\beta}{\sigma_\beta^2} + \frac{1}{\sigma_w^2} \sum_{t=1}^{n} \frac{x_{t-1}}{\lambda_t (1 + x_{t-1}^2)} \left( x_t - \alpha x_{t-1} - \gamma \cos[1.2(t-1)] \right),$$

and for $\gamma$ the values are

$$B^{-1} = \frac{1}{\sigma_\gamma^2} + \frac{1}{\sigma_w^2} \sum_{t=1}^{n} \frac{\cos^2[1.2(t-1)]}{\lambda_t}$$

and

$$b = \frac{\mu_\gamma}{\sigma_\gamma^2} + \frac{1}{\sigma_w^2} \sum_{t=1}^{n} \frac{\cos[1.2(t-1)]}{\lambda_t} \left( x_t - \alpha x_{t-1} - \beta \frac{x_{t-1}}{1 + x_{t-1}^2} \right).$$

In this example, we put $\mu_0 = 0$, $\sigma_0^2 = 10$, and $a_0 = 3$, $b_0 = .05$ (so the prior on $\sigma_w^2$ has mean and standard deviation equal to 10), and $c_0 = 3$, $d_0 = .5$ (so the prior on $\sigma_v^2$ has mean and standard deviation equal to one). The normal prior on $\Theta = (\alpha, \beta, \gamma)'$ had corresponding mean vector equal to $(\mu_\alpha = .5, \mu_\beta = 25, \mu_\gamma = 8)'$ and diagonal variance matrix equal to $\mathrm{diag}\{\sigma_\alpha^2 = .25, \sigma_\beta^2 = 10, \sigma_\gamma^2 = 4\}$. The Gibbs sampler ran for $\ell = 50$ iterations for $G = 500$ parallel replications per iteration. We estimate the marginal posterior density of $x_{101}$ as

$$\widehat{p}(x_{101} \mid Y_{100}) = G^{-1} \sum_{g=1}^{G} \mathrm{N} \left( x_{101} \,\middle|\, [F_t(x_{t-1})]^{(g)}, \lambda_{101}^{(g)} \sigma_w^{2(g)} \right), \quad (4.189)$$

where $\mathrm{N}(\cdot|a, b)$ denotes the normal density with mean $a$ and variance $b$, and

$$[F_t(x_{t-1})]^{(g)} = \alpha^{(g)} x_{t-1}^{(g)} + \beta^{(g)} x_{t-1}^{(g)} / (1 + x_{t-1}^{2(g)}) + \gamma^{(g)} \cos[1.2(t-1)].$$

The estimate, (4.189), with $G = 500$, is shown in Figure 4.15. Other aspects of the analysis, for example, the marginal posteriors of the elements of $\Theta$, can be found in Carlin et al (1992).

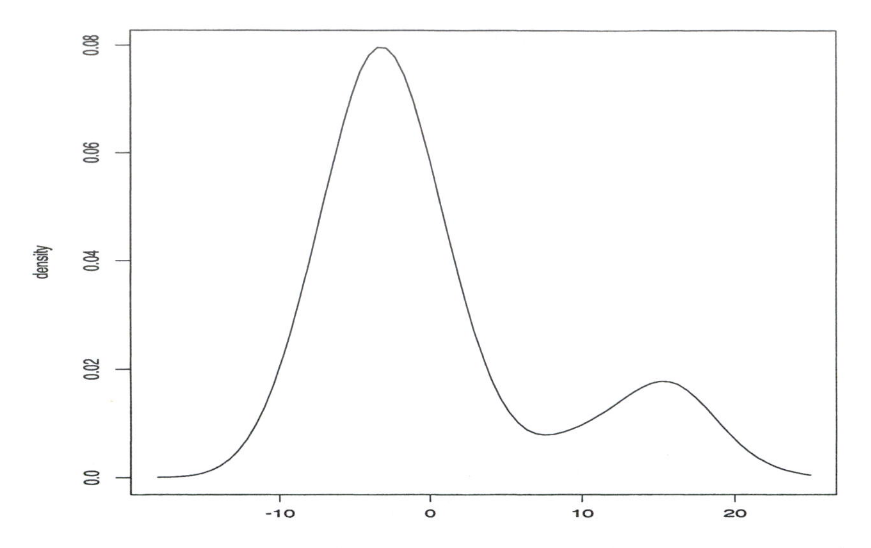


**Figure 4.15:** Estimated one-step-ahead prediction posterior density $\widehat{p}(x_{101}|Y_{100})$ of the state process for the nonlinear and nonnormal model given by (4.185) using Gibbs sampling, $G = 500$.

# 4.10 Stochastic Volatility

Recently, there has been considerable interest in stochastic volatility models. These models are similar to the ARCH models presented in Chapter 2, but they add a stochastic noise term to the equation for $\sigma_t$. Recall from Section 2.15 that a GARCH(1, 1) model for a return, which we denote here by $r_t$, is given by

$$r_t = \sigma_t \epsilon_t \tag{4.190}$$
$$\sigma_t^2 = \alpha_0 + \alpha_1 r_{t-1}^2 + \beta_1 \sigma_{t-1}^2, \tag{4.191}$$

where $\epsilon_t$ is Gaussian white noise. Note that we can rewrite (4.190) as

$$r_t = \exp\left(\frac{1}{2}\log\sigma_t^2\right)\epsilon_t.$$

If we define $h_t = \ln\sigma_t^2$ and $y_t = \ln r_t^2$, (4.190) can be written as

$$y_t = h_t + \ln\epsilon_t^2 \tag{4.192}$$

Equation (4.192) is considered the observation equation, and the stochastic variance $h_t$ is considered to be an unobserved state process. Similar to (4.191), the volatility process follows, in its basic form, an autoregression,

$$h_t = \phi_0 + \phi_1 h_{t-1} + w_t, \tag{4.193}$$

where $w_t$ is white Gaussian noise with variance $\sigma_w^2$.

Together, (4.192) and (4.193) make up the ***stochastic volatility model***. If $\epsilon_t^2$ had a log-normal distribution, (4.192)-(4.193) would form a Gaussian state-space model, and we could then use standard DLM results to fit the model to data. Unfortunately, $y_t = \log r_t^2$ is rarely normal, so we typically keep the ARCH normality assumption on $\epsilon_t$; in which case, $\log \epsilon_t^2$ is distributed as the log of a chi-squared random variable with one degree of freedom. This density is given by

$$f(x) = \frac{1}{\sqrt{2\pi}} \exp\left\{-\frac{1}{2}\left(e^x - x\right)\right\} \quad -\infty < x < \infty, \tag{4.194}$$

and its mean and variance are $-1.27$ and $\pi^2/2$, respectively; the density (4.194) is highly skewed with a long tail on the left (see Figure 4.18).

Various approaches to the fitting of stochastic volatility models have been examined; these methods include a wide range of assumptions on the observational noise process. A good summary of the proposed techniques, both Bayesian (via MCMC, as discussed in Section 4.9) and non-Bayesian approaches (such as quasi-maximum likelihood estimation and the EM algorithm), can be found in Jacquier et al(1994), and Shepard (1995). In an effort to keep matters simple, our method of fitting stochastic volatility models is to retain the Gaussian state equation (4.193), but to write the observation equation, with $y_t = \log r_t^2$, as

$$y_t = h_t + \eta_t, \tag{4.195}$$

where $\eta_t$ is white noise, whose distribution is a mixture of two normals, one centered at zero. In particular, we write

$$\eta_t = u_t z_{t0} + (1 - u_t) z_{t1}, \tag{4.196}$$

where $u_t$ is an iid Bernoulli process, $\Pr\{u_t = 0\} = \pi_0$, $\Pr\{u_t = 1\} = \pi_1$ ($\pi_0 + \pi_1 = 1$), $z_{t0} \sim$ iid $\mathrm{N}(0, \sigma_0^2)$, and $z_{t1} \sim$ iid $\mathrm{N}(\mu_1, \sigma_1^2)$.

The advantage to this model is that it is easy to fit because it uses normality. In fact, the model specified by equations (4.193) and (4.195)-(4.196) is precisely the model presented in Peña and Guttman (1988), and the material presented in Section 4.8 applies here. In particular, the likelihood can be evaluated as in (4.150), but where $m = 2$ and $\pi_j(t)$ is independent of $t$. That is, with $\Theta = (\phi_0, \phi_1, \sigma_0^2, \mu_1, \sigma_1^2, \sigma_w^2, \pi_1)'$, we evaluate the likelihood by

$$\ln L_Y(\Theta) = \sum_{t=1}^{n} \ln\left(\sum_{j=0}^{1} \pi_j f_j(t|t-1)\right), \tag{4.197}$$

where $f_j(t|t-1)$ is approximated by a normal, $\mathrm{N}(h_t^{t-1} + \mu_j,\ \sigma_j^2)$, density ($j = 0, 1$ and $\mu_0 = 0$). Of course, $h_t^{t-1}$ is the state prediction obtained by using the modified filter, (4.135)-(4.141), given in Section 4.8. We may consider

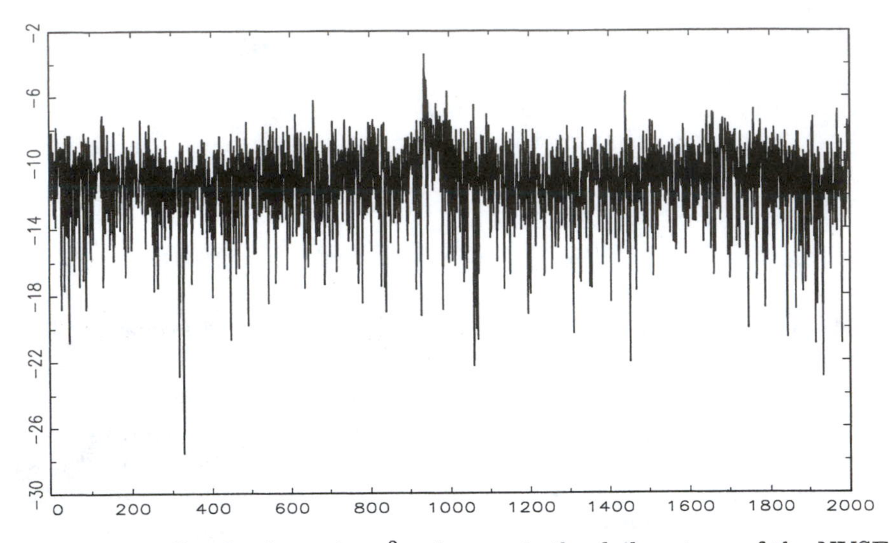


**Figure 4.16:** Graph of $y_t = \log r_t^2$, where $r_t$ is the daily return of the NYSE, 2000 observations.

maximizing (4.197) directly as a function of the parameters $\Theta$ using a Newton method, or we may consider applying the EM algorithm to the complete data likelihood.

**Example 4.21 Analysis of the New York Stock Exchange Returns**

Figure 4.16 shows the log of the squares of returns, $y_t = \log r_t^2$, of 2000 daily observations of the New York Stock Exchange (NYSE). This data set was taken from the S-plus GARCH module available from *MathSoft*.

Model (4.193) and (4.195)-(4.196), with $\pi_1$ fixed at 0.5, was fit to the data using a quasi-Newton–Raphson method to maximize (4.197). The results are given in Table 4.7.

Figure 4.17 shows a histogram of the residuals from the fit, and Figure 4.18 compares the density of the log of a $\chi_1^2$ with the fitted normal mixture.

## 4.11 State-Space and ARMAX Models for Longitudinal Data Analysis

In some studies, we may observe several independent $k$-dimensional time series, say, $\boldsymbol{y}_{t\ell}$, for $\ell = 1, ..., N$. For example, a new treatment may be given to $N$

**Table 4.7:** Estimation Results for the NYSE Fit

| Parameter | Estimate | Estimated Standard Error |
|---|---|---|
| $\phi_0$ | -0.722 | 0.296 |
| $\phi_1$ | 0.928 | 0.029 |
| $\sigma_0$ | 1.189 | 0.066 |
| $\mu_1$ | -2.383 | 0.196 |
| $\sigma_1$ | 2.658 | 0.099 |
| $\sigma_w$ | 0.224 | 0.053 |

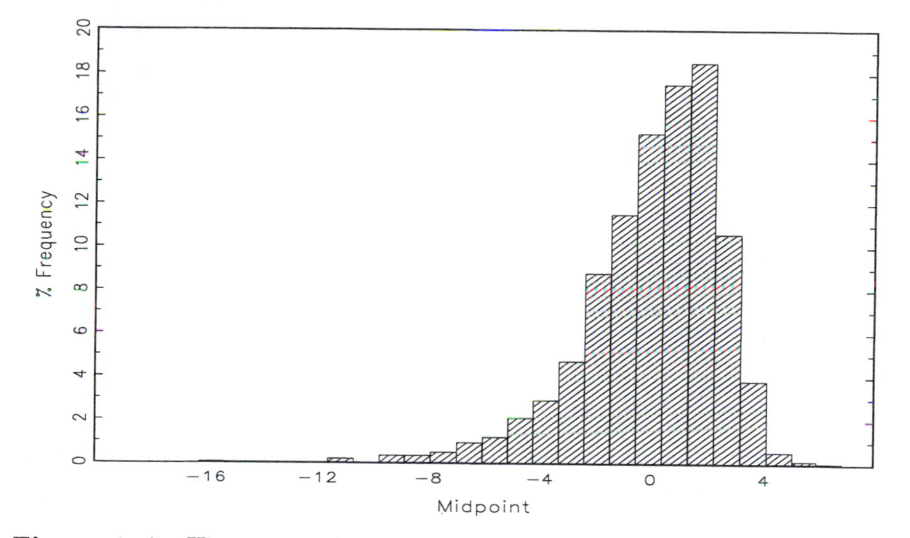


**Figure 4.17:** Histogram of the residuals from the model fit from the NYSE example.

patients with high blood pressure, and the systolic and diastolic blood pressures (SBP and DBP) are recorded at equal time intervals, for some time, using an ambulatory device. We may think of $\boldsymbol{y}_{t\ell}$ as being the bivariate, $k = 2$, recordings of SBP and DBP at time $t$ for person $\ell$. It is also reasonable to assume, in this example, exogenous variables may have been collected on each subject to help explain the variation in blood pressure (for example, gender, race, age, activity, and so on). We might expect to encounter missing data or irregularly spaced observations in this type of experiment; these problems are easier to handle from a state-space perspective.

An extension of the ARMAX model given in (4.16) that might handle the

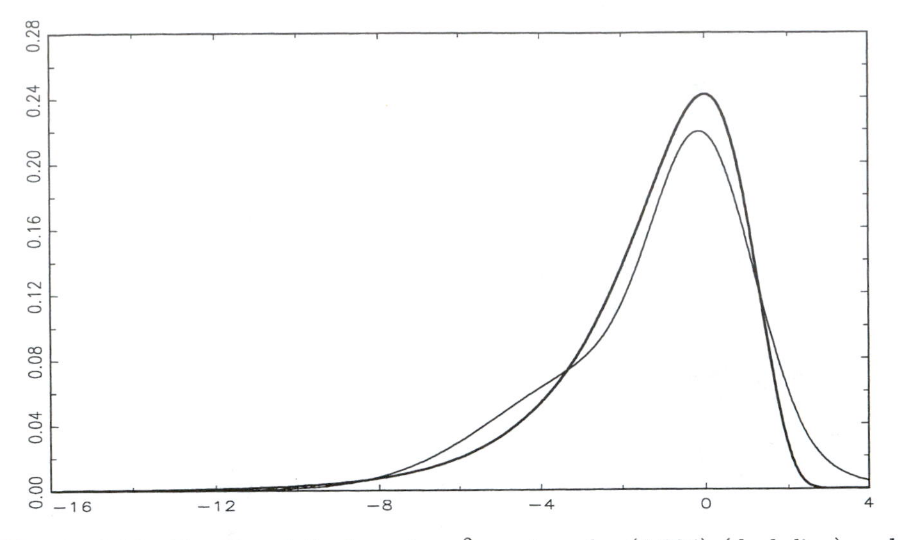


**Figure 4.18:** Density of the log of a $\chi_1^2$ as given by (4.194) (dark line) and the fitted normal mixture (thin line) form the NYSE example.

case of cross-sectional data, $\boldsymbol{y}_{t\ell}$, is

$$\boldsymbol{y}_{t\ell} = \Gamma \boldsymbol{u}_{t\ell} + \sum_{j=1}^{p} \Phi_j \boldsymbol{y}_{t-j,\ell} + \sum_{j=1}^{q} \Theta_j \boldsymbol{w}_{t-j,\ell} + \boldsymbol{w}_{t\ell}, \tag{4.198}$$

where, for $\ell = 1, ..., N$, $\text{var}(\boldsymbol{w}_{t\ell}) = \Sigma_w$ and $\boldsymbol{u}_{t\ell}$ represents the $r \times 1$ vector of exogenous variables. As in Section 4.6, Property P4.6, we can write (4.198) in terms of a state-space model. That is, for $\ell = 1, ..., N$,

$$\boldsymbol{x}_{t+1,\ell} = F\boldsymbol{x}_{t,\ell} + G\boldsymbol{w}_{t,\ell}, \tag{4.199}$$

$$\boldsymbol{y}_{t,\ell} = [I, 0, \cdots, 0]\boldsymbol{x}_{t\ell} + \Gamma \boldsymbol{u}_{t\ell} + \boldsymbol{w}_{t\ell}, \tag{4.200}$$

where matrices $F$ and $G$ are as in (4.109), $\boldsymbol{x}_{t,\ell}$ represents the unobserved state, and $\boldsymbol{y}_{t,\ell}$ is the observation at time $t$, replication $\ell$. Maximum likelihood estimation for state space models with cross-sectional data, such as the example given here, was investigated by Goodrich and Caines (1979), and can be carried out with minor modifications to the methods described in Section 4.3. In particular, given data $\boldsymbol{y}_{t,\ell}$, $t = 1, ..., n$, $\ell = 1, ..., N$, we can use Newton–Raphson to minimize the criterion function, which is, up to a constant term, proportional to the negative of the log likelihood function

$$l(\Theta) = N^{-1} \sum_{\ell=1}^{N} \left( \sum_{t=1}^{n} \log\left|\Sigma_{t,\ell}(\Theta)\right| + \sum_{t=1}^{n} \epsilon_{t,\ell}(\Theta)' \Sigma_{t,\ell}(\Theta)^{-1} \epsilon_{t,\ell}(\Theta) \right), \tag{4.201}$$

where $\epsilon_{t,\ell}(\Theta)$ and $\Sigma_{t,\ell}(\Theta)$ are the innovations and their variance–covariance matrices, respectively. For details, see Goodrich and Caines (1979).

Anderson (1978) did an extensive study of ***replicated ARX*** models, that is, the case in which $q = 0$ in (4.198). We can write this model using regression notation as

$$\boldsymbol{y}_{t\ell} = \mathcal{B}\boldsymbol{z}_{t\ell} + \boldsymbol{w}_{t\ell}, \tag{4.202}$$

for $\ell = 1, ..., N$ and $t = p + 1, ..., n$, where

$$\boldsymbol{z}_{t\ell} = (\boldsymbol{u}'_{t\ell}, \boldsymbol{y}'_{t-1,\ell}, ..., \boldsymbol{y}'_{t-p,\ell})' \tag{4.203}$$

and the matrix of regression coefficients is

$$\mathcal{B} = [\Gamma, \Phi_1, \Phi_2, ..., \Phi_p]. \tag{4.204}$$

The estimate of the regression matrix $\mathcal{B}$ in this case is

$$\widehat{\mathcal{B}} = \left(\sum_{\ell=1}^{N}\sum_{t=p+1}^{n} \boldsymbol{y}_{t\ell}\boldsymbol{z}'_{t\ell}\right)\left(\sum_{\ell=1}^{N}\sum_{t=p+1}^{n} \boldsymbol{z}_{t\ell}\boldsymbol{z}'_{t\ell}\right)^{-1}, \tag{4.205}$$

and an estimate of $\Sigma_w$ is

$$\widehat{\Sigma}_w = \frac{1}{N(n-p)}\sum_{\ell=1}^{N}\sum_{t=p+1}^{n}(\boldsymbol{y}_{t\ell} - \widehat{\mathcal{B}}\boldsymbol{z}_{t\ell})(\boldsymbol{y}_{t\ell} - \widehat{\mathcal{B}}\boldsymbol{z}_{t\ell})'. \tag{4.206}$$

Inference for $\widehat{\mathcal{B}}$ follows as in multivariate regression. That is, the large sample standard error of the $ij$-th element of $\mathcal{B}$ is $\sqrt{\widehat{\sigma}_{jj}c_{ii}}$, where $\widehat{\sigma}_{jj}$ is the $j$-th diagonal element of $\widehat{\Sigma}_w$ and $c_{ii}$ is the $i$-th diagonal element of

$$\left(\sum_{\ell=1}^{N}\sum_{t=p+1}^{n} \boldsymbol{z}_{t\ell}\boldsymbol{z}'_{t\ell}\right)^{-1}.$$

Model (4.198) may be somewhat restrictive in its assumption that the parameters do not change over time. Because replications exist, extending the model to the case of ***time-varying parameters*** is easy. The case of time-varying parameters in (4.202) was also presented in Anderson (1978). In particular, the model is written as

$$\boldsymbol{y}_{t\ell} = \Gamma_t\boldsymbol{u}_{t\ell} + \sum_{j=1}^{p_t}\Phi_{tj}\boldsymbol{y}_{t-j,\ell} + \boldsymbol{w}_{t\ell}, \tag{4.207}$$

and $\text{var}(\boldsymbol{w}_{t\ell}) = \Sigma_t$, for $\ell = 1, ..., N$. The order of the model, $p_t$, is also allowed to vary with time, and the equal spacing of time is not required. Of course, we can still use regression for estimation because the time-varying model can be written as $n$ regressions, one for each point in time,

$$\boldsymbol{y}_{t\ell} = \mathcal{B}_t\boldsymbol{z}_{t\ell} + \boldsymbol{w}_{t\ell}, \tag{4.208}$$

for $\ell = 1, ..., N$, where $z_{t\ell}$ is as in (4.203), but with $p$ replaced by $p_t$, and where now,

$$\mathcal{B}_t = [\Gamma_t, \Phi_{t1}, \Phi_{t2}, ..., \Phi_{tp_t}], \tag{4.209}$$

assuming $t > p_t$. The estimate of $\mathcal{B}_t$, for any time $t$, is now given by

$$\widehat{\mathcal{B}}_t = \left(\sum_{\ell=1}^{N} \boldsymbol{y}_{t\ell}\boldsymbol{z}'_{t\ell}\right)\left(\sum_{\ell=1}^{N} \boldsymbol{z}_{t\ell}\boldsymbol{z}'_{t\ell}\right)^{-1}, \tag{4.210}$$

and an estimate of $\Sigma_t$ is

$$\widehat{\Sigma}_t = \frac{1}{N - p_t - 1}\sum_{\ell=1}^{N}(\boldsymbol{y}_{t\ell} - \widehat{\mathcal{B}}_t\boldsymbol{z}_{t\ell})(\boldsymbol{y}_{t\ell} - \widehat{\mathcal{B}}_t\boldsymbol{z}_{t\ell})'. \tag{4.211}$$

**Example 4.22 The Effect of Prenatal Smoking on Growth**

In this example, we use data taken from an epidemiologic study at the University of Pittsburgh that focused on the effects of substance use during pregnancy. In particular, we focus on the growth of $N = 318$ children followed from birth to six years of age. In this longitudinal study, the children were examined at birth ($t = 0$), and at eight months ($t = 1$), 18 months ($t = 2$), 36 months ($t = 3$), and 72 months ($t = 4$) of age. At times $t = 1, 2, 3, 4$, a growth index, say, $y_{t\ell}$, was calculated for each child $\ell = 1, ..., 318$. The growth index is essentially a standardized score for a child's weight adjusting for that child's age, gender, and height, against the national averages. At birth, $y_{0\ell}$ represents the standardized birthweight of child $\ell$.

We might consider that children not prenatally exposed to teratogens would follow a certain growth curve, whereas exposed children would follow another. To investigate this hypothesis, we propose the following time-varying ARX model for growth:

$$\begin{aligned} y_{t\ell} &= \gamma_{0t} + \gamma_{1t}S_\ell + \gamma_{2t}R_\ell + \gamma_{3t}S_\ell R_\ell \\ &+ \sum_{j=1}^{t}\phi_{tj}\,(y_{t-j,\ell} - \widehat{y}_{t-j,\ell}) + w_{t\ell}, \end{aligned} \tag{4.212}$$

for $t = 0, 1, 2, 3, 4$, where $\text{var}(w_{t\ell}) = \sigma_t^2$, for $\ell = 1, ..., 318$. The exogenous variables in the model are, $S_\ell$, the average number of cigarettes per day the mother smoked during the second trimester of pregnancy, and $R_\ell$, which indicates race (0 = black, 1 = white). The model is written in terms of the innovation sequences, $(y_{t-j,\ell} - \widehat{y}_{t-j,\ell})$, where $\widehat{y}_{t,\ell}$ is the prediction of $y_{t,\ell}$ from the previous model. We did this to remove any effect of smoking or race on previous growth. Figure 4.19 shows the average growth scores over time for four groups: 68 black children not exposed

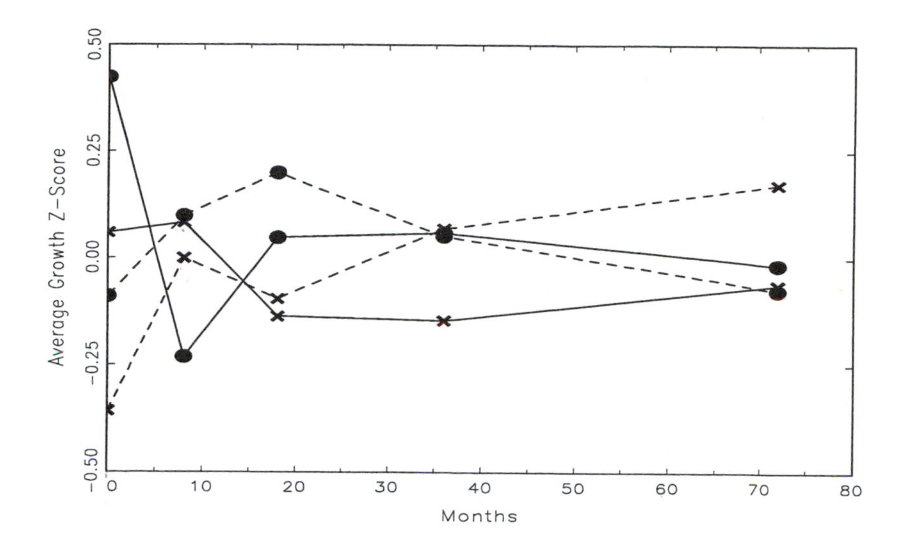


**Figure 4.19:** Average growth scores across time for four groups of children. A solid line represents children not prenatally exposed to cigarette smoke; a dashed line represents children prenatally exposed to cigarette smoke. A circle represents white children, and a cross represents black children.

to smoke prenatally (solid line-cross), 92 white children not exposed to smoke (solid line-circle), 83 black children exposed to smoke (dashed line-cross), and 75 white children exposed to smoke (dashed line-circle). For display purposes in Figure 4.19, smoking has been dichotomized to no exposure versus any exposure, but in the analysis, the smoking variable is in average cigarettes per day.

For example, the model for birthweight, $t = 0$, is

$$y_{0\ell} = \gamma_{00} + \gamma_{10} S_\ell + \gamma_{20} R_\ell + \gamma_{30} S_\ell R_\ell + w_{0\ell}.$$

Once the model has been estimated, the predicted values are calculated

$$\widehat{y}_{0\ell} = \widehat{\gamma}_{00} + \widehat{\gamma}_{10} S_\ell + \widehat{\gamma}_{20} R_\ell + \widehat{\gamma}_{30} S_\ell R_\ell.$$

Then, the model for growth at eight months, $t = 1$, is

$$y_{1\ell} = \gamma_{01} + \gamma_{11} S_\ell + \gamma_{21} R_\ell + \gamma_{31} S_\ell R_\ell + \phi_{11}(y_{0,\ell} - \widehat{y}_{0,\ell}) + w_{1\ell},$$

where $(y_{0,\ell} - \widehat{y}_{0,\ell})$ represents birthweight with the effect of smoking and race removed. In this way, only $S_\ell$ represents smoking and $R_\ell$ represents race, because their effect on birthweight has been removed. The other cases, for $t = 2, 3, 4$ continue in the same way.

The following estimates are the results of the fit; we only report the final models. At ***birth***,

$$\widehat{y}_{0\ell} = 3.295 - 0.011_{(.002)}S_\ell + 0.215_{(.056)}R_\ell,$$

with $\widehat{\sigma}_0 = 0.472$; estimated standard errors are shown in parenthesis. We conclude that prenatal smoking significantly reduces birthweight, white babies are born slightly bigger, and no interaction exists between smoking and race. At ***eight months***,

$$\begin{aligned}\widehat{y}_{1\ell} &= -0.015_{(.011)}S_\ell - 0.335_{(.147)}R_\ell \\ &+ 0.029_{(.012)}S_\ell R_\ell + 0.214_{(.127)}(y_{0,\ell} - \widehat{y}_{0,\ell}),\end{aligned}$$

with $\widehat{\sigma}_1 = 1.066$. The interaction term is significant, indicating that white, unexposed babies are slightly smaller than the others.

The estimated model for ***18 months*** is,

$$\begin{aligned}\widehat{y}_{2\ell} &= 0.340 + 0.278_{(.125)}R_\ell \\ &+ 0.661_{(.056)}(y_{1,\ell} - \widehat{y}_{1,\ell}) + 0.357_{(.126)}(y_{0,\ell} - \widehat{y}_{0,\ell}),\end{aligned}$$

with $\widehat{\sigma}_2 = 1.059$. Now, the effect of prenatal smoking is gone at 18 months, and, at this age, the white kids tend to be larger. The result at ***36 months*** ($t = 3$) is that prenatal smoking becomes significant again, but exposed children are slightly bigger at this age, and race is no longer significant (this result is not as unusual as it might seem; in fact, it has been hypothesized that children exposed prenatally to cigarette smoke tend to become obese as they grow older):

$$\begin{aligned}\widehat{y}_{3\ell} &= 0.334 + 0.008_{(0.004)}S_\ell + 0.310_{(0.044)}(y_{2,\ell} - \widehat{y}_{2,\ell}) \\ &+ 0.450_{(.043)}(y_{1,\ell} - \widehat{y}_{1,\ell}) + 0.465_{(.098)}(y_{0,\ell} - \widehat{y}_{0,\ell}),\end{aligned}$$

with $\widehat{\sigma}_2 = 0.817$. Finally, the result for ***72 months*** is

$$\begin{aligned}\widehat{y}_{4\ell} &= 0.330 + 0.933_{(0.082)}(y_{3,\ell} - \widehat{y}_{3,\ell}) \\ &+ 0.462_{(.063)}(y_{2,\ell} - \widehat{y}_{2,\ell}) + 0.484_{(.062)}(y_{1,\ell} - \widehat{y}_{1,\ell}),\end{aligned}$$

with $\widehat{\sigma}_2 = 1.176$. At this age, the effect of prenatal smoking and the effect of race are gone. Also growth at eight months ($t = 1$) is still a predictor of growth at 72 months, but the effect of birthweight ($t = 0$) is gone.

MIXED LINEAR MODELS IN STATE-SPACE FORM

A widely used general mixed model for longitudinal data was introduced by Laird and Ware (1982). In this case, responses $\boldsymbol{y}_\ell = \{y_{t,\ell}, t = 1, ..., n_\ell\}$ are obtained on $N$ subjects, $\ell = 1, ..., N$. Each response vector is modeled as

$$\boldsymbol{y}_\ell = X_\ell \boldsymbol{\beta} + Z_\ell \boldsymbol{\gamma}_\ell + \boldsymbol{\epsilon}_\ell, \tag{4.213}$$

where $X_\ell$ is an $n_\ell \times b$ design matrix, $\boldsymbol{\beta}$ is a $b \times 1$ vector of fixed parameters, and $Z_\ell$ is an $n_\ell \times g$ design matrix corresponding to the random $g \times 1$ vector of random effects, $\boldsymbol{\gamma}_\ell$, which is assumed to be independent across subject, and distributed as $\boldsymbol{\gamma}_\ell \sim \mathrm{N}(\mathbf{0}, D)$, where $D > 0$ is an arbitrary variance–covariance matrix. The within-subject errors, $\boldsymbol{\epsilon}_\ell$, are independently distributed as $\boldsymbol{\epsilon}_\ell \sim \mathrm{N}(\mathbf{0}, \Sigma_\ell)$; often, $\Sigma_\ell$ is of the form $\sigma^2 I$. A good introduction to these models can be found in many texts; for example, Diggle et al (1994), Jones (1993), and Fahrmeir and Tutz (1994). Jones (1993) focuses on the state-space approach, and so will we.

The model, (4.213), can be written as

$$\boldsymbol{y}_\ell \sim \mathrm{N}\left(X_\ell \boldsymbol{\beta}, V_\ell\right), \tag{4.214}$$

independently, for $\ell = 1, ..., N$, where

$$V_\ell = Z_\ell D Z_\ell' + \Sigma_\ell. \tag{4.215}$$

An example of a typical covariance structure for $V_\ell$ is ***compound symmetry***, wherein $g = 1$, $Z_\ell$ is a vector of ones, $D = \sigma_\gamma^2$ is a scalar, and $\Sigma_\ell = \sigma^2 I$. In this way, $V_\ell$ is an $n_\ell \times n_\ell$ matrix given by

$$V_\ell = \begin{pmatrix} \sigma^2 + \sigma_\gamma^2 & \sigma_\gamma^2 & \dots & \sigma_\gamma^2 \\ \sigma_\gamma^2 & \sigma^2 + \sigma_\gamma^2 & \dots & \sigma_\gamma^2 \\ \vdots & \vdots & \ddots & \vdots \\ \sigma_\gamma^2 & \sigma_\gamma^2 & \dots & \sigma^2 + \sigma_\gamma^2 \end{pmatrix}. \tag{4.216}$$

Another useful covariance structure is the autoregressive structure, where $g = 0$ (that is, no random effects exist) and

$$V_\ell = \Sigma_\ell = \sigma^2 \begin{pmatrix} 1 & \rho & \rho^2 & \dots & \rho^{n_\ell - 1} \\ \rho & 1 & \rho & \dots & \rho^{n_\ell - 2} \\ \vdots & \vdots & \ddots & & \vdots \\ \rho^{n_\ell - 1} & \rho^{n_\ell - 2} & & \dots & 1 \end{pmatrix}, \tag{4.217}$$

with $|\rho| < 1$. This type, and more general types of models were discussed in Section 2.13.

For a particular subject, $\ell$, the vector $\boldsymbol{y}_\ell$ consists of observations, $y_{t\ell}$, taken over time $t = 1, 2, ..., n_\ell$. For subject $\ell$, model (4.213) states

$$y_{t\ell} = \boldsymbol{x}_{t\ell}' \boldsymbol{\beta} + \boldsymbol{z}_{t\ell}' \boldsymbol{\gamma}_\ell + \epsilon_{t\ell}, \tag{4.218}$$

where $\boldsymbol{x}'_{t\ell}$ is the $t$-th row of $X_\ell$ and $z'_{t\ell}$ is the $t$-th row of $Z_\ell$. Using the form of the model given by (4.218), $y_{t\ell}$ is normal with

$$\begin{aligned} E(y_{t\ell}) &= \boldsymbol{x}'_{t\ell}\boldsymbol{\beta}, \\ \text{cov}(y_{t\ell}, y_{s\ell}) &= z'_{t\ell} D z_{s\ell} + \sigma_{\ell,ts}, \\ \text{cov}(y_{t\ell}, y_{sk}) &= 0 \qquad \ell \neq k, \end{aligned}$$

where $\sigma_{\ell,ts}$ is the $ts$-th element of $\Sigma_\ell$. For the example given in (4.216), we would have

$$\text{var}(y_{t\ell}) = \sigma^2 + \sigma^2_\gamma \quad \text{and} \quad \text{cov}(y_{t\ell}, y_{s\ell}) = \sigma^2_\gamma,$$

for any $t \neq s$, so the correlation between two observations on the same subject is given by $\rho = \sigma^2_\gamma/(\sigma^2 + \sigma^2_\gamma)$. In the autoregressive case, (4.217), the correlation between two observations $y_{t\ell}$ and $y_{s\ell}$ on the same subject $t-s$ time units apart is, of course, $\rho^{|t-s|}$.

The Laird–Ware model has a state space formulation; Jones (1993) provides a detailed presentation of these and related topics. If random effects exist, that is $g \geq 1$, and $\Sigma_\ell = \sigma^2 I$, let $\boldsymbol{s}_{t,\ell}$ denote a $g \times 1$ state vector with initial condition $\boldsymbol{s}_{0,\ell} \sim \text{N}(\boldsymbol{0}, D)$. Then, for each $\ell = 1, ..., N$, (4.218) can be written as

$$\boldsymbol{s}_{t,\ell} = \boldsymbol{s}_{t-1,\ell} + \boldsymbol{w}_{t,\ell}, \tag{4.219}$$

$$y_{t\ell} = \boldsymbol{x}'_{t\ell}\boldsymbol{\beta} + z'_{t\ell}\boldsymbol{s}_{t,\ell} + \epsilon_{t\ell}, \tag{4.220}$$

for $t = 1, ..., n_\ell$, where $\boldsymbol{w}_{t,\ell} \equiv \boldsymbol{0}$, or, equivalently, $\boldsymbol{w}_{t,\ell} \sim \text{N}(\boldsymbol{0}, Q)$, where $Q = 0$ is the zero matrix. All other values are as defined in (4.218). The data $y_{t\ell}$ as written in (4.219)-(4.220) have the same properties as the data written in (4.218).

If $g = 0$, that is, no random effects exist, and the variance–covariance structure is autoregressive, as in (4.217), the state-space model can be written as

$$s_{t\ell} = \rho s_{t-1,\ell} + w_{t,\ell}, \tag{4.221}$$

$$y_{t\ell} = \boldsymbol{x}'_{t\ell}\boldsymbol{\beta} + s_{t\ell}, \tag{4.222}$$

where, now, the autoregressive structure is entered into the data via the (scalar, in this example) state, and there is measurement error. In this case, $R = 0$, which does not present a problem in running the Kalman filter, provided $P_0^0 > 0$. To obtain a matrix of the form given in (4.217), $w_{t\ell}$ is white Gaussian noise, with $Q = \sigma^2$, and the initial state satisfies $s_{0,\ell} \sim \text{N}(0, \sigma^2/(1-\rho^2))$. In this case, recall the states, $s_{t\ell}$, for a given subject $\ell$, form a stationary AR(1) process with variance $\sigma^2/(1-\rho^2)$ and ACF given by $\rho(h) = \rho^{|h|}$.

In the more general case in which both random effects, $g > 0$, and an autoregressive error structure exist, we can combine the ideas used to get (4.219)-(4.220) and (4.221)-(4.222). In this case, the state equation would be a $(g+1) \times 1$ process made by stacking (4.219) and (4.221), and the observation equation would be

$$y_{t\ell} = \boldsymbol{x}'_{t\ell}\boldsymbol{\beta} + A_t s_{t\ell},$$

where $A_t = [z'_{t\ell}, 1]$.

We immediately see from (4.219)-(4.220), or from (4.221)-(4.222), that the likelihood of the data is the same as the one given in (4.201), but with $n$ set to $n_\ell$. Consequently, the methods presented in Section 4.3 can be used to estimate the parameters of the Laird–Ware model, namely, $\boldsymbol{\beta}$, and variance components in $V_\ell$, for $\ell = 1, ..., n_\ell$. For simplicity, let $\Theta$ represent the vector of all of the parameters associated with the model.

In the notation of the algorithm presented in Section 4.3, Step 1 is to find initial estimates, $\Theta^{(0)}$, of the parameters $\Theta$. If the $V_\ell$ were known, using a weighted least squares argument (see Section 2.13), the least squares estimate of $\boldsymbol{\beta}$ in the model (4.214)-(4.215) is given by

$$\widehat{\boldsymbol{\beta}} = \left(\sum_{\ell=1}^{N} X'_\ell V_\ell^{-1} X_\ell\right)^{-1} \left(\sum_{\ell=1}^{N} X'_\ell V_\ell^{-1} \boldsymbol{y}_\ell\right). \tag{4.223}$$

Initial guesses for $V_\ell$ should reflect the variance–covariance structure of the model. We can use (4.223) with the the initial values chosen for $V_\ell$ to obtain the initial regression coefficients, $\boldsymbol{\beta}^{(0)}$.

To accomplish Step 2 of the algorithm, for each $\ell = 1, ..., N$, run the Kalman filter (Property P4.1 with the states denoted by $\boldsymbol{s}_t$) for $t = 1, ...n_\ell$ to obtain the initial innovations and their covariance matrices. For example, if the model is of the form given in (4.219)-(4.220), run the Kalman filter with $\Phi = I$, $Q = 0$, $A_t = \boldsymbol{z}'_{t\ell}$, $R = [\sigma^{(0)}]^2$, and initial conditions $\boldsymbol{s}_0^0 = \boldsymbol{0}$, $P_0^0 = D^{(0)} > 0$. In addition, $y_{t\ell}$ replaced by $y_{t\ell} - \boldsymbol{x}'_{t\ell}\boldsymbol{\beta}^{(0)}$; this is also equivalent to running Property P4.6 with uncorrelated noises, wherein the rows of the fixed effects design matrix, $X_\ell$, are the exogenous variables. The Newton–Raphson procedure (steps 3 and 4 of the algorithm in Section 4.3) is performed on the criterion function given in (4.201).

### Example 4.23 Response to Medication

As a simple example of how we can use the state-space formulation of the Laird–Ware model, we analyze the S+ data set *drug.mult*. The data are taken from an experiment in which six subjects are given a dose of medication and then observed immediately and at weekly intervals for three weeks. The data are given in Table 4.8.

We fit model (4.221)-(4.222) to this data using gender as a grouping variable. In particular, if $\boldsymbol{y}_{t\ell}$ is the $4 \times 1$ vector of observations over time for a female ($\ell = 1, 2, 3$), the model is

$$\begin{pmatrix} y_1 \\ y_2 \\ y_3 \\ y_4 \end{pmatrix} = \begin{pmatrix} 1 & 0 \\ 1 & 0 \\ 1 & 0 \\ 1 & 0 \end{pmatrix} \begin{pmatrix} \beta_1 \\ \beta_2 \end{pmatrix} + \begin{pmatrix} \epsilon_1 \\ \epsilon_2 \\ \epsilon_3 \\ \epsilon_4 \end{pmatrix},$$

Table 4.8: Weekly Response to Medication

| | | Week 0 | Week 1 | Week 2 | Week 3 |
|---|---|---|---|---|---|
| $\ell$ | Gender | $y_1$ | $y_2$ | $y_3$ | $y_4$ |
| 1 | F | 75.9 | 74.3 | 80.0 | 78.9 |
| 2 | F | 78.3 | 75.5 | 79.6 | 79.2 |
| 3 | F | 80.3 | 78.2 | 80.4 | 76.2 |
| 4 | M | 80.7 | 77.2 | 82.0 | 83.8 |
| 5 | M | 80.3 | 78.6 | 81.4 | 81.5 |
| 6 | M | 80.1 | 81.1 | 81.9 | 86.4 |

and for a male ($\ell = 4, 5, 6$), the model is

$$\begin{pmatrix} y_1 \\ y_2 \\ y_3 \\ y_4 \end{pmatrix} = \begin{pmatrix} 1 & 1 \\ 1 & 1 \\ 1 & 1 \\ 1 & 1 \end{pmatrix} \begin{pmatrix} \beta_1 \\ \beta_2 \end{pmatrix} + \begin{pmatrix} \epsilon_1 \\ \epsilon_2 \\ \epsilon_3 \\ \epsilon_4 \end{pmatrix},$$

where the $\epsilon_t$, in general, form an AR(1) process given by

$$\begin{aligned} \epsilon_0 &= w_0/\sqrt{1-\rho^2}, \\ \epsilon_t &= \rho\epsilon_{t-1} + w_t \quad t = 1, 2, 3, 4, \end{aligned}$$

where $w_t$ is white Gaussian noise, with $\text{var}(w_t) = \sigma_w^2$. Recall $\text{var}(\epsilon_t) = \sigma_\epsilon^2 = \sigma_w^2/(1-\rho^2)$ and $\rho_\epsilon(h) = \rho^{|h|}$. A different value of $\rho$ was selected for each gender group, say, $\rho_1$ for female subjects and $\rho_2$ for male subjects. We initialized the estimation procedure with $\rho_1^{(0)} = \rho_2^{(0)} = 0$, $\sigma_w^{(0)} = 2$, which, upon using (4.223), yields $\boldsymbol{\beta}^{(0)} = (78.07, 3.18)'$. The final estimates (and their estimated standard errors) were

$$\widehat{\beta}_1 = 78.20(0.56), \quad \widehat{\beta}_2 = 3.24(0.89),$$

$$\widehat{\rho}_1 = -0.47(0.36), \quad \widehat{\rho}_2 = 0.07(0.53), \quad \widehat{\sigma}_w = 2.17(0.36).$$

Because $\widehat{\rho}_1$ and $\widehat{\rho}_2$ are not significantly different from zero, this would suggest either a simple linear regression is sufficient to describe the results, or the model is not correct.

Next, we fit the compound symmetry model using (4.219)-(4.220) with $g = 1$. In this case, the model for a female subject is

$$\begin{pmatrix} y_1 \\ y_2 \\ y_3 \\ y_4 \end{pmatrix} = \begin{pmatrix} 1 & 0 \\ 1 & 0 \\ 1 & 0 \\ 1 & 0 \end{pmatrix} \begin{pmatrix} \beta_1 \\ \beta_2 \end{pmatrix} + \begin{pmatrix} 1 \\ 1 \\ 1 \\ 1 \end{pmatrix} \gamma_1 + \begin{pmatrix} \epsilon_1 \\ \epsilon_2 \\ \epsilon_3 \\ \epsilon_4 \end{pmatrix},$$

and for a male subject, the model is

$$\begin{pmatrix} y_1 \\ y_2 \\ y_3 \\ y_4 \end{pmatrix} = \begin{pmatrix} 1 & 1 \\ 1 & 1 \\ 1 & 1 \\ 1 & 1 \end{pmatrix} \begin{pmatrix} \beta_1 \\ \beta_2 \end{pmatrix} + \begin{pmatrix} 1 \\ 1 \\ 1 \\ 1 \end{pmatrix} \gamma_2 + \begin{pmatrix} \epsilon_1 \\ \epsilon_2 \\ \epsilon_3 \\ \epsilon_4 \end{pmatrix},$$

where $\gamma_1 \sim \mathrm{N}(0, \sigma^2_{\gamma_1})$, $\gamma_2 \sim \mathrm{N}(0, \sigma^2_{\gamma_2})$, and the $\epsilon_t$, for $t = 1, 2, 3, 4$ are uncorrelated with variance $\sigma^2_\epsilon$.

In this case, the state variable is a scalar process with $D = \sigma^2_{\gamma_1}$ for female subjects ($\ell = 1, 2, 3$) and $D = \sigma^2_{\gamma_2}$ for male subjects ($\ell = 4, 5, 6$). Starting the estimation process off with $\sigma^{(0)}_{\gamma_1} = \sigma^{(0)}_{\gamma_2} = 1$, $\sigma^{(0)}_\epsilon = 2$, and $\boldsymbol{\beta}^{(0)} = (78, 3)'$, the final estimates were

$$\widehat{\beta}_1 = 78.03\,(0.67), \quad \widehat{\beta}_2 = 3.51\,(1.05),$$

$$\widehat{\sigma}_{\gamma_1} = 2.05\,(0.45), \quad \widehat{\sigma}_{\gamma_2} = 2.51\,(0.59), \quad \widehat{\sigma}_\epsilon = 2.00\,(0.13).$$

This model fits the data well.

## 4.12 Further Aspects of Multivariate ARMA and ARMAX Models

As discussed in Section 4.1, extending univariate AR (or pure MA) models to the vector case is fairly easy, but extending univariate ARMA models to the multivariate case is not a simple matter. Our discussion will be brief, but interested readers can get more details in Lütkepohl (1993) and Reinsel (1997).

We will change the notation slightly in this section to keep with convention. We will use $p$ and $q$ for the autoregressive and moving-average orders, and we assume we observe a $k$-dimensional vector series $\boldsymbol{x}_t = (x_{t,1}, ..., x_{t,k})'$. Recall a vector-valued time series $\boldsymbol{x}_t$, for $t = 0, \pm 1, \pm 2, ...$, is said to be ARMA($p, q$) if $\boldsymbol{x}_t$ is stationary and

$$\boldsymbol{x}_t = \boldsymbol{\alpha} + \Phi_1 \boldsymbol{x}_{t-1} + \cdots + \Phi_p \boldsymbol{x}_{t-p} + \boldsymbol{w}_t + \Theta_1 \boldsymbol{w}_{t-1} + \cdots + \Theta_q \boldsymbol{w}_{t-q}, \tag{4.224}$$

with $\Phi_p \neq \mathbf{0}$, $\Theta_q \neq \mathbf{0}$, and $\Sigma_w > 0$ (that is, $\Sigma_w$ is positive definite). Here, the coefficient matrices $\Phi_j$; $j = 1, ..., p$ and $\Theta_j$; $j = 1, ..., q$, and $\Sigma_w$ are $k \times k$ matrices. To ease the discussion, we will put $\boldsymbol{\alpha} = \mathbf{0}$ until we talk about estimation.

In the multivariate case, the ***autoregressive operator*** is

$$\Phi(B) = I - \Phi_1 B - \cdots - \Phi_p B^p, \tag{4.225}$$

and the ***moving average operator*** is

$$\Theta(B) = I + \Theta_1 B + \cdots + \Theta_q B^q, \tag{4.226}$$

The ARMA$(p, q)$ model is then written in the concise form as

$$\Phi(B)\boldsymbol{x}_t = \Theta(B)\boldsymbol{w}_t. \tag{4.227}$$

The model is said to be ***causal*** if the roots of $|\Phi(z)|$ (where $|\cdot|$ denotes determinant) are outside the unit circle, $|z| > 1$; that is, $|\Phi(z)| \neq 0$ for any value $z$ such that $|z| \leq 1$. In this case, we can write

$$\boldsymbol{x}_t = \Psi(B)\boldsymbol{w}_t,$$

where $\Psi(B) = \sum_{j=0}^{\infty} \Psi_j B^j$, $\Psi_0 = I$, and $\sum_{j=0}^{\infty} ||\Psi_j|| < \infty$. The model is said to be ***invertible*** if the roots of $|\Theta(z)|$ lie outside the unit circle. Then, we can write

$$\boldsymbol{w}_t = \Pi(B)\boldsymbol{x}_t,$$

where $\Pi(B) = \sum_{j=0}^{\infty} \Pi_j B^j$, $\Pi_0 = I$, and $\sum_{j=0}^{\infty} ||\Pi_j|| < \infty$. Analogous to the univariate case, we can determine the matrices $\Psi_j$ by solving $\Psi(z) = \Phi(z)^{-1}\Theta(z), |z| \leq 1$, and the matrices $\Pi_j$ by solving $\Pi(z) = \Theta(z)^{-1}\Phi(z), |z| \leq 1$.

For a causal model, we can write $\boldsymbol{x}_t = \Psi(B)\boldsymbol{w}_t$ so the general autocovariance structure of an ARMA$(p, q)$ model is

$$\Gamma(h) = \text{cov}(\boldsymbol{x}_{t+h}, \boldsymbol{x}_t) = E(\boldsymbol{x}_{t+h}\boldsymbol{x}_t') = \sum_{j=0}^{\infty} \Psi_{j+h}\Sigma_w \Psi_j'. \tag{4.228}$$

Note, $\Gamma(-h) = \Gamma'(h)$ so we will only exhibit the autocovariances for $h \geq 0$. For pure MA$(q)$ processes, (4.228) becomes

$$\Gamma(h) = \sum_{j=0}^{q-h} \Theta_{j+h}\Sigma_w \Theta_j', \tag{4.229}$$

where $\Theta_0 = I$. Of course, (4.229) implies $\Gamma(h) = 0$ for $h > q$. For pure AR$(p)$ models, the autocovariance structure leads to the multivariate version of the ***Yule–Walker equations***:

$$\Gamma(h) = \sum_{j=1}^{p} \Phi_j \Gamma(h - j), \quad h = 1, 2, ..., \tag{4.230}$$

$$\Gamma(0) = \sum_{j=1}^{p} \Phi_j \Gamma(-j) + \Sigma_w. \tag{4.231}$$

As in the univariate case, we will need conditions for model uniqueness. These conditions are similar to the condition in the univariate case the the autoregressive and moving average polynomials have no common factors. To explore the uniqueness problems that we encounter with multivariate ARMA models, consider a bivariate AR(1) process, $\boldsymbol{x}_t = (x_{t,1}, x_{t,2})'$, given by

$$\begin{aligned} x_{t,1} &= \phi x_{t-1,2} + w_{t,1}, \\ x_{t,2} &= w_{t,2}, \end{aligned}$$

where $w_{t,1}$ and $w_{t,2}$ are independent white noise processes and $|\phi| < 1$. Both processes, $x_{t,1}$ and $x_{t,2}$ are causal and invertible. Moreover, the processes are jointly stationary because $\text{cov}(x_{t+h,1}, x_{t,2}) = \phi\, \text{cov}(x_{t+h-1,2}, x_{t,2}) \equiv \phi\, \gamma_{2,2}(h-1) = \phi \sigma_{w_2}^2 \delta_1^h$ does not depend on $t$; note, $\delta_1^h = 1$ when $h = 1$, otherwise, $\delta_1^h = 0$. In matrix notation, we can write this model as

$$\boldsymbol{x}_t = \Phi \boldsymbol{x}_{t-1} + \boldsymbol{w}_t, \tag{4.232}$$

where

$$\Phi = \begin{bmatrix} 0 & \phi \\ 0 & 0 \end{bmatrix}.$$

We can write (4.232) in operator notation as

$$\Phi(B)\boldsymbol{x}_t = \boldsymbol{w}_t$$

where

$$\Phi(z) = \begin{bmatrix} 1 & -\phi z \\ 0 & 1 \end{bmatrix}.$$

In addition, model (4.232) can be written as a bivariate ARMA(1,1) model

$$\boldsymbol{x}_t = \Phi_1 \boldsymbol{x}_{t-1} + \Theta_1 \boldsymbol{w}_{t-1} + \boldsymbol{w}_t, \tag{4.233}$$

where

$$\Phi_1 = \begin{bmatrix} 0 & \phi + \theta \\ 0 & 0 \end{bmatrix} \quad \text{and} \quad \Theta_1 = \begin{bmatrix} 0 & -\theta \\ 0 & 0 \end{bmatrix},$$

and $\theta$ is arbitrary. To verify this, we write (4.233), as $\Phi_1(B)\boldsymbol{x}_t = \Theta_1(B)\boldsymbol{w}_t$, or

$$\Theta_1(B)^{-1}\Phi_1(B)\boldsymbol{x}_t = \boldsymbol{w}_t,$$

where

$$\Phi_1(z) = \begin{bmatrix} 1 & -(\phi+\theta)z \\ 0 & 1 \end{bmatrix} \quad \text{and} \quad \Theta_1(z) = \begin{bmatrix} 1 & -\theta z \\ 0 & 1 \end{bmatrix}.$$

Then,

$$\Theta_1(z)^{-1}\Phi_1(z) = \begin{bmatrix} 1 & \theta z \\ 0 & 1 \end{bmatrix} \begin{bmatrix} 1 & -(\phi+\theta)z \\ 0 & 1 \end{bmatrix} = \begin{bmatrix} 1 & -\phi z \\ 0 & 1 \end{bmatrix} = \Phi(z),$$

where $\Phi(z)$ is the polynomial associated with the bivariate AR(1) model in (4.232). Because $\theta$ is arbitrary, the parameters of the ARMA(1,1) model given in (4.233) are not identifiable. No problem exists, however, in fitting the AR(1) model given in (4.232).

The problem in the previous discussion was caused by the fact that both $\Theta(B)$ and $\Theta(B)^{-1}$ are finite; such a matrix operator is called ***unimodular***. If $U(B)$ is unimodular, $|U(z)|$ is constant. It is also possible for two seemingly different multivariate ARMA$(p,q)$ models, say, $\Phi(B)\boldsymbol{x}_t = \Theta(B)\boldsymbol{w}_t$ and $\Phi_*(B)\boldsymbol{x}_t = \Theta_*(B)\boldsymbol{w}_t$, to be related through a unimodular operator, $U(B)$ as $\Phi_*(B) = U(B)\Phi(B)$ and $\Theta_*(B) = U(B)\Theta(B)$, in such a way that the orders of $\Phi(B)$ and $\Theta(B)$ are the same as the orders of $\Phi_*(B)$ and $\Theta_*(B)$, respectively. For example, consider the bivariate ARMA(1,1) models given by

$$\Phi\boldsymbol{x}_t \equiv \begin{bmatrix} 1 & -\phi B \\ 0 & 1 \end{bmatrix} \boldsymbol{x}_t = \begin{bmatrix} 1 & \theta B \\ 0 & 1 \end{bmatrix} \boldsymbol{w}_t \equiv \Theta w_t$$

and

$$\Phi_*(B)\boldsymbol{x}_t \equiv \begin{bmatrix} 1 & (\alpha-\phi)B \\ 0 & 1 \end{bmatrix} \boldsymbol{x}_t = \begin{bmatrix} 1 & (\alpha+\theta)B \\ 0 & 1 \end{bmatrix} \boldsymbol{w}_t \equiv \Theta_*(B)\boldsymbol{w}_t,$$

where $\alpha$, $\phi$, and $\theta$ are arbitrary constants. Note,

$$\Phi_*(B) \equiv \begin{bmatrix} 1 & (\alpha-\phi)B \\ 0 & 1 \end{bmatrix} = \begin{bmatrix} 1 & \alpha B \\ 0 & 1 \end{bmatrix} \begin{bmatrix} 1 & -\phi B \\ 0 & 1 \end{bmatrix} \equiv U(B)\Phi(B)$$

and

$$\Theta_*(B) \equiv \begin{bmatrix} 1 & (\alpha+\theta)B \\ 0 & 1 \end{bmatrix} = \begin{bmatrix} 1 & \alpha B \\ 0 & 1 \end{bmatrix} \begin{bmatrix} 1 & \theta B \\ 0 & 1 \end{bmatrix} \equiv U(B)\Theta(B).$$

In this case, both models have the same infinite MA representation $\boldsymbol{x}_t = \Psi(B)\boldsymbol{w}_t$, where

$$\Psi(B) = \Phi(B)^{-1}\Theta(B) = \Phi(B)^{-1}U(B)^{-1}U(B)\Theta(B) = \Phi_*(B)^{-1}\Theta_*(B).$$

This result implies the two models have the same autocovariance function $\Gamma(h)$. Two such ARMA$(p,q)$ models are said to be ***observationally equivalent***.

As previously mentioned, in addition to requiring causality and invertiblity, we will need some additional assumptions in the multivariate case to make sure that the model is unique. To ensure the ***identifiability*** of the parameters of the multivariate ARMA$(p,q)$ model, we need the following additional two conditions: (i) the matrix operators $\Phi(B)$ and $\Theta(B)$ have no common left factors other than unimodular ones; that is, if $\Phi(B) = U(B)\Phi_*(B)$ and $\Theta(B) = U(B)\Theta_*(B)$, the common factor must be unimodular; and (ii) with $q$ as small as possible and $p$ as small as possible for that $q$, the matrix $[\Phi_p, \Theta_q]$ must be full rank, $k$. One suggestion for avoiding most of the aforementioned problems is to fit only vector AR$(p)$ models in multivariate situations. Althought this suggestion might be reasonable for many situations, this philosophy is not in accordance with law of parsimony because we might have to fit a large number of parameters to describe the dynamics of a process.

Analogous to the univariate case, we can define a sequence of matrices, $\Phi_{hh}$, for $h = 1, 2, ...$, called the ***partial autoregression matrices*** at lag $h$. These matrices are obtained by solving the Yule–Walker equations of order $h$, namely,

$$\Gamma(\ell) = \sum_{j=1}^{h} \Phi_{jh} \Gamma(\ell - j), \quad \ell = 1, 2, ..., h. \tag{4.234}$$

The partial autoregression matrices can be viewed as the result of successive AR($h$) fits to the data; that is,

$$\boldsymbol{x}_t = \sum_{j=1}^{h} \Phi_{jh} \boldsymbol{x}_{t-j} + \boldsymbol{w}_t, \quad h = 1, 2, ... \,. \tag{4.235}$$

If the process is truly an AR($p$), the partial autoregression matrices have the property that $\Phi_{pp} = \Phi_p$ and $\Phi_{hh} = 0$ for $h > p$. Unlike the univariate case, however, the elements of these matrices are not partial correlations, or correlations of any kind. As in the univariate case, the $\Phi_{hh}$ can be obtained iteratively using a multivariate extension of the Durbin-Levinson algorithm; details can be found in Reinsel (1997).

The partial canonical correlations can be viewed as the multivariate extension of the PACF in the univariate case. In general, the first ***canonical correlation***, $\lambda_1$, between the $k_1 \times 1$ random vector $\boldsymbol{X}_1$ and the $k_2 \times 1$ random vector $\boldsymbol{X}_2$, $k_1 \leq k_2$, with variance–covariance matrices $\Sigma_{11}$ and $\Sigma_{22}$, respectively, is the largest possible correlation between a linear combination of the components of $\boldsymbol{X}_1$, say, $\boldsymbol{\alpha}'\boldsymbol{X}_1$, and a linear combination of the components of $\boldsymbol{X}_2$, say, $\boldsymbol{\beta}'\boldsymbol{X}_2$, where $\boldsymbol{\alpha}$ is $k_1 \times 1$ and $\boldsymbol{\beta}$ is $k_2 \times 1$. That is,

$$\lambda_1 = \max_{\boldsymbol{\alpha}, \boldsymbol{\beta}} \text{ corr}\left(\boldsymbol{\alpha}'\boldsymbol{X}_1, \boldsymbol{\beta}'\boldsymbol{X}_2\right),$$

subject to the constraints $\text{var}(\boldsymbol{\alpha}'\boldsymbol{X}_1) = \boldsymbol{\alpha}'\Sigma_{11}\boldsymbol{\alpha} = 1$ and $\text{var}(\boldsymbol{\beta}'\boldsymbol{X}_2) = \boldsymbol{\beta}'\Sigma_{22}\boldsymbol{\beta} = 1$. If we let $\Sigma_{ij} = \text{cov}(\boldsymbol{X}_i, \boldsymbol{X}_j)$, for $i, j = 1, 2$, then $\lambda_1^2$ is the largest eigenvalue of the matrix $\Sigma_{11}^{-1}\Sigma_{12}\Sigma_{22}^{-1}\Sigma_{21}$; see Johnson and Wichern (1992, Chapter 10) for details. We call the solutions $U_1 = \boldsymbol{\alpha}_1'\boldsymbol{X}_1$ and $V_1 = \boldsymbol{\beta}_1'\boldsymbol{X}_2$ the first ***canonical variates***, that is, $\lambda_1 = \text{corr}(U_1, V_1)$, and $\boldsymbol{\alpha}_1$ and $\boldsymbol{\beta}_1$ are the coefficients of the linear combinations that maximize the correlation. In a similar fashion, the second canonical correlation, $\lambda_2$, is then the largest possible correlation between $\boldsymbol{\alpha}'\boldsymbol{X}_1$ and $\boldsymbol{\beta}'\boldsymbol{X}_2$ such that $\boldsymbol{\alpha}$ is orthogonal to $\boldsymbol{\alpha}_1$ (that is, $\boldsymbol{\alpha}'\boldsymbol{\alpha}_1 = 0$), and $\boldsymbol{\beta}$ is orthogonal to $\boldsymbol{\beta}_1$ ($\boldsymbol{\beta}'\boldsymbol{\beta}_1 = 0$) . If we call the solutions $U_2 = \boldsymbol{\alpha}_2'\boldsymbol{X}_1$ and $V_2 = \boldsymbol{\beta}_2'\boldsymbol{X}_2$, then $\text{corr}(U_1, U_2) = 0 = \text{corr}(V_1, V_2)$, $\text{corr}(U_i, V_j) = 0$ for $i \neq j$, and by design, $\lambda_1^2 \geq \lambda_2^2$. Also, $\lambda_2^2$ is the second largest eigenvalue of $\Sigma_{11}^{-1}\Sigma_{12}\Sigma_{22}^{-1}\Sigma_{21}$. Continuing this way, we obtain the squared canonical correlations $1 \geq \lambda_1^2 \geq \lambda_2^2 \geq \cdots \geq \lambda_{k_1}^2 \geq 0$ as the ordered eigenvalues of $\Sigma_{11}^{-1}\Sigma_{12}\Sigma_{22}^{-1}\Sigma_{21}$. The canonical correlations, $\lambda_j$, are typically taken to be nonnegative.

We can extend this idea to obtain ***partial canonical correlations*** between $\boldsymbol{X}_1$ and $\boldsymbol{X}_2$ given another random $k_3 \times 1$ vector $\boldsymbol{X}_3$. Let $\Sigma_{ij} = \text{cov}(\boldsymbol{X}_i, \boldsymbol{X}_j)$, for $i, j = 1, 2, 3$. The regression of $\boldsymbol{X}_1$ on $\boldsymbol{X}_3$ is $\Sigma_{13}\Sigma_{33}^{-1}\boldsymbol{X}_3$ so that $\boldsymbol{X}_{1|3} = \boldsymbol{X}_1 - \Sigma_{13}\Sigma_{33}^{-1}\boldsymbol{X}_3$ can be thought of as $\boldsymbol{X}_1$ with the linear effects of $\boldsymbol{X}_3$ removed (*partialled out*). Similarly, $\boldsymbol{X}_{2|3} = \boldsymbol{X}_2 - \Sigma_{23}\Sigma_{33}^{-1}\boldsymbol{X}_3$ can be thought of as $\boldsymbol{X}_2$ with the linear effects of $\boldsymbol{X}_3$ partialled out. The partial variance–covariance matrices are $\Sigma_{ij|3} = \text{cov}(\boldsymbol{X}_{i|3}, \boldsymbol{X}_{j|3}) = \Sigma_{ij} - \Sigma_{i3}\Sigma_{33}^{-1}\Sigma_{3j}$, for $i, j = 1, 2$. The squared partial canonical correlations between $\boldsymbol{X}_1$ and $\boldsymbol{X}_2$ given $\boldsymbol{X}_3$ are the ordered eigenvalues of $\Sigma_{11|3}^{-1}\Sigma_{12|3}\Sigma_{22|3}^{-1}\Sigma_{21|3}$.

For a stationary vector process $\boldsymbol{x}_t$, the partial canonical correlations at lag $h$, for $h = 2, 3, ...,$ denoted $\lambda_1(h) \geq \lambda_2(h) \geq \cdots \geq \lambda_k(h) \geq 0$, are defined to be the partial canonical correlations between $\boldsymbol{x}_h$ and $\boldsymbol{x}_0$ with the effects of $\boldsymbol{X} = (\boldsymbol{x}_{h-1}', ..., \boldsymbol{x}_1')'$ removed. For ease of notation, we put $r = h - 1$. Let $\Sigma_{00|X} = \Gamma(0) - \Gamma_1^{(r)}\Gamma_{r,r}^{-1}\Gamma_1^{(r)'}$, where $\Gamma_{r,r} = \{\Gamma(i-j)\}_{i,j=1}^r$ is a $kr \times kr$ symmetric matrix, and $\Gamma_1^{(r)} = [\Gamma(r)', \Gamma(r-1)', ..., \Gamma(1)']$ is $k \times kr$. Similarly, let $\Sigma_{hh|X} = \Gamma(0) - \Gamma_r^{(1)}\Gamma_{r,r}^{-1}\Gamma_r^{(1)'}$, where $\Gamma_r^{(1)} = [\Gamma(1), \Gamma(2), ..., \Gamma(r)]$ is $k \times kr$. Also needed are $\Sigma_{h0|X} = \Gamma(r) - \Gamma_r^{(1)}\Gamma_{r,r}^{-1}\Gamma_1^{(r)'}$ and $\Sigma_{0h|X} = \Sigma_{h0|X}'$. The squared partial canonical correlations, $\lambda_j^2(h)$, $j = 1, ..., k$ at lag $h$, $h = 2, 3, ...,$ are given by the ordered eigenvalues of $\Sigma_{00|X}^{-1}\Sigma_{0h|X}\Sigma_{hh|X}^{-1}\Sigma_{h0|X}$. The inversion of $\Gamma_{r,r}$, when $h$ is large will, be a problem; see Reinsel (1997) for methods that avoid having to invert $\Gamma_{r,r}$. Finally, we will define the partial canonical correlations between $\boldsymbol{x}_t$ and $\boldsymbol{x}_{t-1}$ to be the lag-one canonical correlations. In this case, $\lambda_j^2(1)$, $j = 1, ..., k$ are the ordered eigenvalues of $\Gamma(0)^{-1}\Gamma(1)\Gamma(0)^{-1}\Gamma(1)'$.

Prediction and estimation for identifiable multivariate ARMA models follow analogously to the univariate case, except in the general case, the estimation of the coefficient parameters and $\Sigma_w$ must be done simultaneously. Preliminary identification of the model uses the sample autocovariance matrices, the sample partial autoregression matrices, and the sample partial canonical correlations. We illustrate the techniques using the mortality data of Examples 2.2, 4.1, and 4.2.

**Example 4.24 Identification, Estimation and Prediction for the Mortality Series**

As in Example 4.2, we consider the trivariate series composed of detrended cardiovascular mortality $x_{t1}$, temperature $x_{t2}$, and particulate levels $x_{t3}$, and set $\boldsymbol{x}_t = (x_{t1}, x_{t2}, x_{t3})'$ as the three-dimensional data vector.

Estimation of the autocovariance matrix is similar to the univariate case, that is, with $\bar{\boldsymbol{x}} = n^{-1}\sum_{t=1}^n \boldsymbol{x}_t$, as an estimate of $\boldsymbol{\mu} = E\boldsymbol{x}_t$,

$$\widehat{\Gamma}(h) = n^{-1}\sum_{t=1}^{n-h}(\boldsymbol{x}_{t+h} - \bar{\boldsymbol{x}})(\boldsymbol{x}_t - \bar{\boldsymbol{x}})', \quad h = 0, 1, 2, .., n-1, \tag{4.236}$$

and $\widehat{\Gamma}(-h) = \widehat{\Gamma}(h)'$. If $\widehat{\gamma}_{i,j}(h)$ denotes the element in the $i$-th row and $j$-th column of $\widehat{\Gamma}(h)$, the cross-correlation functions (CCF), as discussed in (1.35), are estimated by

$$\widehat{\rho}_{i,j}(h) = \frac{\widehat{\gamma}_{i,j}(h)}{\sqrt{\widehat{\gamma}_{i,i}(0)}\sqrt{\widehat{\gamma}_{j,j}(0)}} \qquad h = 0, 1, 2, .., n-1. \tag{4.237}$$

When $i = j$ in (4.237), we get the estimated autocorrelation function (ACF) of the individual series. The first six estimated autocovariance matrices, $\widehat{\Gamma}(h)$, $h = 0, 1, ..., 5$, are (we have rounded the entries to integers to ease the display):

$$\widehat{\Gamma}(0) = \begin{bmatrix} 79 & -37 & 62 \\ -37 & 81 & -2 \\ 62 & -2 & 227 \end{bmatrix} \quad \widehat{\Gamma}(1) = \begin{bmatrix} 56 & -46 & 52 \\ -45 & 49 & -45 \\ 44 & -35 & 125 \end{bmatrix}$$

$$\widehat{\Gamma}(2) = \begin{bmatrix} 56 & -42 & 62 \\ -42 & 50 & -48 \\ 35 & -20 & 136 \end{bmatrix} \quad \widehat{\Gamma}(3) = \begin{bmatrix} 47 & -42 & 59 \\ -41 & 44 & -55 \\ 27 & -18 & 123 \end{bmatrix} \tag{4.238}$$

$$\widehat{\Gamma}(4) = \begin{bmatrix} 44 & -34 & 72 \\ -39 & 46 & -53 \\ 16 & -9 & 120 \end{bmatrix} \quad \widehat{\Gamma}(5) = \begin{bmatrix} 38 & -35 & 68 \\ -39 & 39 & -67 \\ 7 & 3 & 104 \end{bmatrix}.$$

Inspecting the autocovariance matrices, we find mortality, $x_{t1}$, and temperature, $x_{t2}$, are negatively correlated at about the same strength for both positive and negative lags. The strongest cross-correlation occurs at lag $\pm 1$, where $\widehat{\rho}_{12}(-1) \approx -45/\sqrt{79}\sqrt{81} = -0.56$, and $\widehat{\rho}_{12}(1) \approx -46/\sqrt{79}\sqrt{81} = -0.58$. Also, mortality $x_{t1}$ and particulates $x_{t3}$ are positively correlated, the strongest correlation being when particulates leads mortality by about one month, $\widehat{\rho}_{13}(4) \approx 72/\sqrt{79}\sqrt{227} = 0.54$. Finally, we note that particulates and temperature are negatively correlated, the strongest displayed value (which is approximately the strongest overall correlation between the two series) is when particulates leads temperature by about five weeks, $\widehat{\rho}_{23}(5) \approx -67/\sqrt{81}\sqrt{227} = 0.49$. The autocovariance matrices do not cut off at any small lag, and hence a pure moving average model is not indicated.

Replacing $\Gamma(h)$ by $\widehat{\Gamma}(h)$ in (4.234), we can obtain estimates of the partial autoregession matrices. The first four estimated matrices are

$$\widehat{\Phi}_{11} = \begin{bmatrix} 0.47 & -0.36 & 0.10 \\ -0.25 & 0.49 & -0.13 \\ -0.12 & -0.48 & 0.58 \end{bmatrix} \quad \widehat{\Phi}_{22} = \begin{bmatrix} 0.27 & -0.08 & 0.07 \\ -0.04 & 0.35 & -0.09 \\ -0.33 & 0.05 & 0.38 \end{bmatrix}$$

$$\widehat{\Phi}_{33} = \begin{bmatrix} -0.04 & 0.02 & -0.01 \\ 0.00 & 0.11 & -0.03 \\ -0.21 & 0.07 & 0.17 \end{bmatrix} \quad \widehat{\Phi}_{44} = \begin{bmatrix} -0.04 & 0.08 & 0.06 \\ -0.07 & 0.17 & 0.01 \\ -0.26 & 0.12 & 0.13 \end{bmatrix}.$$

As explained above (4.235), we can use (4.234) to estimate successive AR($h$) models with parameter estimates $\widehat{\Phi}_j = \widehat{\Phi}_{jh}$, $j = 1, ..., h$, and $h = 1, 2, ....$ Note, $\widehat{\Phi}_{11}$ is practically the same as $\widehat{\Phi}$ in Example 4.1, and $\widehat{\Phi}_{22}$ is practically the same as $\widehat{\Phi}_2$ in Example 4.2. The only difference in the estimates is that we are using Yule–Walker here, whereas regression was used in the other examples. These matrices contain small components after lag two, indicating the AR(2) relationship, although there is evidence of of some relationship between mortality and particulates at lags of three and four weeks.

The estimated autocovariance matrices can also be used to obtain estimates of the partial canonical correlations. For example, to estimate the lag $h = 3$ partial canonical correlations, $\{\widehat{\lambda}_1^2(3), \widehat{\lambda}_2^2(3), \widehat{\lambda}_3^2(3)\}$, we would put

$$\widehat{\Gamma}_{22} = \begin{bmatrix} \widehat{\Gamma}(0) & \widehat{\Gamma}(1) \\ \widehat{\Gamma}(1)' & \widehat{\Gamma}(0) \end{bmatrix}, \tag{4.239}$$

which represents, in this case, a $6 \times 6$ matrix of the estimated autocovariances that were displayed in (4.238). In addition, we will need the matrices

$$\widehat{\Gamma}_1^{(2)} = \left[\widehat{\Gamma}(2)', \widehat{\Gamma}(1)'\right] \quad \text{and} \quad \widehat{\Gamma}_2^{(1)} = \left[\widehat{\Gamma}(1), \widehat{\Gamma}(2)\right],$$

which are both, in this example, $3 \times 6$ matrices. From these matrices, we construct the $3 \times 3$ matrices

$$\widehat{\Sigma}_{00|21} = \widehat{\Gamma}(0) - \widehat{\Gamma}_1^{(2)} \widehat{\Gamma}_{22}^{-1} \widehat{\Gamma}_1^{(2)'},$$

$$\widehat{\Sigma}_{33|21} = \widehat{\Gamma}(0) - \widehat{\Gamma}_2^{(1)} \widehat{\Gamma}_{22}^{-1} \widehat{\Gamma}_2^{(1)'},$$

and

$$\widehat{\Sigma}_{30|21} = \widehat{\Gamma}(2) - \widehat{\Gamma}_2^{(1)} \widehat{\Gamma}_{22}^{-1} \widehat{\Gamma}_1^{(2)'} = \widehat{\Sigma}'_{03|21}.$$

Finally, the squared partial canonical correlations, $\lambda_j^2(3)$, for $j = 1, 2, 3$, are obtained as the ordered eigenvalues of $\widehat{\Sigma}_{00|21}^{-1} \widehat{\Sigma}_{03|21} \widehat{\Sigma}_{33|21}^{-1} \widehat{\Sigma}_{33|21}$. In this example we obtain

$$\left(\widehat{\lambda}_1^2(h), \widehat{\lambda}_2^2(h), \widehat{\lambda}_3^2(h)\right) = \begin{cases} (0.81, 0.24, 0.02) & h = 1 \\ (0.22, 0.14, 0.06) & h = 2 \\ (0.05, 0.01, 0.00) & h = 3 \\ (0.05, 0.02, 0.00) & h = 4, \end{cases}$$

which also suggests an AR(2) model for the data.

In addition, successive Yule–Walker estimates, for $h = 1, 2, ...,$ of the error variance–covariance matrix can be obtained from (4.231), that is,

$$\widehat{\Sigma}_w^{(h)} = \widehat{\Gamma}(0) - \sum_{j=1}^{h} \widehat{\Phi}_{jh} \widehat{\Gamma}(-j). \tag{4.240}$$

For this data, we obtained (entries are rounded to integers)

$$\widehat{\Sigma}_w^{(1)} = \begin{bmatrix} 31 & 6 & 17 \\ 6 & 41 & 42 \\ 17 & 42 & 144 \end{bmatrix}, \quad \widehat{\Sigma}_w^{(2)} = \begin{bmatrix} 28 & 7 & 16 \\ 7 & 37 & 40 \\ 16 & 40 & 123 \end{bmatrix},$$

$$\widehat{\Sigma}_w^{(3)} = \begin{bmatrix} 28 & 7 & 16 \\ 7 & 37 & 40 \\ 16 & 40 & 118 \end{bmatrix}, \quad \widehat{\Sigma}_w^{(4)} = \begin{bmatrix} 27 & 6 & 14 \\ 6 & 36 & 38 \\ 14 & 38 & 114 \end{bmatrix}.$$

The estimates stabilize (except for perhaps the variance of the particulate series) after $h = 2$, indicating the AR(3) and AR(4) fits do not improve much over the AR(2) fit. Recall the comparison of the autoregressions of order one to five using the SIC, as reported in Table 4.1 also indicated the AR(2) model.

At this point, we would settle on the AR(2) model estimated in Example 4.2 on the detrended data. We will write the estimated model as

$$\widehat{\boldsymbol{x}}_t = \widehat{\Phi}_1 \boldsymbol{x}_{t-1} + \widehat{\Phi}_2 x_{t-2} + \widehat{\boldsymbol{w}}_t, \tag{4.241}$$

where $\widehat{\Phi}_1$ and $\widehat{\Phi}_2$ are given in Example 4.2. The estimate of $\Sigma_w$ for this model is $\widehat{\Sigma}_w^{(2)}$, which is listed below (4.240). Residual analysis, performed on the residuals $\widehat{\boldsymbol{w}}_t = \widehat{\boldsymbol{x}}_t - \widehat{\Phi}_1 \boldsymbol{x}_{t-1} - \widehat{\Phi}_2 \boldsymbol{x}_{t-2}$, for t=3,...,508, suggests the model fits well. Individual residual analyses on the $\widehat{\boldsymbol{w}}_{ti}$, for $i = 1, 2, 3$, show, except for the particulate series, $w_{t3}$, the residuals are Gaussian white noise. For the particualte series, a small, but significant, amount of autocorrelation is still left in that series. In this case, we may wish to fit a higher order (higher than two) model to the particulate series only. In addition, we might be inclined to fit a reduced rank model, and we will discuss this matter later. Inspection of the pairwise CCF between all residual series shows no obvious departures from independence.

Once the model has been estimated, estimated forecasts can be obtained. Analogous to the univariate case, the $m$-step-ahead forecast, $m = 1, 2, ...$, in this example ($n = 508$), is obtained as follows:

$$\widehat{\boldsymbol{x}}_{n+m}^n = \widehat{\Phi}_1 \widehat{\boldsymbol{x}}_{n+m-1}^n + \widehat{\Phi}_2 \widehat{\boldsymbol{x}}_{n+m-2}^n, \tag{4.242}$$

where $\widehat{\boldsymbol{x}}_t^n = \boldsymbol{x}_t$ when $1 \leq t \leq n$. The mean square prediction error matrices can be calculated in a manner similar to the univariate case, (2.100). In the general case of vector ARMA or ARMAX models, forecasts and their mean square prediction errors can be obtained by using the state-space formulation of the model and the Kalman filter (see Section 4.6). Analogous to (2.100), the general form of the $m$-step-ahead mean square prediction error matrix is,

$$\begin{aligned} P_{n+m}^n &= E\left(\boldsymbol{x}_{n+m} - \boldsymbol{x}_{n+m}^n\right)\left(\boldsymbol{x}_{n+m} - \boldsymbol{x}_{n+m}^n\right)' && (4.243) \\ &= \Gamma(0) - \Gamma_n^{(m)} \Gamma_{nn}^{-1} \Gamma_n^{(m)\prime}, && (4.244) \end{aligned}$$

where $\Gamma_n^{(m)} = [\Gamma(m), \Gamma(m+1), ..., \Gamma(m+n-1)]$, is a $k \times nk$ matrix, and $\Gamma_{nn} = \{\Gamma(i-j)\}_{i,j=1}^n$, is an $nk \times nk$ symmetric matrix. Of course, $P_{n+m}^n$ can be estimated by substituting $\widehat{\Gamma}(h)$ for $\Gamma(h)$ in (4.244). The analogue of (2.110) for multivariate ARMA models is

$$P_{n+m}^n = \sum_{j=0}^{m-1} \Psi_j \Sigma_w \Psi_j'. \tag{4.245}$$

When the model is autoregressive, as in this example, a simplification occurs by noticing a $k$-dimensional AR($p$) model can be written as a $kp$-dimensional AR(1) model. For example, we can write the vector AR(2) model as

$$\boldsymbol{X}_t = \boldsymbol{\alpha} + A(\boldsymbol{X}_{t-1} - \boldsymbol{\alpha}) + \boldsymbol{\eta}_t, \tag{4.246}$$

where

$$\boldsymbol{X}_t = \begin{bmatrix} \boldsymbol{x}_t \\ \boldsymbol{x}_{t-1} \end{bmatrix} \quad \boldsymbol{\alpha} = \begin{bmatrix} \boldsymbol{\mu} \\ \boldsymbol{\mu} \end{bmatrix} \quad A = \begin{bmatrix} \Phi_1 & \Phi_2 \\ I & 0 \end{bmatrix} \quad \boldsymbol{\eta}_t = \begin{bmatrix} \boldsymbol{w}_t \\ \boldsymbol{0} \end{bmatrix}.$$

Of course, this technique generalizes to any dimension $k$ and any order $p$. From (4.246) we immediately obtain the forecasts and mean square prediction errors as

$$\boldsymbol{X}_{n+m}^n = \boldsymbol{\alpha} + A^m(\boldsymbol{X}_n - \boldsymbol{\alpha})$$

and

$$\begin{aligned} Q_{n+m}^n &= E\left(\boldsymbol{X}_{n+m} - \boldsymbol{X}_{n+m}^n\right)\left(\boldsymbol{X}_{n+m} - \boldsymbol{X}_{n+m}^n\right)' \\ &= \Gamma_X(0) - A^m \Gamma_X(0) A'^m, \end{aligned}$$

where

$$\Gamma_X(0) = \begin{bmatrix} \Gamma(0) & \Gamma(1) \\ \Gamma(1)' & \Gamma(0) \end{bmatrix}.$$

We can then obtain the desired mean square prediction error matrices $P_{n+m}^n$ as submatrices of $Q_{n+m}^n$. In addition, Yule–Walker estimation and forecasting can be accomplished by substituting autocovariance matrices by their sample equivalents obtained via (4.236).

For this numerical example,

$$\widehat{A} = \begin{bmatrix} \widehat{\Gamma}(1) & \widehat{\Gamma}(2) \\ \widehat{\Gamma}(0) & \widehat{\Gamma}(1) \end{bmatrix} \begin{bmatrix} \widehat{\Gamma}(0) & \widehat{\Gamma}(1) \\ \widehat{\Gamma}(1)' & \widehat{\Gamma}(0) \end{bmatrix}^{-1} = \begin{bmatrix} \widehat{\Phi}_1 & \widehat{\Phi}_2 \\ I & 0 \end{bmatrix},$$

where $\widehat{\Phi}_1$ and $\widehat{\Phi}_2$ are as given in Example 4.2. In the general case, we obtain the coefficient estimates from the top $k$ rows of $\widehat{A}$. Similarly, estimated forecasts in this example are found as follows:

$$\begin{bmatrix} \widehat{\boldsymbol{x}}_{n+m}^n \\ \widehat{\boldsymbol{x}}_{n+m-1}^n \end{bmatrix} = \widehat{A}^m \begin{bmatrix} \boldsymbol{x}_n \\ \boldsymbol{x}_{n-1} \end{bmatrix}.$$

Because $\boldsymbol{x}_{507} = (8.62, -1.85, 12.16)'$ and $\boldsymbol{x}_{508} = (4.71, -4.67, 17.20)'$, we can, for example, calculate the the one-step-ahead and two-step-ahead forecasts by putting $m = 2$ and using the numerical values given in Example 4.2 to construct $\widehat{A}^2$,

$$\begin{bmatrix} \widehat{\boldsymbol{x}}_{510}^{508} \\ \\ \widehat{\boldsymbol{x}}_{509}^{508} \end{bmatrix} = \widehat{A}^2 \begin{bmatrix} \widehat{\boldsymbol{x}}_{508} \\ \widehat{\boldsymbol{x}}_{507} \end{bmatrix} = \begin{bmatrix} 6.13 \\ -5.94 \\ 11.23 \\ \\ 6.43 \\ -4.77 \\ 10.53 \end{bmatrix}.$$

Substituting autocovariance matries with their estimates, we may write

$$\begin{aligned} \widehat{Q}_{510}^{508} &= \begin{bmatrix} \widehat{\Gamma}(0) & \widehat{\Gamma}(1) \\ \widehat{\Gamma}(1)' & \widehat{\Gamma}(0) \end{bmatrix} - \widehat{A}^2 \begin{bmatrix} \widehat{\Gamma}(0) & \widehat{\Gamma}(1) \\ \widehat{\Gamma}(1)' & \widehat{\Gamma}(0) \end{bmatrix} \widehat{A}'^2 \\ &= \begin{bmatrix} \widehat{P}_{510}^{508} & \widehat{P}_{510,509}^{508} \\ \\ \widehat{P}_{509,510}^{508} & \widehat{P}_{509}^{508} \end{bmatrix}, \end{aligned}$$

where we have written $\widehat{P}_{s,t}^n$ to be the estimate of $E\{(\boldsymbol{x}_s - \boldsymbol{x}_s^n)\,(\boldsymbol{x}_t - \boldsymbol{x}_t^n)'\}$. In this example, we found (entries are rounded)

$$\widehat{Q}_{510}^{508} = \begin{bmatrix} 31 & 5 & 19 & 8 & -4 & 2 \\ 5 & 39 & 38 & -2 & 7 & 2 \\ 19 & 38 & 135 & 6 & 2 & 33 \\ \\ 8 & -2 & 6 & 28 & 7 & 16 \\ -4 & 7 & 2 & 7 & 37 & 40 \\ 2 & 2 & 33 & 16 & 40 & 123 \end{bmatrix}.$$

Note, $\widehat{P}_{509}^{508} = \widehat{\Sigma}_w = \widehat{\Sigma}_w^{(2)}$. The diagonal elements of $\widehat{Q}_{510}^{508}$ give the individual mean-square prediction errors. For example, an approximate 95% prediction interval for $x_{510,1}^{508}$ is $6.13 \pm 2\sqrt{31}$ or (-5.0, 17.2 ).

Although the estimation in Example 4.24 was performed using Yule–Walker estimation, we could have also used conditional or unconditional maximum likelihood estimation, or conditional (as in Example 4.2) or unconditional least squares estimation. Because, as we have seen, any $k$-dimensional AR($p$) model can be written as a $kp$-dimensional AR(1) model, any of these estimation techniques are straightforward multivariate extensions to the univariate case presented in equations (2.124)-(2.133). Also, as in the univariate case, the Yule–Walker estimators, the maximum likelihood estimators, and the least squares estimators are asymptotically equivalent. To exhibit the asymptotic distribution of the autoregression parameter estimators, we write

$$\boldsymbol{\phi} = \text{vec}\,(\Phi_1, ..., \Phi_p)\,,$$

where the ***vec operator*** stacks the columns of a matrix into a vector. For example, for a bivariate AR(2) model,

$$\boldsymbol{\phi} = \text{vec}\,(\Phi_1, \Phi_2) = (\Phi_{1_{11}}, \Phi_{1_{21}}, \Phi_{1_{12}}, \Phi_{1_{22}} \Phi_{2_{11}}, \Phi_{2_{21}}, \Phi_{2_{12}}, \Phi_{2_{22}})'\,,$$

where $\Phi_{\ell_{ij}}$ is the $ij$-th element of $\Phi_\ell$, $\ell = 1, 2$. Because $(\Phi_1, ..., \Phi_p)$ is a $k \times kp$ matrix, $\boldsymbol{\phi}$ is a $k^2p \times 1$ vector. We now state the following property.

***Property P4.7: Large Sample Distribution of the Vector Autoregression Estimators***
*Let $\widehat{\boldsymbol{\phi}}$ denote the vector of parameter estimators (obtained via Yule–Walker, least squares, or maximum likelihood) for a k-dimensional AR(p) model. Then,*

$$\sqrt{n}\left(\widehat{\boldsymbol{\phi}} - \boldsymbol{\phi}\right) \sim \text{AN}(\mathbf{0}, \Sigma_w \otimes \Gamma_{pp}^{-1}), \tag{4.247}$$

*where $\Gamma_{pp} = \{\Gamma(i-j)\}_{i,j=1}^{p}$ is a $kp \times kp$ matrix, $\Sigma_w \otimes \Gamma_{pp}^{-1} = \{\sigma_{ij}\Gamma_{pp}^{-1}\}_{i,j=1}^{k}$ is a $k^2p \times k^2p$ matrix, and $\sigma_{ij}$ is the $ij$-th element of $\Sigma_w$.*

The variance–covariance matrix of the estimator $\widehat{\boldsymbol{\phi}}$ is approximated by replacing $\Sigma_w$ by $\widehat{\Sigma}_w$, and replacing $\Gamma(h)$ by $\widehat{\Gamma}(h)$ in $\Gamma_{pp}$. The square root of the diagonal elements of $\widehat{\Sigma}_w \otimes \widehat{\Gamma}_{pp}^{-1}$ divided by $\sqrt{n}$ gives the individual standard errors. For the mortality data example, the estimated standard errors for the VAR(2) fit are listed in Example 4.2; although those standard errors were taken from a regression run, they could have also been calculated using Property P4.7 along with the numerical values taken from $\widehat{\Sigma}_w^{(2)}$ given below (4.240) and $\widehat{\Gamma}_{22}$ given in (4.239).

Asymptotic inference for the general case of vector ARMA models is more complicated than pure AR models; details can be found in Reinsel (1997) or Lütkepohl (1993), for example. In view of Section 4.6, however, the results of Section 4.3 still apply because the vector ARMA model can be written as a state-space model. Thus, estimation for vector ARMA can be recast into the problem of estimation for state-space models that was discussed in Section 4.3.

A simple algorithm for fitting multivariate ARMA models from Spliid (1983) is worth mentioning because it repeatedly uses the multivariate regression equations. Consider a general ARMA$(p, q)$ model for a time series with a nonzero mean

$$\boldsymbol{x}_t = \boldsymbol{\alpha} + \Phi_1\boldsymbol{x}_{t-1} + \cdots + \Phi_p\boldsymbol{x}_{t-p} + \boldsymbol{w}_t + \Theta_1\boldsymbol{w}_{t-1} + \cdots + \Theta_q\boldsymbol{w}_{t-q}. \tag{4.248}$$

If $\boldsymbol{\mu} = E\boldsymbol{x}_t$, then $\boldsymbol{\alpha} = (I - \Phi_1 - \cdots - \Phi_p)\boldsymbol{\mu}$. If $\boldsymbol{w}_{t-1}, ..., \boldsymbol{w}_{t-q}$ were observed, we could rearrange (4.248) as a multivariate regression model

$$\boldsymbol{x}_t = \mathcal{B}\boldsymbol{z}_t + \boldsymbol{w}_t, \tag{4.249}$$

with

$$\boldsymbol{z}_t = (1, \boldsymbol{x}'_{t-1}, ..., \boldsymbol{x}'_{t-p}, \boldsymbol{w}'_{t-1}, ..., \boldsymbol{w}'_{t-q})' \tag{4.250}$$

and

$$\mathcal{B} = [\boldsymbol{\alpha}, \Phi_1, ..., \Phi_p, \Theta_1, ..., \Theta_q], \tag{4.251}$$

for $t = p+1, ..., n$. Given an initial estimator $\mathcal{B}_0$, of $\mathcal{B}$, we can reconstruct $\{\boldsymbol{w}_{t-1}, ..., \boldsymbol{w}_{t-q}\}$ by setting

$$\boldsymbol{w}_{t-j} = \boldsymbol{x}_{t-j} - \mathcal{B}_0 \boldsymbol{z}_{t-j}, \quad t = p+1, ..., n, \quad j = 1, ..., q, \tag{4.252}$$

where, if $q > p$, we put $\boldsymbol{w}_{t-j} = \boldsymbol{0}$ for $t - j \leq 0$. The new values of $\{\boldsymbol{w}_{t-1}, ..., \boldsymbol{w}_{t-q}\}$ are then put into the regressors $\boldsymbol{z}_t$ and a new estimate, say, $\mathcal{B}_1$, is obtained. The initial value, $\mathcal{B}_0$, can be computed by fitting a pure autoregression of order $p$ or higher, and taking $\Theta_1 = \cdots = \Theta_q = \boldsymbol{0}$. The procedure is then iterated until the parameter estimates stabilize. The algorithm usually converges, but not to the maximum likelihood estimators. Experience suggests the estimators are reasonably close to the maximum likelihood estimators.

As discussed in Section 4.1, the special form assumed for the constant component, $\boldsymbol{\alpha}$, of the general ARMA model in (4.248) can be generalized to include a fixed $r \times 1$ vector of inputs, say, $\boldsymbol{u}_t$. In this case we have a $k$-dimensional ARMAX model:

$$\boldsymbol{x}_t = \Gamma \boldsymbol{u}_t + \sum_{j=1}^{p} \Phi_j \boldsymbol{x}_{t-j} + \sum_{j=1}^{q} \Theta_j \boldsymbol{w}_{t-j} + \boldsymbol{w}_t, \tag{4.253}$$

where $\Gamma$ is a $k \times r$ parameter matrix. Recall the X in ARMAX refers to the exogenous vector process we have denoted here by $\boldsymbol{u}_t$ and the introduction of exogenous variables through setting $\boldsymbol{\alpha} = \Gamma \boldsymbol{u}_t$ does not present any special problems in making inferences.

### Example 4.25 An ARMAX Model for Cardiovascular Mortality

In Example 2.2, we regressed the cardiovascular mortality series, $M_t$, on time $t$, temperature $T_t$, and particulate pollution $P_t$. There, the interest was an analysis of the effect of temperature and pollution on cardiovascular mortality. In Example 4.2, we fit a multivariate ARMA model to the trivariate vector $(M_t, T_t, P_t)$, as if modeling the behavior of temperature and pollution was equally as important as modeling the behavior of mortality. In this example, we are interested in using temperature and pollution to explain some of the variation in the mortality series.

To examine the CCF between mortality and temperature, and between mortality and pollution, we first prewhitened mortality by fitting an AR(2) to the detrended data. That is, we first fit the model

$$M_t = \beta_0 + \beta_1 t + \phi_1 M_{t-1} + \phi_2 M_{t-2} + \epsilon_t.$$

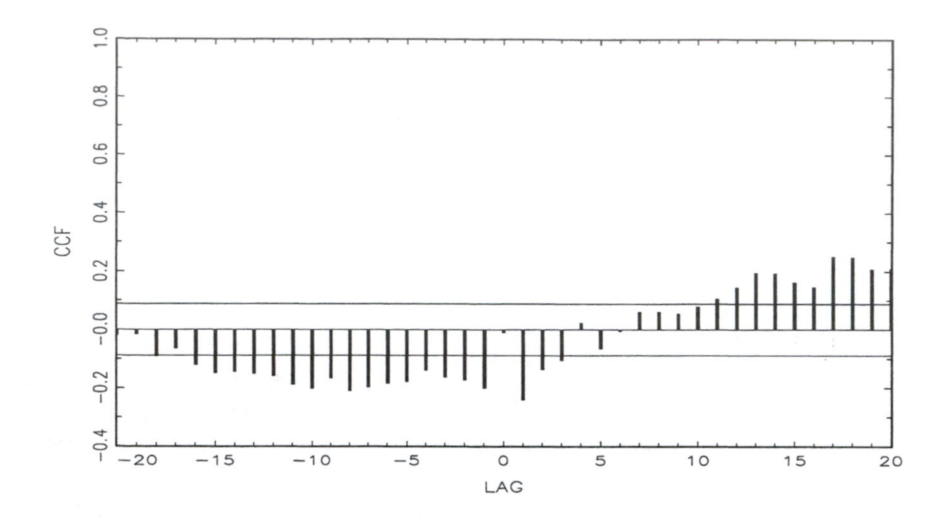


**Figure 4.20:** CCF between prewhitened mortality and temperature (positive lag means temperature leads mortality).

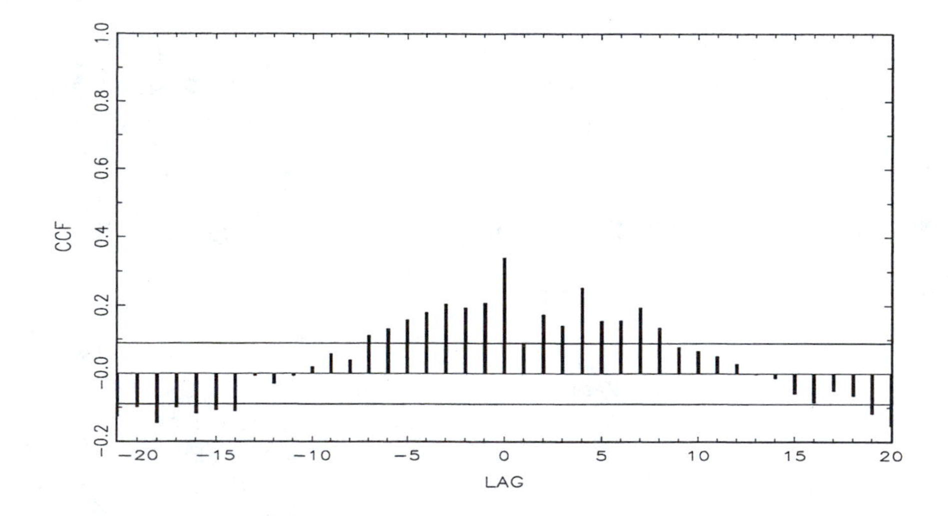


**Figure 4.21:** CCF between prewhitened mortality and particulate pollution (positive lag means pollution leads mortality).

Using the residuals of the fit, say, $\widehat{\epsilon}_t$, we then calculated the CCF between $\widehat{\epsilon}_t$ and $T_t$, and between $\widehat{\epsilon}_t$ and $P_t$. Figure 4.20 shows the cross-correlation of prewhitened mortality and temperature (positive lag means temperature leads mortality) and a significant correlation is seen at lag $h = 1$. Figure 4.21 shows a similar plot for the CCF of prewhitened mortality and pollution, and significant correlations are seen at lags $h = 0, 2, 4, 7$. After some preliminary fitting, the final model uses the exogenous variables $\boldsymbol{u}_t = (1, t, T_{t-1}, T_{t-1}^2, P_t, P_{t-4})'$, along with an AR(2) on mortality, $M_t$; the inclusion of particulate pollution at lags two and seven were not significant when lags zero and four are in the model. In this case, the ARMAX model is

$$M_t = \Gamma \boldsymbol{u}_t + \phi_1 M_{t-1} + \phi_2 M_{t-2} + w_t,$$

where $\Gamma = [\gamma_0, \gamma_1, \gamma_2, \gamma_3, \gamma_4]$.

Estimation was accomplished using the regression approach described in (4.17)and (4.18). In this case, the fitted model was (values are rounded)

$$\begin{aligned} \widehat{M_t} &= 42.9 - 0.01_{(.002)} t - 0.18_{(.03)} T_{t-1} + 0.11_{(.02)} P_t + 0.05_{(.02)} P_{t-4} \\ &+ 0.31_{(.04)} M_{t-1} + 0.30_{(.04)} M_{t-2} + \widehat{w}_t, \end{aligned}$$

where $\widehat{\sigma}_w^2 = 25.7$ and $R^2 = 74.3\%$. Each coefficient is highly significant, as seen from the estimated standard errors listed below each parameter estimate. Finally, an analysis of the residuals, $\widehat{w}_t$, shows, except for a few outliers, the model fits well. The value of the Ljung–Box–Pierce statistic for H=24 was Q=25.7, which when compared to a $\chi^2_{22}$, is not significant. In addition, a Q-Q plot shows no departure from the Gaussian assumption, except for the few outliers. Our general conclusions are that decrease in cardiovascular mortality occurred during the period studied, and an increase in mortality is associated with lower temperatures the previous week and higher particulate pollution both currently and one month prior.

## Contemporaneous Dependence and Reduced Rank Models

Example 4.25 suggests we may be interested in addressing zero-order (contemporaneous) dependence among time series. That is, particulate pollution $P_t$, as it evolves over a week, is highly correlated with cardiovascular mortality $M_t$ in the same week. For a simple example, consider bivariate data $\boldsymbol{x}_t = (x_{t,1}, x_{t,2})'$, evolving as

$$\begin{aligned} x_{t,1} &= \alpha_1 x_{t-1,1} + \epsilon_{t,1}, \\ x_{t,2} &= \beta x_{t,1} + \alpha_2 x_{t-1,1} + \alpha_3 x_{t-1,2} + \epsilon_{t,2}, \end{aligned} \tag{4.254}$$

where the white noise terms, $\epsilon_{t,1}$ and $\epsilon_{t,2}$ are independent with respective variances $\sigma_1^2$ and $\sigma_2^2$. This model implies the first series $x_{t,1}$ is generated by an AR(1) process, and the current and previous values of the first series, $x_{t,1}$ and $x_{t-1,1}$, and the previous value of the second series, $x_{t-1,2}$, can be used to predict the second component, $x_{t,2}$. In this case, the model has the general form

$$L^{-1}\boldsymbol{x}_t = A\boldsymbol{x}_{t-1} + \boldsymbol{\epsilon}_t, \tag{4.255}$$

where $L$ is lower triangular with ones on the diagonal, and the variance–covariance matrix of $\boldsymbol{\epsilon}_t$ is diagonal, say, $D_\epsilon = \text{diag}\{\sigma_1^2, \sigma_2^2\}$. In this particular example,

$$L = \begin{bmatrix} 1 & 0 \\ \beta & 1 \end{bmatrix}, \quad A = \begin{bmatrix} \alpha_1 & 0 \\ \alpha_2 & \alpha_3 \end{bmatrix}.$$

The model is an identifiable bivariate AR(1) model, and we can write (4.255) as

$$\boldsymbol{x}_t = \Phi_1 \boldsymbol{x}_{t-1} + \boldsymbol{w}_t, \tag{4.256}$$

where $\Phi_1 = LA$ and $\Sigma_w = LD_\epsilon L'$.

Because, for the multivariate ARMA$(p,q)$ model given in (4.224) with $\boldsymbol{\alpha} = \boldsymbol{0}$, we assume $\Sigma_w$ is positive definite, a lower triangular matrix exists with ones along the diagonal, say, $\widetilde{\Phi}_0$, such that $\widetilde{\Phi}_0 \Sigma_w \widetilde{\Phi}_0' = D_\epsilon$, where $D_\epsilon$ is a diagonal, positive definite matrix; this is based on the Cholesky decomposition of $\Sigma_w$. Thus, the multivariate ARMA model, (4.224), can also be written as

$$\widetilde{\Phi}_0 \boldsymbol{x}_t = \widetilde{\Phi}_1 \boldsymbol{x}_{t-1} + \cdots + \widetilde{\Phi}_p \boldsymbol{x}_{t-p} + \boldsymbol{\epsilon}_t + \widetilde{\Theta}_1 \boldsymbol{\epsilon}_{t-1} + \cdots + \widetilde{\Theta}_q \boldsymbol{\epsilon}_{t-q}, \tag{4.257}$$

where $\boldsymbol{\epsilon}_t$ has uncorrelated components. In particular, $\widetilde{\Phi}_j = \widetilde{\Phi}_0 \Phi_j$, $\widetilde{\Theta}_j = \widetilde{\Phi}_0 \Theta_j \widetilde{\Phi}_0^{-1}$, and the noise sequence $\boldsymbol{\epsilon}_t = \widetilde{\Phi}_0 \boldsymbol{w}_t$ has variance–covariance matrix $D_\epsilon$. This representation is referred to as the ***echelon canonical form*** of the multivariate ARMA model.

### Example 4.26 Contemporaneous Dependence

Consider a bivariate process given by

$$\boldsymbol{x}_t = \begin{bmatrix} 1.5 & 0 \\ 0 & -.45 \end{bmatrix} \boldsymbol{x}_{t-1} + \begin{bmatrix} -.75 & 0 \\ .7 & 0 \end{bmatrix} \boldsymbol{x}_{t-2} + \boldsymbol{w}_t, \tag{4.258}$$

where

$$\Sigma_w = \begin{bmatrix} 1 & -0.5 \\ -0.5 & 25 \end{bmatrix}.$$

In terms of the individual components, we can write (4.258) as

$$\begin{aligned} x_{t,1} &= 1.5x_{t-1,1} - 0.75x_{t-2,1} + w_{t,1}, \\ x_{t,2} &= 0.45x_{t-1,2} + 0.7x_{t-2,1} + w_{t,2}, \end{aligned} \tag{4.259}$$

where $(w_{t,1}, w_{t,2})'$ is a bivariate iid Gaussian processes, with $\text{var}(w_{t,1}) = 1$, $\text{var}(w_{t,2}) = 25$, and $\text{cov}(w_{t,1}, w_{t,2}) = -0.5$.

In this case, we put

$$D_\epsilon = \begin{bmatrix} 1 & 0 \\ 0.5 & 1 \end{bmatrix} \begin{bmatrix} 1 & -0.5 \\ -0.5 & 25 \end{bmatrix} \begin{bmatrix} 1 & 0.5 \\ 0 & 1 \end{bmatrix} = \begin{bmatrix} 1 & 0 \\ 0 & 24.75 \end{bmatrix}.$$

Also, let

$$\widetilde{\Phi}_0 = \begin{bmatrix} 1 & 0 \\ 0.5 & 1 \end{bmatrix}^{-1} = \begin{bmatrix} 1 & 0 \\ -0.5 & 1 \end{bmatrix},$$

$$\widetilde{\Phi}_1 = \widetilde{\Phi}_0 \Phi_1 = \begin{bmatrix} 1 & 0 \\ -0.5 & 1 \end{bmatrix} \begin{bmatrix} 1.5 & 0 \\ 0 & -0.45 \end{bmatrix} = \begin{bmatrix} 1.5 & 0 \\ -0.75 & -0.45 \end{bmatrix},$$

and

$$\widetilde{\Phi}_2 = \widetilde{\Phi}_0 \Phi_2 = \begin{bmatrix} 1 & 0 \\ -0.5 & 1 \end{bmatrix} \begin{bmatrix} -.75 & 0 \\ .7 & 0 \end{bmatrix} = \begin{bmatrix} -.75 & 0 \\ 1.075 & 0 \end{bmatrix}.$$

Then, we can write (4.258) in echelon canonical form as

$$\widetilde{\Phi}_0 \boldsymbol{x}_t = \widetilde{\Phi}_1 \boldsymbol{x}_{t-1} + \widetilde{\Phi}_2 \boldsymbol{x}_{t-2} + \boldsymbol{\epsilon}_t, \tag{4.260}$$

where $\text{var}(\boldsymbol{\epsilon}_t) = D_\epsilon$. In terms of the individual components, we can write (4.260) as

$$x_{t,1} = 1.5x_{t-1,1} - 0.75x_{t-2,1} + \epsilon_{t,1}, \tag{4.261}$$

$$\begin{aligned} x_{t,2} = {} & -0.45x_{t-1,2} + 0.5x_{t,1} - 0.75x_{t-1,1} \\ & + 1.075x_{t-2,1} + \epsilon_{t,2}, \end{aligned} \tag{4.262}$$

where $\epsilon_{t,1}$ and $\epsilon_{t,2}$ are independent iid Gaussian processes, with $\text{var}(\epsilon_{t,1}) = 1$ and $\text{var}(\epsilon_{t,2}) = 24.75$. Comparing (4.261) and (4.259), we see from (4.261) that the first component $x_{t,1}$ is still an AR(2), as in (4.259), but now the second component $x_{t,2}$ is contemporaneously dependent on the first component. Of course, both models (4.261) and (4.259) are equivalent.

To estimate the parameters in model (4.261), we could first estimate the model in the form of (4.259), and then convert back to the echelon canonical form of (4.261). For example, we simulated $n = 144$ observations from (4.259) and then estimated the parameters using Yule–Walker. The first series is shown in Figure 2.5. We found

$$\widehat{\Sigma}_w = \begin{bmatrix} 1.28 & -0.17 \\ -0.17 & 23.54 \end{bmatrix},$$

so we estimate $D_\epsilon$ by calculating

$$\widehat{D}_\epsilon = \begin{bmatrix} 1 & 0 \\ 0.13 & 1 \end{bmatrix} \begin{bmatrix} 1.28 & -0.17 \\ -0.17 & 23.54 \end{bmatrix} \begin{bmatrix} 1 & 0.13 \\ 0 & 1 \end{bmatrix} = \begin{bmatrix} 1.28 & 0 \\ 0 & 23.52 \end{bmatrix}.$$

Similarly, the estimate of $\widetilde{\Phi}_0$ is

$$\widehat{\widetilde{\Phi}}_0 = \begin{bmatrix} 1 & 0 \\ -0.13 & 1 \end{bmatrix},$$

and so on. Of course, if we did not model the process as having contemporaneous dependence, but the dynamics of the process was given by (4.261), we would have arrived at the equivalent AR(2) model given in (4.259).

When fitting multivariate models to data, we have to be concerned with the large number of parameters involved. With no restrictions on the parameters in the $k$-dimensional ARMA$(p, q)$ model given by (4.224), there are $pk^2$ parameters in $\{\Phi_1, ..., \Phi_p\}$, $qk^2$ parameters in $\{\Theta_1, ..., \Theta_q\}$, and $k(k+1)/2$ parameters in $\Sigma_w$. Thus, for example, with bivariate data ($k = 2$), an ARMA(1,1) will have 11 parameters that must be estimated; for trivariate data ($k = 3$), an ARMA(1,1) will have 24 parameters that must be estimated. It is of interest then to investigate the use of models with restrictions on the parameters. One example of this type of parameter constraints was the multiplicative models used in univariate seasonal ARIMA models that were discussed in Section 2.10. For example, in the seasonal ARIMA $(1,0,0) \times (1,0,0)_{12}$ model we have $x_t = \phi x_{t-1} + \Phi x_{t-12} + \Phi\phi x_{t-13} + w_t$ so that the coefficient of $x_{t-13}$ is constrained to be the product of $\Phi$ and $\phi$. A more general model would be $x_t = \beta_1 x_{t-1} + \beta_2 x_{t-12} + \beta_3 x_{t-13} + w_t$, and this would require estimation of an additional parameter.

Two models that allow for a reduction in the number of parameters and have been of recent interest are ***nested reduced-rank models*** (see Reinsel, 1997) and ***scalar component models*** (SCM) from Tiao and Tsay (1989). We will give a brief introduction to these techniques; more detailed discussions can be found in Reinsel (1997) and Tiao and Tsay (1989).

We begin with nested reduced-rank AR$(p)$ models. Suppose a $k$-dimensional process $\boldsymbol{x}_t$ follows an AR$(p)$ model

$$\boldsymbol{x}_t = \sum_{j=1}^{p} \Phi_j \boldsymbol{x}_{t-j} + \boldsymbol{w}_t, \tag{4.263}$$

but the regression parameters $\Phi_j$ have the reduced-rank structure that $r_j = \text{rank}(\Phi_j) \geq \text{rank}(\Phi_{j+1}) = r_{j+1}$, for $j = 1, 2, ..., p-1$. It is possible to show (4.263) can be written as

$$\boldsymbol{x}_t = \sum_{j=1}^{p} A_j B_j \boldsymbol{x}_{t-j} + \boldsymbol{w}_t, \tag{4.264}$$

where $A_j$ is a $k \times r_j$, rank $r_j$, matrix having the special form $A_j = A_1 D_j$, where $D_j = [I_{r_j}, 0]'$ is an $r_1 \times r_j$ matrix, where $I_{r_j}$ is the $r_j \times r_j$ identity matrix. The matrix $B_j$ is $r_j \times k$, of rank $r_j$ (see Reinsel, 1997, Chapter 6). Although this decomposition is not unique, we can put further restrictions on $A_1$ for uniqueness. To this end, consider the model written in canonical form, that is

$$z_t = \sum_{j=1}^{p} \begin{bmatrix} \widetilde{\Phi}_{j,1} \\ 0 \end{bmatrix} z_{t-j} + e_t, \tag{4.265}$$

where $z_t = L\boldsymbol{x}_t$, $e_t = L\boldsymbol{w}_t$, and the $k \times k$ matrix $L$ is lower triangular with ones along the diagonal. The coefficient matrices have the form $\widetilde{\Phi}_j = L\Phi_j L^{-1} = [\widetilde{\Phi}'_{j,1}, 0']$, where $\widetilde{\Phi}_{j,1}$ is a $r_j \times k$, rank $r_j$ matrix, so the number of corresponding zero rows is increasing in $j$. The matrices $B_j$ are found by setting $B_j = D'_j L\Phi_j$. Details on the existence and construction of such a matrix $L$ can be found in Reinsel (1997). The unique decomposition is formed by requiring the columns of $A_1$ in (4.264) to be first $r_1$ columns of $L$ (this assumes the processes have been arranged so the upper $r_j \times r_j$ block matrix of $A_j$ is full rank.

### Example 4.27 A Reduced Rank Model

Consider the model given in (4.258), and note the model has the nested reduced-rank structure with rank$(\Phi_1) = 2$ and rank$(\Phi_2) = 1$. Let

$$L = \begin{bmatrix} 1 & 0 \\ \frac{.70}{.75} & 1 \end{bmatrix},$$

in which case, $z_t = L\boldsymbol{x}_t$ can be written as

$$z_t = \begin{bmatrix} 1.50 & 0 \\ 1.82 & -0.45 \end{bmatrix} z_{t-1} + \begin{bmatrix} -0.75 & 0 \\ 0 & 0 \end{bmatrix} z_{t-1} + e_t, \tag{4.266}$$

where $\text{var}(e_t) = L\Sigma_w L'$. In this case, we have simply left-multiplied the model in (4.258) by the matrix $L$; that is, (4.266) is simply

$$L\boldsymbol{x}_t = L\Phi_1 L^{-1} L\boldsymbol{x}_{t-1} + L\Phi_2 L^{-1} L\boldsymbol{x}_{t-2} + L\boldsymbol{w}_t,$$

where $\Phi_1, \Phi_2$ and the distribution of $\boldsymbol{w}_t$ are given in (4.258).

From the canonical form (4.266), we can obtain $A_j$ and $B_j$ as previously discussed. Because $r_1 = 2$ and $r_2 = 1$, we have $D_1 = I_2$, and $D_2 = (1, 0)'$. Then, $A_1 = L^{-1}D_1 = L^{-1}$ and $B_j = D'_j\widetilde{\Phi}_j$. In this example,

$$A_1 = \begin{bmatrix} 1 & 0 \\ -\frac{.70}{.75} & 1 \end{bmatrix}, \quad B_1 = \begin{bmatrix} 1.50 & 0 \\ 1.40 & -0.45 \end{bmatrix},$$

and

$$A_2 = A_1 D_2 = \begin{bmatrix} 1 \\ -\frac{.70}{.75} \end{bmatrix}, \quad B_2 = [\,-0.75 \quad 0\,].$$

The reader should verify $A_1 B_1 = \Phi_1$, and $A_1 D_2 B_2 = A_2 B_2 = \Phi_2$, where $\Phi_1$ and $\Phi_2$ are given in (4.258). This, gives the desired representation of (2.214) in terms of the decomposition (2.220).

Preliminary identification of a reduced-rank model can be obtained via the partial canonical correlations, $\{\lambda_i(j);\ i = 1, ..., k;\ j = 1, 2...\}$. Because of the particular structure of the nested reduced-rank model, at least $k - r_j$ zero partial canonical correlations will exist between $\boldsymbol{x}_t$ and $\boldsymbol{x}_{t-j}$ given $\{\boldsymbol{x}_{t-1}, ..., \boldsymbol{x}_{t-j+1}\}$, $j = 1, 2, ...$ (see Reinsel, 1997, § 6.1.1 for details). The following test statistic can be used for preliminary identification of the ranks:

$$C(j,h) = -(n-j-1) \sum_{i=(j-h)+1}^{k} \log\left(1 - \widehat{\lambda}_i^2(j)\right), \quad h = 1, ..., k. \tag{4.267}$$

In the reduced rank model, under the null hypothesis of $\text{rank}(\Phi_j) \le k - h$, the test statistic $C(j, h)$ has an asymptotic $\chi^2$ distribution with $h^2$ degrees of freedom (see Tiao and Tsay, 1989).

**Example 4.28 Identification of the Ranks in a Reduced Model**

In Example 4.26, we generated $n = 144$ observations from the bivariate model (4.258). Continuing with Examples 4.26 and 4.27, we estimated the partial canonical correlations from the simulated data to be

$$\{\widehat{\lambda}_1^2(j), \widehat{\lambda}_2^2(j)\} = \{0.76, 0.07\}, \{0.58, 0.00\}, \{0.03, 0.00\}, \{0.03, 0.00\}$$

for $j = 1, 2, 3, 4$. Thus, with $n = 144$, we find

$$\begin{array}{rr} C(1,1) = 10.82, & C(1,2) = 210.99, \\ C(2,1) = 1.44, & C(2,2) = 124.19, \\ C(3,1) = 0.08, & C(3,2) = 4.64, \\ C(4,1) = 0.55, & C(4,2) = 2.05. \end{array}$$

Because $\chi_1^2(0.95) = 3.84$ and $\chi_4^2(0.95) = 9.49$, we are lead to the appropriate conclusion that the model is an AR(2) with $\text{rank}(\Phi_1) = 2$ and $\text{rank}(\Phi_2) = 1$.

Maximum (conditional) likelihood estimation of the parameters in the reduced-rank model is accomplished via Newton–Raphson. The reason we have to resort to a numerical method is that the constraints on the parameter matrices are nonlinear. Let $\boldsymbol{\beta}$ be the elements of $A_1$ and $B_j$, for $j = 1, ..., p$. Then, the MLEs of $\boldsymbol{\beta}$ and $\Sigma$ are found by minimizing the criterion function (which, up to a constant, is -2 log likelihood),

$$l(\boldsymbol{\beta}, \Sigma) = n \log|\Sigma| + \sum_{t=p+1}^{n} \boldsymbol{w}_t' \Sigma^{-1} \boldsymbol{w}_t,$$

with respect to $\boldsymbol{\beta}$ and $\Sigma$. The form of $\boldsymbol{w}_t$ is given in (4.264); that is, $\boldsymbol{w}_t = \boldsymbol{x}_t - \sum_{j=1}^{p} A_j B_j \boldsymbol{x}_{t-j}$. Reinsel (1997, §6.1.3) gives an explicit expression for an approximate Newton–Raphson iterative procedure for estimating the coefficient parameters $\boldsymbol{\beta}$. Also, the asymptotic (normal) distribution of these estimators, as well as numerous examples, can be found in Reinsel (1997, Chapter 6).

SCMs are a type of canonical variates approach to vector ARMA modeling. In this brief introduction to SCMs, we will focus on causal AR($p$) models; the interested reader can see Tiao and Tsay (1989) for details on the general approach. For a comparison of nested reduced-rank methods and SCMs, see Reinsel (1997, Chapter 3). An SCM of order $p^* \le p$ is said to exist if a linear combination of the components of the data vector exists, say, $z_t = \boldsymbol{a}'\boldsymbol{x}_t$, where $\boldsymbol{a}$ is a $k \times 1$ vector of constants, such that

$$z_t = \sum_{j=1}^{p^*} \boldsymbol{a}'\Phi_j \boldsymbol{x}_{t-j} + \boldsymbol{a}'\boldsymbol{w}_t, \tag{4.268}$$

and $u_t = \boldsymbol{a}'\boldsymbol{w}_t$ is uncorrelated with $\{\boldsymbol{w}_{t-1}, \boldsymbol{w}_{t-2}, ...\}$.

Detection of SCMs can be accomplished by looking at certain canonical correlations. For example, suppose $\boldsymbol{x}_t$ is a $k \times 1$ vector AR(2) process, and an SCM with $p^* = 1$ exists. Then, there exists a $k \times 1$ vector, $\boldsymbol{a}$, such that $u_t = \boldsymbol{a}'\boldsymbol{x}_t - \boldsymbol{a}'\Phi_1\boldsymbol{x}_{t-1}$ is uncorrelated with $\boldsymbol{x}_{t-s}$, for $s \ge 2$. If we consider the $2k \times 1$ vector process $\boldsymbol{y}_{t,1} = (\boldsymbol{x}_t', \boldsymbol{x}_{t-1}')'$ and let $\boldsymbol{b} = (\boldsymbol{a}', -\boldsymbol{a}'\Phi_1)'$ be a $2k \times 1$ vector, then, for any arbitrary $k \times 1$ vector $\boldsymbol{c}$, and any $s \ge 2$, $\text{corr}(\boldsymbol{b}'\boldsymbol{y}_{t,1}, \boldsymbol{c}'\boldsymbol{x}_{t-s}) = \text{corr}(u_t, \boldsymbol{c}'\boldsymbol{x}_{t-s}) = 0$. From this result we can conclude there will be at least one zero canonical correlation between $\boldsymbol{y}_{t,1}$ and $\boldsymbol{x}_{t-s}$, $s \ge 2$. In general, the fitting of SCMs involves the inspection of the canonical correlations between the data vectors $\boldsymbol{y}_{t,m_1} = (\boldsymbol{x}_t', \boldsymbol{x}_{t-1}', ..., \boldsymbol{x}_{t-m_1}')'$ and $\boldsymbol{y}_{t-j,m_2} = (\boldsymbol{x}_{t-j}', \boldsymbol{x}_{t-j-1}', ..., \boldsymbol{x}_{t-j-m_2}')'$ for various values of $j = 1, 2, ...$ and $m_1, m_2 = 0, 1, ...$, with $m_1 \le m_2$.

In the $k$-dimensional vector AR approach of Tiao and Tsay (1989), a linearly independent set of $k$ SCMs, say, $z_{ti} = \boldsymbol{a}_i'\boldsymbol{x}_t$, for $i = 1, ..., k$, are found such that the orders of the models, say, $p_i$, for $i = 1, ..., k$, are as small as possible. Once a set of SCMs has been specified, a model of the form

$$A\boldsymbol{x}_t = \sum_{j=1}^{p} B_j \boldsymbol{x}_{t-j} + A\boldsymbol{w}_t \tag{4.269}$$

is fit, where the $i$-th row of the $k \times k$ matrix $A$ is $\boldsymbol{a}_i'$, and $B_j = A\Phi_j$. The relationship between reduced-rank AR models and SCMs can be seen by comparing (4.265) with (4.269). In fact, the two models are identical. To show this, in (4.269), set $A = L$ and $\boldsymbol{z}_t = A\boldsymbol{x}_t = L\boldsymbol{x}_t$, where $L$ is the lower triangular matrix defined in (4.265). Then, (4.269) becomes

$$\boldsymbol{z}_t = \sum_{j=1}^{p} B_j L^{-1} L \boldsymbol{x}_{t-j} + A\boldsymbol{w}_t = \sum_{j=1}^{p} \widetilde{\Phi}_j \boldsymbol{z}_{t-j} + \boldsymbol{e}_t,$$

where $\widetilde{\Phi}_j$ and $\boldsymbol{e}_t$ are as defined in (4.265).

Although the models are the same, the approaches to nested reduced-rank modeling and SCM modeling differ in how the matrix $L$ is treated. In the SCM approach, the matrix $L$, or, equivalently, the transformation $z_t = L\boldsymbol{x}_t$, is obtained first from information obtained via the canonical correlation analysis. Once the transformation has been selected, a model is estimated for the transformed process $z_t$. The lower diagonal matrix $L$ is not considered a parameter of the model. In the nested reduced-rank approach, the matrix $L$ is considered a parameter to be estimated via maximum likelihood.

# Problems

*Section 4.1*

**4.1** Consider a system process given by $x_t = -.9x_{t-2} + w_t$ for $t = 1, ..., n$, where $x_0 \sim \mathrm{N}(0, \sigma_0^2)$ and $w_t$ is Gaussian white noise with variance $\sigma_w^2$. The system process is observed with noise, say, $y_t = x_t + v_t$, where $v_t$ is Gaussian white noise with variance $\sigma_v^2$. Further, suppose $x_0$, $\{w_t\}$ and $\{v_t\}$ are independent processes.

(a) Write the system and observation equations in the form of a state space model.

(b) Find the value of $\sigma_0^2$ that makes the observations, $y_t$, stationary.

(c) Generate $n = 100$ observations with $\sigma_w = 1$, $\sigma_v = 1$ and using the value of $\sigma_0$ found in (b). Do a time plot of $x_t$ and of $y_t$ and compare the two processes. Also, compare the sample ACF and PACF of $x_t$ and of $y_t$.

(d) Repeat (c), but with $\sigma_v = 10$.

**4.2** Consider the state-space model presented in Example 4.5. Let $x_t^{t-1} = E(x_t|y_{t-1}, ..., y_1)$ and let $P_t^{t-1} = E(x_t - x_t^{t-1})^2$. The innovation sequence or residuals are $\epsilon_t = y_t - y_t^{t-1}$, where $y_t^{t-1} = E(y_t|y_{t-1}, ..., y_1)$. Find $\mathrm{cov}(\epsilon_s, \epsilon_t)$ in terms of $x_t^{t-1}$ and $P_t^{t-1}$ for (i) $s \neq t$ and (ii) $s = t$.

*Section 4.2*

**4.3** The data $y_1, y_2, ..., y_{10}$ listed in Table 4.2 are $n = 10$ observations generated from the state-space model presented in Examples 4.5 and 4.6. That is, $x_t = 0.8x_{t-1} + w_t$ and $y_t = x_t + v_t$, where $x_0 \sim \mathrm{N}(0, 2.78)$, $w_t \sim$ iid $\mathrm{N}(0, 1)$, $v_t \sim$ iid $\mathrm{N}(0, 1)$ are all mutually independent. Use Properties P4.1 and P4.2 to calculate the predictors, $x_t^{t-1}$, the filters, $x_t^t$, and the smoothers, $x_t^{10}$, for $t = 1, ..., 10$.

**4.4** Suppose the vector $\boldsymbol{z} = (\boldsymbol{x}', \boldsymbol{y}')'$, where $\boldsymbol{x}$ $(p \times 1)$ and $\boldsymbol{y}$ $(q \times 1)$ are jointly distributed with mean vectors $\boldsymbol{\mu}_x$ and $\boldsymbol{\mu}_y$ and with covariance matrix

$$\text{cov}(\boldsymbol{z}) = \begin{pmatrix} \Sigma_{xx} & \Sigma_{xy} \\ \Sigma_{yx} & \Sigma_{yy} \end{pmatrix}.$$

Consider projecting $\boldsymbol{x}$ on $\mathcal{M} = \overline{\text{sp}}\{\boldsymbol{1}, \boldsymbol{y}\}$, say, $\widehat{\boldsymbol{x}} = \boldsymbol{b} + B\boldsymbol{y}$.

(a) Show the orthogonality conditions can be written as

$$E(\boldsymbol{x} - \boldsymbol{b} - B\boldsymbol{y}) = 0,$$

$$E[(\boldsymbol{x} - \boldsymbol{b} - B\boldsymbol{y})\boldsymbol{y}'] = 0,$$

leading to the solutions

$$\boldsymbol{b} = \boldsymbol{\mu}_x - B\boldsymbol{\mu}_y \quad \text{and} \quad B = \Sigma_{xy}\Sigma_{yy}^{-1}.$$

(b) Prove the mean square error matrix is

$$MSE = E[(\boldsymbol{x} - \boldsymbol{b} - B\boldsymbol{y})\boldsymbol{x}'] = \Sigma_{xx} - \Sigma_{xy}\Sigma_{yy}^{-1}\Sigma_{yx}.$$

(c) How can these results be used to justify the claim that, in the absence of normality, Property P4.1 yields the best linear estimate of the state $\boldsymbol{x}_t$ given the data $Y_t$, namely, $\boldsymbol{x}_t^t$, and its corresponding MSE, namely, $P_t^t$?

**4.5** Verify (4.54) and (4.57).

**4.6** ***Derivation of Property P4.2 Based on the Projection Theorem.*** Throughout this problem, we use the notation of Property P4.2 and of the Projection Theorem given in Section T2.15, Theorem 2.1, where $\mathcal{H}$ is $L^2$. We assume $P_0^0 > 0$ and $R > 0$.

(a) Let $\mathcal{L}_{k+1} = \overline{\text{sp}}\{\boldsymbol{y}_1, ..., \boldsymbol{y}_{k+1}\}$, and let $\mathcal{V}_{k+1} = \overline{\text{sp}}\{\boldsymbol{y}_{k+1} - \boldsymbol{y}_{k+1}^k\}$, for $k = 0, 1, ..., n-1$, where $\boldsymbol{y}_{k+1}^k$ is the projection of $\boldsymbol{y}_{k+1}$ on $\mathcal{L}_k$. Show $\mathcal{L}_{k+1} = \mathcal{L}_k \oplus \mathcal{V}_{k+1}$.

(b) Show the projection of $\boldsymbol{x}_k$ on $\mathcal{L}_{k+1}$, that is, $\boldsymbol{x}_k^{k+1}$, is given by

$$\boldsymbol{x}_k^{k+1} = \boldsymbol{x}_k^k + H_{k+1}(\boldsymbol{y}_{k+1} - \boldsymbol{y}_{k+1}^k),$$

where $H_{k+1}$ can be determined by the orthogonality property

$$E\left\{ \left(\boldsymbol{x}_k - H_{k+1}(\boldsymbol{y}_{k+1} - \boldsymbol{y}_{k+1}^k)\right) \left(\boldsymbol{y}_{k+1} - \boldsymbol{y}_{k+1}^k\right)' \right\} = 0.$$

Show

$$H_{k+1} = P_k^k \Phi' A_{k+1} \left[A_{k+1} P_{k+1}^k A_{k+1}' + R\right]^{-1}.$$

(c) Define $J_k = P_k^k \Phi' [P_{k+1}^k]^{-1}$, and show

$$\boldsymbol{x}_k^{k+1} = \boldsymbol{x}_k^k + J_k(\boldsymbol{x}_{k+1}^{k+1} - \boldsymbol{x}_{k+1}^k).$$

(d) Repeating the process, show

$$\boldsymbol{x}_k^{k+2} = \boldsymbol{x}_k^k + J_k(\boldsymbol{x}_{k+1}^{k+1} - \boldsymbol{x}_{k+1}^k) + H_{k+2}(\boldsymbol{y}_{k+2} - \boldsymbol{y}_{k+2}^{k+1}),$$

solving for $H_{k+2}$. Simplify and show

$$\boldsymbol{x}_k^{k+2} = \boldsymbol{x}_k^k + J_k(\boldsymbol{x}_{k+1}^{k+2} - \boldsymbol{x}_{k+1}^k).$$

(e) Using induction, conclude

$$\boldsymbol{x}_k^n = \boldsymbol{x}_k^k + J_k(\boldsymbol{x}_{k+1}^n - \boldsymbol{x}_{k+1}^k),$$

which yields the smoother with $k = t - 1$.

*Section 4.3*

**4.7** (a) Consider the univariate state-space model given by state conditions $x_0 = w_0$, $x_t = x_{t-1} + w_t$ and observations $y_t = x_t + v_t$, $t = 1, 2, ...$, where $w_t$ and $v_t$ are independent, Gaussian, white noise processes with $\text{var}(w_t) = \sigma_w^2$ and $\text{var}(v_t) = \sigma_v^2$. Show the data follow an IMA(1,1) model, that is, $\nabla y_t$ follows an MA(1) model.

(b) Fit the model specified in part (a) to the logarithm of the glacial varve series and compare the results to those presented in Example 2.41.

**4.8** Let $y_t$ represent the global temperature data first presented in Chapter 1, Figure 1.2.

(a) Using regression, fit a third-degree polynomial in time to $y_t$, that is, fit the model

$$y_t = \beta_0 + \beta_1 t + \beta_2 t^2 + \beta_3 t^3 + \epsilon_t,$$

where $\epsilon_t$ is white noise. Do a time plot of the data fit, $\widehat{y}_t$, superimposed on the data, $y_t$, for t=1,...,108.

(b) Write the model $y_t = x_t + v_t$ with $\nabla^3 x_t = w_t$, where $w_t$ and $v_t$ are independent white noise processes, in state-space form. Hint: The state will be a $3 \times 1$ vector, say, $\boldsymbol{x}_t = (x_t, x_{t-1}, x_{t-2})'$. Fit the state-space model to the data, and do a time plot of the estimated filter, $\widehat{x}_t^{t-1}$, and the estimated smoother, $\widehat{x}_t^n$, superimposed on the data, $y_t$, for t=1,...,108. Compare these results with the results of part (a).

**4.9** Consider the model

$$y_t = x_t + v_t,$$

where $v_t$ is Gaussian white noise with variance $\sigma_v^2$, $x_t$ are independent Gaussian random variables with mean zero and $\text{var}(x_t) = r_t\sigma_x^2$ with $x_t$ independent of $v_t$, and $r_1, \dots, r_n$ are known constants. Show that applying the EM algorithm to the problem of estimating $\sigma_x^2$ and $\sigma_v^2$ leads to updates (represented by hats)

$$\widehat{\sigma}_x^2 = \frac{1}{n}\sum_{t=1}^n \frac{\sigma_t^2 + \mu_t^2}{r_t} \quad \text{and} \quad \widehat{\sigma}_v^2 = \frac{1}{n}\sum_{t=1}^n [(y_t - \mu_t)^2 + \sigma_t^2],$$

where, based on the current estimates (represented by tildes),

$$\mu_t = \frac{r_t\widetilde{\sigma}_x^2}{r_t\widetilde{\sigma}_x^2 + \widetilde{\sigma}_v^2}\, y_t \quad \text{and} \quad \sigma_t^2 = \frac{r_t\widetilde{\sigma}_x^2\widetilde{\sigma}_v^2}{r_t\widetilde{\sigma}_x^2 + \widetilde{\sigma}_v^2}.$$

**4.10** To explore the stability of the filter, consider a univariate state-space model. That is, for $t = 1, 2, ...$, the observations are $y_t = x_t + v_t$ and the state equation is $x_t = \phi x_{t-1} + w_t$, where $\sigma_w = \sigma_v = 1$ and $|\phi| < 1$. The initial state, $x_0$, has zero mean and variance one.

(a) Exhibit the recursion for $P_t^{t-1}$ in Property P4.1 in terms of $P_{t-1}^{t-2}$.

(b) Use the result of (a) to verify $P_t^{t-1}$ approaches a limit ($t \to \infty$) $P$ that is the positive solution of $P^2 + (1-\phi)P - 1 = 0$.

(c) With $K = \lim_{t\to\infty} K_t$ as given in Property P4.1, show $|1 - K| < 1$.

(d) Show, in steady-state, the one-step-ahead predictor, $y_{n+1}^n = E(y_{n+1} \mid y_n, y_{n-1}, ...)$, of a future observation satisfies

$$y_{n+1}^n = \sum_{j=0}^\infty \phi^j (1-K)^j y_{n-j}.$$

**4.11** In Section 4.3, we discussed that it is possible to obtain a recursion for the gradient vector, $-\partial \ln L_Y(\Theta)/\partial\Theta$. Assume the model is given by (4.19) and (4.20) and $A_t$ is a known design matrix that does not depend on $\Theta$, in which case Property P4.1 applies. For the gradient vector, show

$$\begin{aligned}\partial \ln L_Y(\Theta)/\partial\Theta_i &= \sum_{t=1}^n \left\{ \epsilon_t'\Sigma_t^{-1}\frac{\partial\epsilon_t}{\partial\Theta_i} - \frac{1}{2}\epsilon_t'\Sigma_t^{-1}\frac{\partial\Sigma_t}{\partial\Theta_i}\Sigma_t^{-1}\epsilon_t \right.\\ &\qquad \left. + \frac{1}{2}\text{tr}\left(\Sigma_t^{-1}\frac{\partial\Sigma_t}{\partial\Theta_i}\right)\right\},\end{aligned}$$

where the dependence of the innovation values on $\Theta$ is understood. In addition, with the general definition $\partial_i g = \partial g(\Theta)/\partial\Theta_i$, show the following recursions, for $t = 2, ..., n$ apply:

- $\partial_i \epsilon_t = -A_t \, \partial_i \boldsymbol{x}_t^{t-1}$,
- $\partial_i \boldsymbol{x}_t^{t-1} = \partial_i \Phi \, \boldsymbol{x}_{t-1}^{t-2} + \Phi \, \partial_i \boldsymbol{x}_{t-1}^{t-2} + \partial_i K_{t-1} \, \epsilon_{t-1} + K_{t-1} \, \partial_i \epsilon_{t-1}$,
- $\partial_i \Sigma_t = A_t \, \partial_i P_t^{t-1} A_t' + \partial_i R$,
- $\partial_i K_t = \left[ \partial_i \Phi \, P_t^{t-1} A_t' + \Phi \, \partial_i P_t^{t-1} \, A_t' - K_t \, \partial_i \Sigma_t \right] \Sigma_t^{-1}$,
- $\partial_i P_t^{t-1} = \partial_i \Phi \, P_{t-1}^{t-2} \Phi' + \Phi \, \partial_i P_{t-1}^{t-2} \, \Phi' + \Phi \, P_{t-1}^{t-2} \, \partial_i \Phi' + \partial_i Q,$ $\quad - \partial_i K_{t-1} \, \Sigma_t K_{t-1}' - K_{t-1} \, \partial_i \Sigma_t \, K_{t-1}' - K_{t-1} \Sigma_t \, \partial_i K_{t-1}'$,

using the fact that $P_t^{t-1} = \Phi P_{t-1}^{t-2} \Phi' + Q - K_{t-1} \Sigma_t K_{t-1}'$.

**4.12** Continuing with the previous problem, consider the evaluation of the Hessian matrix and the numerical evaluation of the asymptotic variance–covariance matrix of the parameter estimates. The information matrix satisfies

$$E\left\{ -\frac{\partial^2 \ln L_Y(\Theta)}{\partial \Theta \, \partial \Theta'} \right\} = E\left\{ \left( \frac{\partial \ln L_Y(\Theta)}{\partial \Theta} \right) \left( \frac{\partial \ln L_Y(\Theta)}{\partial \Theta} \right)' \right\};$$

see Anderson (1984, Section 4.4), for example. Show the $(i,j)$-th element of the information matrix, say, $\mathcal{I}_{ij}(\Theta) = E\left\{ -\partial^2 \ln L_Y(\Theta) / \partial \Theta_i \, \partial \Theta_j \right\}$, is

$$\begin{aligned} \mathcal{I}_{ij}(\Theta) \;&=\; \sum_{t=1}^{n} E\Big\{ \partial_i \epsilon_t' \, \Sigma_t^{-1} \;\, \partial_j \epsilon_t + \frac{1}{2} \mathrm{tr}\big( \Sigma_t^{-1} \, \partial_i \Sigma_t \, \Sigma_t^{-1} \, \partial_j \Sigma_t \big) \\ &\qquad + \frac{1}{4} \mathrm{tr}\left( \Sigma_t^{-1} \, \partial_i \Sigma_t \right) \mathrm{tr}\big( \Sigma_t^{-1} \, \partial_j \Sigma_t \big) \Big\}. \end{aligned}$$

Consequently, an approximate Hessian matrix can be obtained from the sample by dropping the expectation, $E$, in the above result and using only the recursions needed to calculate the gradient vector.

*Section 4.4*

**4.13** As an example of the way the state-space model handles the missing data problem, suppose the first-order autoregressive process

$$x_t = \phi x_{t-1} + w_t$$

has an observation missing at $t = m$, leading to the observations $y_t = A_t x_t$, where $A_t = 1$ for all $t$, except $t = m$ wherein $A_t = 0$. Assume $x_0 = 0$ with variance $\sigma_w^2/(1 - \phi^2)$, where the variance of $w_t$ is $\sigma_w^2$. Show the Kalman smoother estimators in this case are

$$x_t^n = \begin{cases} \phi y_1, & t = 0, \\ \frac{\phi}{1+\phi^2}(y_{m-1} + y_{m+1}), & t = m, \\ y_t, & t \neq 0, m, \end{cases}$$

with mean square covariances determined by

$$P_t^n = \begin{cases} \sigma_w^2, & t = 0, \\ \frac{\sigma_w^2}{1+\phi^2}, & t = m, \\ 0 & t \neq 0, m. \end{cases}$$

**4.14** The data set labeled `ar1miss.dat` is $n = 100$ observations generated from an AR(1) process, $x_t = \phi x_{t-1} + w_t$, with $\phi = .9$ and $\sigma_w = 1$, where 10% of the data has been zeroed out at random. Considering the zeroed out data to be missing data, use the results of Problem 4.13 to estimate the parameters of the model, $\phi$ and $\sigma_w$, using the EM algorithm, and then estimate the missing values.

*Section 4.5*

**4.15** Using Example 4.10 as a guide, fit a structural model to the Federal Reserve Board Production Index data and compare it with the model fit in Example 2.40.

*Section 4.6*

**4.16** Use Property P4.6 to complete the following exercises.

(a) Write a univariate AR(1) model, $y_t = \phi y_{t-1} + v_t$, in state-space form. Verify your answer is indeed an AR(1).

(b) Repeat (a) for an MA(1) model, $y_t = v_t + \theta v_{t-1}$.

(c) Write an IMA(1,1) model, $y_t = y_{t-1} + v_t + \theta v_{t-1}$, in state-space form.

**4.17** Verify Property P4.5.

**4.18** Verify Property P4.6.

*Section 4.7*

**4.19** Repeat the bootstrap analysis of Example 4.12 on the entire three-month treasury bills and rate of inflation data set of 110 observations. Do the conclusions of Example 4.12—that the dynamics of the data is best described in terms of a fixed, rather than stochastic, regression—still hold?

*Section 4.8*

**4.20** Argue that a switching model is reasonable in explaining the behavior of the number of sunspots (see Figure 3.20) and then fit a switching model to the sunspot data.

*Section 4.9*

**4.21** Use the material presented in Example 4.18 to perform a Bayesian analysis of the model for the Johnson & Johnson data presented in Example 4.10.

**4.22** Verify (4.174) and (4.175).

**4.23** Verify (4.180) and (4.187).

*Section 4.10*

**4.24** Fit a stochastic volatility model to the monthly returns of a stock dividend yield analyzed in Example 2.46. Compare the results with those of the ARCH model fit of Example 2.46.

*Section 4.11*

**4.25** In a small pilot study, a psychiatrist wanted to examine the effects of the drug lithium on bulimics (bulimics have continuous abnormal hunger and frequently go on eating binges). Although evidence of the effectiveness of lithium on bulimics has been shown, he was not sure if depressed subjects would respond differently than those without depression. He treated eight teenage female patients with lithium for 12 weeks; four of the subjects were diagnosed with depression, and half of the subjects received behavioral therapy. At the end of each four-week period, he recorded the number of binges each subject had during that week. The following are the results:

Weekly Number of Binges

| Subject | Depression | Week 0 | Week 4 | Week 8 | Week 12 |
|---|---|---|---|---|---|
| 1 | No | 13 | 3 | 0 | 0 |
| 2 | No | 15 | 4 | 3 | 1 |
| 3 | No | 16 | 4 | 3 | 2 |
| 4 | No | 14 | 2 | 1 | 2 |
| 5 | Yes | 10 | 7 | 4 | 3 |
| 6 | Yes | 18 | 7 | 2 | 4 |
| 7 | Yes | 16 | 6 | 5 | 4 |
| 8 | Yes | 19 | 8 | 5 | 7 |

Fit a longitudinal model that addresses the concerns of the psychiatrist. Because the data are counts (number of occurrences), consider a square root transformation prior to the analysis.

*Section 4.12*

**4.26** Consider the data set containing quarterly U.S. unemployment, U.S. GNP, consumption, and government and private investment from 1948-III to 1988-II. The seasonal component has been removed from the data. Concentrating on unemployment ($U_t$), GNP ($G_t$), and consumption ($C_t$), fit a vector ARMA model to the data after first logging each series, and then removing the linear trend. That is, fit a vector ARMA model to $\boldsymbol{x}_t = (x_{1t}, x_{2t}, x_{3t})'$, where, for example, $x_{1t} = \log(U_t) - \widehat{\beta}_0 - \widehat{\beta}_1 t$, where $\widehat{\beta}_0$ and $\widehat{\beta}_1$ are the least squares estimates for the regression of $\log(U_t)$ on time, $t$. Run a complete set of diagnostics on the residuals. Discuss whether the data lend themselves to fitting a reduced-rank model.

# CHAPTER 5

# Statistical Methods in the Frequency Domain

## 5.1 Introduction

In Chapters 3 and 4, we saw many applied time series problems that involved relating series to each other or to evaluating the effects of treatments or design parameters that arise when time-varying phenomena are subjected to periodic stimuli. In many cases, the nature of the physical or biological phenomena under study are best described by their Fourier components rather than by the difference equations involved in ARIMA or state-space models. The fundamental tools we use in studying periodic phenomena are the discrete Fourier transforms (DFTs) of the processes and their statistical properties. Hence, in Section 5.2, we review the properties of the DFT of a multivariate time series and discuss various approximations to the likelihood function based on the large-sample properties and the properties of the complex multivariate normal distribution. This enables extension of the classical techniques discussed in the following paragraphs to the multivariate time series case.

An extremely important class of problems in classical statistics develops when we are interested in relating a collection of input series to some output series. For example, in Chapter 1, we have previously considered relating temperature and various pollutant levels to daily mortality, but have not investigated the frequencies that appear to be driving the relation and have not looked at the possibility of leading or lagging effects. In Chapter 3, we isolated a definite lag structure that could be used to relate sea surface temperature to the number of new recruits. In Problem 3.23 of Chapter 3, the possible driving processes that could be used to explain inflow to Shasta Lake were hypothesized in terms of the possible inputs precipitation, cloud cover, temperature,

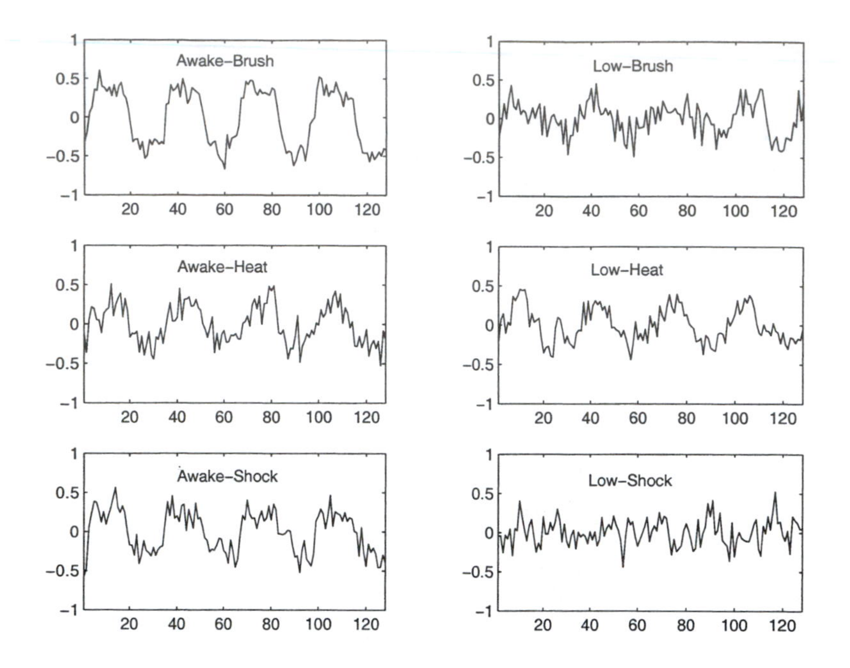


**Figure 5.1:** Mean response of subjects to various combinations of periodic stimulae measured at the cortex (primary somatosensory, contralateral).

and other variables. Identifying the combination of input factors in Figure 3.21 that produce the best prediction for inflow is an example of ***multiple regression in the frequency domain***, with the models treated theoretically by considering the regression, conditional on the random input processes.

A situation somewhat different from that above would be one in which the input series are regarded as fixed and known. In this case, we have a model analogous to that occurring in ***analysis of variance***, in which the analysis now can be performed on a frequency by frequency basis. This analysis works especially well when the inputs are dummy variables, depending on some configuration of treatment and other design effects and when effects are largely dependent on periodic stimuli. As an example, we will look at a designed experiment measuring the fMRI brain responses of a number of awake and mildly anesthetized subjects to several levels of periodic brushing, heat, and shock effects. Some limited data from this experiment have been discussed previously in Example 1.5 of Chapter 1. Figure 5.1 shows mean responses to various levels of periodic heat, brushing, and shock stimuli for subjects awake and subjects under mild anesthesia. The stimuli were periodic in nature, applied alternately for 32 seconds (16 points) and then stopped for 32 seconds. The periodic input signal comes through under all three design conditions when the subjects are awake, but is somewhat attenuated under anesthesia. The mean shock level response hardly shows on the input signal; shock levels were designed to simulate surgical incision without inflicting tissue damage. The means in Figure 5.1 are from a single location. Actually, for each individual, some nine series were recorded at various locations in the brain. It is natural to consider testing the effects of brushing, heat, and shock under the two levels of consciousness, using a time series generalization of analysis of variance.

A generalization to random coefficient regression is also considered, paralleling the univariate approach to signal extraction and detection presented in Section 3.9. This method enables a treatment of multivariate ***ridge***-type regressions and ***inversion problems***. Also, the usual random effects analysis of variance in the frequency domain becomes a special case of the random coefficient model.

The extension of frequency domain methodology to more classical approaches to multivariate discrimination and clustering is of interest in the frequency dependent case. Many time series differ in their means and in their autocovariance functions, making the use of both the mean function and the spectral density matrices relevant. As an example of such data, consider the bivariate series consisting of the P and S components derived from several earthquakes and explosions, such as those shown in Figure 5.2, where the P and S components, representing different arrivals have been separated from from the first and second halves, respectively, of wave forms like those shown originally in Figure 1.6 of Chapter 1.

Two earthquakes and two explosions from a set of eight earthquakes and explosions are shown in Figure 5.2 and some essential differences exist that might be used to characterize the two classes of events. Also, the frequency content of the two components of the earthquakes appears to be lower than those of the explosions, and relative amplitudes of the two classes appear to differ. For example, the ratio of the S to P amplitudes in the earthquake group is much higher for this restricted subset. Spectral differences were also noticed in Chapter 3, Figure 3.10, where the explosion processes had a stronger high-frequency component relative to the low-frequency contributions. Examples like these are typical of applications in which the essential differences between multivariate time series can be expressed by the behavior of either the frequency-dependent mean value functions or the spectral matrix. In ***discriminant analysis***, these types of differences are exploited to develop combinations of linear and quadratic classification criteria. Such functions can then be used to classify events of unknown origin, such as the Novaya Zemyla event shown in Figure 5.2, which tends to bear a visual resemblance to the explosion group.

Finally, for multivariate processes, the structure of the spectral matrix is also of great interest. We might reduce the dimension of the underlying process to a smaller set of input processes that explain most of the variability in the cross-spectral matrix as a function of frequency. ***Principal component analysis*** can be used to decompose the spectral matrix into a smaller subset of component factors that explain decreasing amounts of power. For example, the hydrological data might be explained in terms of a component process

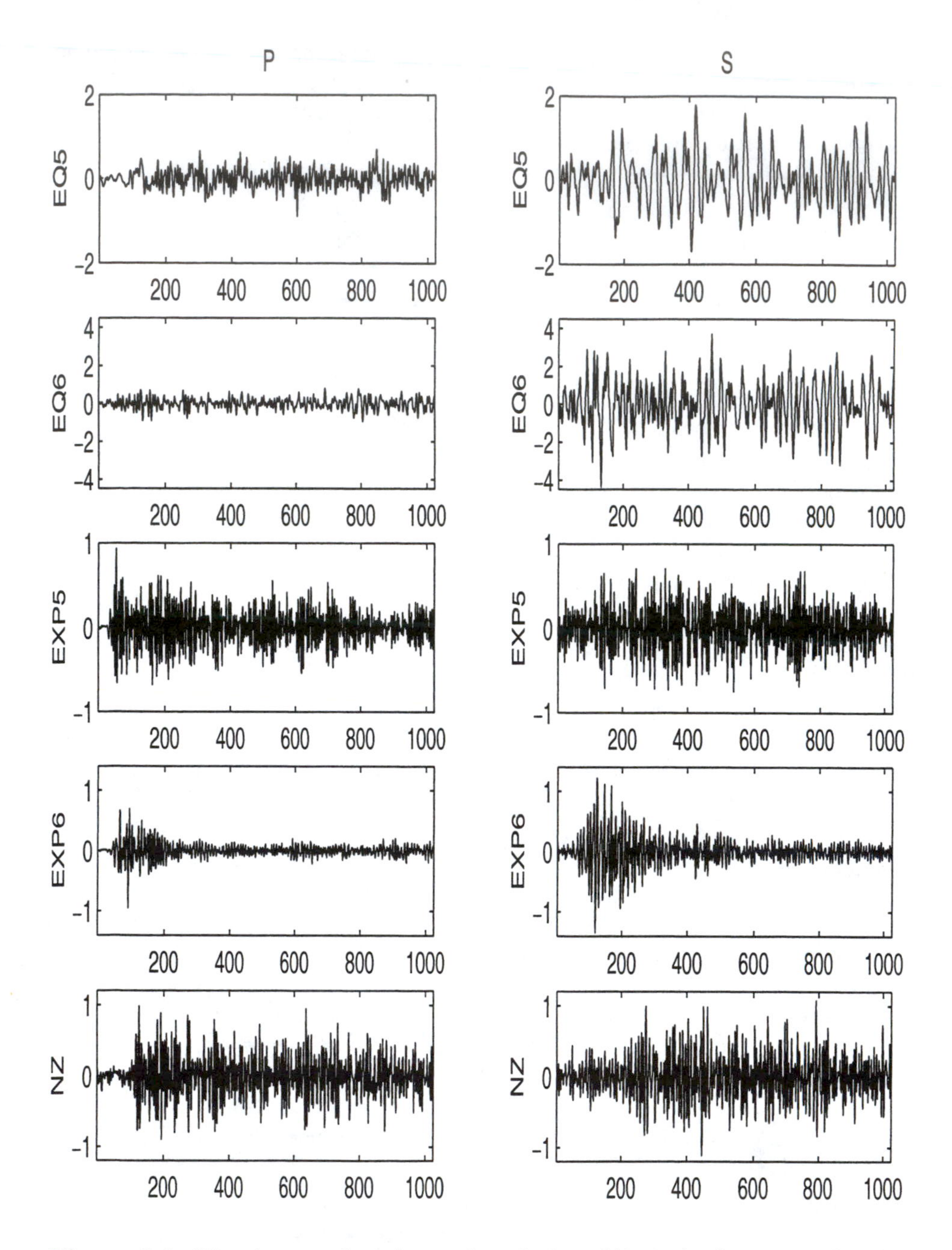


**Figure 5.2:** Bivariate earthquakes and explosions (40 pts/sec) compared with an event NZ (Novaya Zemlya) of unknown origin.

that weights heavily on precipitation and inflow and one that weights heavily on temperature and cloud cover. Perhaps these two components could explain most of the power in the spectral matrix at a given frequency. The ideas behind principal component analysis can also be generalized to include an optimal scaling methodology for categorical data called the ***spectral envelope*** (see Stoffer et al 1993). In succeeding sections, we also give an introduction to ***dynamic Fourier analysis*** and to ***wavelet analysis***.

## 5.2 Spectral Matrices and Likelihood Functions

We have previously argued for an approximation to the log likelihood based on the joint distribution of the DFTs in (3.89), where we used approximation as an aid in estimating parameters for certain parameterized spectra. In this chapter, we make heavy use of the fact that the sine and cosine transforms of the $p \times 1$ vector process $\boldsymbol{x}_t = (x_{t1}, x_{t2}, \ldots, x_{tp})'$ with mean $E\boldsymbol{x}_t = \boldsymbol{\mu}_t$, say, with DFT

$$\begin{aligned} \boldsymbol{X}(\nu_k) &= n^{-1/2} \sum_{t=1}^{n} \boldsymbol{x}_t \, \mathrm{e}^{-2\pi i \nu_k t} \\ &= \boldsymbol{X}_c(\nu_k) - i\boldsymbol{X}_s(\nu_k) \end{aligned} \tag{5.1}$$

and mean

$$\begin{aligned} \boldsymbol{M}(\nu_k) &= n^{-1/2} \sum_{t=1}^{n} \boldsymbol{\mu}_t \, \mathrm{e}^{-2\pi i \nu_k t} \\ &= \boldsymbol{M}_c(\nu_k) - i\boldsymbol{M}_s(\nu_k) \end{aligned} \tag{5.2}$$

will be approximately uncorrelated, where we evaluate at the usual Fourier frequencies $\{\nu_k = k/n, 0 < |\nu_k| < 1/2\}$. By Theorem 3.4, the approximate $2p \times 2p$ covariance matrix of the cosine and sine transforms, say, $\boldsymbol{Z}(\nu_k) = (\boldsymbol{X}_c(\nu_k)', \boldsymbol{X}_s(\nu_k)')'$, is

$$\Sigma(\nu_k) = \frac{1}{2} \begin{pmatrix} C(\nu_k) & -Q(\nu_k) \\ Q(\nu_k) & C(\nu_k) \end{pmatrix}, \tag{5.3}$$

and the real and imaginary parts are jointly normal. This result implies by Section T3.13 the density function of the vector DFT, say, $\boldsymbol{X}(\nu_k)$, can be approximated as

$$p(\nu_k) \approx |\boldsymbol{f}(\nu_k)|^{-1} \exp\{-(\boldsymbol{X}(\nu_k) - \boldsymbol{M}(\nu_k))^* f^{-1}(\nu_k)(\boldsymbol{X}(\nu_k) - \boldsymbol{M}(\nu_k))\},$$

where the spectral matrix is the usual

$$f(\nu_k) = C(\nu_k) - iQ(\nu_k). \tag{5.4}$$

Certain computations that we do in the section on discriminant analysis will involve approximating the joint likelihood by the product of densities like the one given above over subsets of the frequency band $0 < \nu_k < 1/2$.

To use the likelihood function for estimating the spectral matrix, for example, we appeal to the limiting result implied by Theorem 3.5 and again choose $L$ frequencies in the neighborhood of some target frequency $\nu$, say, $\boldsymbol{X}(\nu_k + \ell/n), \ell = -(L-1)/2, \ldots, (L-1)/2$. Then, let $\boldsymbol{X}_\ell, \ell = 1, \ldots, L$ denote the indexed values, and note the DFTs of the mean adjusted vector process are approximately jointly normal with mean zero and complex covariance matrix $\boldsymbol{f} = \boldsymbol{f}(\nu)$. Then, write the log likelihood over the $L$ sub-frequencies as

$$\ln L(\boldsymbol{X}_1, \ldots, \boldsymbol{X}_L; f) \approx -L \ln |f| - \sum_{\ell=1}^{L} (\boldsymbol{X}_\ell - \boldsymbol{M}_\ell)^* f^{-1} (\boldsymbol{X}_\ell - \boldsymbol{M}_\ell), \tag{5.5}$$

where we have suppressed the argument of $f = f(\nu)$ for ease of notation. The use of spectral approximations to the likelihood has been fairly standard, beginning with the work of Whittle (1961) and continuing in Brillinger (1981) and Hannan (1970). In this case, assuming the mean adjusted series are available, i.e., that $\boldsymbol{M}_\ell$ is known, so that we may assume that $\boldsymbol{X}_\ell$ is the mean-adjusted series. We may obtain the maximum likelihood estimator for $f$ by writing the joint log likelihood of the real and imaginary parts in terms of $\boldsymbol{Z}_\ell = (\boldsymbol{X}'_{c\ell}, \boldsymbol{X}'_{s\ell})'$ and obtaining the maximum likelihood estimators for $C$ and $Q$, the real and imaginary parts of $f$. Problem 5.2 shows we will obtain

$$\widehat{f} = L^{-1} \sum_{\ell=1}^{L} (\boldsymbol{X}_\ell - \boldsymbol{M}_\ell)(\boldsymbol{X}_\ell - \boldsymbol{M}_\ell)^*, \tag{5.6}$$

which is just the usual mean-adjusted estimator for the spectral matrix.

## 5.3 Regression for Jointly Stationary Series

In Section 3.8, we considered a model of the form

$$y_t = \sum_{r=-\infty}^{\infty} \beta_{1r} x_{t-r,1} + v_t, \tag{5.7}$$

where $x_{t1}$ is a single observed input series and $y_t$ is the observed output series, and we are interested in estimating the filter coefficients $\beta_{1r}$ relating the adjacent lagged values of $x_{t1}$ to the output series $y_t$. In the case of the SOI and recruitment series, we identified the El Niño driving series as $x_{t1}$, the input and $y_t$, the recruitment series, as the output. In general, more than a single plausible input series may exist. For example, the hydrological data shown in Figure 3.21 suggests there may be at least five possible series driving the inflow. Hence, we may envision a $q \times 1$ input vector of driving series, say, $\boldsymbol{x}_t = (x_{t1}, x_{t2}, \ldots, x_{tq})'$, and a set of $q \times 1$ vector of regression functions $\boldsymbol{\beta}_r = (\beta_{1r}, \beta_{2r,}, \ldots, \beta_{qr})'$, which are related as

$$y_t = \sum_{r=-\infty}^{\infty} \boldsymbol{\beta}_r' \boldsymbol{x}_{t-r} + v_t. \tag{5.8}$$

Writing the matrix form out as

$$y_t = \sum_{j=1}^{q} \sum_{r=-\infty}^{\infty} \beta_{jr} x_{t-r,j} + v_t \tag{5.9}$$

shows the output is basically a sum of linearly filtered versions of the input processes and a stationary noise process $v_t$, assumed to be uncorrelated with $\boldsymbol{x}_t$. Each filtered component in the sum over $j$ gives the contribution of lagged values of the $j$-th input series to the output series. We assume the regression functions $\beta_{jr}$ are fixed and unknown.

The model given by (5.8) is useful under several different scenarios, corresponding to a number of different assumptions that can be made about the components. Assuming the input and output processes are jointly stationary with zero means leads to the conventional regression analysis given in this section. The analysis depends on theory that assumes we observe the output process $y_t$ conditional on fixed values of the input vector $\boldsymbol{x}_t$; this is the same as the assumptions made in conventional regression analysis. Assumptions considered later involve letting the coefficient vector $\boldsymbol{\beta}_t$ be a random unknown signal vector that can be estimated by Bayesian arguments, using the conditional expectation given the data. The answers to this approach, given in Section 5.5, allow signal extraction and deconvolution problems to be handled. Assuming the inputs are fixed allows various experimental designs and analysis of variance to be done for both fixed and random effects models. Estimation of the frequency-dependent random effects variance components in the analysis of variance model is also considered in Section 5.5.

For the approach in this section, assume the inputs and outputs have zero means and are jointly stationary with the $(q+1) \times 1$ vector process $(\boldsymbol{x}_t', y_t)'$ of inputs $\boldsymbol{x}_t$ and outputs $y_t$ assumed to have a spectral matrix of the form

$$f(\nu) = \begin{pmatrix} f_x(\nu) & \boldsymbol{f}_{xy}(\nu) \\ \boldsymbol{f}_{yx}'(\nu) & f_y(\nu) \end{pmatrix}, \tag{5.10}$$

where $\boldsymbol{f}_{yx}(\nu) = (f_{yx_1}(\nu), f_{yx_2}(\nu), \ldots, f_{yx_q}(\nu))'$ is the $1 \times q$ vector of cross-spectra relating the $q$ inputs to the output and $f_x(\nu)$ is the $q \times q$ spectral matrix of the inputs. Generally, we observe the inputs and search for the vector of regression functions $\boldsymbol{\beta}_t$ relating the inputs to the outputs. We assume all autocovariance functions satisfy the absolute summability conditions of the form

$$\sum_{h=-\infty}^{\infty} |h||\gamma_{jk}(h)| < \infty. \tag{5.11}$$

($j, k = 1, \ldots, q+1$), where $\gamma_{jk}(h)$ is the autocovariance corresponding to the cross-spectrum $f_{jk}(\nu)$ in (5.10). We also need to assume a linear process of the form (3.164) as a condition for using Theorem 3.5 on the joint distribution of the discrete Fourier transforms in the neighborhood of some fixed frequency.

ESTIMATION OF THE REGRESSION FUNCTION

In order to estimate the regression function $\boldsymbol{\beta}_r$, the Projection theorem applied to minimizing

$$MSE = E\big[(y_t - \sum_{r=-\infty}^{\infty} \boldsymbol{\beta}_r' \boldsymbol{x}_{t-r})^2\big] \tag{5.12}$$

leads to the orthogonality conditions

$$E\big[(y_t - \sum_{r=-\infty}^{\infty} \boldsymbol{\beta}_r' \boldsymbol{x}_{t-r})\boldsymbol{x}_{t-s}'\big] = \mathbf{0}' \tag{5.13}$$

for all $s = 0, \pm1, \pm2, \ldots$, where $\mathbf{0}'$ denotes the $1 \times q$ zero vector. Taking the expectations inside and substituting for the definitions of the autocovariance functions appearing and leads to the normal equations

$$\sum_{r=-\infty}^{\infty} \boldsymbol{\beta}_r' \, \Gamma_x(s-r) = \boldsymbol{\gamma}_{yx}'(s), \tag{5.14}$$

for $s = 0, \pm1, \pm2, \ldots$, where $\Gamma_x(s)$ denotes the $q \times q$ autocovariance matrix of the vector series $\boldsymbol{x}_t$ at lag $s$ and $\boldsymbol{\gamma}_{yx}(s) = (\gamma_{yx_1}(s), \ldots, \gamma_{yx_q}(s))'$ is a vector containing the lagged covariances between $y_t$ and $\boldsymbol{x}_t$ . Again, a frequency domain approximate solution is easier in this case because the computations can be done frequency by frequency using cross-spectra that can be estimated from sample data using the DFT. In order to develop the frequency domain solution, substitute the representation into the normal equations, using the same approach as used in the simple case derived in Section 3.8. This approach yields

$$\int_{-1/2}^{1/2} \sum_{r=-\infty}^{\infty} \boldsymbol{\beta}_r' \, e^{2\pi i\nu(s-r)} \, f_{xx}(\nu) \, d\nu = \boldsymbol{\gamma}_{yx}'(s).$$

Now, because $\boldsymbol{\gamma}_{yx}'(s)$ is the Fourier transform of the cross-spectral vector $\boldsymbol{f}_{yx}'(\nu) = \boldsymbol{f}_{xy}^*(\nu)$, we might write the system of equations in the frequency domain, using the uniqueness of the Fourier transform, as

$$\boldsymbol{B}'(\nu) f_x(\nu) = \boldsymbol{f}_{xy}^*(\nu), \tag{5.15}$$

where $f_x(\nu)$ is the $q \times q$ spectral matrix of the inputs and $\boldsymbol{B}(\nu)$ is the $q \times 1$ vector Fourier transform of $\boldsymbol{\beta}_t$. Multiplying (5.15) on the right by $f_x^{-1}(\nu)$, assuming $f_x(\nu)$ is nonsingular at $\nu$, leads to the ***frequency domain estimator***

$$\boldsymbol{B}'(\nu) = \boldsymbol{f}_{xy}^*(\nu) f_x^{-1}(\nu). \tag{5.16}$$

Note, (5.16) implies the regression function would take the form

$$\boldsymbol{\beta}_t = \int_{-1/2}^{1/2} \boldsymbol{B}(\nu)\, e^{2\pi i \nu t}\, d\nu. \tag{5.17}$$

As before, it is conventional to introduce the DFT as the approximate estimator for the integral (5.17) and write

$$\boldsymbol{\beta}_t^M = M^{-1} \sum_{k=0}^{M-1} \boldsymbol{B}(\omega_k)\, e^{2\pi i \omega_k t}, \tag{5.18}$$

where $\omega_k = k/M, M << n$. The approximation was shown in Problem 3.21 to hold exactly as long as $\boldsymbol{\beta}_t = \boldsymbol{0}$ for $|t| \geq M$ and to have a mean squared error bounded by a function of the zero-lag autocovariance and the absolute sum of the neglected coefficients.

The mean squared error (5.12) can be written using the orthogonality principle, giving

$$MSE = \int_{-1/2}^{1/2} f_{y\cdot x}(\nu)\, d\nu, \tag{5.19}$$

where

$$f_{y\cdot x}(\nu) = f_y(\nu) - \boldsymbol{f}_{xy}^*(\nu) f_x^{-1}(\nu) \boldsymbol{f}_{xy}(\nu) \tag{5.20}$$

denotes the residual or error spectrum The resemblance of (5.20) to the usual equations in regression analysis is striking. It is useful to pursue the multiple regression analogy further by noting a ***squared multiple coherence*** can be defined as

$$\rho_{y\cdot x}^2(\nu) = \frac{\boldsymbol{f}_{xy}^*(\nu) f_x^{-1}(\nu) \boldsymbol{f}_{xy}(\nu)}{f_y(\nu)}. \tag{5.21}$$

This expression leads to the mean squared error in the form

$$MSE = \int_{-1/2}^{1/2} f_y(\nu)[1 - \rho_{y\cdot x}^2(\nu)]\, d\nu, \tag{5.22}$$

and we have an interpretation of $\rho_{y\cdot x}^2(\nu)$ as the ***proportion of power*** accounted for by the lagged regression on $\boldsymbol{x}_t$ at frequency $\nu$. If $\rho_{y\cdot x}^2(\nu) = 0$ for all $\nu$, we have

$$MSE = \int_{-1/2}^{1/2} f_y(\nu)\, d\nu = E[y_t^2],$$

which is the mean squared error when no predictive power exists. As long as $f_x(\nu)$ is positive definite at all frequencies, $MSE \geq 0$, and we will have

$$0 \leq \rho_{y\cdot x}^2(\nu) \leq 1 \tag{5.23}$$

for all $\nu$. If the multiple coherence is unity for all frequencies, the mean squared error in (5.22) is zero and the output series is perfectly predicted by a linearly filtered combination of the inputs. Problem 5.3 shows the ordinary squared coherence between the series $y_t$ and the linearly filtered combinations of the inputs appearing in (5.12) is exactly (5.21).

### Estimation Using Sampled Data

Clearly, the matrices of spectra and cross-spectra will not ordinarily be known, so the regression computations need to be based on sampled data. We assume, therefore, the inputs $x_{t1}, x_{t2}, \ldots, x_{tq}$ and output $y_t$ series are available at the time points $t = 1, 2, \ldots, n$, as in Chapter 3. In order to develop reasonable estimates for the spectral quantities, some replication must be assumed. Often, only one replication of each of the inputs and the output will exist, so it is necessary to assume a band exists over which the spectra and cross-spectra are approximately equal to $f_x(\nu)$ and $\boldsymbol{f}_{xy}(\nu)$, respectively. Then, let $Y(\nu_k + \ell/n)$ and $\boldsymbol{X}(\nu_k + \ell/n)$ be the DFTs of $y_t$ and $\boldsymbol{x}_t$ over the band, say, at frequencies of the form

$$\nu_k + \ell/n, \; \ell = -(L-1)/2, \ldots, 0 \ldots, (L-1)/2,$$

as before. Then, simply substitute the sample spectral matrix

$$\widehat{f}_x(\nu) = L^{-1} \sum_{\ell=-(L-1)/2}^{(L-1)/2} \boldsymbol{X}(\nu_k + \ell/n) \boldsymbol{X}^*(\nu_k + \ell/n) \tag{5.24}$$

and the vector of sample cross-spectra

$$\widehat{\boldsymbol{f}}_{xy}(\nu) = L^{-1} \sum_{\ell=-(L-1)/2}^{(L-1)/2} \boldsymbol{X}(\nu_k + \ell/n) \overline{Y(\nu_k + \ell/n)} \tag{5.25}$$

for the respective terms in (5.16) to get the regression estimator $\widehat{\boldsymbol{B}}(\nu)$. For the regression estimator (5.18), we may use

$$\widehat{\beta}_t^M = \frac{1}{M} \sum_{k=0}^{M-1} \widehat{\boldsymbol{f}}_{xy}^*(\omega_k) \widehat{f}_x^{-1}(\omega_k) \, e^{2\pi i \omega_k t} \tag{5.26}$$

for $t = 0, \pm 1, \pm 2, \ldots, \pm(M/2 - 1)$, as the estimated regression function.

### Tests of Hypotheses

The estimated squared multiple coherence, corresponding to the theoretical coherence (5.21), becomes

$$\widehat{\rho}_{y \cdot x}^2(\nu) = \frac{\widehat{\boldsymbol{f}}_{xy}^*(\nu) \widehat{f}_x^{-1}(\nu) \widehat{\boldsymbol{f}}_{xy}(\nu)}{\widehat{f}_y(\nu)}. \tag{5.27}$$

We may obtain a distributional result for the multiple coherence function analogous to that obtained in the univariate case by writing the multiple regression model in the frequency domain, as was done in Example 3.22 of Chapter 3. We obtain the statistic

$$F_{2q,2(L-q)} = \frac{(L-q)}{q}\frac{\widehat{\rho}^2_{y\cdot x}(\nu)}{[1-\widehat{\rho}^2_{y\cdot x}(\nu)]}, \tag{5.28}$$

which has an $F$-distribution with $2q$ and $2(L-q)$ degrees of freedom under the null hypothesis that $\rho^2_{y\cdot x}(\nu) = 0$, or equivalently, that $\boldsymbol{B}(\nu) = 0$, in the model

$$Y(\nu_k + \ell/n) = \boldsymbol{B}'(\nu)X(\nu_k + \ell/n) + V(\nu_k + \ell/n), \tag{5.29}$$

where the spectral density of the error $V(\nu_k + \ell/n)$ is $f_{y\cdot x}(\nu)$. Problem 5.5 sketches a derivation of this result.

A second kind of hypothesis of interest is one that might be used to test whether a full model with $q$ inputs is significantly better than some submodel with $q_1 < q$ components. In the time domain, this hypothesis implies, for a partition of the vector of inputs into $q_1$ and $q_2$ components ($q_1 + q_2 = q$), say, $\boldsymbol{x}_t = (\boldsymbol{x}'_{t1}, \boldsymbol{x}'_{t2})'$, and the similarly partitioned vector of regression functions $\boldsymbol{\beta}_t = (\boldsymbol{\beta}'_{1t}, \boldsymbol{\beta}'_{2t}))'$, we would be interested in testing whether $\boldsymbol{\beta}_{2t} = \mathbf{0}$ in the partitioned regression model

$$y_t = \sum_{r=-\infty}^{\infty} \boldsymbol{\beta}'_{1r}\boldsymbol{x}_{t-r,1} + \sum_{r=-\infty}^{\infty} \boldsymbol{\beta}'_{2r}\boldsymbol{x}_{t-r,2} + v_t. \tag{5.30}$$

Rewriting the regression model (5.30) in the frequency domain in a form that is similar to (5.29) establishes that, under the partitions of the spectral matrix into its $q_i \times q_j$ $(i,j = 1,2)$ submatrices, say,

$$\widehat{f}_x(\nu) = \begin{pmatrix} \widehat{f}_{11}(\nu) & \widehat{f}_{12}(\nu) \\ \widehat{f}_{21}(\nu) & \widehat{f}_{22}(\nu) \end{pmatrix}, \tag{5.31}$$

and the cross-spectral vector into its $q_i \times 1$ $(i = 1,2)$ subvectors,

$$\widehat{\boldsymbol{f}}_{xy}(\nu) = \begin{pmatrix} \widehat{\boldsymbol{f}}_{1y}(\nu) \\ \widehat{\boldsymbol{f}}_{2y}(\nu) \end{pmatrix}, \tag{5.32}$$

we may test the hypothesis $\boldsymbol{\beta}_{2t} = \mathbf{0}$ at frequency $\nu$ by comparing the estimated residual power

$$\widehat{f}_{y\cdot x}(\nu) = \widehat{f}_y(\nu) - \widehat{\boldsymbol{f}}^*_{xy}(\nu)\widehat{f}_x^{-1}(\nu)\widehat{\boldsymbol{f}}_{xy}(\nu) \tag{5.33}$$

under the full model with that under the reduced model, given by

$$\widehat{f}_{y\cdot 1}(\nu) = \widehat{f}_y(\nu) - \widehat{\boldsymbol{f}}^*_{1y}(\nu)\widehat{f}_{11}^{-1}(\nu)\widehat{\boldsymbol{f}}_{1y}(\nu). \tag{5.34}$$

**Table 5.1:** Analysis of Power (ANOPOW) for Testing No Contribution from the Subset $\boldsymbol{x}_{t2}$ in the Partitioned Regression Model

| Source | Power | Degrees of Freedom |
|---|---|---|
| $x_{t,q_1+1},\ldots,x_{t,q_1+q_2}$ | SSR($\nu$)(5.35) | $2q_2$ |
| Error | SSE($\nu$)(5.36) | $2(L-q_1-q_2)$ |
| Total | $L\widehat{f}_{y\cdot 1}(\nu)$ | $2(L-q_1)$ |

The power due to regression can be written as

$$\text{SSR}(\nu) = L[\widehat{f}_{y\cdot 1}(\nu) - \widehat{f}_{y\cdot x}(\nu)], \tag{5.35}$$

with the usual error power given by

$$\text{SSE}(\nu) = L\widehat{f}_{y\cdot x}(\nu). \tag{5.36}$$

The test of no regression proceeds using the $F$-statistic

$$F_{2q_2,2(L-q)} = \frac{(L-q)}{q_2}\frac{\text{SSR}(\nu))}{\text{SSE}(\nu)}. \tag{5.37}$$

The distribution of this $F$-statistic with $q_2$ numerator degrees of freedom and $2(L-q)$ denominator degrees of freedom follows from an argument paralleling that given in in Example 3.22 for the case of a single input. The test results can be summarized in an ***Analysis of Power*** (ANOPOW) table that parallels the usual analysis of variance (ANOVA) table. Table 5.1 shows the components of power for testing $\boldsymbol{\beta}_{2t} = \mathbf{0}$ at a particular frequency $\nu$. The ratio of the two components divided by their respective degrees of freedom just yields the $F$-statistic (5.33) used for testing whether the $q_2$ add significantly to the predictive power of the regression on the $q_1$ series.

**Example 5.1 Predicting Shasta Lake Inflow**

We illustrate some of the preceding ideas by considering the problem of predicting the transformed inflow series shown in Figure 3.21 from some combination of the inputs. First, look for the best single input predictor using the squared coherence function (5.27). The results, exhibited in Figure 5.3, show transformed precipitation produces the most consistently high squared coherence values at all frequencies ($L = 41$), with the seasonal frequencies $.08, .17, .25$, and $.33$ cycles per month corresponding to 12-month, six-month, four-month, and three-month periods contributing most significantly at the $\alpha = .001$ level.

Other inputs, with the exception of wind speed, also appear to be plausible contributors. In order to evaluate the other contributors, we consider partitioned tests with models including each of the other variables and

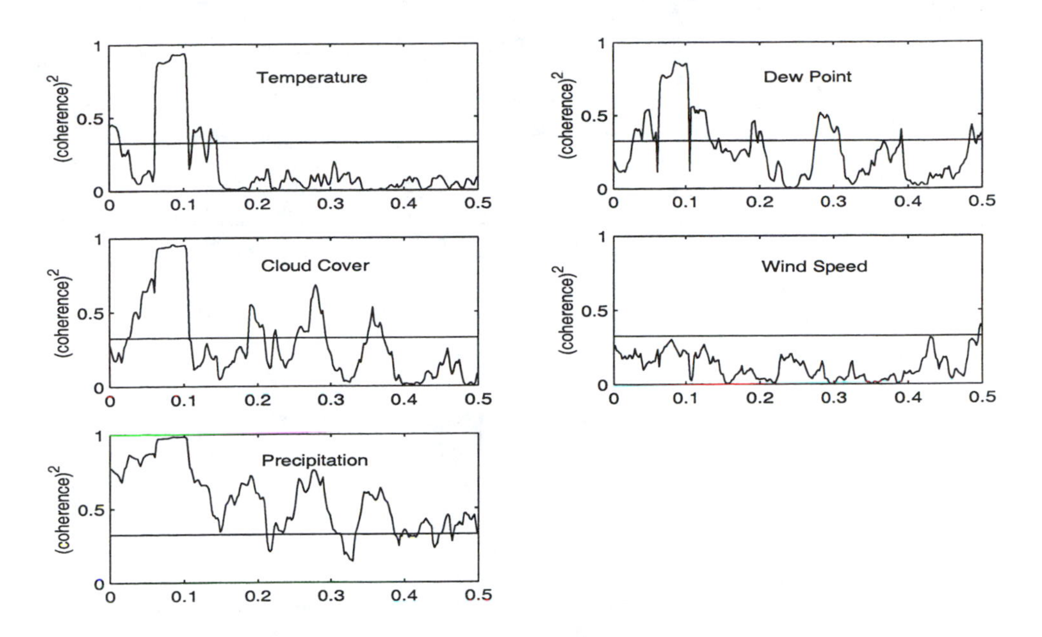


**Figure 5.3:** Univariate coherence functions relating Shasta Lake inflow to various inputs (frequency scale is cycles per month).

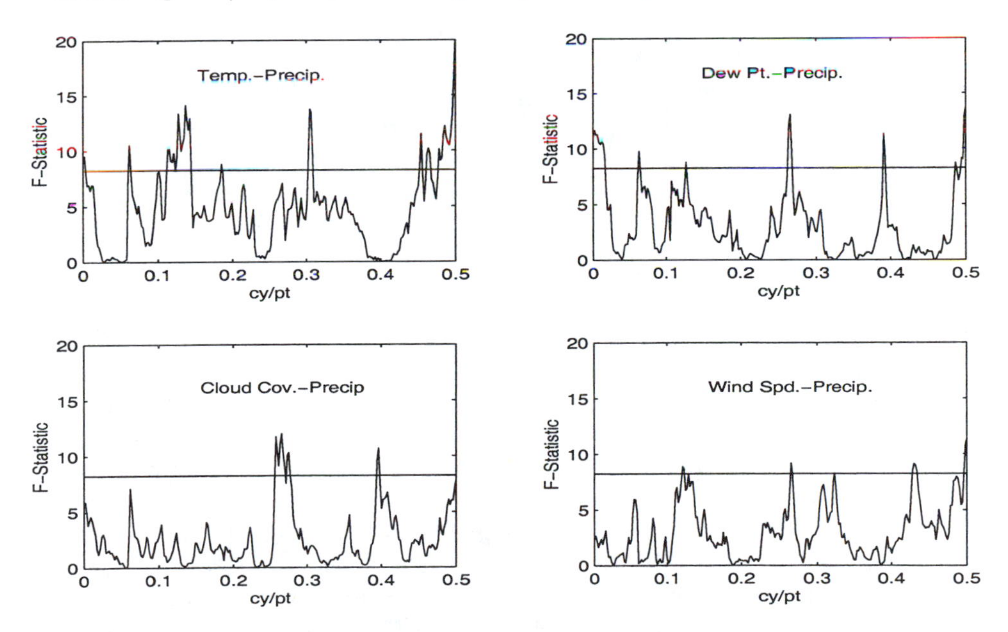


**Figure 5.4:** $F$-statistics for testing whether various inputs combined with precipitation add to the ability to predict Shasta Lake inflow.

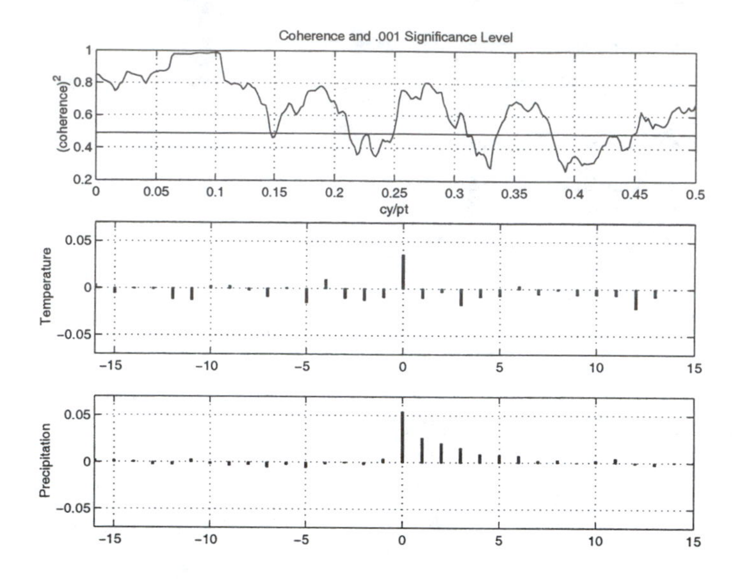


**Figure 5.5:** Multiple coherence between inflow and combined precipitation and temperature along with multiple impulse response functions for the regression relations.

precipitation tested against models including precipitation alone. Figure 5.4 shows a plot of the $F$-statistic (5.28) as a function of frequency for testing each of the inputs as a possible additional component. We see here some isolated significance points, particularly in the temperature series at some of the higher seasonal components, although the strong coherence at the 12-month frequency seems to have been essentially eliminated by the incorporation of precipitation.

The additional contribution of temperature to the model seems somewhat marginal because the multiple coherence (5.27), shown in the top panel of Figure 5.5, seems only slightly better than the univariate coherence with precipitation shown in Figure 5.3. It is, however, instructive to produce the multiple regression functions, using (5.26) to see if a simple model for inflow exists that would involve some regression combination of inputs temperature and precipitation that would be useful for predicting inflow to Shasta Lake. With this in mind, denoting the possible inputs $P_t$ for transformed precipitation and $T_t$ for transformed temperature, the regression function has been plotted in the lower two panels of Figure 5.5. The time axes run over both positive and negative values and are centered at time $t = 0$. Hence, the relation with temperature seems to be instantaneous and positive and an exponentially decaying relation to precipitation exists that has been noticed previously in the analysis in Problem 3.23 of Chapter 3. The plots suggest a transfer function model of the general form fitted to the recruit and SOI series in Example 2.45 of Chapter 2. We might propose fitting the inflow output, say, $I_t$, using the model

$$I_t = \alpha_0 + \frac{\delta_0}{(1 - \omega_1 B)} P_t + \alpha_2 T_t + \eta_t,$$

which is the transfer function model, without the temperature component, considered in that section.

## 5.4 Regression with Deterministic Inputs

The previous section considered the case in which the input and output series were jointly stationary, but there are many circumstances where in which we might want to assume that the input functions are fixed and have a known functional form. This case happens in the analysis of data from designed experiments. For example, we may want to take a collection of earthquakes and explosions such as are shown in Figure 5.2 and test whether the mean functions are the same for either the P or S components or, perhaps, for them jointly. In certain other signal detection problems using arrays, the inputs are used as dummy variables to express lags corresponding to the arrival times of the signal at various elements, under a model corresponding to that of a plane wave from a fixed source propagating across the array. In Figure 5.1, we plotted the mean responses of the cortex as a function of various underlying design configurations corresponding to various stimuli applied to awake and mildly anesthetized subjects.

It is necessary to introduce a replicated version of the underlying model to handle even the univariate situation, and we replace (5.8) by

$$y_{jt} = \sum_{r=-\infty}^{\infty} \boldsymbol{\beta}_r' \boldsymbol{z}_{j,t-r} + v_{jt} \tag{5.38}$$

for $j = 1, 2, \ldots, N$ series, where we assume the vector of known deterministic inputs, $\boldsymbol{z}_{jt} = (z_{jt1}, \ldots, z_{jtq})'$, satisfies

$$\sum_{t=-\infty}^{\infty} |t||z_{jtk}| < \infty$$

for $j = 1, \ldots, N$ replicates of an underlying process involving $k = 1, \ldots, q$ regression functions. The model can also be treated under the assumption that the deterministic function satisfy Grenanders' conditions, as in Hannan (1970), but we do not need those conditions here and simply follow the approach in Shumway (1983, 1988).

It will sometimes be convenient in what follows to represent the model in matrix notation, writing (5.38) as

$$\boldsymbol{y}_t = \sum_{r=-\infty}^{\infty} z_{t-r}\, \boldsymbol{\beta}_r + \boldsymbol{v}_t, \tag{5.39}$$

where $z_t = (\boldsymbol{z}_{1t}, \ldots, \boldsymbol{z}_{Nt})'$ are the $N \times q$ matrices of independent inputs and $\boldsymbol{y}_t$ and $\boldsymbol{v}_t$ are the $N \times 1$ output and error vectors. The error vector $\boldsymbol{v}_t = (v_{1t}, \ldots, v_{Nt})'$ is assumed to be a multivariate, zero-mean, stationary, normal process with spectral matrix $f_v(\nu) I_N$ that is proportional to the $N \times N$ identity matrix. That is, we assume the error series $v_{jt}$ are independently and identically distributed with spectral densities $f_v(\nu)$.

**Example 5.2 An Infrasonic Signal From a Nuclear Explosion**

Often, we will observe a common signal, say, $\beta_t$ on an array of sensors, with the response at the $j$-th sensor denoted by $y_{jt}, j = 1, \ldots, N$ For example, Figure 5.6 shows an infrasonic or low-frequency acoustic signal from a nuclear explosion, as observed on a small triangular array of $N = 3$ acoustic sensors. These signals appear at slightly different times. Because of the way signals propagate, a plane wave signal of this kind, from a given source, traveling at a given velocity, will arrive at elements in the array at predictable time delays. In the case of the infrasonic signal in Figure 5.6, the delays were approximated by computing the cross-correlation between elements and simply reading off the time delay corresponding to the maximum. For a detailed discussion of the statistical analysis of array signals, see Shumway et al (1999).

A simple additive signal plus noise model of the form

$$y_{jt} = \beta_{t-\tau_j} + v_{jt} \tag{5.40}$$

can be assumed, where $\tau_j, j = 1, 2, \ldots, N$ are the time delays that determine the start point of the signal at each element of the array. The model (5.40) is written in the form (5.38) by letting $z_{jt} = \delta_{t-\tau_j}$, where $\delta_t = 0$ for $t = 0$ and is zero otherwise. In this case, we are interested in both the problem of detecting the presence of the signal and in estimating its waveform $\beta_t$. In this case, a plausible estimator of the waveform would be the unbiased ***beam***, say,

$$\widehat{\beta}_t = \sum_{j=1}^{N} y_{j,t+\tau_j}, \tag{5.41}$$

where time delays in this case were measured as $\tau_1 = -17, \tau_2 = 0$, and $\tau_3 = 22$ from the cross-correlation function. The bottom panel of Figure 5.6 shows the computed beam in this case, and the noise in the individual channels has been reduced and the essential characteristics of the common signal are retained in the average.

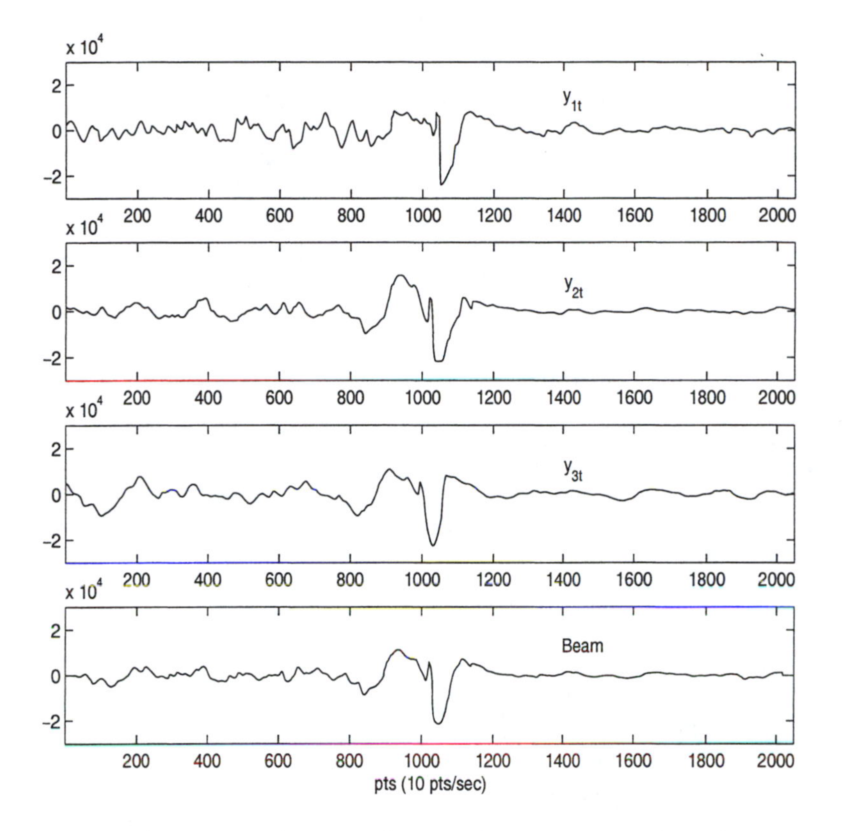


**Figure 5.6:** Three series for a nuclear explosion detonated 25 km south of Christmas Island and the delayed average or beam.

The above discussion and example serve to motivate a more detailed look at the estimation and detection problems in the case in which the input series $z_{jt}$ are fixed and known. We consider the modifications needed for this case in the following sections.

## Estimation of the Regression Relation

Because the regression model (5.38) involves fixed functions, we may parallel the usual approach using the Gauss–Markov theorem to search for linear-filtered estimators of the form

$$\widehat{\boldsymbol{\beta}}_t = \sum_{j=1}^{N} \sum_{r=-\infty}^{\infty} \boldsymbol{h}_{jr} y_{j,t-r}, \tag{5.42}$$

where $\boldsymbol{h}_{jt} = (h_{jt1} \ldots, h_{jtq})'$ is a vector of filter coefficients, determined so the estimators are unbiased and have minimum variance. The equivalent matrix form is

$$\widehat{\beta}_t = \sum_{r=-\infty}^{\infty} h_r \, \boldsymbol{y}_{t-r}, \tag{5.43}$$

where $h_t = (\boldsymbol{h}_{1t}, \ldots, \boldsymbol{h}_{Nt})$ is a $q \times N$ matrix of filter functions. The matrix form resembles the usual classical regression case and is more convenient for extending the the Gauss–Markov theorem to lagged regression. The unbiased condition is considered in Problem 5.6. It can be shown (see Shumway and Dean, 1968) that $\boldsymbol{h}_{js}$ can be taken as the Fourier transform of

$$\boldsymbol{H}_j(\nu) = S_z^{-1}(\nu)\overline{\boldsymbol{Z}_j(\nu)}, \tag{5.44}$$

where

$$\boldsymbol{Z}_j(\nu) = \sum_{t=-\infty}^{\infty} \boldsymbol{z}_{jt} \mathrm{e}^{-2\pi i\nu t} \tag{5.45}$$

is the infinite Fourier transform of $\boldsymbol{z}_{jt}$. The matrix

$$S_z(\nu) = \sum_{j=1}^{N} \overline{\boldsymbol{Z}_j(\nu)} \boldsymbol{Z}_j'(\nu) \tag{5.46}$$

can be written in the form

$$S_z(\nu) = Z^*(\nu)Z(\nu), \tag{5.47}$$

where the $N \times q$ matrix $Z(\nu)$ is defined by $Z(\nu) = (\boldsymbol{Z}_1(\nu), \ldots, \boldsymbol{Z}_N(\nu))'$. In matrix notation, the Fourier transform of the optimal filter becomes

$$H(\nu) = S_z^{-1}(\nu)Z^*(\nu), \tag{5.48}$$

where $H(\nu) = (\boldsymbol{H}_1(\nu), \ldots, \boldsymbol{H}_N(\nu))$ is the $q \times N$ matrix of frequency response functions. The optimal filter then becomes the Fourier transform

$$h_t = \int_{-1/2}^{1/2} H(\nu)\mathrm{e}^{2\pi i\nu t} \, d\nu. \tag{5.49}$$

If the transform is not tractable to compute, an approximation analogous to (5.26) may be used.

**Example 5.3 Estimation of the Infrasonic Signal in Example 5.2**

We consider the problem of producing a best linearly filtered unbiased estimator for the infrasonic signal in Example 5.2. In this case, $q = 1$ and (5.45) becomes

$$Z_j(\nu) = \sum_{t=-\infty}^{\infty} \delta_{t-\tau_j} \mathrm{e}^{-2\pi i\nu t} = \mathrm{e}^{-2\pi i\nu\tau_j}$$

and $S_z(\nu) = N$. Hence, we have

$$\overline{H_j(\nu)} = \frac{1}{N} e^{2\pi i \nu \tau_j}.$$

Using (5.49), we obtain $h_{jt} = \delta(t + \tau_j)$. Substituting in (5.42), we obtain the best linear unbiased estimator as the beam, computed as in (5.41).

### Tests of Hypotheses

We consider first testing the hypothesis that the complete vector $\boldsymbol{\beta}_t$ is zero, i.e., that the vector signal is absent. We develop a test at each frequency $\nu$ by taking single adjacent frequencies of the form $\nu_k = k/n$, as in the initial section. We may approximate the DFT of the observed vector in the model (5.38) using a representation of the form

$$Y_j(\nu_k) = \boldsymbol{B}'(\nu_k)\boldsymbol{Z}_j(\nu_k) + V_j(\nu_k) \tag{5.50}$$

for $j = 1, \ldots, N$, where the error terms will be uncorrelated with common variance $f(\nu_k)$, the spectral density of the error term. The independent variables $\boldsymbol{Z}_j(\nu_k)$ can either be the infinite Fourier transform, or they can be approximated by the DFT. Hence, we can obtain the matrix version of a complex regression model, written in the form

$$\boldsymbol{Y}(\nu_k) = Z(\nu_k)\boldsymbol{B}(\nu_k) + \boldsymbol{V}(\nu_k), \tag{5.51}$$

where the $N \times q$ matrix $Z(\nu_k)$ has been defined previously below (5.47) and $\boldsymbol{Y}(\nu_k)$ and $\boldsymbol{V}(\nu_k)$ are $N \times 1$ vectors with the error vector $\boldsymbol{V}(\nu_k)$ having mean zero, with covariance matrix $f(\nu_k)I_N$. The usual regression arguments show that the maximum likelihood estimator for the regression coefficient will be

$$\widehat{\boldsymbol{B}}(\nu_k) = S_z^{-1}(\nu_k)\boldsymbol{s}_{zy}(\nu_k), \tag{5.52}$$

where $S_z(\nu_k)$ is given by (5.47) and

$$\begin{aligned}
\boldsymbol{s}_{zy}(\nu_k) &= Z^*(\nu_k)\boldsymbol{Y}(\nu_k) \\
&= \sum_{j=1}^{N} \overline{\boldsymbol{Z}_j(\nu_k)} Y_j(\nu_k).
\end{aligned} \tag{5.53}$$

Also, the maximum likelihood estimator for the error spectral matrix is proportional to

$$\begin{aligned}
s_{y\cdot z}^2(\nu_k) &= \sum_{j=1}^{N} |Y_j(\nu_k) - \widehat{\boldsymbol{B}}(k)'\boldsymbol{Z}_j(\nu_k)|^2 \\
&= \boldsymbol{Y}^*(\nu_k)\boldsymbol{Y}(\nu_k) - \boldsymbol{Y}^*(\nu_k)Z(\nu_k)[Z^*(\nu_k)Z(\nu_k)]^{-1}Z^*(\nu_k)\boldsymbol{Y}(\nu_k) \\
&= s_y^2(\nu_k) - \boldsymbol{s}_{zy}^*(\nu_k)S_z^{-1}(\nu_k)\boldsymbol{s}_{zy}(\nu_k),
\end{aligned} \tag{5.54}$$

**Table 5.2:** Analysis of Power (ANOPOW) for Testing No Contribution from the Independent Series at Frequency $\nu$ in the Fixed Input Case

| Source | Power | Degrees of Freedom |
|---|---|---|
| Regression | SSR($\nu$)(5.56) | $2Lq$ |
| Error | SSE($\nu$) (5.57) | $2L(N-q)$ |
| Total | SST($\nu$) | $2LN$ |

where

$$s_y^2(\nu_k) = \sum_{j=1}^{N} |Y_j(\nu_k)|^2. \tag{5.55}$$

Under the null hypothesis that the regression coefficient $\boldsymbol{B}(\nu_k) = \boldsymbol{0}$, the estimator for the error power is just $s_y^2(\nu_k)$ If smoothing is needed, we may replace the (5.54) and (5.55) by smoothed components over the frequencies $\nu_k + \ell/n, \ell = -(L-1)/2, \dots (L-1)/2$ close to $\nu$. In that case, we obtain the regression and error spectral components as

$$\text{SSR}(\nu) = \sum_{\ell=-(L-1)/2}^{(L-1)/2} \boldsymbol{s}_{zy}^*(\nu_k + \ell/n) S_z^{-1}(\nu_k + \ell/n) \boldsymbol{s}_{zy}(\nu_k + \ell/n) \tag{5.56}$$

and

$$\text{SSE}(\nu) = \sum_{\ell=-(L-1)/2}^{(L-1)/2} s_{y\cdot z}^2(\nu_k + \ell/n). \tag{5.57}$$

The $F$-statistic for testing no regression relation is

$$F_{2Lq,2L(N-q)} = \frac{q}{N-q} \frac{\text{SSR}(\nu)}{\text{SSE}(\nu)}. \tag{5.58}$$

The analysis of power pertaining to this situation appears in Table 5.2.

In the fixed regression case, the partitioned hypothesis that is the analog of $\boldsymbol{\beta}_{2t} = 0$ in (5.30) with $\boldsymbol{x}_{t1}, \boldsymbol{x}_{t2}$ replaced by $\boldsymbol{z}_{t1}, \boldsymbol{z}_{t2}$. Here, we partition $S_z(\nu)$ into $q_i \times q_j$ $(i, j = 1, 2)$ submatrices, say,

$$S_z(\nu_k) = \begin{pmatrix} S_{11}(\nu_k) & S_{12}(\nu_k) \\ S_{21}(\nu_k) & S_{22}(\nu_k) \end{pmatrix}, \tag{5.59}$$

and the cross-spectral vector into its $q_i \times 1$, for $i = 1, 2$, subvectors

$$\boldsymbol{s}_{zy}(\nu_k) = \begin{pmatrix} \boldsymbol{s}_{1y}(\nu_k) \\ \boldsymbol{s}_{2y}(\nu_k) \end{pmatrix}. \tag{5.60}$$

Here, we test the hypothesis $\boldsymbol{\beta}_{2t} = \boldsymbol{0}$ at frequency $\nu$ by comparing the residual power (5.54) under the full model with the residual power under the reduced

**Table 5.3:** Analysis of Power (ANOPOW) for Testing No Contribution from the Last $q_2$ Inputs in the Fixed Input Case

| Source | Power | Degrees of Freedom |
|---|---|---|
| Regression | SSR($\nu$)(5.62) | $2Lq_2$ |
| Error | SSE($\nu$) (5.63) | $2L(N-q)$ |
| Total | SST($\nu$) | $2LNq_1$ |

model, given by

$$s_{y\cdot 1}^2(\nu_k) = s_y^2(\nu_k) - \boldsymbol{s}_{1y}^*(\nu_k) S_{11}^{-1}(\nu_k)\boldsymbol{s}_{1y}(\nu_k). \tag{5.61}$$

Again, it is desirable to add over adjacent frequencies with roughly comparable spectra so the regression and error power components can be taken as

$$\text{SSR}(\nu) = \sum_{\ell=-(L-1)/2}^{(L-1)/2} \boldsymbol{s}_{1y}^*(\nu_k + \ell/n) S_{11}^{-1}(\nu_k + \ell/n)\boldsymbol{s}_{1y}(\nu_k + \ell/n) \tag{5.62}$$

and

$$\text{SSE}(\nu) = \sum_{\ell=-(L-1)/2}^{(L-1)/2} s_{y\cdot z}^2(\nu_k + \ell/n). \tag{5.63}$$

The information can again be summarized as in Table 5.3, where the ratio of mean power regression and error components leads to the $F$-statistic

$$F_{2Lq_2, 2L(N-q)} = \frac{(N-q)}{q_2} \frac{\text{SSR}(\nu)}{\text{SSE}(\nu)}. \tag{5.64}$$

We illustrate the analysis of power procedure using the infrasonic signal detection procedure of Example 5.2.

### Example 5.4 Detecting the Infrasonic Signal Using ANOPOW

We consider the problem of detecting the common signal for the three infrasonic series observing the common signal, as shown in Figure 5.3. The presence of the signal is obvious in the waveforms shown, so the test here mainly confirms the statistical significance and isolates the frequencies containing the strongest signal components. Each series contained $n = 1024$ points, sampled at 10 points per second. We use the model in (5.40) so $Z_j(\nu) = \mathrm{e}^{-2\pi i\nu\tau_j}$ and $S_z(\nu) = 1/N$ as in Example 5.3, with $s_{zy}(\nu_k)$ given as

$$s_{zy}(\nu_k) = \sum_{j=1}^{N} \mathrm{e}^{2\pi i\nu\tau_j} Y_j(\nu_k),$$

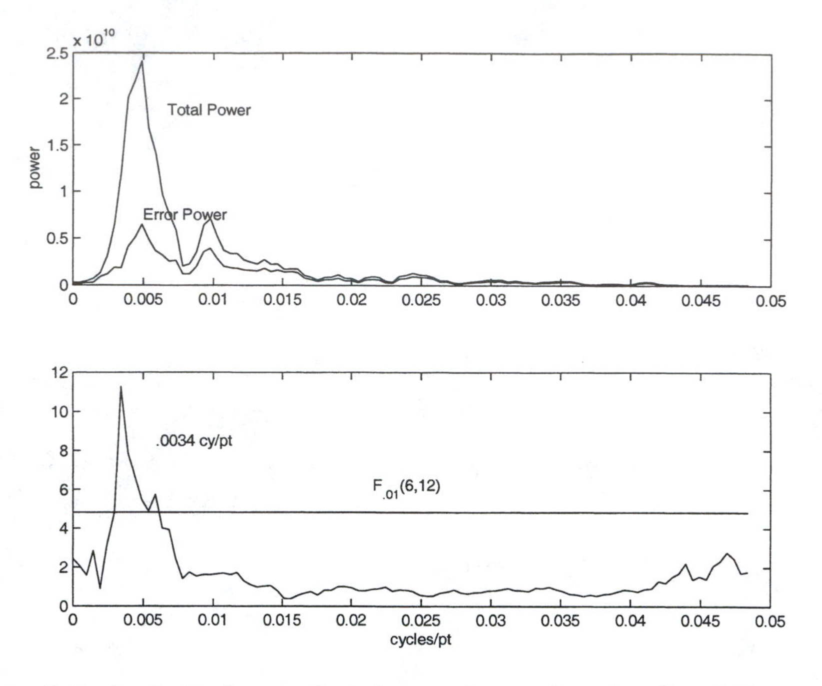


**Figure 5.7:** Analysis of power for infrasound array (top panel) and $F$-statistic (bottom panel) showing detection at .033 cy/sec (10 pts/sec).

using (5.46)and (5.53). The above expression can be interpreted as being proportional to the weighted mean or ***beam***, computed in frequency, and we introduce the notation

$$B_w(\nu_k) = \frac{1}{N} \sum_{j=1}^{N} e^{2\pi i \nu \tau_j} Y_j(\nu_k) \tag{5.65}$$

for that term. Substituting for the power components in Table 5.3 yields

$$\boldsymbol{s}_{zy}^*(\nu_k) S_z^{-1}(\nu_k) \boldsymbol{s}_{zy}(\nu_k) = N|B_w(\nu_k)|^2$$

and

$$\begin{aligned} s_{y\cdot z}^2(\nu_k) &= \sum_{j=1}^{N} |Y_j(\nu_k) - B_w(\nu_k)|^2 \\ &= \sum_{j=1}^{N} |Y_j(\nu_k)|^2 - N|B_w(\nu_k)|^2 \end{aligned}$$

for the regression signal and error components, respectively. Because only three elements in the array and a reasonable number of points in time exist, it seems advisable to employ some smoothing over frequency to obtain additional degrees of freedom. In this case, $L = 3$, yielding $2(3) = 6$ and $2(3)(3-1) = 12$ degrees of freedom for the numerator and denominator of the $F$-statistic (5.58). Figure 5.7 shows the analysis of power components due to error and the total power. The power is maximum at about .0044 cycles per point or about .044 cycles per second. The $F$-statistic is compared with the 1% significance level $F_{.01}(6,12) = 4.82$ in the bottom panel and has the strongest detection at about .034 cycles per second, a result mainly because the error power is decreasing more quickly than the regression or signal power in that band. Little power of consequence appears to exist in the higher range (.3-5 cycles per second).

Although there are examples of detecting multiple regression functions of the general type considered above (see, for example, Shumway, 1983), we do not consider additional examples of partitioning in the fixed input case here. The reason is that several examples exist in the section on designed experiments that illustrate the partitioned approach.

## 5.5 Random Coefficient Regression

The lagged regression models considered so far have assumed the input process is either stochastic or fixed and the components of the vector of regression function $\boldsymbol{\beta}_t$ are fixed and unknown parameters to be estimated. There are many cases in time series analysis in which it is more natural to regard the regression vector as an unknown stochastic signal. For example, we have studied the state-space model in Chapter 4, where the state equation can be considered as involving a random parameter vector that is essentially a multivariate autoregressive process. In Section 3.9, we considered estimating the univariate regression function $\beta_t$ as a signal extraction problem.

In this section, we consider a ***random coefficient regression model*** of (5.39) in the equivalent form

$$\boldsymbol{y}_t = \sum_{r=-\infty}^{\infty} z_{t-r}\, \boldsymbol{\beta}_r + \boldsymbol{v}_t, \tag{5.66}$$

where $\boldsymbol{y}_t = (y_{1t}, \dots, y_{Nt})'$ is the $N \times 1$ response vector and $z_t = (\boldsymbol{z}_{1t}, \dots, \boldsymbol{z}_{Nt})'$ are the $N \times q$ matrices containing the fixed input processes. Here, the components of the $q \times 1$ regression vector $\boldsymbol{\beta}_t$ are zero-mean, uncorrelated, stationary series with common spectral matrix $f_\beta(\nu) I_q$ and the error series $\boldsymbol{v}_t$ have zero-means and spectral matrix $f_v(\nu) I_N$, where $I_N$ is the $N \times N$ identity matrix. Then, defining the $N \times q$ matrix $Z(\nu) = (\boldsymbol{Z}_1(\nu), \boldsymbol{Z}_2(\nu), \dots, \boldsymbol{Z}_N(\nu))'$ of Fourier transforms of $z_t$, as in (5.45), it is easy to show the spectral matrix of the response vector $\boldsymbol{y}_t$ is given by

$$f_y(\nu) = f_\beta(\nu) Z(\nu) Z^*(\nu) + f_v(\nu) I_N. \tag{5.67}$$

The regression model with a stochastic stationary signal component is a general version of the simple additive noise model

$$y_t = \beta_t + v_t,$$

considered by Wiener (1949) and Kolmogorov (1941), who derived the minimum mean squared error estimators for $\beta_t$, as in Section 3.9. The more general multivariate version (5.66) represents the series as a convolution of the signal vector $\boldsymbol{\beta}_t$ and a known set of vector input series contained in the matrix $\boldsymbol{z}_t$. Restricting the the covariance matrices of signal and noise to diagonal form is consistent with what is done in statistics using random effects models, which we consider here in a later section. The problem of estimating the regression function $\boldsymbol{\beta}_t$ is often called ***deconvolution*** in the engineering and geophysical literature.

## Estimation of the Regression Relation

The regression function $\boldsymbol{\beta}_t$ can be estimated by a general filter of the form (5.43), where we write that estimator in matrix form

$$\widehat{\boldsymbol{\beta}}_t = \sum_{r=-\infty}^{\infty} h_t \, \boldsymbol{y}_{t-r}, \tag{5.68}$$

where $h_t = (\boldsymbol{h}_{1t}, \dots, \boldsymbol{h}_{Nt})$, and apply the orthogonality principle, as in Section 3.9. A generalization of the argument in that section (see Problem 5.8) leads to the estimator

$$H(\nu) = [S_z(\nu) + \theta(\nu) I_q]^{-1} Z^*(\nu) \tag{5.69}$$

for the Fourier transform of the minimum mean-squared error filter, where the parameter

$$\theta(\nu) = \frac{f_v(\nu)}{f_\beta(\nu)} \tag{5.70}$$

is the inverse of the signal-to-noise ratio. It is clear from the frequency domain version of the linear model (5.51), the comparable version of the estimator (5.52) can be written as

$$\widehat{\boldsymbol{B}}(\nu) = [S_z(\nu) + \theta(\nu) I_q]^{-1} \boldsymbol{s}_{zy}(\nu). \tag{5.71}$$

This version exhibits the estimator in the stochastic regressor case as the usual estimator, with a ***ridge correction***, $\theta(\nu)$, that is proportional to the inverse of the signal-to-noise ratio.

The mean-squared covariance of the estimator is shown to be

$$E[(\widehat{\boldsymbol{B}} - \boldsymbol{B})(\widehat{\boldsymbol{B}} - \boldsymbol{B})^*] = f_v(\nu)[S_z(\nu) + \theta(\nu)I_q]^{-1}, \tag{5.72}$$

which again exhibits the close connection between this case and the variance of the estimator (5.52), which can be shown to be $f_v(\nu)S_z^{-1}(\nu)$.

**Example 5.5 Estimating the Random Infrasonic Signal**

In Example 5.4, we have already determined the components needed in (5.69) and (5.70) to obtain the estimators for the random signal. The Fourier transform of the optimum filter at series $j$ has the form

$$H_j(\nu) = \frac{e^{2\pi i\nu\tau_j}}{N + \theta(\nu)} \tag{5.73}$$

with the mean-squared error given by $f_\beta(\nu)/[N + \theta(\nu)]$ from (5.72). The net effect of applying the filters will be the same as filtering the beam with the frequency response function

$$\begin{aligned} H_0(\nu) &= \frac{N}{N + \theta(\nu)} \\ &= \frac{N f_\beta(\nu)}{f_v(\nu) + N f_\beta(\nu)}, \end{aligned} \tag{5.74}$$

where the last form is more convenient in cases in which portions of the signal spectrum are essentially zero.

The optimal filters $h_t$ have frequency response functions that depend on the signal spectrum $f_\beta(\nu)$ and noise spectrum $f_v(\nu)$, so we will need estimators for these parameters to apply the optimal filters. Sometimes, there will be values, suggested from experience, for the signal-to-noise ratio $1/\theta(\nu)$ as a function of frequency. The analogy between the model here and the usual variance components model in statistics, however, suggests we try an approach along those lines as in the next section.

### Detection and Parameter Estimation

The analogy to the usual variance components situation suggests looking at the regression and error components of Table 5.2 under the stochastic signal assumptions. We consider the components of (5.56) and (5.57) at a single frequency $\nu_k$. In order to estimate the spectral components $f_\beta(\nu)$ and $f_v(\nu)$, we reconsider the linear model (5.51) under the assumption that $\boldsymbol{B}(\nu_k)$ is a random process with spectral matrix $f_\beta(\nu_k)I_q$. Then, the spectral matrix of the observed process is (5.67), evaluated at frequency $\nu_k$.

Consider first the component of the regression power, defined as

$$
\begin{aligned}
SSR(\nu_k) &= \boldsymbol{s}^*_{zy}(\nu_k)S_z^{-1}(\nu_k)\boldsymbol{s}_{zy}(\nu_k) \\
&= \boldsymbol{Y}^*(\nu_k)Z(\nu_k)S_z^{-1}(\nu_k)Z^*(\nu_k)\boldsymbol{Y}(\nu_k).
\end{aligned}
$$

A computation shows

$$
E[SSR(\nu_k)] = f_\beta(\nu_k)\ \mathrm{tr}\{S_z(\nu_k)\} + qf_v(\nu_k),
$$

where tr denotes the trace of a matix. If we can find a set of frequencies of the form $\nu_k + \ell/n$, where the spectra and the Fourier transforms $S_z(\nu_k + \ell/n) \approx S_z(\nu)$ are relatively constant, the expectation of the averaged values in (5.56) yields

$$
E[SSR(\nu)] = Lf_\beta(\nu)\mathrm{tr}\ [S_z(\nu)] + Lqf_v(\nu). \tag{5.75}
$$

A similar computation establishes

$$
E[SSE(\nu)] = L(N-q)f_v(\nu). \tag{5.76}
$$

We may obtain an approximately unbiased estimator for the spectra $f_v(\nu)$ and $f_\beta(\nu)$ by replacing the expected power components by their values and solving (5.75) and (5.76).

**Example 5.6 Estimating the Power Components and the Random Infrasonic Signal**

In order to provide an optimum estimator for the infrasonic signal, we need to have estimators for the signal and noise spectra $f_\beta(\nu)$ and $f_v(\nu)$ for the case considered in Example 5.5. The form of the filter is $H_0(\nu)$, given in (5.74), and with $q = 1$ and the matrix $S_z(\nu) = N$ at all frequencies in this example simplifies the computations considerably. We may estimate

$$
\widehat{f}_v(\nu) = \frac{SSE(\nu)}{L(N-1)} \tag{5.77}
$$

and

$$
\widehat{f}_\beta(\nu) = (LN)^{-1}\left(SSR(\nu) - \frac{SSE(\nu)}{(N-1)}\right), \tag{5.78}
$$

using (5.75) and (5.76) for this special case. Cases will exist in which (5.78) is negative and the estimated signal spectrum can be set to zero for those frequencies. The estimators can be substituted into the optimal filters to apply to the beam, say, $H_0(\nu)$ in (5.74), or to use in the filter applied to each level (5.73).

The analysis of variance estimators can be computed using the analysis of power given in Figure 5.7, and the results of that computation and

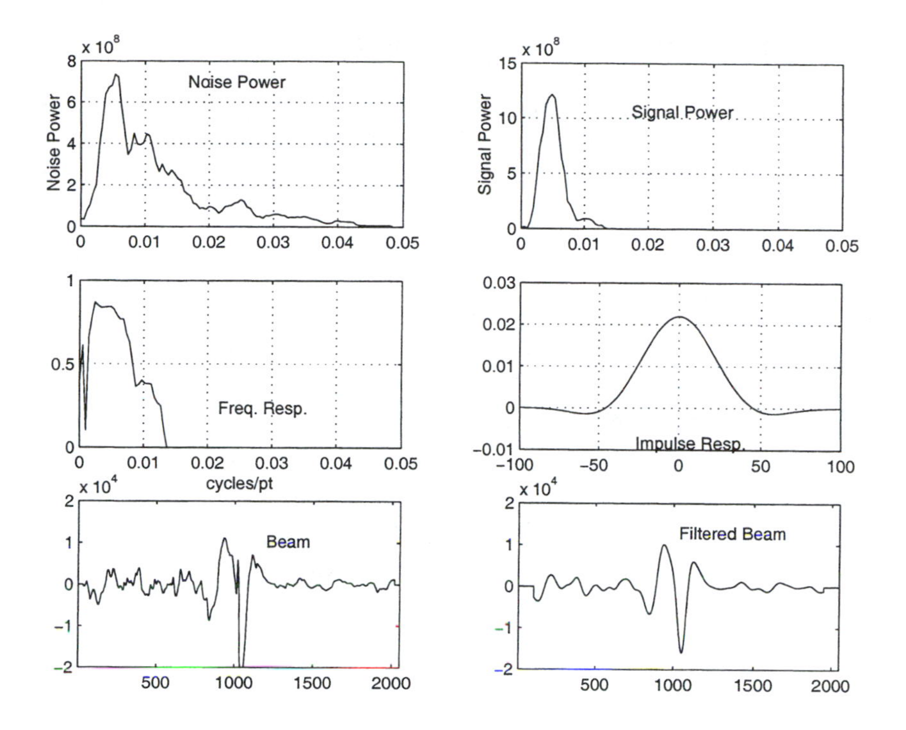


**Figure 5.8:** Estimated signal and noise spectra, filter responses, and beams.

applying (5.77) and (5.78) are shown in the top panel of Figure 5.8 for a bandwidth of $B = 7/2048 =$ cycles per point or about .03 cycles per second (Hz). Neither spectrum contains any significant power for frequencies greater than .04 cycles per point or about .4 Hz. As expected, the signal spectral estimator is substantial over a narrow band, and this leads to an estimated filter, with estimated frequency response function $\widehat{H}_0(\nu)$, shown on the left-hand side of the second panel. The estimated optimal filter essentially deletes frequencies above .014 Hz and, subject to slight modification, differs little from a standard low-pass filter with that cutoff. Computing the time version with a cutoff at $M = 201$ points and using a taper leads to the estimated impulse response function $\widehat{h}_0(t)$, as shown on the right-hand side of the middle panel. Finally, we apply the optimal filter to the beam and get the filtered beam $\widehat{\beta}_t$ shown in the bottom right-hand panel. It is smoother than the left-hand bottom panel, where we have reproduced the beam shown earlier in Figure 5.3. The analysis shows the primary signal as basically a low-frequency signal with primary power at about .05 Hz or, essentially, a wave with a 20-second period.

## 5.6 Analysis of Designed Experiments

An important special case (see Brillinger, 1973, 1980) of the regression model (5.50) occurs when the regression (5.39) is of the form

$$\boldsymbol{y}_t = z\boldsymbol{\beta}_t + \boldsymbol{v}_t, \tag{5.79}$$

where $z = (z_1, z_2, \ldots, z_N)'$ is a matrix that determines what is observed by the $j$-th series; i.e.,

$$y_{jt} = \boldsymbol{z}_j'\boldsymbol{\beta}_t + v_{jt}. \tag{5.80}$$

In this case, the the matrix $\boldsymbol{z}$ of independent variables is constant and we will have the frequency domain model.

$$\boldsymbol{Y}(\nu_k) = Z\boldsymbol{B}(\nu_k) + \boldsymbol{V}(\nu_k) \tag{5.81}$$

corresponding to (5.51), where the matrix $Z(\nu_k)$ was a function of frequency $\nu_k$. The matrix is purely real, in this case, but the equations (5.52)-(5.58) can be applied with $Z(\nu_k)$ replaced by the constant matrix $Z$.

EQUALITY OF MEANS

A typical general problem that we encounter in analyzing real data is a simple ***equality of means test*** in which there might be a collection of time series $y_{ijt}, i = 1, \ldots, I, j = 1, \ldots, N_i$, belonging to $I$ possible groups, with $N_i$ series in group $i$. To test equality of means, we may write the regression model in the form

$$y_{ijt} = \mu_t + \alpha_{it} + v_{ijt}, \tag{5.82}$$

where $\mu_t$ denotes the overall mean and $\alpha_{it}$ denotes the effect of the $i$-th group at time $t$ and we require that $\sum_i \alpha_{it} = 0$ for all $t$. In this case, the full model can be written in the general regression notation as

$$y_{ijt} = \boldsymbol{z}_{ij}'\boldsymbol{\beta}_t + v_{ijt}$$

where

$$\boldsymbol{\beta}_t = (\mu_t, \alpha_{1t}, \alpha_{2t}, \ldots, \alpha_{I-1,t})'$$

denotes the regression vector, subject to the constraint. The reduced model becomes

$$y_{ijt} = \mu_t + v_{ijt} \tag{5.83}$$

under the assumption that the group means are equal. In the full model, there are $I$ possible values for the $I \times 1$ design vectors $\boldsymbol{z}_{ij}$; the first component is always one for the mean, and the rest have a one in the $i$-th position for $i = 1, \ldots, I-1$ and zeros elsewhere. The vectors for the last group take the value $-1$ for $i = 2, 3, \ldots, I-1$. Under the reduced model, each $\boldsymbol{z}_{ij}$ is a single column of ones. The rest of the analysis follows the approach summarized in (5.52)-(5.58). In this particular case, the power components in Table 5.3 (before smoothing) simplify to

$$SSR(\nu_k) = \sum_{i=1}^{I} \sum_{j=1}^{N_i} |Y_{i\cdot}(\nu_k) - Y_{\cdot\cdot}(\nu_k)|^2 \tag{5.84}$$

and

$$SSE(\nu_k) = \sum_{i=1}^{I} \sum_{j=1}^{N_i} |Y_{ij}(\nu_k) - Y_{i\cdot}(\nu_k)|^2, \tag{5.85}$$

which are analogous to the usual sums of squares in analysis of variance. Note, $\cdot$ stands for a mean, taken over the appropriate subscript, so the regression power component $SSR(\nu_k)$ is basically the power in the residuals of the group means from the overall mean and the error power component $SSE(\nu_k)$ reflects the departures of the group means from the original data values. Smoothing each component over $L$ frequencies leads to the usual $F$-statistic (5.64) with $2L(I-1)$ and $2L(\sum_i N_i - I)$ degrees of freedom at each frequency $\nu$ of interest.

**Example 5.7 Means Test for the Magnetic Resonance Imaging Data**

Figure 5.1 showed the mean responses of subjects to various levels of periodic stimulation while awake and while under anesthesia, as collected in a pain perception experiment of Antognini et al (1997). Three types of periodic stimuli were presented to awake and anesthetized subjects, namely, brushing, heat, and shock. The periodicity was introduced by applying the stimuli, brushing, heat, and shocks in on-off sequences lasting 32 seconds each and the sampling rate was one point every two seconds. The blood oxygenation level (BOLD) signal intensity (Ogawa et al, 1990) was measured at nine locations in the brain. Areas of activation were determined using a technique first described by Bandettini et al (1993). The specfic locations of the brain where the signal was measured were Cortex 1: Primary Somatosensory, Contralateral, Cortex 2: Primary Somatosensory, Ipsilateral, Cortex 3: Secondary Somatosensory, Contralateral, Cortex 4: Secondary Somatosensory, Ipsilateral, Caudate, Thalamus 1: Contralateral, Thalamus 2: Ipsilateral, Cerebellum 1: Contralateral and Cerebellum 2: Ipsilateral. Figure 5.1 shows the mean response of subjects at Cortex 1 for each of the six treatment combinations, 1: Awake-Brush (5 subjects), 2: Awake-Heat (4 subjects), 3: Awake-Shock (5 subjects), 4: Low-Brush (3 subjects), 5: Low-Heat (5 subjects), and 6: Low-Shock( 4 subjects). The objective of this first analysis is to test equality of these six group means, paying special attention to the 64-second period band (1/64 cycles per second) expected from the periodic driving stimuli. Because a test of equality is needed

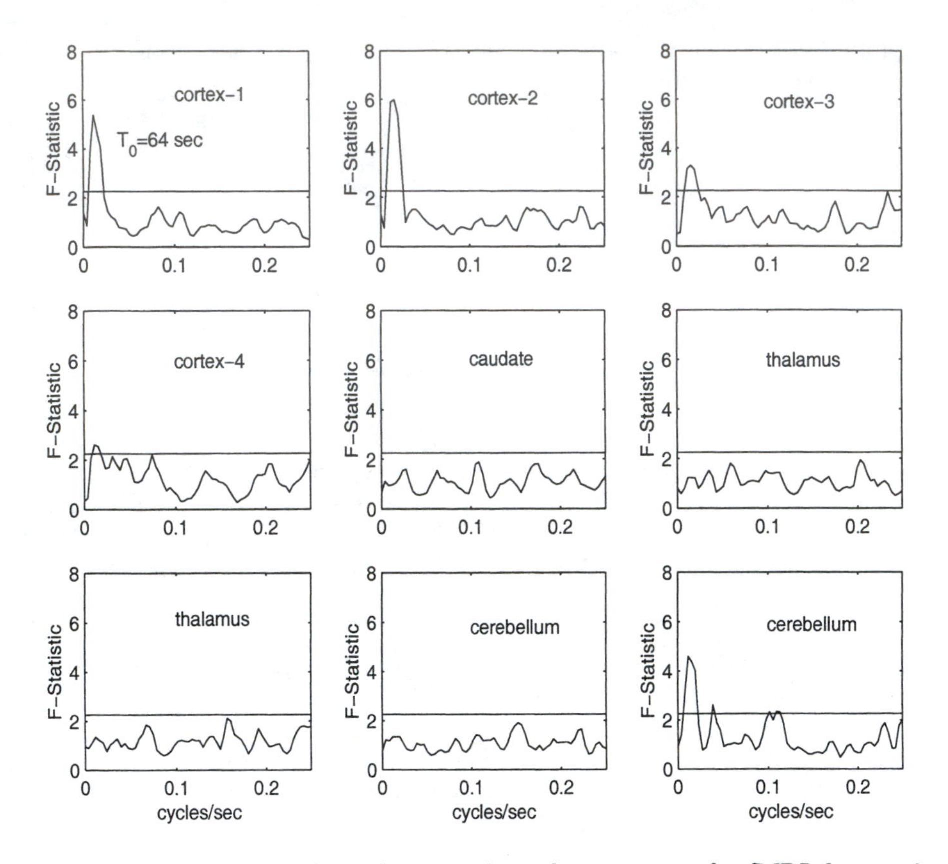


**Figure 5.9:** Frequency-dependent equality of means tests for fMRI data at 9 brain locations. $L = 3$ and critical value $F_{.001}(30, 120) = 2.26$.

at each of the nine brain locations, we took $\alpha = .001$ to control for the overall error rate. Figure 5.9 shows $F$-statistics, computed from (5.64), with $L = 3$, and we see substantial signals for the four cortex locations and for the second cerebellum trace, but the effects are nonsignificant in the caudate and thalamus regions. Hence, we will retain the four cortex locations and the second cerebellum location for further analysis.

### An Analysis of Variance Model

The arrangement of treatments for the fMRI data in Figure 5.1 suggests more information might be available than was obtained from the simple equality of means test. Separate effects caused by state of consciousness as well as the separate treatments brush, heat, and shock might exist. The reduced signal present in the low shock mean suggests a possible interaction between the treatments and level of consciousness. The arrangement in the classical two-way table suggests looking at the analog of the two factor analysis of variance as a function of frequency. In this case, we would obtain a different version of the regression model (5.82) of the form

$$y_{ijkt} = \mu_t + \alpha_{it} + \beta_{jt} + \gamma_{ijt} + v_{ijkt} \tag{5.86}$$

for $k$-th individual undergoing the $i$-th level of some factor A and the $j$-th level of some other factor B, $i = 1, \ldots I, j = 1 \ldots, J, k = 1, \ldots n_{ij}$. The number of individuals in each cell can be different, as for the fMRI data in the next example. In the above model, we assume the response can be modeled as the sum of a mean, $\mu_t$, a ***row effect*** (type of stimulus), $\alpha_{it}$, a ***column effect*** (level of consciousness), $\beta_{jt}$ and an ***interaction***, $\gamma_{ijt}$, with the usual restrictions

$$\sum_i \alpha_{it} = \sum_j \beta_{jt} = \sum_i \gamma_{ijt} = \sum_j \gamma_{ijt} = 0$$

required for a full rank design matrix $Z$ in the overall regression model (5.81). If the number of observations in each cell were the same, the usual simple analogous version of the power components (5.84) and (5.85) would exist for testing various hypotheses. In the case of (5.86), we are interested in testing hypotheses obtained by dropping one set of terms at a time out of (5.86), so an A factor (testing $\alpha_{it} = 0$), a B factor ($\beta_{jt} = 0$), and an interaction term ($\gamma_{ijt} = 0$) will appear as components in the analysis of power. Because of the unequal numbers of observations in each cell, we often put the model in the form of the regression model (5.79)-(5.81).

**Example 5.8 Analysis of Power Tests for the Magnetic Resonance Imaging Data**

For the fMRI data given as the means in Figure 5.1, a model of the form (5.86) is plausible and will yield more detailed information than the simple equality of means test described earlier. The results of that test, shown in Figure 5.9, were that the means were different for the four cortex locations and for the second cerebellum location. We may examine these differences further by testing whether the mean differences are because of the nature of the stimulus or the consciousness level, or perhaps due to an interaction between the two factors. Unequal numbers of observations exist in the cells that contributed the means in Figure 5.1. For the regression vector,

$$(\mu_t, \alpha_{1t}, \beta_{1t}, \beta_{2t}, \gamma_{11t}, \gamma_{21t})',$$

the rows of the design matrix are as specified in Table 5.4. Note the restrictions given above for the parameters.

The results of testing the three hypotheses are shown in Figure 5.10 for the four cortex locations and the cerebellum, the components that showed some significant differences in the means in Figure 5.9. Again,

**Table 5.4:** Rows of the Design Matrix $z_j'$ for fMRI Data. Number of Observations per Cell in Parentheses

| | Awake | Low Anesthesia |
|---|---|---|
| Brush | 1 1 0 1 1 0 (5) | 1 1 0 -1 -1 0 (3) |
| Heat | 1 0 1 1 0 1 (4) | 1 0 1 -1 0 -1 (5) |
| Shock | 1 -1 -1 1 -1 -1 (5) | 1 -1 -1 -1 1 1 (4) |

the regression power components were smoothed over $L = 3$ frequencies. Appealing to the ANOPOW results summarized in Table 5.3 for each of the subhypotheses, $q_2 = 1$ when the stimulus effect is dropped, and $q_2 = 2$ when either the conciousness effect or the interaction terms are dropped. Hence, $2Lq_2 = 6, 12$ for the two cases, with $N = \sum_{ij} n_{ij} = 26$ total observations. Here, the form of the stimulus has the major effect, with the brushing, heat, and shock means substantially different at the probe frequency in four out of five cases. The level of consciousness was less significant and did not show the strong component at the signal frequency. A significant interaction occurred, however, at the ipsilateral component of the primary somatosensory cortex location. The more detailed model does separate the stimuli as having the major effect, but does not isolate which of the three might be more substantial than the other two.

### Simultaneous Inference

In the previous examples involving the fMRI data, it would be helpful to focus on the components that contributed most to the rejection of the equal means hypothesis. One way to accomplish this is to develop a test for the significance of an arbitrary ***linear compound*** of the form

$$\Psi(\nu_k) = \boldsymbol{A}^*(\nu_k)\boldsymbol{B}(\nu_k), \tag{5.87}$$

where the components of the vector $\boldsymbol{A}(\nu_k) = (A_1(\nu_k), A_2(\nu_k), \ldots, A_q(\nu_k))'$ are chosen in such a way as to isolate particular linear functions of parameters in the regression vector $\boldsymbol{B}(\nu_k)$ in the regression model (5.81). This argument suggests developing a test of the hypothesis $\Psi(\nu_k) = 0$ for ***all possible*** values of the linear coefficients in the compound (5.87) as is done in the conventional analysis of variance approach (see, for example, Scheffé, 1959).

Recalling the material involving the regression models of the form (5.51), the linear compound (5.87) can be estimated by

$$\widehat{\Psi}(\nu_k) = \boldsymbol{A}^*(\nu_k)\widehat{\boldsymbol{B}}(\nu_k), \tag{5.88}$$

where $\widehat{\boldsymbol{B}}(\nu_k)$ is the estimated vector of regression coefficients given by (5.52) and independent of the error spectrum $s^2_{y\cdot z}(\nu_k)$ in (5.54). It is possible to show

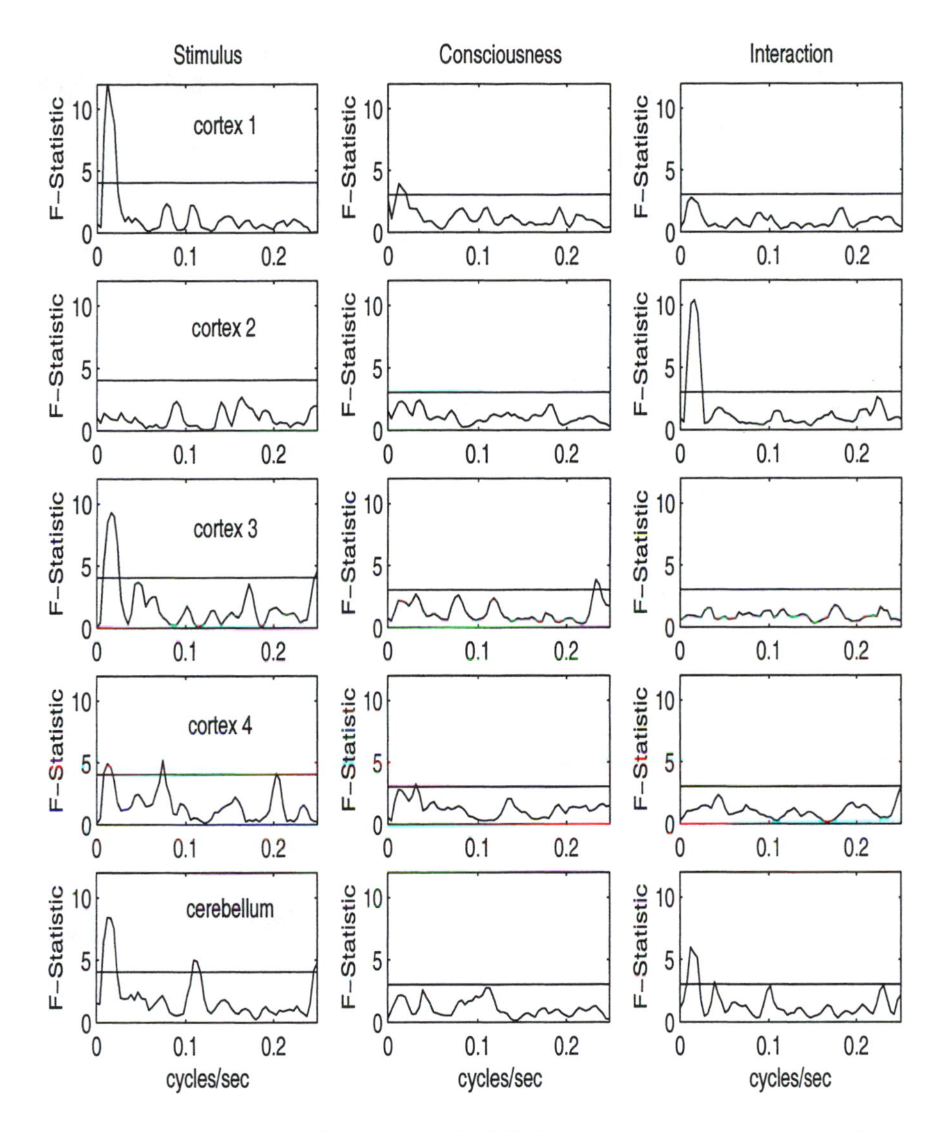


**Figure 5.10:** Analysis of power for fMRI data at five locations, $L = 3$ and critical values $F_{.001}(6, 120) = 4.04$ for stimulus and $F_{.001}(12, 120) = 3.02$ for consciousness and interaction.

the maximum of the ratio

$$F(\boldsymbol{A}) = \frac{N-q}{q} \, \frac{|\widehat{\Psi}(\nu_k) - \Psi(\nu_k)|^2}{s^2_{y\cdot z}(\nu_k) Q(\boldsymbol{A})}, \tag{5.89}$$

where

$$Q(\boldsymbol{A}) = \boldsymbol{A}^*(\nu_k) S_z^{-1}(\nu_k) \boldsymbol{A}(\nu_k) \tag{5.90}$$

is bounded by a statistic that has an $F$-distribution with $2q$ and $2(N-q)$ degrees of freedom. Testing the hypothesis that the compound has a particular value, usually $\Psi(\nu_k) = 0$, then proceeds naturally, by comparing the statistic (5.89) evaluated at the hypothesized value with the $\alpha$ level point on an $F_{2q,2(N-q)}$ distribution. We can choose an infinite number of compounds of the form (5.87) and the test will still be valid at level $\alpha$. As before, arguing the error spectrum is relatively constant over a band enables us to smooth the numerator and denominator of (5.89) separately over $L$ frequencies so distribution involving the smooth components is $F_{2Lq,2L(N-q)}$.

**Example 5.9 Simultaneous Inference for Magnetic Resonance Imaging Data**

As an example, consider the previous tests for significance of the fMRI factors, in which we have indicated the primary effects are among the stimuli but have not investigated which of the stimuli, heat, brushing, or shock, had the most effect. To analyze this further, consider the means model (5.82) and a $6 \times 1$ contrast vector of the form

$$\widehat{\Psi} = \boldsymbol{A}^*(\nu_k)\widehat{\boldsymbol{B}}(\nu_k) = \sum_{i=1}^{6} A_i^*(\nu_k)\boldsymbol{Y}_{i\cdot}(\nu_k), \tag{5.91}$$

where the means are easily shown to be the regression coefficients in this particular case. In this case, the means are ordered by columns; the first three means are the the three levels of stimuli for the awake state, and the last three means are the levels for the anesthetized state. In this special case, the denominator terms are

$$Q = \sum_{i=1}^{6} \frac{|A_i(\nu_k)|^2}{N_i}, \tag{5.92}$$

with $SSE(\nu_k)$ available in (5.85). In order to evaluate the effect of a particular stimulus, like brushing over the two levels of consciousness, we may take $A_1(\nu_k) = A_4(\nu_k) = 1$ for the two brush levels and $A(\nu_k) = 0$ zero otherwise. From Figure 5.11, we see that, at the first and third cortex locations, brush and heat are both significant, whereas the fourth cortex shows only brush and the second cerebellum shows only heat. Shock appears to be transmitted relatively weakly, when averaged over the awake and mildly anesthetized states.

### Multivariate Tests

Although it is possible to develop multivariate regression along lines analogous to the usual real valued case, we will only look at tests involving equality

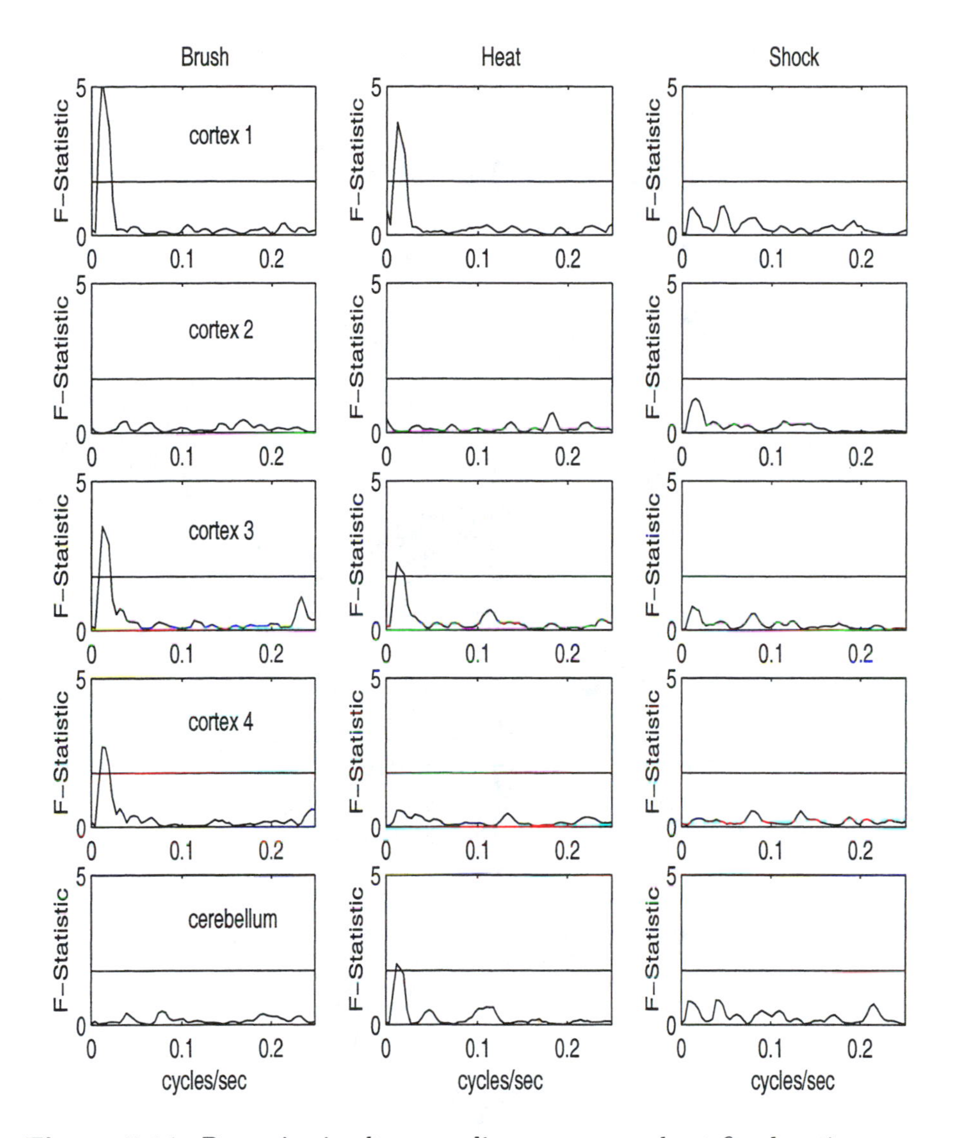


**Figure 5.11:** Power in simultaneous linear compounds at five locations, enhancing brush, heat, and shock effects, $L = 3, F_{.001}(36, 120) = 1.80$.

of group means and spectral matrices, because these tests appear to be used most often in applications. For these results, consider the $p$-variate time series $\boldsymbol{y}_{ijt} = (y_{ijt1}, \ldots, y_{ijtp})'$ to have arisen from observations on $j = 1, \ldots, N_i$ individuals in group $i$, all having mean $\boldsymbol{\mu}_{it}$ and stationary autocovariance matrix $\Gamma_i(h)$. Denote the DFTs of the group mean vectors as $\boldsymbol{Y}_{i\cdot}(\nu_k)$ and the $p \times p$ spectral matrices as $\widehat{f}_i(\nu_k)$ for the $i = 1, 2, \ldots, I$ groups. Assume the same general properties as for the vector series considered in Section 5.3.

In the multivariate case, we obtain the analogous versions of (5.84) and (5.85) as the ***between cross-power*** and ***within cross-power*** matrices

$$SPR(\nu_k) = \sum_{i=1}^{I}\sum_{j=1}^{N_i}\big(\boldsymbol{Y}_{i\cdot}(\nu_k) - \boldsymbol{Y}_{\cdot\cdot}(\nu_k)\big)\big(\boldsymbol{Y}_{i\cdot}(\nu_k) - \boldsymbol{Y}_{\cdot\cdot}(\nu_k)\big)^* \tag{5.93}$$

and

$$SPE(\nu_k) = \sum_{i=1}^{I}\sum_{j=1}^{N_i}\big(\boldsymbol{Y}_{ij}(\nu_k) - \boldsymbol{Y}_{i\cdot}(\nu_k)\big)\big(\boldsymbol{Y}_{ij}(\nu_k) - \boldsymbol{Y}_{i\cdot}(\nu_k)\big)^*. \tag{5.94}$$

The equality of means test is rejected using the fact that the likelihood ratio test yields a monotone function of

$$\Lambda(\nu_k) = \frac{|SPE(\nu_k)|}{|SPE(\nu_k) + SPR(\nu_k)|}. \tag{5.95}$$

Khatri (1965) and Hannan (1970) give the approximate distribution of the statistic

$$\chi^2_{2(I-1)p} = -2\Big(\sum N_i - I - p - 1\Big)\log\Lambda(\nu_k) \tag{5.96}$$

as chi-squared with $2(I-1)p$ degrees of freedom when the group means are equal.

The case of $I = 2$ groups reduces to Hotelling's $T^2$, as has been shown by Giri (1965), where

$$T^2 = \frac{N_1N_2}{(N_1+N_2)}\big[\boldsymbol{Y}_{1\cdot}(\nu_k) - \boldsymbol{Y}_{2\cdot}(\nu_k)\big]^* \widehat{f}_v^{-1}(\nu_k)\big[\boldsymbol{Y}_{1\cdot}(\nu_k) - \boldsymbol{Y}_{2\cdot}(\nu_k)\big], \tag{5.97}$$

where

$$\widehat{f}_v(\nu_k) = \frac{SPE(\nu_k)}{\sum_i N_i - I} \tag{5.98}$$

is the pooled error spectrum given in (5.94),with $I = 2$. The test statistic, in this case, is

$$F_{2p,2(N_1+N_2-p-1)} = \frac{(N_1+N_2-2)p}{(N_1+N_2-p-1)}T^2, \tag{5.99}$$

which was shown by Giri (1965) to have the indicated limiting $F$-distribution with $2p$ and $2(N_1 + N_2 - p - 1)$ degrees of freedom when the means are the same. The classical $t$-test for inequality of two univariate means will be just (5.98) and (5.99) with $p = 1$.

Testing equality of the spectral matrices is also of interest, not only for discrimination and pattern recognition, as considered in the next section, but also as a test indicating whether the equality of means test, which assumes equal spectral matrices, is valid. The test evolves from the likelihood ration criterion, which compares the single group spectral matrices

$$\widehat{f}_i(\nu_k) = \frac{1}{N_i - 1} \sum_{j=1}^{N_i} \left(\boldsymbol{Y}_{ij}(\nu_k) - \boldsymbol{Y}_{i\cdot}(\nu_k)\right)^* \left(\boldsymbol{Y}_{ij}(\nu_k) - \boldsymbol{Y}_{i\cdot}(\nu_k)\right) \tag{5.100}$$

with the pooled spectral matrix (5.98). A modification of the likelihood ratio test, which incorporates the degrees of freedom $M_i = N_i - 1$ and $M = \sum M_i$ rather than the sample sizes into the likelihood ratio statistic, uses

$$L'(\nu_k) = \frac{M^{Mp}}{\prod_{i=1}^{I} M_i^{M_i p}} \frac{\prod |M_i \widehat{f}_i(\nu_k)|^{M_i}}{|M \widehat{f}_v(\nu_k)|^M}. \tag{5.101}$$

Krishnaiah et al (1976) have given the moments of $L'(\nu_k)$ and calculated 95% critical points for $p = 3, 4$ using a Pearson Type I approximation. For reasonably large samples involving smoothed spectral estimators, the approximation involving the first term of the usual chi-squared series will suffice and Shumway (1982) has given

$$\chi^2_{(I-1)p^2} = -2r \log L'(\nu_k), \tag{5.102}$$

where

$$1 - r = \frac{(p+1)(r+1)}{6p(I-1)} \left( \sum_i M_i^{-1} - M^{-1} \right), \tag{5.103}$$

with an approximate chi-squared distribution with $(I-1)p^2$ degrees of freedom when the spectral matrices are equal. Introduction of smoothing over $L$ frequencies leads to replacing $M_j$ and $M$ by $LM_j$ and $LM$ in the equations above.

Of course, it is often of great interest to use the above result for testing equality of two univariate spectra, and it is obvious from the material in Chapter 3

$$F_{2LM_1, 2LM_2} = \frac{\widehat{f}_1(\nu)}{\widehat{f}_2(\nu)} \tag{5.104}$$

will have the requisite $F$-distribution with $2LM_1$ and $2LM_2$ degrees of freedom.

**Example 5.10 Equality of Means and Spectral Matrices for Earthquakes and Explosions**

An interesting problem arises when attempting to develop a methodology for discriminating between waveforms originating from explosions and those that came from the more commonly occurring earthquakes. Figure 5.2 shows a small subset of a larger population of bivariate series consisting of two phases from each of eight earthquakes and eight explosions. If the large–sample approximations to normality hold for the DFTs of these series, it is of interest to known whether the differences between the two classes are better represented by the mean functions or by the spectral matrices. The tests described above can be applied to look at these two questions. The upper left panel of Figure 5.12 shows the test statistic (5.99) with the straight line denoting the critical level for $\alpha = .001$, i.e., $F_{.001}(4, 26) = 7.36$, for equal means using $L = 1$, and the test statistic remains well below its critical value at all frequencies, implying that the means of the two classes of series are not significantly different. Checking Figure 5.2 shows little reason exists to suspect that either the earthquakes or explosions have a nonzero mean signal. Checking the equality of the spectra and the spectral matrices, however, leads to a different conclusion. Some smoothing ($L = 21$) is useful here, and univariate tests on both the P and S components using (5.104) and $N_1 = N_2 = 8$ lead to strong rejections of the equal spectra hypotheses, with $F_{.001}(\infty, \infty) = 1.00$ exceeded at almost all frequencies. The rejection seems stronger for the S component and we might tentatively identify that component as being dominant. Testing equality of the spectral matrices using (5.102) and $\chi^2_{.001}(4) = 18.47$ shows a similar strong rejection of the equality of spectral matrices. We use these results to suggest optimal discriminant functions based on spectral differences in the next section.

## 5.7 Discrimination and Cluster Analysis

The extension of classical pattern-recognition techniques to experimental time series is a problem of great practical interest. A series of observations indexed in time often produces a pattern that may form a basis for discriminating between different classes of events. As an example, consider Figure 5.2, which shows regional (100-2000 km) recordings of several typical Scandinavian earthquakes and mining explosions measured by stations in Scandinavia. A listing of the events is given in Kakizawa et al (1998). The problem of discriminating between mining explosions and earthquakes is a reasonable proxy for the problem of discriminating between nuclear explosions and earthquakes. This latter problem is one of critical importance for monitoring a comprehensive test-ban treaty. Time series classification problems are not restricted to geophysical applications, but occur under many and varied circumstances in other fields. Traditionally, the detecting of a signal embedded in a noise series has been analyzed in the engineering literature by statistical pattern recognition techniques (see Problems 5.14 and 5.15) .

The historical approaches to the problem of discriminating among different classes of time series can be divided into two distinct categories. The ***optimality*** approach, as found in the engineering and statistics literature, makes specific Gaussian assumptions about the probability density functions of the

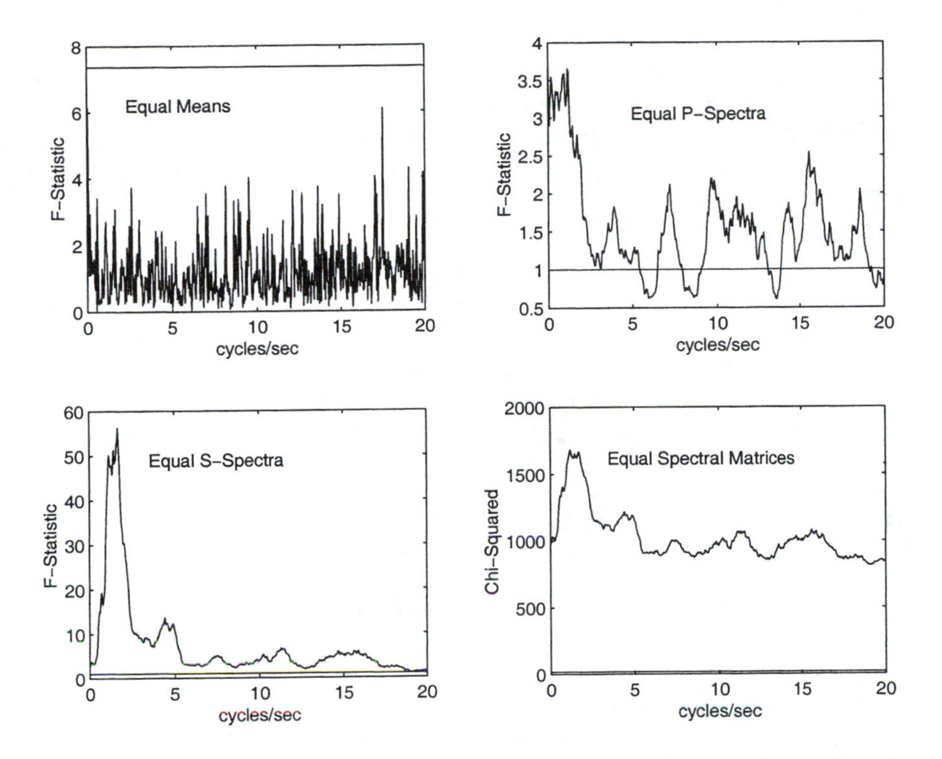


**Figure 5.12:** Tests for equality of means, spectra, and spectral matrices for the earthquake and explosion data $p = 2, L = 21, n = 1024$ pts at 40 points per second.

separate groups and then develops solutions that satisfy well-defined minimum error criteria. Typically, in the time series case, we might assume the difference between classes is expressed through differences in the theoretical mean and covariance functions and use likelihood methods to develop an optimal classification function. A second class of techniques, which might be described as a ***feature extraction*** approach, proceeds more heuristically by looking at quantities that tend to be good visual discriminators for well-separated populations and have some basis in physical theory or intuition Less attention is paid to finding functions that are approximations to some well-defined optimality criterion.

As in the case of regression, both time domain and frequency domain approaches to discrimination will exist. For relatively short univariate series, a time domain approach that follows conventional multivariate discriminant analysis as described in conventional multivariate texts, such as Anderson (1984) or Johnson and Wichern (1992) may be preferable. We might even characterize differences by the autocovariance functions generated by different ARMA or state-space models. For longer multivariate time series that can be regarded as stationary after the common mean has been subtracted, the frequency domain approach will be easier computationally because the $np$ dimensional vector in the time domain, represented here as $\boldsymbol{x} = (\boldsymbol{x}_1', \boldsymbol{x}_t', \ldots, \boldsymbol{x}_n')'$, with $\boldsymbol{x}_t = (x_{t1}, \ldots, x_{tp})'$, will reduced to separate computations made on the $p$-dimensional DFTs. This happens because of the approximate independence of the DFTs, $\boldsymbol{X}(\nu_k), 0 \leq \nu_k \leq 1$, a property that we have often used in preceding chapters.

Finally, the grouping properties of measures like the discrimination information and likelihood-based statistics can be used to develop measures of ***disparity*** for clustering multivariate time series. In this section, we define a measure of disparity between two multivariate times series by the spectral matrices of the two processes and then apply hierarchical clustering and partitioning techniques to identify natural groupings within the bivariate earthquake and explosion populations.

## The General Discrimination Problem

The general problem of classifying a vector time series $\boldsymbol{x}$ occurs in the following way. We observe a time series $\boldsymbol{x}$ known to belong to one of $g$ populations, denoted by $\Pi_1, \Pi_2, \ldots, \Pi_g$. The general problem is to assign or ***classify*** this observation into one of the $g$ groups in some optimal fashion. An example might be the $g = 2$ populations of earthquakes and explosions shown in Figure 5.2. We would like to classify the unknown event, shown as NZ in the bottom two panels, as belonging to either the earthquake ($\Pi_1$) or explosion ($\Pi_2$) populations. To solve this problem, we need an optimality criterion that leads to a statistic $T(\boldsymbol{x})$ that can be used to assign the NZ event to either the earthquake or explosion populations. To measure the success of the classification, we need to evaluate errors that can be expected in the future relating to the number of earthquakes classified as explosions (false alarms) and the number of explosions classified as earthquakes (missed signals).

The problem can be formulated by assuming the observed series $\boldsymbol{x}$ has a probability density $p_i(\boldsymbol{x})$ when the observed series is from population $\Pi_i$ for $i = 1, \ldots, g$. Then, partition the space spanned by the $np$-dimensional process $\boldsymbol{x}$ into $g$ mutually exclusive regions $R_1, R_2, \ldots, R_g$ such that, if $\boldsymbol{x}$ falls in $R_i$, we assign $\boldsymbol{x}$ to population $\Pi_i$. The ***misclassification probability*** is defined as the probability of classifying the observation into population $\Pi_j$ when it belongs to $\Pi_i$, for $j \neq i$ and would be given by the expression

$$P(j|i) = \int_{R_j} p_i(\boldsymbol{x}) \, d\boldsymbol{x}. \tag{5.105}$$

The overall ***total error probability*** depends also on the ***prior probabilities***, say, $\pi_1, \pi_2, \ldots, \pi_g$, of belonging to one of the $g$ groups. For example, the probability that an observation $\boldsymbol{x}$ originates from $\Pi_i$ and is then classified into

$\Pi_j$ is obviously $\pi_i P(j|i)$, and the total error probability becomes

$$P_e = \sum_{i=1}^{g} \pi_i \sum_{j \neq i} P(j|i). \tag{5.106}$$

Although costs have not been incorporated into (5.106), it is easy to do so by multiplying $P(j|i)$ by $C(j|i)$, the cost of assigning a series from population $\Pi_i$ to $\Pi_j$.

The overall error $P_e$ is minimized by classifying $\boldsymbol{x}$ into $\Pi_i$ if

$$\frac{p_i(\boldsymbol{x})}{p_j(\boldsymbol{x})} > \frac{\pi_j}{\pi_i} \tag{5.107}$$

for all $j \neq i$ (see, for example, Anderson, 1984). A quantity of interest, from the Bayesian perspective, is the ***posterior probability*** an observation belongs to population $\Pi_i$, conditional on observing $\boldsymbol{x}$, say,

$$P(\Pi_i|\boldsymbol{x}) = \frac{\pi_i p_i(\boldsymbol{x})}{\sum_j \pi_j(\boldsymbol{x}) p_j(\boldsymbol{x})}. \tag{5.108}$$

The procedure that classifies $\boldsymbol{x}$ into the population $\Pi_i$ for which the posterior probability is largest is equivalent to that implied by using the criterion (5.107). The posterior probabilities give an intuitive idea of the relative odds of belonging to each of the plausible populations.

Many situations occur, such as in the classification of earthquakes and explosions, in which there are only $g = 2$ populations of interest. For two populations, the ***Neyman–Pearson lemma*** implies, in the absence of prior probabilities, classifying an observation into $\Pi_1$ when

$$\frac{p_1(\boldsymbol{x})}{p_2(\boldsymbol{x})} > K \tag{5.109}$$

minimizes each of the error probabilities for a fixed value of the other. The rule is identical to the Bayes rule (5.107) when $K = \pi_2/\pi_1$.

The theory given above takes a simple form when the vector $\boldsymbol{x}$ has a $p$-variate normal distribution with mean vectors $\boldsymbol{\mu}_j$ and covariance matrices $\Sigma_j$ under $\Pi_j$ for $j = 1, 2, \ldots, g$. In this case, simply use

$$p_j(\boldsymbol{x}) = (2\pi)^{-p/2}|\Sigma_j|^{-1/2} \exp\left\{-\frac{1}{2}(\boldsymbol{x} - \boldsymbol{\mu}_j)'\Sigma_j^{-1}(\boldsymbol{x} - \boldsymbol{\mu}_j)\right\}. \tag{5.110}$$

The classification functions are conveniently expressed by quantities that are proportional to the logarithms of the densities, say,

$$g_j(\boldsymbol{x}) = -\frac{1}{2}\ln|\Sigma_j| - \frac{1}{2}\boldsymbol{x}'\Sigma_j^{-1}\boldsymbol{x} + \boldsymbol{\mu}_j'\Sigma_j^{-1}\boldsymbol{x} - \frac{1}{2}\boldsymbol{\mu}_j'\Sigma_j^{-1}\boldsymbol{\mu}_j + \ln \pi_j. \tag{5.111}$$

In expressions involving the log likelihood, we will generally ignore terms involving the constant $-\ln 2\pi$. For this case, we may assign an observation $\boldsymbol{x}$ to population $\Pi_i$ whenever

$$g_i(\boldsymbol{x}) > g_j(\boldsymbol{x}) \tag{5.112}$$

for $j \neq i, j = 1, \ldots, g$ and the posterior probability (5.108) has the form

$$P(\Pi_i|\boldsymbol{x}) = \frac{\exp\{g_i(\boldsymbol{x})\}}{\sum_j \exp\{g_j(\boldsymbol{x})\}}.$$

A common situation occurring in applications involves classification for $g = 2$ groups under the assumption of multivariate normality and equal covariance matrices; i.e., $\Sigma_1 = \Sigma_2 = \Sigma$. Then, the criterion (5.112) can be expressed in terms of the ***linear discriminant function***

$$\begin{aligned} d_l(\boldsymbol{x}) &= g_1(\boldsymbol{x}) - g_2(\boldsymbol{x}) \\ &= (\boldsymbol{\mu}_1 - \boldsymbol{\mu}_2)'\Sigma^{-1}\boldsymbol{x} - \frac{1}{2}(\boldsymbol{\mu}_1 - \boldsymbol{\mu}_2)'\Sigma^{-1}(\boldsymbol{\mu}_1 + \boldsymbol{\mu}_2) + \ln\frac{\pi_1}{\pi_2}, \end{aligned} \tag{5.113}$$

where we classify into $\Pi_1$ or $\Pi_2$ according to whether $d_l(\boldsymbol{x}) \geq 0$ or $d_l(\boldsymbol{x}) < 0$. The linear discriminant function is clearly a combination of normal variables and, for the case $\pi_1 = \pi_2 = .5$, will have mean $D^2/2$ under $\Pi_1$ and mean $-D^2/2$ under $\Pi_2$, with variances given by $D^2$ under both hypotheses, where

$$D^2 = (\boldsymbol{\mu}_1 - \boldsymbol{\mu}_2)'\Sigma^{-1}(\boldsymbol{\mu}_1 - \boldsymbol{\mu}_2) \tag{5.114}$$

is the ***Mahalanobis distance*** between the mean vectors $\boldsymbol{\mu}_1$ and $\boldsymbol{\mu}_2$. In this case, the two misclassification probabilities (5.1) are

$$\begin{aligned} P(1|2) &= P(2|1) \\ &= \Phi\left(-\frac{D}{2}\right), \end{aligned} \tag{5.115}$$

and the performance is directly related to the Mahalanobis distance (5.114).

For the case in which the covariance matrices cannot be assumed to be the the same, the discriminant function takes a different form, with the difference $g_1(\boldsymbol{x}) - g_2(\boldsymbol{x})$ taking the form

$$\begin{aligned} d_q(\boldsymbol{x}) &= -\frac{1}{2}\ln\frac{|\Sigma_1|}{|\Sigma_2|} - \frac{1}{2}\boldsymbol{x}'(\Sigma_1^{-1} - \Sigma_2^{-1})\boldsymbol{x} \\ &\quad + (\boldsymbol{\mu}_1'\Sigma_1^{-1} - \boldsymbol{\mu}_2'\Sigma_2^{-1})\boldsymbol{x} + \ln\frac{\pi_1}{\pi_2} \end{aligned} \tag{5.116}$$

for $g = 2$ groups. This discriminant function differs from the equal covariance case in the linear term and in a nonlinear quadratic term involving the differing covariance matrices. The distribution theory is not tractable for the quadratic case so no convenient expression like (5.115) is available for the error probabilities for the quadratic discriminant function.

A difficulty in applying the above theory to real data is that the group mean vectors $\boldsymbol{\mu}_j$ and covariance matrices $\Sigma_j$ are seldom known. Some engineering problems, such as the detection of a signal in white noise, assume the means and covariance parameters are known exactly, and this can lead to an optimal solution (see Problems 5.14 and 5.15). In the classical multivariate situation, it is possible to collect a sample of $N_i$ ***training*** vectors from from group $\Pi_i$, say, $\boldsymbol{x}_{ij}$, for $j = 1, \ldots, N_i$, and use them to estimate the mean vectors and covariance matrices for each of the groups $i = 1, 2, \ldots, g$; i.e., simply choose $\boldsymbol{x}_{i\cdot}$ and

$$S_i = (N_i - 1)^{-1} \sum_{j=1}^{N_i} (\boldsymbol{x}_{ij} - \boldsymbol{x}_{i\cdot})(\boldsymbol{x}_{ij} - \boldsymbol{x}_{i\cdot})' \tag{5.117}$$

as the estimators for $\boldsymbol{\mu}_i$ and $\Sigma_i$, respectively. In the case in which the covariance matrices are assumed to be equal, simply use the pooled estimator

$$S = \left( \sum_i N_i - g \right)^{-1} \sum_i (N_i - 1) S_i. \tag{5.118}$$

For the case of a linear discriminant function, we may use

$$\widehat{g_i(\boldsymbol{x})} = \boldsymbol{x}_{i\cdot}' S^{-1} \boldsymbol{x} - \frac{1}{2}\, \boldsymbol{x}_{i\cdot}' S^{-1} \boldsymbol{x}_{i\cdot} + \log \pi_i \tag{5.119}$$

as a simple estimator for $g_i(\boldsymbol{x})$. For large samples, $\boldsymbol{x}_{i\cdot}$ and $S$ converge to $\boldsymbol{\mu}_i$ and $\Sigma$ in probability so $\widehat{g_i(\boldsymbol{x})}$ converges in distribution to $g_i(\boldsymbol{x})$ in that case. The procedure works reasonably well for the case in which $N_i, i = 1, \ldots g$ are large, relative to the length of the series $n$, a case that is relatively rare in time series analysis. For this reason, we will resort to using spectral approximations for the case in which data are given as long time series.

The performance of sample discriminant functions can be evaluated in several different ways. If the population parameters are known, (5.114) and (5.115) can be evaluated directly. If the parameters are estimated, the estimated Mahalanobis distance $\widehat{D^2}$ can be substituted for the theoretical value in very large samples. Another approach is to calculate the ***apparent error rates*** using the result of applying the classification procedure to the training samples. If $n_{ij}$ denotes the number of observations from population $\Pi_j$ classified into $\Pi_i$, the sample error rates can be estimated by the ratio

$$\widehat{P(i|j)} = \frac{n_{ij}}{\sum_i n_{ij}} \tag{5.120}$$

for $i \neq j$. If the training samples are not large, this procedure may be biased and a resampling option like cross validation or the bootstrap can be employed. A simple version of cross validation is the jacknife procedure proposed by Lachenbruch and Mickey (1968), which holds out the observation to be classified, deriving the classification function from the remaining observations.

**Table 5.5:** Logarithms of Maximum Peak-to-Peak Amplitudes from P and S Components for Eight Earthquakes and Eight Explosions

| EQ | $\log_{10} P$ | $\log_{10} S$ | EXP | $\log_{10} P$ | $\log_{10} S$ |
|---|---|---|---|---|---|
| 1 | 3.91 | 4.67 | 1 | 4.55 | 4.88 |
| 2 | 4.78 | 5.71 | 2 | 4.74 | 4.43 |
| 3 | 3.98 | 4.86 | 3 | 4.90 | 5.09 |
| 4 | 3.76 | 4.14 | 3 | 4.60 | 4.86 |
| 5 | 3.80 | 4.14 | 5 | 4.81 | 4.76 |
| 6 | 4.88 | 5.56 | 6 | 4.36 | 4.55 |
| 7 | 5.06 | 6.03 | 6 | 5.04 | 5.06 |
| 8 | 3.80 | 4.45 | 8 | 4.08 | 4.14 |
| NZ | 3.18 | 3.27 | | | |

Repeating this procedure for each of the members of the training sample and computing (5.120) for the ***holdout*** samples leads to better estimators of the error rates.

**Example 5.11 Discriminant Analysis Using Amplitudes from Earthquakes and Explosions**

We can give a simple example of applying the above procedures to the logarithms of the amplitudes of the separate P and S components of the original earthquake and explosion traces. The logarithms (base 10) of the maximum peak-to-peak amplitudes of the P and S components, denoted by $\log_{10} P$ and $\log_{10} S$, can be considered as two-dimensional feature vectors, say, $\boldsymbol{x} = (x_1, x_2)' = (\log_{10} P, \log_{10} S)'$, from a bivariate normal population with differering means and covariances. The original data, from Kakizawa et al (1998), are shown in Table 5.5 and in the left-hand panel of Figure 5.13. The table includes the Novaya Zemlya (NZ) event of unknown origin. The tendency of the earthquakes to have higher values for $\log_{10} S$, relative to $\log_{10} P$ has been noted by many and the use of the logarithm of the ratio, i.e., $\log_{10} P - \log_{10} S$ in some references (see Lay, 1997, pp. 40-41) is a tacit indicator that a linear function of the two parameters will be a useful discriminant.

The sample means $\boldsymbol{x}_{1\cdot} = (4.25, 4.95)'$ and $\boldsymbol{x}_{2\cdot} = (4.64, 4.73)'$, and covariance matrices

$$S_1 = \begin{pmatrix} .3096 & .3954 \\ .3954 & .5378 \end{pmatrix}$$

and

$$S_2 = \begin{pmatrix} .0954 & .0804 \\ .0804 & .1070 \end{pmatrix}$$

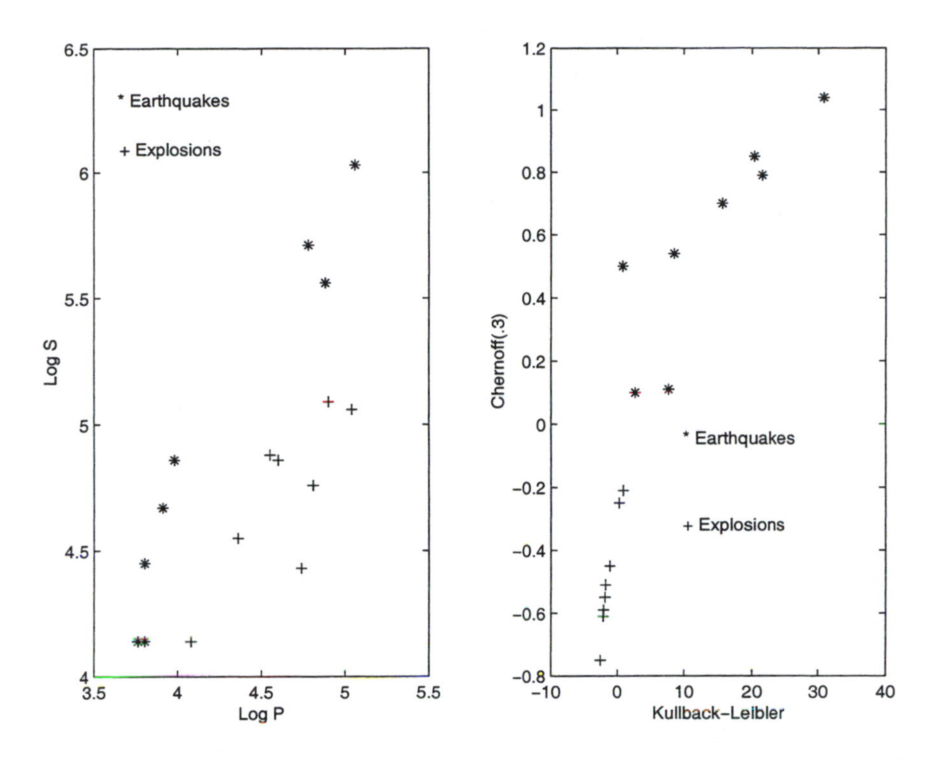


**Figure 5.13:** Classification of earthquakes and explosions using the magnitude features (left panel) and the K-L and Chernoff disparity measures (right panel).

are immediate from (5.117), with the pooled covariance matrix given by

$$S = \begin{pmatrix} .2025 & .2379 \\ .2379 & .3238 \end{pmatrix}$$

from (5.118). Although the covariance matrices are not equal, we try the linear discriminant function anyway, which yields (with equal prior probabilities $\pi_1 = \pi_2 = .5$) the sample discriminant functions

$$\widehat{g_1(\boldsymbol{x})} = 22.12x_1 - .98x_2 - 45.23$$

and

$$\widehat{g_2(\boldsymbol{x})} = 42.61x_2 - 16.8x_2 - 59.80$$

from (5.119), with the estimated linear discriminant function (5.113) as

$$\widehat{d_l(\boldsymbol{x})} = -20.49x_1 + 15.82x_2 + 14.57,$$

indicating $\log_{10} S - \log_{10} P = x_2 - x_1$ is not far from the optimal linear discriminant function. The jacknifed posterior probabilities of being an earthquake for the earthquake group ranged from .791 to 1.000, whereas the explosion probabilities for the explosion group ranged from .814 to .998, except for the first explosion, which was classified as an earthquake with a posterior probability of .949. Hence, $n_{12} = 1$ for this particular example. The unknown event, NZ, was classified as an earthquake, with posterior probability .753. Components of the vector for the unknown event NZ were well outside the range of the values spanned by the training set, so the classification here is somewhat suspect. The quadratic discriminant might be more appropriate here, given the observed differences in the two covariance matrices. Applying the sample version of (5.116) leads to essentially the same results, namely, the misclassification of the first earthquake as an explosion with a posterior probability of .807 and the classification of the unknown NZ event into the earthquake group.

FREQUENCY DOMAIN DISCRIMINATION

The feature extraction approach often works well for discriminating between classes of univariate or multivariate series when there is a simple low-dimensional vector that seems to capture the essence of the differences between the classes. It still seems sensible, however, to develop optimal methods for classification that exploit the differences between the multivariate means and covariance matrices in the time series case. Such methods can be based on the Whittle approximation to the log likelihood given in Section 5.2. In this case, the vector DFTs, say, $\boldsymbol{X}(\nu_k)$, are assumed to be approximately normal, with means $\boldsymbol{M}_j(\nu_k)$ and spectral matrices $f_j(\nu_k)$ for population $\Pi_j$ at frequencies $\nu_k = k/n, k = 0, 1, \ldots n/2$ and are approximately uncorrelated at different frequencies, say, $\nu_k$ and $\nu_\ell$ for $k \neq \ell$. Then, writing the complex normal densities as in Section 5.2 leads to a criterion similar to (5.111); namely,

$$\begin{aligned} g_j(\boldsymbol{X}) &= \ln \pi_j - \sum_{0<\nu_k<1/2} \Big[ \ln |f_j(\nu_k)| + \boldsymbol{X}^*(\nu_k) f_j^{-1}(\nu_k) \boldsymbol{X}(\nu_k) \\ &\qquad -2\boldsymbol{M}_j^*(\nu_k) f_j^{-1}(\nu_k) \boldsymbol{X}(\nu_k) + \boldsymbol{M}_j^*(k) f_j^{-1}(\nu_k) \boldsymbol{M}_j(\nu_k) \Big], \end{aligned} \tag{5.121}$$

where the sum goes over frequencies for which $|f_j(\nu_k)| \neq 0$. The periodicity of the spectral density matrix and DFT allows adding over $0 < k < 1/2$. The classification rule is as in (5.112).

In the time series case, it is more likely the discriminant analysis involves assuming the covariance matrices are different and the means are equal. For example, the tests, shown in Figure 5.12, imply, for the earthquakes and explosions, the primary differences are in the bivariate spectral matrices and the means are essentially the same. For this case, it will be convenient to write the Whittle approximation to the log likelihood in the form

$$\ln p_j(\boldsymbol{X}) = \sum_{0<\nu_k<1/2} \Big[ -\ln |f_j(\nu_k)| - \boldsymbol{X}^*(\nu_k) f_j^{-1}(\nu_k) \boldsymbol{X}(\nu_k) \Big], \tag{5.122}$$

where we have omitted the prior probabilities from the equation. The quadratic detector in this case can be written in the form

$$\ln p_j(\boldsymbol{X}) = \sum_{0<\nu_k<1/2} \Big[ -\ln |f_j(\nu_k)| - \mathrm{tr}\big\{ I(\nu_k) f_j^{-1}(\nu_k) \big\} \Big], \tag{5.123}$$

where

$$I(\nu_k) = \boldsymbol{X}(\nu_k)\boldsymbol{X}^*(\nu_k) \tag{5.124}$$

denotes the ***periodogram matrix***. For equal prior probabilities, we may assign an observation $\boldsymbol{x}$ into population $\Pi_i$ whenever

$$\ln p_i(\boldsymbol{X}) > \ln p_j(\boldsymbol{X}) \tag{5.125}$$

for $j \neq i, j = 1, 2, \dots, g$.

Numerous authors have considered various versions of discriminant analysis in the frequency domain. Shumway and Unger (1974) considered (5.121) for $p = 1$ and equal covariance matrices, so the criterion reduces to a simple linear one. They apply the criterion to discriminating between earthquakes and explosions using teleseismic P wave data in which the means over the two groups might be considered as fixed. Alagón (1989) and Dargahi-Noubary and Laycock (1981) considered discriminant functions of the form (5.121) in the univariate case when the means are zero and the spectra for the two groups are different. Taniguchi et al (1994) adopted (5.122) as a criterion and discussed its ***non-Gaussian robustness***. Shumway (1982) reviews general discriminant functions in both the univariate and multivariate time series cases.

MEASURES OF DISPARITY

Before proceeding to examples of discriminant and cluster analysis, it is useful to consider the relation to the Kullback–Leibler (K-L) ***discrimination information***, as defined in Problem 1.29 of Chapter 1. Using the spectral approximation and noting the periodogram matrix has the approximate expectation

$$E_j I(\nu_k) = f_j(\nu_k)$$

under the assumption that the data come from population $\Pi_j$, and approximating the ratio of the densities by

$$\ln \frac{p_1(\boldsymbol{X})}{p_2(\boldsymbol{X})} = \sum_{0<\nu_k<1/2} \left[ -\ln \frac{|f_1(\nu_k)|}{|f_2(\nu_k)|} - \mathrm{tr}\Big\{ \big(f_2^{-1}(\nu_k) - f_1^{-1}(\nu_k)\big) I(\nu_k) \Big\} \right],$$

we may write the approximate discrimination information as

$$\begin{aligned} I(f_1; f_2) &= \frac{1}{n} E_1 \ln \frac{p_1(\boldsymbol{X})}{p_2(\boldsymbol{X})} \\ &= \frac{1}{n} \sum_{0<\nu_k<1/2} \left[ \mathrm{tr}\left\{ f_1(\nu_k) f_2^{-1}(\nu_k) \right\} - \ln \frac{|f_1(\nu_k)|}{|f_2(\nu_k)|} - p \right]. \end{aligned} \tag{5.126}$$

The approximation may be carefully justified by noting the multivatiate normal time series $\boldsymbol{x} = (\boldsymbol{x}_1', \boldsymbol{x}_2' \ldots, \boldsymbol{x}_n')$ with zero means and $np \times np$ stationary covariance matrices $\Gamma_1$ and $\Gamma_2$ will have $p$, $n \times n$ blocks, with elements of the form $\gamma_{ij}^{(l)}(s-t), s, t = 1, \ldots, n, i, j = 1, \ldots, p$ for population $\Pi_\ell, \ell = 1, 2$. The discrimination information, under these conditions, becomes

$$\begin{aligned} I(1;2:\boldsymbol{x}) &= \frac{1}{n} E_1 \ln \frac{p_1(\boldsymbol{x})}{p_2(\boldsymbol{x})} \\ &= \frac{1}{2n}\left[\operatorname{tr}\{\Gamma_1\Gamma_2^{-1}\} - \ln\frac{|\Gamma_1|}{|\Gamma_2|} - np\right]. \end{aligned} \tag{5.127}$$

The limiting result

$$\lim_{n\to\infty} I(1;2:\boldsymbol{x}) = \frac{1}{2}\int_{-1/2}^{1/2}\left[\operatorname{tr}\{f_1(\nu)f_2^{-1}(\nu)\} - \ln\frac{|f_1(\nu)|}{|f_2(\nu)|} - p\right] d\nu$$

has been shown, in various forms, by Pinsker (1964), Hannan (1970), and Kazakos and Papantoni-Kazakos (1980). The discrete version of (5.126) is just the approximation to the integral of the limiting form. The K-L measure of disparity is not a true distance, but it can be shown that $I(1;2) \geq 0$, with equality if and only if $f_1(\nu) = f_2(\nu)$ almost everywhere. This result makes it potentially suitable as a measure of disparity between the two densities.

A connection exists, of course, between the discrimination information number, which is just the expectation of the likelihood criterion and the likelihood itself. For example, we may measure the disparity between the sample and the process defined by the theoretical spectrum $f_j(\nu_k)$ corresponding to population $\Pi_j$ in the sense of Kullback (1978), as $I(\widehat{f}; f_j)$, where

$$\widehat{f}(\nu_k) = L^{-1} \sum_{\ell=-(L-1)/2}^{(L-1)/2} I(\nu_k + \ell/n) \tag{5.128}$$

denotes the smoothed spectral matrix. The likelihood ratio criterion can be thought of as measuring the disparity between the periodogram and the theoretical spectrum for each of the populations. To make the discrimination information finite, we replace the periodogram implied by the log likelihood by the sample spectrum. In this case, the classification procedure can be regarded as finding the population closest, in the sense of minimizing disparity between the sample and theoretical spectral matrices. The classification in this case proceeds by simply choosing the population $\Pi_j$ that minimizes $I(\widehat{f}; f_j)$, i.e., assigning $\boldsymbol{x}$ to population $\Pi_i$ whenever

$$I(\widehat{f}; f_i) < I(\widehat{f}; f_j) \tag{5.129}$$

for $j \neq i, j = 1, 2, \ldots, g$.

Kakizawa et al (1998) proposed using the ***Chernoff (CH) information measure*** (Chernoff, 1952, Renyi, 1961), defined as

$$B_\alpha(1;2) = -\ln E_2\left\{\left(\frac{p_2(\boldsymbol{x})}{p_1(\boldsymbol{x})}\right)^\alpha\right\}, \tag{5.130}$$

where the measure is indexed by a ***regularizing parameter*** $\alpha$, for $0 < \alpha < 1$. When $\alpha = .5$, the Chernoff measure is the ***symmetric divergence*** proposed by Bhattacharya (1943). For the multivariate normal case,

$$B_\alpha(1;2:\boldsymbol{x}) = \frac{1}{n}\left[\ln\frac{|\alpha\Gamma_1 + (1-\alpha)\Gamma_2|}{|\Gamma_2|} - \alpha\ln\frac{|\Gamma_1|}{|\Gamma_2|}\right]. \tag{5.131}$$

The large sample spectral approximation to the Chernoff information measure is analogous to that for the discrimination information, namely,

$$\begin{aligned} B_\alpha(f_1;f_2) &= \frac{1}{2n}\sum_{0<\nu_k<1/2}\left[\ln\frac{|\alpha f_1(\nu_k) + (1-\alpha)f_2(\nu_k)|}{|f_2(\nu_k)|}\right. \\ &\qquad \left. -\alpha\ln\frac{|f_1(\nu_k)|}{|f_2(\nu_k)|}\right]. \end{aligned} \tag{5.132}$$

The Chernoff measure, when divided by $\alpha(1-\alpha)$, behaves like the discrimination information in the limit in the sense that it converges to $I(1;2:\boldsymbol{x})$ for $\alpha \to 0$ and to $I(2;1:\boldsymbol{x})$ for $\alpha \to 1$. Hence, near the boundaries of the parameter $\alpha$, it tends to behave like discrimination information and for other values represents a compromise between the two information measures. The classification rule for the Chernoff measure reduces to assigning $\boldsymbol{x}$ to population $\Pi_i$ whenever

$$B_\alpha(\widehat{f};f_i) < B_\alpha(\widehat{f};f_j) \tag{5.133}$$

for $j \neq i, j = 1, 2, \ldots, g$.

Although the classification rules above are well defined if the group spectral matrices are known, this will not be the case in general. If there are $g$ training samples, $\boldsymbol{x}_{ij}, j = 1, \ldots, N_i, i = 1\ldots, g$, with $N_i$ vector observations available in each group, the natural estimator for the spectral matrix of the group $i$ is just the single-group spectral matrix (5.100), namely, with $\boldsymbol{X}_{ij}(\nu_k)$ denoting the vector DFTs,

$$\widehat{f}_i(\nu_k) = \frac{1}{N_i - 1}\sum_{j=1}^{N_i}\left(\boldsymbol{X}_{ij}(\nu_k) - \boldsymbol{X}_{i\cdot}(\nu_k)\right)^*\left(\boldsymbol{X}_{ij}(\nu_k) - \boldsymbol{X}_{i\cdot}(\nu_k)\right), \tag{5.134}$$

A second consideration is the choice of the regularization parameter $\alpha$ for the Chernoff criterion, (5.132). For the case of $g = 2$ groups, it should be chosen to maximize the disparity between the two group spectra, as defined in (5.132). Kakizawa et al (1998) simply plot (5.132) as a function of $\alpha$, using the estimated group spectra in (5.134), choosing the value that gives the maximum disparity between the two groups.

**Example 5.12 Discriminant Analysis for Earthquakes and Explosions**

The simplest approaches to discriminating between the earthquake and explosion groups have been based on either the relative amplitudes of the P and S phases, as in Figure 5.4 or on relative power components in various frequency bands. Considerable effort has been expended on using various spectral ratios involving the bivariate P and S phases as discrimination features. Kakizawa et al (1998) mention a number of measures that have be used in the seismological literature as features. These features include ratios of power for the two phases and ratios of power components in high- and low-frequency bands. The use of such features of the spectrum suggests an optimal procedure based on discriminating between the spectral matrices of two stationary processes would be reasonable. The fact that the hypothesis that the spectral matrices were equal, tested in Example 5.10, was also soundly rejected suggests the use of a discriminant function based on spectral differences. Recall the sampling rate is 40 points per second, leading to a folding frequency of 20 Hz. To avoid numerical problems, we used a broad band (2Hz, $L = 51$) and the criteria (5.126) and (5.132), summed over the interval from 0 to 8 Hz, where the spectra were both positive. Narrowing the bandwidth and summing over a broader interval did not substantially change the results. The maximum value of the estimated Chernoff disparity $B_\alpha(\widehat{f}_1; \widehat{f}_2)$ occurs for $\alpha = .3$, and we use that value in the discriminant criterion (5.132). Discriminant scores using the holdout classification functions are shown in Table 5.6 for both criteria. We note the generally good performance of the Chernoff measure, which separates the two populations well and makes no errors; the discrimination information misclassified explosions one and eight as earthquakes. The values for the two sets of scores are plotted in the right-hand panel of Figure 5.13, and the earthquake variances of the discrimination information have larger variances than do those for the explosions (the standard deviations were 9.34 and 1.25, respectively). The Chernoff discriminant scores are distributed on either side of the decision point 0, with means .58 and -.48 for the earthquake and explosion groups, respectively; the standard deviations of the two samples were .34 and .20. The NZ event was also classified using the average spectral matrices of the eight earthquakes and explosions, giving the value -.49 for the discimination information and -.31 for the Chernoff measure, putting the event in the explosion population by this criterion. Previously, in Example 5.11, the extracted log amplitudes classified this event in the earthquake group. The Russians have asserted no mine blasting or nuclear testing occurred in the area in question, so the event remains as somewhat of a mystery. The fact that it was relatively removed geographically from the test set may also have introduced some uncertainties into the procedure.

**Table 5.6:** Discriminant Scores $I = I(\widehat{f}; f_1) - I(\widehat{f}; f_2)$ and $B = B_{.3}(\widehat{f}; f_1) - B_{.3}(\widehat{f}; f_2)$ for Earthquakes and Explosions

| EQ | $I$ | $B$ | EXP | $I$ | $B$ |
|---|---|---|---|---|---|
| 1 | 8.51 | .54 | 1 | .29 | -.25 |
| 2 | .81 | .50 | 2 | -2.55 | -.75 |
| 3 | 30.80 | 1.04 | 4 | -1.82 | -.61 |
| 4 | 2.73 | .10 | 4 | -1.89 | -.44 |
| 5 | 7.69 | .11 | 5 | -1.16 | -.45 |
| 6 | 21.50 | .79 | 6 | -2.12 | -.61 |
| 7 | 20.31 | .85 | 7 | -2.10 | -.59 |
| 8 | 15.54 | .70 | 8 | .93 | -.21 |

### Cluster Analysis

For the purpose of clustering, it may be more useful to consider a ***symmetric disparity measures*** and we introduce the ***J-Divergence*** measure

$$J(f_1; f_2) = I(f_1; f_2) + I(f_2; f_1) \tag{5.135}$$

and the symmetric Chernoff number

$$JB_\alpha(f_1; f_2) = B_\alpha(f_1; f_2) + B_\alpha(f_2; f_1) \tag{5.136}$$

for that purpose. In this case, we define the disparity between the sample spectral matrix of a single vector, $\boldsymbol{x}$, and the population $\Pi_j$ as

$$J(\widehat{f}; f_j) = I(\widehat{f}; f_j) + I(f_j; \widehat{f}) \tag{5.137}$$

and

$$JB_\alpha(\widehat{f}; f_j) = B_\alpha(\widehat{f}; f_j) + B_\alpha(f_j; \widehat{f}), \tag{5.138}$$

respectively and use these as quasi-distances between the vector and population $\Pi_j$.

The measures of disparity can be used to cluster multivariate time series. The symmetric measures of disparity, as defined above ensure that the disparity between $f_i$ and $f_j$ is the same as the disparity between $f_j$ and $f_i$. Hence, we will consider the symmetric forms (5.137) and (5.138) as quasi-distances for the purpose of defining a distance matrix for input into one of the standard clustering procedures (see Johnson and Wichern, 1992). In general, we may consider either ***hierarchical*** or ***partitioned*** clustering methods using the quasi-distance matrix as an input.

For purposes of illustration, we may use the symmetric divergence (5.137), which implies the quasi-distance between sample series with estimated spectral matrices $\widehat{f}_i$ and $\widehat{f}_j$ would be (5.137); i.e.,

$$J(\widehat{f}_i; \widehat{f}_j) = \frac{1}{n} \sum_{0<\nu_k<1/2} \left[ \operatorname{tr}\{\widehat{f}_i(\nu_k) \widehat{f}_j^{-1}(\nu_k)\} + \operatorname{tr}\{\widehat{f}_j(\nu_k) \widehat{f}_i^{-1}(\nu_k)\} - 2p \right], \tag{5.139}$$

for $i \neq j$. We can also use the comparable form for the Chernoff divergence, but we may not want to make an assumption for the regularization parameter $\alpha$.

For hierarchical clustering, we begin by clustering the two members of the population that minimize the disparity measure (5.139). Then, these two items form a cluster, and we can compute distances between unclustered items as before. The distance between unnclustered items and a current cluster is defined here as the average of the distances to elements in the cluster. Again, we combine objects that are closest together. We may also compute the distance between the unclustered items and clustered items as the closest distance, rather than the average. Once a series is in a cluster, it stays there. At each stage, we have a fixed number of clusters, depending on the merging stage.

Alternatively, we may think of clustering as a partitioning of the sample into a prespecified number of groups. MacQueen (1967) has proposed this using ***k-means clustering***, using the Mahalonobis distance between an observation and the group mean vectors. At each stage, a reassignment of an observation into its closest affinity group is possible. To see how this procedure applies in the current context, consider a preliminary partition into a fixed number of groups and define the disparity between the spectral matrix of the observation, say, $\widehat{f}$, and the average spectral matrix of the group, say, $\widehat{f}_i$, as $J(\widehat{f}; \widehat{f}_i)$, where the group spectral matrix can be estimated by (5.134). At any pass, a single series is reassigned to the group for which its disparity is minimized. The reassignment procedure is repeated until all observations stay in their current groups. Of course, the number of groups must be specified for each repetition of the partitioning algorithm and a starting partition must be chosen. This assignment can either be random or chosen from a preliminary hierarchical clustering, as described above. kip

**Example 5.13 Cluster Analysis for Earthquakes and Explosions**

It is instructive to try the clustering procedure on the population of known earthquakes and explosions. Table 5.7 shows the results of applying partitioned clustering under the assumption that either two or three groups are appropriate. Two groups would be simple assuming the vectors classified naturally into the earthquake and explosion classes, whereas three groups would imply possible outliers from the two primary groups. The starting partitions were defined by either randomly assigning observations to groups or using the result of the hierarchichal clustering procedure. The two-group partition with the hierarchical start configuration tends to produce a final partition that agrees closely with the known configuration, assuming the NZ event is an explosion. The random starting partition puts two of the earthquakes into the explosion group. For the three-group partitions, one or two earthquakes and the last explosion join the third cluster that we have designated as the outlying group.

**Table 5.7:** Clustering Results for Earthquakes and Explosions

| Beginning | Cluster 1 | Cluster 2 | Cluster 3 |
|---|---|---|---|
| **Two Groups:** | | | |
| Random | EQ 123678 | EX 12345678<br>EQ 45 NZ | |
| Hierarchical | EQ 12345678 | EX 12345678<br>NZ | |
| **Three Groups:** | | | |
| Random | EQ 123678 | EX 1234567<br>EQ 4 NZ | EQ 5 EX 8 |
| Hierarchical | EQ 123678 | EX 1234567<br>NZ | EQ 45 EX 8 |

## 5.8 Principal Components, Canonical, and Factor Analysis

In this section, we introduce the related topics of spectral domain ***principal components***, ***canonical analysis***, and ***factor analysis*** for time series. The topics of principal components and canonical analysis in the frequency domain are rigorously presented in Brillinger (1981, Chapters 9 and 10) and many of the details concerning these concepts can be found there.

The techniques presented here are related to each other in that they focus on extracting pertinent information from spectral matrices. This information is important because dealing directly with a high-dimensional spectral matrix $f(\nu)$ itself is somewhat cumbersome because it is a function into the set of complex, nonnegative-definite, Hermitian matrices. We can view these techniques as easily understood, parsimonious tools for exploring the behavior of vector-valued time series in the frequency domain with minimal loss of information. Because our focus is on spectral matrices, we assume for convenience that the time series of interest have zero means; the techniques are easily adjusted in the case of nonzero means.

In this and subsequent sections, it will be convenient to work occasionally with ***complex-valued time series***. A $p\times 1$ complex-valued time series can be represented as $\boldsymbol{x}_t = \boldsymbol{x}_{1t} - i\boldsymbol{x}_{2t}$, where $\boldsymbol{x}_{1t}$ is the real part and $\boldsymbol{x}_{2t}$ is the imaginary part of $\boldsymbol{x}_t$. The process is said to be stationary if $E(\boldsymbol{x}_t)$ and $E(\boldsymbol{x}_{t+h}\boldsymbol{x}_t^*)$ exist and are independent of time $t$. The $p \times p$ autocovariance function,

$$\Gamma_x(h) = E(\boldsymbol{x}_{t+h}\boldsymbol{x}_t^*) - E(\boldsymbol{x}_{t+h})E(\boldsymbol{x}_t^*),$$

of $\boldsymbol{x}_t$ satisfies conditions similar to those of the real-valued case. Writing $\Gamma_x(h) = \{\gamma_{ij}(h)\}$, for $i, j = 1, ..., p$, we have (i) $\gamma_{ii}(0) \geq 0$ is real, (ii) $|\gamma_{ij}(h)|^2 \leq \gamma_{ii}(0)\gamma_{jj}(0)$ for all integers $h$, and (iii) $\Gamma_x(h)$ is Hermitian, that is, $\Gamma_x(h) = \Gamma_x(h)^*$. The spectral theory of complex-valued vector time series is analogous to the real-valued case. For example, $\Gamma_x(h)$ is a nonnegative-definite function on the integers, and if $\sum_h ||\Gamma_x(h)|| < \infty$, the spectral density matrix of the complex series $\boldsymbol{x}_t$ is given by

$$f_x(\nu) = \sum_{h=-\infty}^{\infty} \Gamma_x(h) \exp(-2\pi i h \nu).$$

### Principal Components

Classical principal component analysis is concerned with explaining the variance–covariance structure among $p$ variables, $\boldsymbol{x} = (x_1, ..., x_p)'$, through a few linear combinations of the components of $\boldsymbol{x}$. Suppose we wish to find a linear combination

$$y = \boldsymbol{c}'\boldsymbol{x} = c_1 x_1 + \cdots + c_p x_p \tag{5.140}$$

of the components of $\boldsymbol{x}$ such that var$(y)$ is as large as possible. Because var$(y)$ can be increased by simply multiplying $\boldsymbol{c}$ by a constant, it is common to restrict $\boldsymbol{c}$ to be of unit length; that is, $\boldsymbol{c}'\boldsymbol{c} = 1$. Noting that var$(y) = \boldsymbol{c}'\Sigma_x \boldsymbol{c}$, where $\Sigma_x$ is the $p \times p$ variance–covariance matrix of $\boldsymbol{x}$, another way of stating the problem is to find $\boldsymbol{c}$ such that

$$\max_{\boldsymbol{c} \neq \boldsymbol{0}} \frac{\boldsymbol{c}'\Sigma_x \boldsymbol{c}}{\boldsymbol{c}'\boldsymbol{c}}. \tag{5.141}$$

Denote the ***eigenvalue–eigenvector pairs*** of $\Sigma_x$ by $\{(\lambda_1, \boldsymbol{e}_1), ..., (\lambda_p, \boldsymbol{e}_p)\}$, where $\lambda_1 \geq \lambda_2 \geq \cdots \geq \lambda_p \geq 0$, and the eigenvectors are of unit length. The solution to (5.141) is to choose $\boldsymbol{c} = \boldsymbol{e}_1$, in which case the linear combination $y_1 = \boldsymbol{e}_1'\boldsymbol{x}$ has maximum variance, var$(y_1) = \lambda_1$. In other words,

$$\max_{\boldsymbol{c} \neq \boldsymbol{0}} \frac{\boldsymbol{c}'\Sigma_x \boldsymbol{c}}{\boldsymbol{c}'\boldsymbol{c}} = \frac{\boldsymbol{e}_1'\Sigma_x \boldsymbol{e}_1}{\boldsymbol{e}_1'\boldsymbol{e}_1} = \lambda_1. \tag{5.142}$$

The linear combination, $y_1 = \boldsymbol{e}_1'\boldsymbol{x}$, is called the ***first principal component***. Because the eigenvalues of $\Sigma_x$ are not necessarily unique, the first principal component is not necessarily unique.

The ***second principal component*** is defined to be the linear combination $y_2 = \boldsymbol{c}'\boldsymbol{x}$ that maximizes var$(y_2)$ subject to $\boldsymbol{c}'\boldsymbol{c} = 1$ and such that cov$(y_1, y_2) = 0$. The solution is to choose $\boldsymbol{c} = \boldsymbol{e}_2$; in which case, var$(y_2) = \lambda_2$. In general, the ***k-th principal component***, for $k = 1, 2, ..., p$, is the the linear combination $y_k = \boldsymbol{c}'\boldsymbol{x}$ that maximizes var$(y_k)$ subject to $\boldsymbol{c}'\boldsymbol{c} = 1$ and such that cov$(y_k, y_j) = 0$, for $j = 1, 2, ..., k-1$. The solution is to choose $\boldsymbol{c} = \boldsymbol{e}_k$; in which case var$(y_k) = \lambda_k$.

One measure of the importance of a principal component is to assess the proportion of the total variance attributed to that principal component. The ***total variance*** of $\boldsymbol{x}$ is defined to be the sum of the variances of the individual components; that is, var$(x_1) + \cdots +$ var$(x_p) = \sigma_{11} + \cdots + \sigma_{pp}$, where $\sigma_{jj}$ is the $j$-th diagonal element of $\Sigma_x$. This sum is also denoted as $\mathrm{tr}(\Sigma_x)$, or the ***trace*** of $\Sigma_x$. Because $\mathrm{tr}(\Sigma_x) = \lambda_1 + \cdots + \lambda_p$, the ***proportion of the total variance attributed to the k-th principal component*** is given simply by $\mathrm{var}(y_k) \;/\; \mathrm{tr}(\Sigma_x) = \lambda_k \;/\; \sum_{j=1}^{p} \lambda_j$.

Given a random sample $\boldsymbol{x}_1, ..., \boldsymbol{x}_n$, the ***sample principal components*** are defined as above, but with $\Sigma_x$ replaced by the sample variance–covariance matrix, $S_x = (n-1)^{-1} \sum_{i=1}^{n} (\boldsymbol{x}_i - \bar{\boldsymbol{x}})(\boldsymbol{x}_i - \bar{\boldsymbol{x}})'$. Further details can be found in the introduction to classical principal component analysis in Johnson and Wichern (1992, Chapter 9).

For the case of time series, suppose we have a zero mean, $p \times 1$, stationary vector process $\boldsymbol{x}_t$ that has a $p \times p$ spectral density matrix given by $f_x(\nu)$. Recall $f_x(\nu)$ is a complex-valued, nonnegative-definite, Hermitian matrix. Using the analogy of classical principal components, and in particular (5.140) and (5.141), suppose, for a fixed value of $\nu$, we want to find a complex-valued univariate process $y_t(\nu) = \boldsymbol{c}(\nu)^* x_t$, where $\boldsymbol{c}(\nu)$ is complex, such that the spectral density of $y_t(\nu)$ is maximized at frequency $\nu$, and $\boldsymbol{c}(\nu)$ is of unit length, $\boldsymbol{c}(\nu)^*\boldsymbol{c}(\nu) = 1$. Because, at frequency $\nu$, the spectral density of $y_t(\nu)$ is $f_y(\nu) = \boldsymbol{c}(\nu)^* f_x(\nu)\boldsymbol{c}(\nu)$, the problem can be restated as: Find complex vector $\boldsymbol{c}(\nu)$ such that

$$\max_{\boldsymbol{c}(\nu) \neq \boldsymbol{0}} \frac{\boldsymbol{c}(\nu)^* f_x(\nu)\boldsymbol{c}(\nu)}{\boldsymbol{c}(\nu)^*\boldsymbol{c}(\nu)}. \tag{5.143}$$

Let $\{(\lambda_1(\nu), \boldsymbol{e}_1(\nu)) \;, ..., \; (\lambda_p(\nu), \boldsymbol{e}_p(\nu))\}$ denote the eigenvalue–eigenvector pairs of $f_x(\nu)$, where $\lambda_1(\nu) \geq \lambda_2(\nu) \geq \cdots \geq \lambda_p(\nu) \geq 0$, and the eigenvectors are of unit length. The solution to (5.143) is to choose $\boldsymbol{c}(\nu) = \boldsymbol{e}_1(\nu)$; in which case the desired linear combination is $y_t(\nu) = \boldsymbol{e}_1(\nu)^*\boldsymbol{x}_t$. For this choice,

$$\max_{\boldsymbol{c}(\nu) \neq \boldsymbol{0}} \frac{\boldsymbol{c}(\nu)^* f_x(\nu)\boldsymbol{c}(\nu)}{\boldsymbol{c}(\nu)^*\boldsymbol{c}(\nu)} = \frac{\boldsymbol{e}_1(\nu)^* f_x(\nu)\boldsymbol{e}_1(\nu)}{\boldsymbol{e}_1(\nu)^*\boldsymbol{e}_1(\nu)} = \lambda_1(\nu). \tag{5.144}$$

This process may be repeated for any frequency $\nu$, and the complex-valued process, $y_{t1}(\nu) = \boldsymbol{e}_1(\nu)^*\boldsymbol{x}_t$, is called the ***first principal component at frequency*** $\nu$. The $k$-th principal component at frequency $\nu$, for $k = 1, 2, ..., p$, is the complex-valued time series $y_{tk}(\nu) = \boldsymbol{e}_k(\nu)^*\boldsymbol{x}_t$, in analogy to the classical case. In this case, the spectral density of $y_{tk}(\nu)$ at frequency $\nu$ is $f_{y_k}(\nu) = \boldsymbol{e}_k(\nu)^* f_x(\nu)\boldsymbol{e}_k(\nu) = \lambda_k(\nu)$.

The previous development of spectral domain principal components is related to the ***spectral envelope*** methodology first discussed in Stoffer et al (1993). We will present the spectral envelope in the next section, where we motivate the use of principal components as it is presented above. Another way to motivate the use of principal components in the frequency domain was given in Brillinger (1981, Chapter 9). Although this technique leads to the same analysis, the motivation may be more satisfactory to the reader at this point. In this case, we suppose we have a stationary, $p$-dimensional, vector-valued process $\boldsymbol{x}_t$ and we are only able to keep a univariate process $y_t$ such that, when needed, we may reconstruct the vector-valued process, $\boldsymbol{x}_t$, according to an optimality criterion.

Specifically, we suppose we want to approximate a mean-zero, stationary, vector-valued time series, $\boldsymbol{x}_t$, with spectral matrix $f_x(\nu)$, by a univariate process $y_t$ defined by

$$y_t = \sum_{j=-\infty}^{\infty} \boldsymbol{c}_{t-j}^* \boldsymbol{x}_j, \tag{5.145}$$

where $\{\boldsymbol{c}_j\}$ is a $p \times 1$ vector-valued filter, such that $\{\boldsymbol{c}_j\}$ is absolutely summable; that is, $\sum_{j=-\infty}^{\infty} |\boldsymbol{c}_j| < \infty$. The approximation is accomplished so the reconstruction of $\boldsymbol{x}_t$ from $y_t$, say,

$$\widehat{\boldsymbol{x}}_t = \sum_{j=-\infty}^{\infty} \boldsymbol{b}_{t-j} y_j, \tag{5.146}$$

where $\{\boldsymbol{b}_j\}$ is an absolutely summable $p \times 1$ filter, is such that the mean square approximation error

$$E\{(\boldsymbol{x}_t - \widehat{\boldsymbol{x}}_t)^*(\boldsymbol{x}_t - \widehat{\boldsymbol{x}}_t)\} \tag{5.147}$$

is minimized.

Let $\boldsymbol{b}(\nu)$ and $\boldsymbol{c}(\nu)$ be the transforms of $\{\boldsymbol{b}_j\}$ and $\{\boldsymbol{c}_j\}$, respectively. For example,

$$\boldsymbol{c}(\nu) = \sum_{j=-\infty}^{\infty} \boldsymbol{c}_j \exp(-2\pi i j \nu), \tag{5.148}$$

and, consequently,

$$\boldsymbol{c}_j = \int_{-1/2}^{1/2} \boldsymbol{c}(\nu) \exp(2\pi i j \nu) d\nu. \tag{5.149}$$

Brillinger (1981, Theorem 9.3.1) shows the solution to the problem is to choose $\boldsymbol{c}(\nu)$ to satisfy (5.143) and to set $\boldsymbol{b}(\nu) = \overline{\boldsymbol{c}(\nu)}$. This is precisely the previous problem, with the solution given by (5.144). That is, we choose $\boldsymbol{c}(\nu) = \boldsymbol{e}_1(\nu)$ and $\boldsymbol{b}(\nu) = \overline{\boldsymbol{e}_1(\nu)}$; the filter values can be obtained via the inversion formula given by (5.149). Using these results, in view of (5.145), we may form the ***first principal component series***, say $y_{t1}$.

This technique may be extended by requesting another series, say, $y_{t2}$, for approximating $\boldsymbol{x}_t$ with respect to minimum mean square error, but where the coherency between $y_{t2}$ and $y_{t1}$ is zero. In this case, we choose $\boldsymbol{c}(\nu) = \boldsymbol{e}_2(\nu)$. Continuing this way, we can obtain the first $q \leq p$ principal components series, say, $\boldsymbol{y}_t = (y_{t1}, ..., y_{tq})'$, having spectral density $f_q(\nu) = \text{diag}\{\lambda_1(\nu), ..., \lambda_q(\nu)\}$. The series $y_{tk}$ is the ***k-th principal component series.***

As in the classical case, given observations, $\boldsymbol{x}_1, \boldsymbol{x}_2, ..., \boldsymbol{x}_n$, from the process $\boldsymbol{x}_t$, we can form an estimate $\widehat{f}_x(\nu)$ of $f_x(\nu)$ and define the ***sample principal component series*** by replacing $f_x(\nu)$ with $\widehat{f}_x(\nu)$ in the previous discussion. Precise details pertaining to the asymptotic ($n \to \infty$) behavior of the principal component series and their spectra can be found in Brillinger (1981, ch 9).

To give a basic idea of what we can expect, we focus on the first principal component series and on the spectral estimator obtained by smoothing the periodogram matrix, $I_n(\nu_j)$; that is

$$\widehat{f}_x(\nu_j) = \sum_{\ell=-(L-1)/2}^{(L-1)/2} h_\ell I_n(\nu_j + \ell/n), \tag{5.150}$$

where $L$ is odd and the weights are chosen so $h_\ell = h_{-\ell}$ are positive and $\sum_\ell h_\ell = 1$. Under the conditions for which $\widehat{f}_x(\nu_j)$ is a well-behaved estimator of $f_x(\nu_j)$, and for which the largest eigenvalue of $f_x(\nu_j)$ is unique,

$$\left\{\eta_n \left[\widehat{\lambda}_1(\nu_j) - \lambda_1(\nu_j)\right] \Big/ \lambda_1(\nu_j), \quad \eta_n \left[\widehat{\boldsymbol{e}}_1(\nu_j) - \boldsymbol{e}_1(\nu_j)\right];\ j = 1, ..., J\right\} \tag{5.151}$$

converges ($n \to \infty$) jointly in distribution to independent, zero-mean normal distributions, the first of which is standard normal. In (5.151), $\eta_n^{-2} = \sum_{\ell=-(L-1)/2}^{(L-1)/2} h_\ell^2$, noting we must have $L \to \infty$ and $\eta_n \to \infty$, but $L/n \to 0$ as $n \to \infty$. The asymptotic variance–covariance matrix of $\widehat{\boldsymbol{e}}_1(\nu)$, say, $\Sigma_{e_1}(\nu)$, is given by

$$\Sigma_{e_1}(\nu) = \eta_n^{-2}\lambda_1(\nu) \sum_{\ell=2}^{p} \lambda_\ell(\nu) \left\{\lambda_1(\nu) - \lambda_\ell(\nu)\right\}^{-2} \boldsymbol{e}_\ell(\nu)\boldsymbol{e}_\ell^*(\nu). \tag{5.152}$$

The distribution of $\widehat{\boldsymbol{e}}_1(\nu)$ depends on the other latent roots and vectors of $f_x(\nu)$. Writing $\widehat{\boldsymbol{e}}_1(\nu) = (\widehat{e}_{11}(\nu), \widehat{e}_{12}(\nu), ..., \widehat{e}_{1p}(\nu))'$, we may use this result to form confidence regions for the components of $\widehat{\boldsymbol{e}}_1$ by approximating the distribution of

$$\frac{2\left|\widehat{\boldsymbol{e}}_{1,j}(\nu) - \boldsymbol{e}_{1,j}(\nu)\right|^2}{s_j^2(\nu)}, \tag{5.153}$$

for $j = 1, ..., p$, by a $\chi^2$ distribution with two degrees of freedom. In (5.153), $s_j^2(\nu)$ is the $j$-th diagonal element of $\widehat{\Sigma}_{e_1}(\nu)$, the estimate of $\Sigma_{e_1}(\nu)$. We can use (5.153) to check whether the value of zero is in the confidence region by comparing $2|\widehat{\boldsymbol{e}}_{1,j}(\nu)|^2/s_j^2(\nu)$ with $\chi_2^2(1-\alpha)$, the $1-\alpha$ upper tail cutoff of the $\chi_2^2$ distribution.

**Example 5.14 Principal Component Analysis of the fMRI Data**

Recall Example 1.5 of Chapter 1, where the vector time series $\boldsymbol{x}_t = (x_{t1}, ..., x_{t8})'$, $t = 1, ..., 128$, represents consecutive measures of average blood oxygenation level dependent (BOLD) signal intensity, which measures areas of activation in the brain. Recall subjects were given a non-painful brush on the hand and the stimulus was applied for 32 seconds and then stopped for 32 seconds; thus, the signal period is 64 seconds (the sampling rate was one observation every two seconds for 256 seconds). The series $x_{tk}$ for $k = 1, 2, 3, 4$ represent locations in cortex, series $x_{t5}$

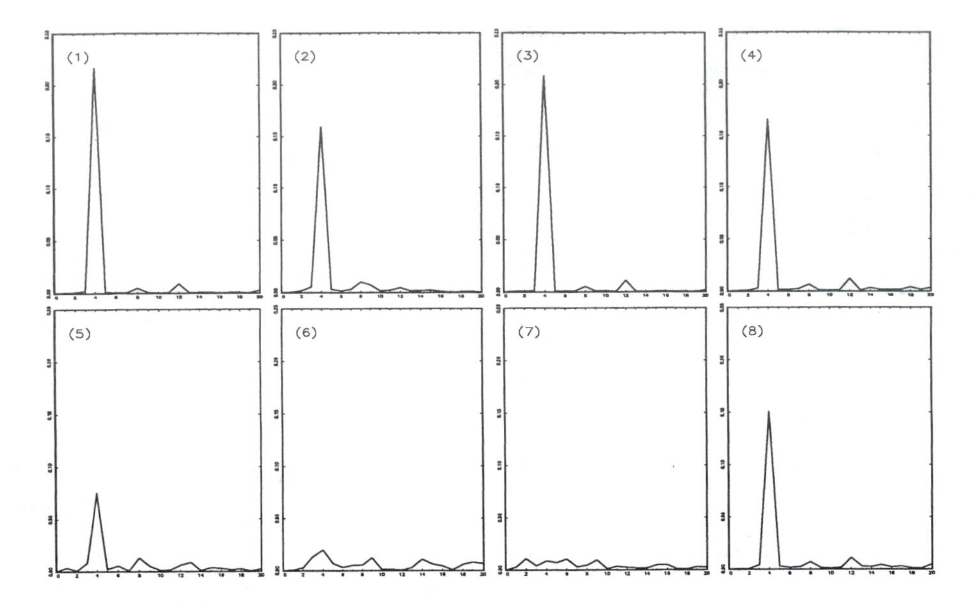


**Figure 5.14:** The individual periodograms of $x_{tk}$, for $k = 1, ..., 8$, in Example 5.14.

**Table 5.8:** Magnitudes of the PC Vector at the Stimulus Frequency in Example 5.14

| Location | 1 | 2 | 3 | 4 | 5 | 6 | 7 | 8 |
|---|---|---|---|---|---|---|---|---|
| $\mid \widehat{e}_1(\frac{4}{128}) \mid$ | 0.46 | 0.40 | 0.45 | 0.40 | 0.28 | 0.15 | 0.09* | 0.39 |

*The value of zero is in an approximate 99% confidence region for this component.

and $x_{t6}$ represent locations in the thalamus, and $x_{t7}$ and $x_{t8}$ represent locations in the cerebellum.

As is evident from Figure 1.5 in Chapter 1, different areas of the brain are responding differently, and a principal component analysis may help in indicating which locations are responding with the most spectral power, and which locations do not contribute to the spectral power at the stimulus signal period. In this analysis, we will focus primarily on the signal period of 64 seconds, which translates to four cycles in 256 seconds or $\nu = 4/128$ cycles per time point. In addition, all calculations were performed using the standardized series; that is, we used $x_{tk}/s_k$, for $k = 1, ..., 8$, where $s_k$ is the sample standard deviation of the the $k$-th series, in the computations.

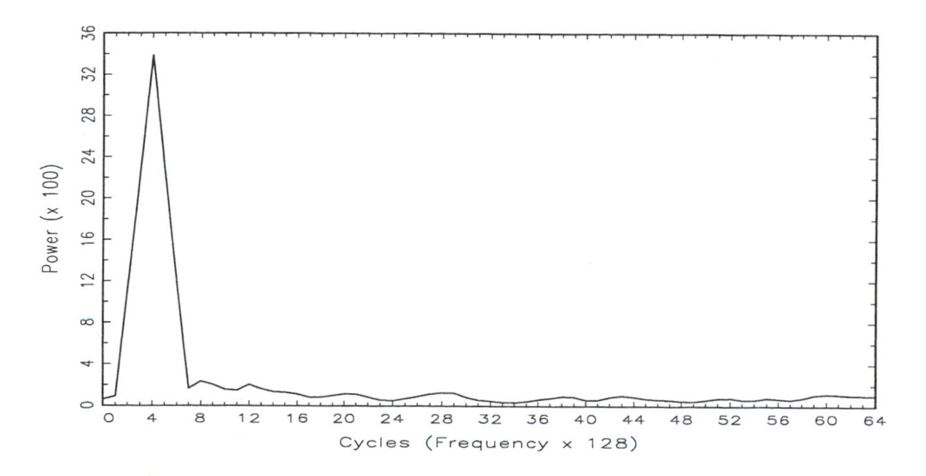


**Figure 5.15:** The estimated spectral density, $\widehat{\lambda}_1(j/128)$, of the first principal component series in Example 5.14.

Figure 5.14 shows individual periodograms of the series $x_{tk}$ for $k = 1, ..., 8$. As was evident from Figure 1.5, a strong response to the brush stimulus occurred in areas of the cortex. To estimate the spectral density of $\boldsymbol{x}_t$, we used (5.150) with $L = 5$ and $\{h_0 = 3/9, h_{\pm 1} = 2/9, h_{\pm 2} = 1/9\}$. Calling the estimated spectrum $\widehat{f}_x(j/128)$, for $j = 0, 1, ..., 64$, we can obtain the estimated spectrum of the first principal component series $y_{t1}$ by calculating the largest eigenvalue, $\widehat{\lambda}_1(j/128)$, of $\widehat{f}_x(j/128)$ for each $j = 0, 1, ..., 64$. The result, $\widehat{\lambda}_1(j/128)$, is shown in Figure 5.15. As expected, there is a large peak at the stimulus frequency 4/128, wherein $\widehat{\lambda}_1(4/128) = 0.339$. The total power at the stimulus frequency is $\operatorname{tr}\left(\widehat{f}_x(4/128)\right) = 0.353$, so the proportion of the power at frequency 4/128 attributed to the first principal component series is 0.339/0.353 = 96%. Because the first principal component explains nearly all of the total power at the stimulus frequency there is no need to explore the other principal component series at this frequency.

The estimated first principal component series at frequency 4/128 is given by $\widehat{y}_{t1}(4/128) = \widehat{\boldsymbol{e}}_1^*(4/128)\boldsymbol{x}_t$, and the components of $\widehat{\boldsymbol{e}}_1(4/128)$ can give insight as to which locations of the brain are responding to the brush stimulus. Table 5.8 shows the magnitudes of $\widehat{\boldsymbol{e}}_1(4/128)$. In addition, an approximate 99% confidence interval was obtained for each component using (5.153). As expected, the analysis indicates that location 7 is not contributing to the power at this frequency, but surprisingly, the analysis suggests location 6 is responding to the stimulus.

CANONICAL CORRELATION ANALYSIS

The concept of classical canonical correlation analysis was first presented in Chapter 4, Section 12. Recall the first ***canonical correlation***, $\lambda_1$, between a $k_1 \times 1$ random vector $\boldsymbol{x}_1$ and a $k_2 \times 1$ random vector $\boldsymbol{x}_2$, $k_1 \le k_2$, with nonsingular variance–covariance matrices $\Sigma_{11}$ and $\Sigma_{22}$, respectively, is the largest possible correlation between a linear combination of the components of $\boldsymbol{x}_1$, say, $\boldsymbol{\alpha}'\boldsymbol{x}_1$, and a linear combination of the components of $\boldsymbol{x}_2$, say, $\boldsymbol{\beta}'\boldsymbol{x}_2$, where $\boldsymbol{\alpha}$ is $k_1 \times 1$ and $\boldsymbol{\beta}$ is $k_2 \times 1$. That is,

$$\lambda_1 = \max_{\boldsymbol{\alpha},\boldsymbol{\beta}} \; \text{corr}\left(\boldsymbol{\alpha}'\boldsymbol{x}_1, \boldsymbol{\beta}'\boldsymbol{x}_2\right),$$

subject to the constraints $\text{var}(\boldsymbol{\alpha}'\boldsymbol{x}_1) = \boldsymbol{\alpha}'\Sigma_{11}\boldsymbol{\alpha} = 1$ and $\text{var}(\boldsymbol{\beta}'\boldsymbol{x}_2) = \boldsymbol{\beta}'\Sigma_{22}\boldsymbol{\beta} = 1$. If we let $\Sigma_{ij} = \text{cov}(\boldsymbol{x}_i, \boldsymbol{x}_j)$, for $i, j = 1, 2$, then $\lambda_1^2$ is the largest eigenvalue of the matrix $\Sigma_{11}^{-1}\Sigma_{12}\Sigma_{22}^{-1}\Sigma_{21}$.

We call the solutions $u_1 = \boldsymbol{\alpha}_1'\boldsymbol{x}_1$ and $v_1 = \boldsymbol{\beta}_1'\boldsymbol{x}_2$ the first ***canonical variates***, that is, $\lambda_1 = \text{corr}(u_1, v_1)$, and $\boldsymbol{\alpha}_1$ and $\boldsymbol{\beta}_1$ are the coefficients of the linear combinations that maximize the correlation. In particular, $\boldsymbol{\alpha}_1$ and $\boldsymbol{\beta}_1$ are taken proportional to the first eigenvectors of $\Sigma_{11}^{-1/2}\Sigma_{12}\Sigma_{22}^{-1}\Sigma_{21}\Sigma_{11}^{-1/2}$ and $\Sigma_{22}^{-1/2}\Sigma_{21}\Sigma_{11}^{-1}\Sigma_{12}\Sigma_{22}^{-1/2}$, respectively.

In a similar fashion, the second canonical correlation, $\lambda_2$, is the largest possible correlation between $\boldsymbol{\alpha}'\boldsymbol{x}_1$ and $\boldsymbol{\beta}'\boldsymbol{x}_2$ such that $\boldsymbol{\alpha}$ is orthogonal to $\boldsymbol{\alpha}_1$ (that is, $\boldsymbol{\alpha}'\boldsymbol{\alpha}_1 = 0$), and $\boldsymbol{\beta}$ is orthogonal to $\boldsymbol{\beta}_1$ $(\boldsymbol{\beta}'\boldsymbol{\beta}_1 = 0)$ . If we call the solutions $u_2 = \boldsymbol{\alpha}_2'\boldsymbol{x}_1$ and $v_2 = \boldsymbol{\beta}_2'\boldsymbol{x}_2$, then $\text{corr}(u_1, u_2) = 0 = \text{corr}(v_1, v_2)$, $\text{corr}(u_i, v_j) = 0$ for $i \ne j$, and by design, $\lambda_1^2 \ge \lambda_2^2$. Also, $\lambda_2^2$ is the second largest eigenvalue of $\Sigma_{11}^{-1}\Sigma_{12}\Sigma_{22}^{-1}\Sigma_{21}$ and $\boldsymbol{\alpha}_2$ and $\boldsymbol{\beta}_2$ are taken proportional to the second eigenvectors of $\Sigma_{11}^{-1/2}\Sigma_{12}\Sigma_{22}^{-1}\Sigma_{21}\Sigma_{11}^{-1/2}$ and $\Sigma_{22}^{-1/2}\Sigma_{21}\Sigma_{11}^{-1}\Sigma_{12}\Sigma_{22}^{-1/2}$, respectively. Continuing this way, we obtain the squared canonical correlations $1 \ge \lambda_1^2 \ge \lambda_2^2 \ge \cdots \ge \lambda_{k_1}^2 \ge 0$ as the ordered eigenvalues of $\Sigma_{11}^{-1}\Sigma_{12}\Sigma_{22}^{-1}\Sigma_{21}$. The canonical correlations, $\lambda_j$, are typically taken to be nonnegative. See, for example, Johnson and Wichern (1992, Chapter 10) for details.

Brillinger (1981, Chapter 10) discusses a time series extension of canonical correlation analysis. Here, we suppose we have stationary, mean-zero, $k_1 \times 1$ time series $\boldsymbol{x}_{t1}$ and $k_2 \times 1$ time series $\boldsymbol{x}_{t2}$, with respective nonsingular spectral density matrices, $f_{11}(\nu)$ and $f_{22}(\nu)$. The cross-spectral matrix between $\boldsymbol{x}_{t1}$ and $\boldsymbol{x}_{t2}$ is the $k_1 \times k_2$ matrix containing the cross-spectra between the components of $\boldsymbol{x}_{t1}$ and $\boldsymbol{x}_{t2}$. We will denote this matrix by $f_{12}(\nu)$ and note $f_{21}(\nu) = f_{12}^*(\nu)$.

In analogy to the classical case, we suppose we want to find, at a specific frequency $\nu$, the complex linear combinations, $u_t(\nu) = \boldsymbol{\alpha}^*\boldsymbol{x}_{t1}$, and $v_t(\nu) = \boldsymbol{\beta}^*\boldsymbol{x}_{t1}$, where $\boldsymbol{\alpha}$ and $\boldsymbol{\beta}$ are $k_1 \times 1$ and $k_2 \times 1$ complex vectors, respectively, such that the squared coherency $\rho_{uv}^2(\nu)$ between $u_t(\nu)$ and $v_t(\nu)$ is maximum. Noting the spectral density of $u_t$ at $\nu$ is $f_{uu}(\nu) = \boldsymbol{\alpha}^* f_{11}(\nu)\boldsymbol{\alpha}$, the spectral density of $v_t(\nu)$ at $\nu$ is $f_{vv}(\nu) = \boldsymbol{\beta}^* f_{11}(\nu)\boldsymbol{\beta}$, and the cross-spectrum between

$u_t(\nu)$ and $v_t(\nu)$ is $f_{uv}(\nu) = \boldsymbol{\alpha}^* f_{12}(\nu)\boldsymbol{\beta}$, we have

$$\rho_{uv}^2(\nu) = \frac{|f_{uv}(\nu)|^2}{f_{uu}(\nu)\ f_{vv}(\nu)} = \frac{|\boldsymbol{\alpha}^* f_{12}(\nu)\boldsymbol{\beta}|^2}{[\boldsymbol{\alpha}^* f_{11}(\nu)\boldsymbol{\alpha}]\ [\boldsymbol{\beta}^* f_{22}(\nu)\boldsymbol{\beta}]}. \tag{5.154}$$

Calling the solutions $\boldsymbol{\alpha} = \boldsymbol{\alpha}_1(\nu)$ and $\boldsymbol{\beta} = \boldsymbol{\beta}_1(\nu)$, we choose $\boldsymbol{\alpha}_1(\nu)$ to be proportional to the first eigenvector of $f_{11}^{-1/2}(\nu) f_{12}(\nu) f_{22}^{-1}(\nu) f_{21}(\nu) f_{11}^{-1/2}(\nu)$ and choose $\boldsymbol{\beta}_1(\nu)$ to be proportional to the first eigenvector of $f_{22}^{-1/2}(\nu) f_{21}(\nu)$ $f_{11}^{-1}(\nu) f_{12}(\nu) f_{22}^{-1/2}(\nu)$. The maximum squared coherency at $\nu$ is the largest eigenvalue, $\lambda_1^2(\nu)$, of $f_{11}^{-1}(\nu) f_{12}(\nu) f_{22}^{-1}(\nu) f_{21}(\nu)$. Typically, $\boldsymbol{\alpha}_1(\nu)$ and $\boldsymbol{\beta}_1(\nu)$ are subject to the constraints

$$\boldsymbol{\alpha}_1(\nu)^* f_{11}(\nu)\boldsymbol{\alpha}_1(\nu) = 1 \quad \text{and} \quad \boldsymbol{\beta}_1(\nu)^* f_{22}(\nu)\boldsymbol{\beta}_1(\nu) = 1,$$

respectively. In this case,

$$\max \rho_{uv}^2(\nu) = |\boldsymbol{\alpha}_1^*(\nu) f_{12}(\nu)\boldsymbol{\beta}_1(\nu)|^2 = \lambda_1^2(\nu). \tag{5.155}$$

The other canonical series are selected in an obvious fashion by analogy to the classical case.

As in principal components, another view of canonical analysis exists, and this is the approach taken in Brillinger (1981, Chapter 10). Here, consider $k_i \times 1$ linear filters $\{\boldsymbol{b}_{ti}\}$ such that $\sum_t |\boldsymbol{b}_{ti}| < \infty$, $i = 1, 2$. The real-valued univariate series

$$u_t = \sum_{j=-\infty}^{\infty} \boldsymbol{b}_{t-j,1}^* \boldsymbol{x}_{j1} \quad \text{and} \quad v_t = \sum_{j=-\infty}^{\infty} \boldsymbol{b}_{t-j,2}^* \boldsymbol{x}_{j2},$$

having maximum squared coherency, $\rho_{uv}^2(\nu)$, at each $\nu$, and subject to the constraints $\boldsymbol{b}_i^*(\nu) f_{ii}(\nu)\boldsymbol{b}_i(\nu) = 1$, for $i = 1, 2$, where $\boldsymbol{b}_i(\nu)$ is the transform of $\{\boldsymbol{b}_{ti}\}$, are given by finding the largest scalar $\lambda(\nu)$ such that

$$f_{11}(\nu)^{-1/2} f_{12}(\nu) f_{22}(\nu)^{-1} f_{21}(\nu) f_{11}(\nu)^{-1/2}\boldsymbol{\alpha}(\nu) = \lambda^2(\nu)\boldsymbol{\alpha}(\nu) \tag{5.156}$$

and

$$f_{22}(\nu)^{-1/2} f_{21}(\nu) f_{11}(\nu)^{-1} f_{12}(\nu) f_{22}(\nu)^{-1/2}\boldsymbol{\beta}(\nu) = \lambda^2(\nu)\boldsymbol{\beta}(\nu). \tag{5.157}$$

The maximum squared coherency achieved between $u_t$ and $v_t$ is $\lambda^2(\nu)$, and $\boldsymbol{b}_1(\nu)$ and $\boldsymbol{b}_2(\nu)$ are taken proportional to first eigenvectors of $f_{11}^{-1/2}(\nu) f_{12}(\nu)$ $f_{22}^{-1}(\nu) f_{21}(\nu) f_{11}^{-1/2}(\nu)$ and of $f_{22}^{-1/2}(\nu) f_{21}(\nu)$ $f_{11}^{-1}(\nu) f_{12}(\nu) f_{22}^{-1/2}(\nu)$, respectively. The required filters can be obtained by inverting $\boldsymbol{b}_1(\nu)$ and $\boldsymbol{b}_2(\nu)$ using a relationship such as (5.149). Again, the other canonical variate series are obtained in an obvious way, and estimation proceeds by replacing the spectra $f_{ij}(\nu)$ by their respective estimates $\widehat{f}_{ij}(\nu)$, for $i, j = 1, 2$. An example of canonical variates will be given in Section 5.9, Example 5.21, where we discuss matching sequences. Also, see Problem 5.16.

FACTOR ANALYSIS

Classical factor analysis is similar to classical principal component analysis. Suppose $\boldsymbol{x}$ is a mean-zero, $p\times 1$, random vector with variance–covariance matrix $\Sigma_x$. The factor model proposes that $\boldsymbol{x}$ is dependent on a few unobserved common factors, $z_1, ..., z_q$, plus error. In this model, one hopes that $q$ will be much smaller than $p$. The ***factor model*** is given by

$$\boldsymbol{x} = \mathcal{B}\boldsymbol{z} + \boldsymbol{\epsilon}, \tag{5.158}$$

where $\mathcal{B}$ is a $p \times q$ matrix of ***factor loadings***, $\boldsymbol{z} = (z_1, ..., z_q)'$ is a random $q \times 1$ vector of ***factors*** such that $E(\boldsymbol{z}) = \boldsymbol{0}$ and $E(\boldsymbol{z}\boldsymbol{z}') = I_q$, the $q \times q$ identity matrix. The $p \times 1$ unobserved error vector $\boldsymbol{\epsilon}$ is assumed to be independent of the factors, with zero mean and diagonal variance–covariance matrix $D = \text{diag}\{\delta_1^2, ..., \delta_p^2\}$. Note, (5.158) differs from the multivariate regression model, (4.2), because the factors, $\boldsymbol{z}$, are unobserved. Equivalently, the factor model, (5.158), can be written in terms of the covariance structure of $\boldsymbol{x}$,

$$\Sigma_x = \mathcal{B}\mathcal{B}' + D; \tag{5.159}$$

that is, the variance–covariance matrix of $\boldsymbol{x}$ is the sum of a symmetric, nonnegative-definite rank $q \le p$ matrix and a nonnegative-definite diagonal matrix. If $q = p$, then $\Sigma_x$ can be reproduced exactly as $\mathcal{B}\mathcal{B}'$, using the fact that $\Sigma_x = \lambda_1 \boldsymbol{e}_1 \boldsymbol{e}_1' + \cdots + \lambda_p \boldsymbol{e}_p \boldsymbol{e}_p'$, where $(\lambda_i, \boldsymbol{e}_i)$ are the eigenvalue–eigenvector pairs of $\Sigma_x$. As previously indicated, however, we hope $q$ will be much smaller than $p$. Unfortunately, most covariance matrices cannot be factored as (5.159) when $q$ is much smaller than $p$.

To motivate factor analysis, suppose the components of $\boldsymbol{x}$ can be grouped into meaningful groups. Within each group, the components are highly correlated, but the correlation between variables that are not in the same group is small. A group is supposedly formed by a single construct, represented as an unobservable factor, responsible for the high correlations within a group. For example, a person competing in a decathlon performs $p = 10$ athletic events, and we may represent the outcome of the decathlon as a $10 \times 1$ vector of scores. The events in a decathlon involve running, jumping, or throwing, and it is conceivable the $10 \times 1$ vector of scores might be able to be factored into $q = 4$ factors, (1) arm strength, (2) leg strength, (3) running speed, and (4) running endurance. The model (5.158) specifies that $\text{cov}(\boldsymbol{x}, \boldsymbol{z}) = \mathcal{B}$, or $\text{cov}(x_i, z_j) = b_{ij}$ where $b_{ij}$ is the $ij$-th component of the ***factor loading matrix*** $\mathcal{B}$, for $i = 1, ..., p$ and $j = 1, ..., q$. Thus, the elements of $\mathcal{B}$ are used to identify which hypothetical factors the components of $\boldsymbol{x}$ belong to, or load on.

At this point, some ambiguity is still associated with the factor model. Let $Q$ be a $q \times q$ orthogonal matrix; that is $Q'Q = QQ' = I_q$. Let $\mathcal{B}_* = \mathcal{B}Q$ and $\boldsymbol{z}_* = Q'\boldsymbol{z}$ so (5.158) can be written as

$$\boldsymbol{x} = \mathcal{B}\boldsymbol{z} + \boldsymbol{\epsilon} = \mathcal{B}QQ'\boldsymbol{z} + \boldsymbol{\epsilon} = \mathcal{B}_*\boldsymbol{z}_* + \boldsymbol{\epsilon}. \tag{5.160}$$

The model in terms of $\mathcal{B}_*$ and $z_*$ fulfills all of the factor model requirements, for example, $\text{cov}(z_*) = Q'\text{cov}(z)Q = QQ' = I_q$, so

$$\Sigma_x = \mathcal{B}_*\text{cov}(z_*)\mathcal{B}_*' + D = \mathcal{B}QQ'\mathcal{B}' + D = \mathcal{B}\mathcal{B}' + D. \tag{5.161}$$

Hence, on the basis of observations on $x$, we cannot distinguish between the loadings $\mathcal{B}$ and the rotated loadings $\mathcal{B}_* = \mathcal{B}Q$. Typically, $Q$ is chosen so the matrix $\mathcal{B}$ is easy to interpret, and this is the basis of what is called ***factor rotation***.

Given a sample $x_1, ..., x_n$, a number of methods are used to estimate the parameters of the factor model, and we discuss two of them here. The first method is the ***principal component method***. Let $S_x$ denote the sample variance–covariance matrix, and let $(\widehat{\lambda}_i, \widehat{e}_i)$ be the eigenvalue–eigenvector pairs of $S_x$. The $p \times q$ matrix of estimated factor loadings is found by setting

$$\widehat{\mathcal{B}} = \left[\widehat{\lambda}_1^{1/2}\, \widehat{e}_1 \,\middle|\, \widehat{\lambda}_2^{1/2}\, \widehat{e}_2 \,\middle|\, \cdots \,\middle|\, \widehat{\lambda}_q^{1/2}\, \widehat{e}_q\right]. \tag{5.162}$$

The argument here is that if $q$ factors exist, then

$$S_x \approx \widehat{\lambda}_1 \widehat{e}_1 \widehat{e}_1' + \cdots + \widehat{\lambda}_q \widehat{e}_q \widehat{e}_q' = \widehat{\mathcal{B}}\widehat{\mathcal{B}}', \tag{5.163}$$

because the remaining eigenvalues, $\widehat{\lambda}_{q+1}, ..., \widehat{\lambda}_p$, will be negligible. The estimated diagonal matrix of error variances is then obtained by setting $\widehat{D} = \text{diag}\{\widehat{\delta}_1^2, ..., \widehat{\delta}_p^2\}$, where $\widehat{\delta}_j^2$ is the $j$-th diagonal element of $S_x - \widehat{\mathcal{B}}\widehat{\mathcal{B}}'$.

The second method, which can give answers that are considerably different from the principal component method is maximum likelihood. Upon further assumption that in (5.158), $z$ and $\epsilon$ are multivariate normal, the log likelihood of $\mathcal{B}$ and $D$ ignoring a constant is

$$-2\ln L(\mathcal{B}, D) = n \ln |\Sigma_x| + \sum_{j=1}^{n} x_j' \Sigma_x^{-1} x_j. \tag{5.164}$$

The likelihood depends on $\mathcal{B}$ and $D$ through (5.159), $\Sigma_x = \mathcal{B}\mathcal{B}' + D$. As discussed in (5.160)-(5.161), the likelihood is not well defined because $\mathcal{B}$ can be rotated. Typically, restricting $\mathcal{B}D^{-1}\mathcal{B}'$ to be a diagonal matrix is a computationally convenient uniqueness condition. The actual maximization of the likelihood is accomplished using numerical methods.

One obvious method of performing maximum likelihood for the Gaussian factor model is the EM algorithm. For example, suppose the factor vector $z$ is known. Then, the factor model is simply the multivariate regression model given by (4.2). Following (4.3) and (4.4), write $X' = [x_1, x_2, ..., x_n]$ and $Z' = [z_1, z_2, ..., z_n]$, and note that $X$ is $n \times p$ and $Z$ is $n \times q$. Then, the MLE of $\mathcal{B}$ is

$$\widehat{\mathcal{B}} = X'Z(Z'Z)^{-1} = \left(n^{-1}\sum_{j=1}^{n} x_j z_j'\right)\left(n^{-1}\sum_{j=1}^{n} z_j z_j'\right)^{-1} \stackrel{\text{def}}{=} C_{xz}C_{zz}^{-1}, \tag{5.165}$$

and the MLE of $D$ is

$$\widehat{D} = \mathrm{Diag}\left\{ n^{-1} \sum_{j=1}^{n} \left(\boldsymbol{x}_j - \widehat{\mathcal{B}}\boldsymbol{z}_j\right)\left(\boldsymbol{x}_j - \widehat{\mathcal{B}}\boldsymbol{z}_j\right)' \right\}; \tag{5.166}$$

that is, only the diagonal elements of the right-hand-side of (5.166) are used. The bracketed quantity in (5.166) reduces to

$$C_{xx} - C_{xz} C_{zz}^{-1} C_{xz}', \tag{5.167}$$

where $C_{xx} = n^{-1} \sum_{j=1}^{n} \boldsymbol{x}_j \boldsymbol{x}_j'$.

Based on the derivation of the EM algorithm for the state-space model, (4.66)-(4.75), we conclude that, to employ the EM algorithm here, given the current parameter estimates, in $C_{xz}$, we replace $\boldsymbol{x}_j \boldsymbol{z}_j'$ by $\boldsymbol{x}_j \widetilde{\boldsymbol{z}}_j'$, where $\widetilde{\boldsymbol{z}}_j = E(\boldsymbol{z}_j \mid \boldsymbol{x}_j)$, and in $C_{zz}$, we replace $\boldsymbol{z}_j \boldsymbol{z}_j'$ by $P_z + \widetilde{\boldsymbol{z}}_j \widetilde{\boldsymbol{z}}_j'$, where $P_z = \mathrm{var}(\boldsymbol{z}_j \mid \boldsymbol{x}_j)$. Using the fact that the $(p+q) \times 1$ vector $(\boldsymbol{x}_j', \boldsymbol{z}_j')'$ is multivariate normal with mean-zero, and variance–covariance matrix given by

$$\begin{pmatrix} \mathcal{B}\mathcal{B}' + D & \mathcal{B} \\ \mathcal{B}' & I_q \end{pmatrix}, \tag{5.168}$$

we have

$$\widetilde{\boldsymbol{z}}_j \equiv E(\boldsymbol{z}_j \mid \boldsymbol{x}_j) = \mathcal{B}'(\mathcal{B}'\mathcal{B} + D)^{-1} \boldsymbol{x}_j \tag{5.169}$$

and

$$P_z \equiv \mathrm{var}(\boldsymbol{z}_j \mid \boldsymbol{x}_j) = I_q - \mathcal{B}'(\mathcal{B}'\mathcal{B} + D)^{-1}\mathcal{B}. \tag{5.170}$$

For time series, suppose $\boldsymbol{x}_t$ is a stationary $p \times 1$ process with $p \times p$ spectral matrix $f_x(\nu)$. Analogous to the classical model displayed in (5.159), we may postulate that at a given frequency of interest, $\nu$, the spectral matrix of $\boldsymbol{x}_t$ satisfies

$$f_x(\nu) = \mathcal{B}(\nu)\mathcal{B}(\nu)^* + D(\nu), \tag{5.171}$$

where $\mathcal{B}(\nu)$ is a complex-valued $p \times q$ matrix with $\mathrm{rank}\big(\mathcal{B}(\nu)\big) = q \le p$ and $D(\nu)$ is a real, nonnegative-definite, diagonal matrix. Typically, we expect $q$ will be much smaller than $p$.

As an example of a model that gives rise to (5.171), let $\boldsymbol{x}_t = (x_{t1}, ..., x_{tp})'$, and suppose

$$x_{tj} = c_j s_{t-\tau_j} + \epsilon_{tj}, \quad j = 1, ..., p, \tag{5.172}$$

where $c_j \ge 0$ are individual amplitudes and $s_t$ is a common unobserved signal (factor) with spectral density $f_s(\nu)$. The values $\tau_j$ are the individual phase shifts. Assume $s_t$ is independent of $\boldsymbol{\epsilon}_t = (\epsilon_{t1}, ..., \epsilon_{tp})'$ and the spectral matrix of $\boldsymbol{\epsilon}_t$, $D_\epsilon(\nu)$, is diagonal. The DFT of $x_{tj}$ is given by

$$X_j(\nu) = n^{-1/2} \sum_{t=1}^{n} x_{tj} \exp(-2\pi i t \nu)$$

and, in terms of the model (5.172),

$$X_j(\nu) = a_j(\nu)X_s(\nu) + X_{\epsilon_j}(\nu), \tag{5.173}$$

where $a_j(\nu) = c_j \exp(-2\pi i \tau_j \nu)$, and $X_s(\nu)$ and $X_{\epsilon_j}(\nu)$ are the respective DFTs of the signal $s_t$ and the noise $\epsilon_{tj}$. Stacking the individual elements of (5.173), we obtain a complex version of the classical factor model with one factor,

$$\begin{pmatrix} X_1(\nu) \\ \vdots \\ X_p(\nu) \end{pmatrix} = \begin{pmatrix} a_1(\nu) \\ \vdots \\ a_p(\nu) \end{pmatrix} X_s(\nu) + \begin{pmatrix} X_{\epsilon_1}(\nu) \\ \vdots \\ X_{\epsilon_p}(\nu) \end{pmatrix},$$

or more succinctly,

$$\boldsymbol{X}(\nu) = \boldsymbol{a}(\nu)X_s(\nu) + \boldsymbol{X}_\epsilon(\nu). \tag{5.174}$$

From (5.174), we can identify the spectral components of the model; that is,

$$f_x(\nu) = \boldsymbol{b}(\nu)\boldsymbol{b}(\nu)^* + D_\epsilon(\nu), \tag{5.175}$$

where $\boldsymbol{b}(\nu)$ is a $p \times 1$ complex-valued vector such that $\boldsymbol{b}(\nu)\boldsymbol{b}(\nu)^* = \boldsymbol{a}(\nu)f_s(\nu)\boldsymbol{a}(\nu)^*$. Model (5.175) could be considered the one-factor model for time series. This model can be extended to more than one factor by adding other independent signals into the original model (5.172). More details regarding this and related models can be found in Stoffer (1999).

**Example 5.15 Single Factor Analysis of the fMRI Data**

The fMRI data analyzed in Example 5.14 is well suited for a single factor analysis using the model (5.172), or, equivalently, the complex-valued, single factor model (5.174). In terms of (5.172), we can think of the signal $s_t$ as representing the brush stimulus signal. As before, the frequency of interest is $\nu = 4/128$, which corresponds to a period of 32 time points, or 64 seconds.

A simple way to estimate the components $\boldsymbol{b}(\nu)$ and $D_\epsilon(\nu)$, as specified in (5.175), is to use the principal components method. Let $\widehat{f}_x(\nu)$ denote the estimate of the spectral density of $\boldsymbol{x}_t = (x_{t1}, ..., x_{t8})'$ obtained in Example 5.14. Then, analogous to (5.162) and (5.163), we set

$$\widehat{\boldsymbol{b}}(\nu) = \sqrt{\widehat{\lambda}_1(\nu)}\, \widehat{\boldsymbol{e}}_1(\nu),$$

where $\left(\widehat{\lambda}_1(\nu), \widehat{\boldsymbol{e}}_1(\nu)\right)$ is the first eigenvalue–eigenvector pair of $\widehat{f}_x(\nu)$. The diagonal elements of $\widehat{D}_\epsilon(\nu)$ are obtained from the diagonal elements of $\widehat{f}_x(\nu) - \widehat{\boldsymbol{b}}(\nu)\widehat{\boldsymbol{b}}(\nu)^*$. The appropriateness of the model can be assessed by checking the elements of the residual matrix, $\widehat{f}_x(\nu) - [\widehat{\boldsymbol{b}}(\nu)\widehat{\boldsymbol{b}}(\nu)^* + \widehat{D}_\epsilon(\nu)]$, are negligible in magnitude.

Concentrating on the stimulus frequency, recall $\widehat{\lambda}_1(4/128) = 0.339$. The magnitudes of $\widehat{\boldsymbol{e}}_1(4/128)$ are displayed in Table 5.8, indicating all locations load on the stimulus factor except for location 7, and location 6 could be considered borderline. The diagonal elements of $\widehat{f}_x(\nu) - \widehat{\boldsymbol{b}}(\nu)\widehat{\boldsymbol{b}}(\nu)^*$ yield

$$\widehat{D}_\epsilon(4/128) = 0.001 \times \text{diag}\{0.27, 1.06, 0.45, 1.26, 1.64, 4.22, 4.38, 1.08\}.$$

The magnitudes of the elements of residual matrix at $\nu = 4/128$ are

$$0.001 \times \begin{pmatrix} 0.00 & 0.19 & 0.14 & 0.19 & 0.49 & 0.49 & 0.65 & 0.46 \\ 0.19 & 0.00 & 0.49 & 0.86 & 0.71 & 1.11 & 1.80 & 0.58 \\ 0.14 & 0.49 & 0.00 & 0.62 & 0.67 & 0.65 & 0.39 & 0.22 \\ 0.19 & 0.86 & 0.62 & 0.00 & 1.02 & 1.33 & 1.16 & 0.14 \\ 0.49 & 0.71 & 0.67 & 1.02 & 0.00 & 0.85 & 1.11 & 0.57 \\ 0.49 & 1.11 & 0.65 & 1.33 & 0.85 & 0.00 & 1.81 & 1.36 \\ 0.65 & 1.80 & 0.39 & 1.16 & 1.11 & 1.81 & 0.00 & 1.57 \\ 0.46 & 0.58 & 0.22 & 0.14 & 0.57 & 1.36 & 1.57 & 0.00 \end{pmatrix},$$

indicating the model fit is good.

A number of authors have considered factor analysis in the spectral domain, for example Priestley et al (1974), Priestley & Subba Rao (1975), Geweke (1977) and Geweke and Singleton (1981), to mention a few. An obvious extension of simple model (5.172) is the factor model

$$\boldsymbol{x}_t = \sum_{j=-\infty}^{\infty} \Lambda_j \boldsymbol{s}_{t-j} + \boldsymbol{\epsilon}_t, \tag{5.176}$$

where $\{\Lambda_j\}$ is a real-valued $p \times q$ filter, $\boldsymbol{s}_t$ is a $q \times 1$ stationary, unobserved signal, with independent components, and $\boldsymbol{\epsilon}_t$ is white noise. We assume the signal and noise process are independent, $\boldsymbol{s}_t$ has $q \times q$ real, diagonal spectral matrix $f_s(\nu) = \text{diag}\{f_{s1}(\nu), ..., f_{sq}(\nu)\}$, and $\boldsymbol{\epsilon}_t$ has a real, diagonal, $p \times p$ spectral matrix given by $D_\epsilon(\nu) = \text{diag}\{f_{\epsilon 1}(\nu), ..., f_{\epsilon p}(\nu)\}$. If, in addition, $\sum ||\Lambda_j|| < \infty$, the spectral matrix of $\boldsymbol{x}_t$ can be written as

$$f_x(\nu) = \Lambda(\nu) f_s(\nu) \Lambda(\nu)^* + D_\epsilon(\nu) = \mathcal{B}(\nu)\mathcal{B}(\nu)^* + D_\epsilon(\nu), \tag{5.177}$$

where

$$\Lambda(\nu) = \sum_{t=-\infty}^{\infty} \Lambda_t \exp(-2\pi i t \nu) \tag{5.178}$$

and $\mathcal{B}(\nu) = \Lambda(\nu) f_s^{1/2}(\nu)$. Thus, by (5.177), the model (5.176) is seen to satisfy the basic requirement of the spectral domain factor analysis model; that is, the $p \times p$ spectral density matrix of the process of interest, $f_x(\nu)$, is the sum of a rank $q \leq p$ matrix, $\mathcal{B}(\nu)\mathcal{B}(\nu)^*$, and a real, diagonal matrix, $D_\epsilon(\nu)$. For the purpose of identifiability we set $f_s(\nu) = I_q$ for all $\nu$; in which case, $\mathcal{B}(\nu) = \Lambda(\nu)$. As in the classical case [see (5.161)], the model is specified only up to rotations; for details, see Bloomfield and Davis (1994).

Parameter estimation for the model (5.176), or equivalently (5.177), can be accomplished using the principal component method. Let $\widehat{f}_x(\nu)$ be an estimate of $f_x(\nu)$, and let $\big(\widehat{\lambda}_j(\nu), \widehat{\boldsymbol{e}}_j(\nu)\big)$, for $j = 1, ..., p$, be the eigenvalue–eigenvector pairs, in the usual order, of $\widehat{f}_x(\nu)$. Then, as in the classical case, the $p \times q$ matrix $\mathcal{B}$ is estimated by

$$\widehat{\mathcal{B}}(\nu) = \Big[\widehat{\lambda}_1(\nu)^{1/2}\, \widehat{\boldsymbol{e}}_1(\nu) \,\Big|\, \widehat{\lambda}_2(\nu)^{1/2}\, \widehat{\boldsymbol{e}}_2(\nu) \,\Big|\, \cdots \,\Big|\, \widehat{\lambda}_q(\nu)^{1/2}\, \widehat{\boldsymbol{e}}_q(\nu)\Big]. \qquad (5.179)$$

The estimated diagonal spectral density matrix of errors is then obtained by setting $\widehat{D}_\epsilon(\nu) = \text{diag}\{\widehat{f}_{\epsilon 1}(\nu), ..., \widehat{f}_{\epsilon p}(\nu)\}$, where $\widehat{f}_{\epsilon j}(\nu)$ is the $j$-th diagonal element of $\widehat{f}_x(\nu) - \widehat{\mathcal{B}}(\nu)\widehat{\mathcal{B}}(\nu)^*$.

Alternatively, we can estimate the parameters by approximate likelihood methods. As in (5.174), let $\boldsymbol{X}(\nu_j)$ denote the DFT of the data $\boldsymbol{x}_1, ..., \boldsymbol{x}_n$ at frequency $\nu_j = j/n$. Similarly, let $\boldsymbol{X}_s(\nu_j)$ and $\boldsymbol{X}_\epsilon(\nu_j)$ be the DFTs of the signal and of the noise processes, respectively. Then, under certain conditions (see Pawitan and Shumway, 1989), for $\ell = 0, \pm 1, ..., \pm(L-1)/2$,

$$\boldsymbol{X}(\nu_j + \ell/n) = \Lambda(\nu_j)\boldsymbol{X}_s(\nu_j + \ell/n) + \boldsymbol{X}_\epsilon(\nu_j + \ell/n) + o_{as}(n^{-\alpha}), \qquad (5.180)$$

where $\Lambda(\nu_j)$ is given by (5.178) and $o_{as}(n^{-\alpha}) \to 0$ almost surely for some $0 \le \alpha < 1/2$ as $n \to \infty$. In (5.180), the $\boldsymbol{X}(\nu_j + \ell/n)$ are the DFTs of the data at the $L$ odd frequencies $\{\nu_j + \ell/n;\ \ell = 0, \pm 1, ..., \pm(L-1)/2\}$ surrounding the central frequency of interest $\nu_j = j/n$.

Under appropriate conditions $\{\boldsymbol{X}(\nu_j + \ell/n);\ m = 0, \pm 1, ..., \pm(L-1)/2\}$ in (5.180) are approximately ($n \to \infty$) independent, complex Gaussian random vectors with variance–covariance matrix $f_x(\nu_j)$. The approximate likelihood is given by

$$\begin{aligned} &-2\ln L\big(\mathcal{B}(\nu_j), D_\epsilon(\nu_j)\big) \\ &\quad = n\ln\big|f_x(\nu_j)\big| + \sum_{\ell=-(L-1)/2}^{(L-1)/2} \boldsymbol{X}^*(\nu_j + \ell/n) f_x^{-1}(\nu_j)\boldsymbol{X}(\nu_j + \ell/n), \end{aligned} \qquad (5.181)$$

with the constraint $f_x(\nu_j) = \mathcal{B}(\nu_j)\mathcal{B}(\nu_j)^* + D_\epsilon(\nu_j)$. As in the classical case, we can use various numerical methods to maximize $L\big(\mathcal{B}(\nu_j), D_\epsilon(\nu_j)\big)$ at every frequency, $\nu_j$, of interest. For example, the EM algorithm discussed for the classical case, (5.165)-(5.170), can easily be extended to this case.

Assuming $f_s(\nu) = I_q$, the estimate of $\mathcal{B}(\nu_j)$ is also the estimate of $\Lambda(\nu_j)$. Calling this estimate $\widehat{\Lambda}(\nu_j)$, the time domain filter can be estimated by

$$\widehat{\Lambda}_t^M = M^{-1} \sum_{j=0}^{M-1} \widehat{\Lambda}(\nu_j) \exp(2\pi i j t/n), \qquad (5.182)$$

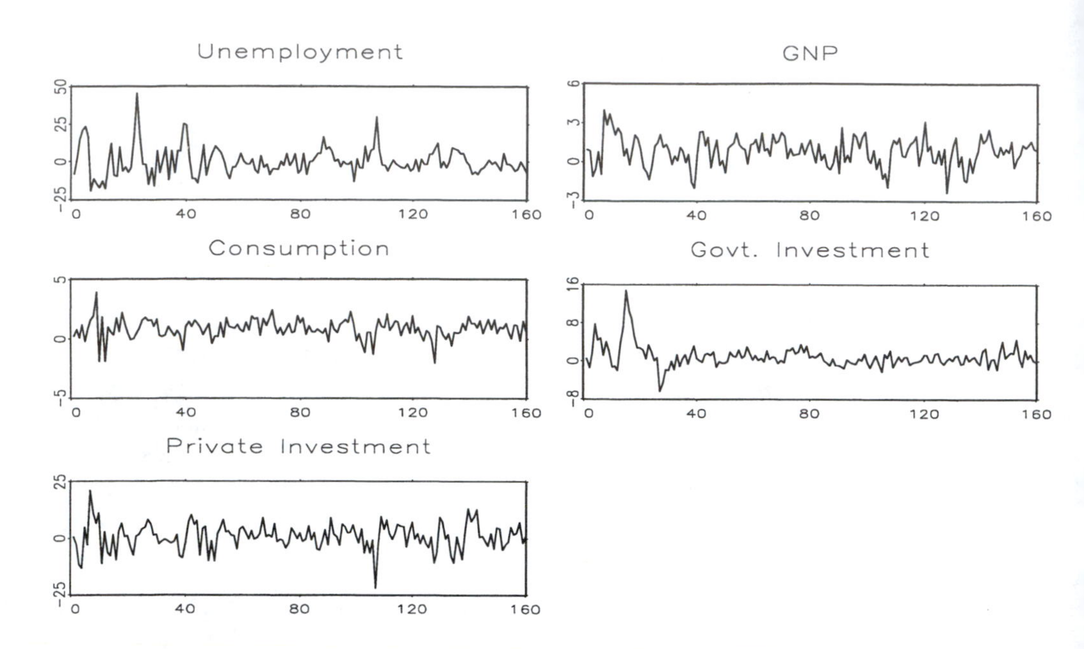


**Figure 5.16:** The seasonally adjusted, quarterly growth rate (as percentages) of five macroeconomic series, Unemployment, GNP, Consumption, Government Investment, and Private Investment in the U.S. between 1948 and 1988, $n = 160$ values.

for some $0 < M \leq n$, which is the discrete and finite version of the inversion formula given by

$$\Lambda_t = \int_{-1/2}^{1/2} \Lambda(\nu) \exp(2\pi i \nu t) d\nu. \tag{5.183}$$

Note that we have used this approximation earlier in Chapter 3, (3.109), for estimating the time response of a frequency response function defined over a finite number of frequencies. A bound for the mean-squared error of the approximation was given in Problem 3.21.

**Example 5.16 Government Spending, Private Investment, and Unemployment in the U.S.**

Figure 5.16 shows the seasonally adjusted, quarterly growth rate (as percentages) of five macroeconomic series, Unemployment, GNP, Consumption, Government Investment, and Private Investment in the U.S. between 1948 and 1988, $n = 160$ values. These data are analyzed in the

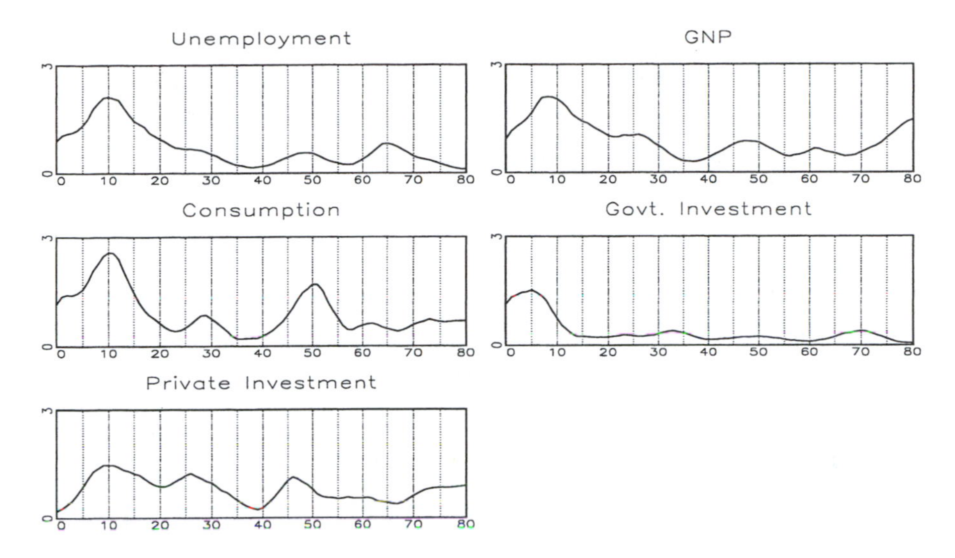


**Figure 5.17:** The individual estimated spectra (scaled by 1000) of each series show in Figure 5.16 in terms of the number of cycles in 160 quarters.

time domain by Young and Pedregal (1998) who were investigating how government spending and private capital investment influenced the rate of unemployment.

Spectral estimation was performed on the detrended, standardized, and tapered (using a cosine bell) growth rate values. Then, as described in (5.150), a set of $L = 11$ triangular weights, $\{h_0 = 6/36, h_{\pm1} = 5/36, h_{\pm2} = 4/36, h_{\pm3} = 3/36, h_{\pm4} = 2/36, h_{\pm5} = 1/36\}$, were used to smooth in $5 \times 5$ periodogram matrices. Figure 5.17 shows the individual estimated spectra (scaled by 1000) of each series in terms of the number of cycles. We focus on three interesting frequencies. First, we note the lack of spectral power near 40 cycles ($\nu = 40/160 = 1/4$; one cycle every four quarters, or one year), indicating the data have been seasonally adjusted. In addition, because of the seasonal adjustment, some spectral power appears near the seasonal frequency; this is a distortion apparently caused by the method of seasonally adjusting the data. Next, we note spectral power appears near 10 cycles ($\nu = 10/160 = 1/16$; one cycle every four years) in Unemployment, GNP, Consumption, and, to lesser degree, in Private Investment. Finally, spectral power appears near five cycles ($\nu = 5/160 = 1/32$; one cycle every 8 years) in Government Investment, and perhaps to lesser degrees in Unemployment, GNP, and Consumption.

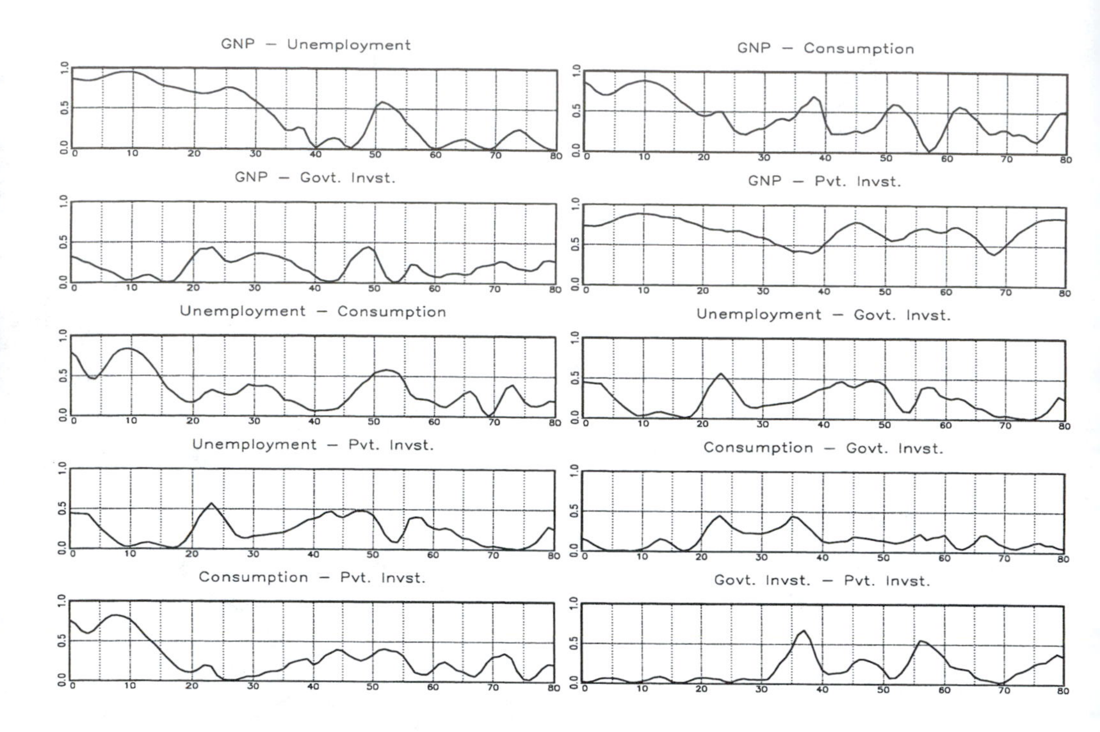


**Figure 5.18:** The squared coherencies between the various series displayed in Figure 5.16 in terms of the number of cycles in 160 quarters.

Figure 5.18 shows the coherences among various series. At the frequencies of interest ($\nu = 5/160$ and $10/160$), pairwise, GNP, Unemployment, Consumption, and Private Investment (except for Unemployment and Private Investment) are coherent. Government Investment is either not coherent or minimally coherent with the other series.

Figure 5.19 shows $\widehat{\lambda}_1(\nu)$ and $\widehat{\lambda}_2(\nu)$, the first and second eigenvalues of the estimated spectral matrix $\widehat{f}_x(\nu)$. These eigenvalues suggest the first factor is identified by the frequency of one cycle every four years, whereas the second factor is identified by the frequency of one cycle every eight years. The modulus of the corresponding eigenvectors at the frequencies of interest, $\widehat{\boldsymbol{e}}_1(10/160)$ and $\widehat{\boldsymbol{e}}_2(5/160)$, are shown in Table 5.9. These values confirm Unemployment, GNP, Consumption, and Private Investment load on the first factor, and Government Investment loads on the second factor. The remainder of the details involving the factor analysis of these data is left as an exercise.

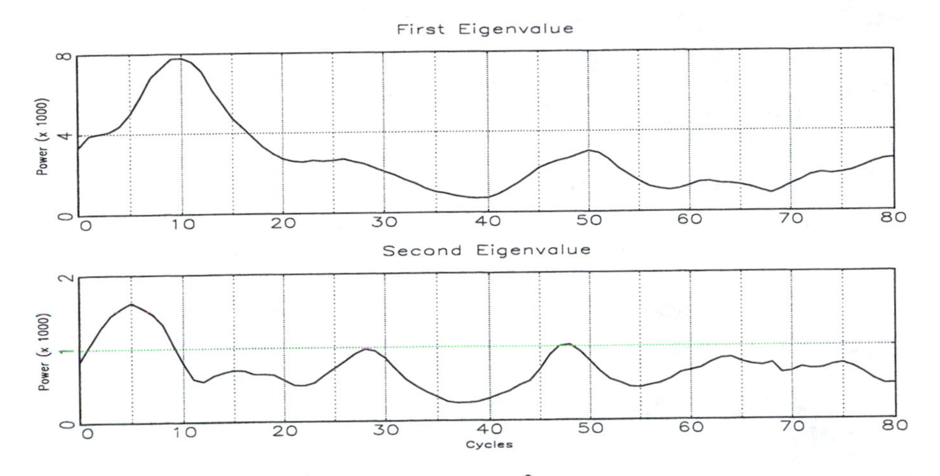


**Figure 5.19:** The first, $\widehat{\lambda}_1(\nu)$, and second, $\widehat{\lambda}_2(\nu)$, eigenvalues (scaled by 1000) of the estimated spectral matrix $\widehat{f}_x(\nu)$ in terms of the number of cycles in 160 quarters.

**Table 5.9:** Magnitudes of the Eigenvectors in Example 5.16

| Series | Unemp | GNP | Cons | G. Inv. | P. Inv. |
|---|---|---|---|---|---|
| $\mid \widehat{e}_1(\frac{10}{160}) \mid$ | 0.51 | 0.51 | 0.57 | 0.05 | 0.41 |
| $\mid \widehat{e}_2(\frac{5}{160}) \mid$ | 0.17 | 0.03 | 0.39 | 0.87 | 0.27 |

## 5.9 The Spectral Envelope

The concept of spectral envelope for the spectral analysis and ***scaling*** of categorical time series was first introduced in Stoffer et al (1993). Since then, the idea has been extended in various directions (not only restricted to categorical time series), and we will explore these problems as well. First, we give a brief introduction to the concept of scaling time series.

The spectral envelope was motivated by collaborations with researchers who collected categorical-valued time series with an interest in the cyclic behavior of the data. For example, Table 5.10 shows the per-minute sleep state of an infant taken from a study on the effects of prenatal exposure to alcohol. Details can be found in Stoffer et al (1988), but, briefly, an electroencephalographic

(EEG) sleep recording of approximately two hours is obtained on a full-term infant 24 to 36 hours after birth, and the recording is scored by a pediatric neurologist for sleep state. Sleep state is categorized, per minute, into one of six possible states: `qt`: quiet sleep - trace alternant, `qh`: quiet sleep - high voltage, `tr`: transitional sleep, `al`: active sleep - low voltage, `ah`: active sleep - high voltage, and `aw`: awake. This particular infant was never awake during the study.

It is not difficult to notice a pattern in the data if we concentrate on active vs. quiet sleep (that is, focus on the first letter). But, it would be difficult to try to assess patterns in a longer sequence, or if more categories were present, without some graphical aid. One simple method would be to *scale* the data, that is, *assign numerical values to the categories* and then draw a time plot of the scaled series. Because the states have an order, one obvious scaling is

$$1 = \texttt{qt} \quad 2 = \texttt{qh} \quad 3 = \texttt{tr} \quad 4 = \texttt{al} \quad 5 = \texttt{ah} \quad 6 = \texttt{aw}, \tag{5.184}$$

and Figure 5.20 shows the time plot using this scaling. Another interesting scaling might be to combine the quiet states and the active states:

$$1 = \texttt{qt} \quad 1 = \texttt{qh} \quad 2 = \texttt{tr} \quad 3 = \texttt{al} \quad 3 = \texttt{ah} \quad 4 = \texttt{aw}. \tag{5.185}$$

The time plot using (5.185) would be similar to Figure 5.20 as far as the cyclic (in and out of quiet sleep) behavior of this infant's sleep pattern. Figure 5.21 shows the periodogram of the sleep data using the scaling in (5.184). A large peak exists at the frequency corresponding to one cycle every 60 minutes. As we might imagine, the general appearance of the periodogram using the scaling (5.185) (not shown) is similar to Figure 5.20. Most of us would feel

**Table 5.10:** Infant EEG Sleep-States (per minute)
(read down and across)

| | | | | | | | |
|---|---|---|---|---|---|---|---|
| ah | qt | qt | al | tr | qt | al | ah |
| ah | qt | qt | ah | tr | qt | al | ah |
| ah | qt | tr | ah | tr | qt | al | ah |
| ah | qt | al | ah | qh | qt | al | ah |
| ah | qt | al | ah | qh | qt | al | ah |
| ah | tr | al | ah | qt | qt | al | ah |
| ah | qt | al | ah | qt | qt | al | ah |
| ah | qt | al | ah | qt | qt | al | ah |
| tr | qt | tr | tr | qt | qt | al | tr |
| ah | qt | ah | tr | qt | tr | al | |
| tr | qt | al | ah | qt | al | al | |
| ah | qt | al | ah | qt | al | al | |
| ah | qt | al | ah | qt | al | al | |
| qh | qt | al | ah | qt | al | ah | |

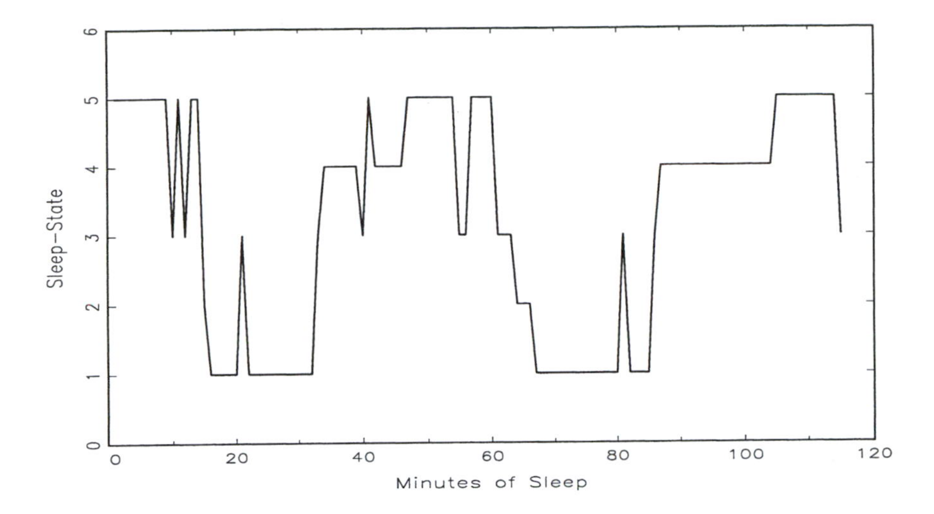


**Figure 5.20:** Time plot of the EEG sleep state data in Table 5.10 using the scaling in (5.184).

comfortable with this analysis even though we made an arbitrary and ad hoc choice about the particular scaling. It is evident from the data (without any scaling) that if the interest is in infant sleep cycling, this particular sleep study indicates an infant cycles between active and quiet sleep at a rate of about one cycle per hour.

The intuition used in the previous example is lost when we consider a long DNA sequence. Briefly, a DNA strand can be viewed as a long string of linked nucleotides. Each nucleotide is composed of a nitrogenous base, a five carbon sugar, and a phosphate group. There are four different bases, and they can be grouped by size; the pyrimidines, thymine (T) and cytosine (C), and the purines, adenine (A) and guanine (G). The nucleotides are linked together by a backbone of alternating sugar and phosphate groups with the $5'$ carbon of one sugar linked to the $3'$ carbon of the next, giving the string direction. DNA molecules occur naturally as a double helix composed of polynucleotide strands with the bases facing inwards. The two strands are complementary, so it is sufficient to represent a DNA molecule by a sequence of bases on a single strand. Thus, a strand of DNA can be represented as a sequence of letters, termed base pairs (bp), from the finite alphabet $\{\mathtt{A}, \mathtt{C}, \mathtt{G}, \mathtt{T}\}$. The order of the nucleotides contains the genetic information specific to the organism. Expression of information stored in these molecules is a complex multistage process. One important task is to translate the information stored in the protein-coding sequences (CDS) of the DNA. A common problem in analyzing long DNA sequence data is in identifying CDS dispersed throughout the sequence and separated by regions

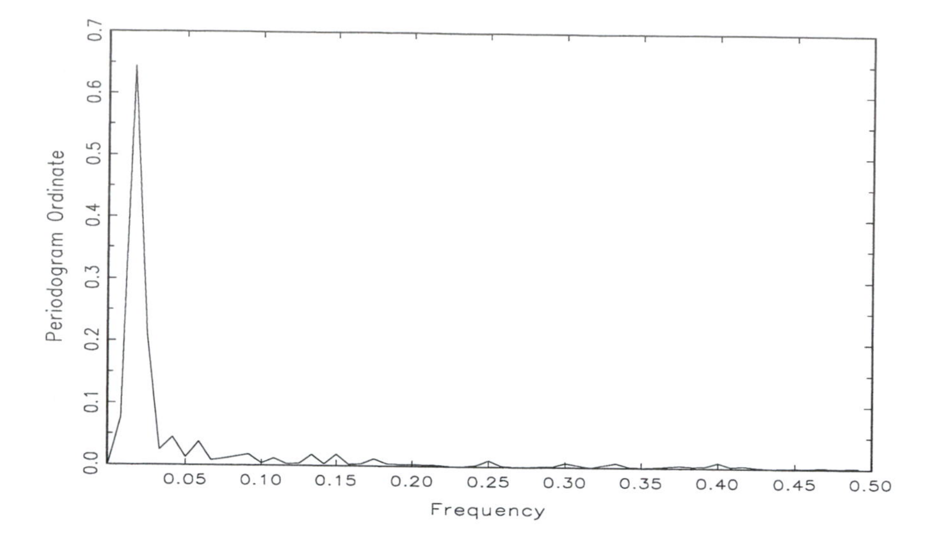


**Figure 5.21:** Periodogram of the EEG sleep state data in Figure 5.20 based on the scaling in (5.184). The peak corresponds to a frequency of approximately one cycle every 60 minutes.

of noncoding (which makes up most of the DNA). Table 5.11 shows part of the Epstein–Barr virus (EBV) DNA sequence. The entire EBV DNA sequence consists of approximately 172,000 bp.

We could try scaling according to the purine–pyrimidine alphabet, that is $\mathtt{A} = \mathtt{G} = 0$ and $\mathtt{C} = \mathtt{T} = 1$, but this is not necessarily of interest for every CDS of EBV. Numerous possible alphabets of interest exist. For example, we might focus on the strong–weak hydrogen-bonding alphabet $\mathtt{C} = \mathtt{G} = 0$ and $\mathtt{A} = \mathtt{T} = 1$. Although model calculations as well as experimental data strongly agree that some kind of periodic signal exists in certain DNA sequences, a large disagreement about the exact type of periodicity exists. In addition, a disagreement exists about which nucleotide alphabets are involved in the signals.

If we consider the naive approach of arbitrarily assigning numerical values (scales) to the categories and then proceeding with a spectral analysis, the result will depend on the particular assignment of numerical values. For example, consider the artificial sequence ACGTACGTACGT... . Then, setting $\mathtt{A} = \mathtt{G} = 0$ and $\mathtt{C} = \mathtt{T} = 1$ yields the numerical sequence 010101010101..., or one cycle every two base pairs. Another interesting scaling is $\mathtt{A} = 1, \mathtt{C} = 2, \mathtt{G} = 3$, and $\mathtt{T} = 4$, which results in the sequence 123412341234..., or one cycle every four bp. In this example, both scalings (that is, $\{\mathtt{A}, \mathtt{C}, \mathtt{G}, \mathtt{T}\} = \{0, 1, 0, 1\}$ and $\{\mathtt{A}, \mathtt{C}, \mathtt{G}, \mathtt{T}\} = \{1, 2, 3, 4\}$) of the nucleotides are interesting and bring out different

**Table 5.11:** Part of the Epstein-Barr Virus DNA Sequence (read across and down)

| AGAATTCGTC | TTGCTCTATT | CACCCTTACT | TTTCTTCTTG | CCCGTTCTCT | TTCTTAGTAT |
|---|---|---|---|---|---|
| GAATCCAGTA | TGCCTGCCTG | TAATTGTTGC | GCCCTACCTC | TTTTGGCTGG | CGGCTATTGC |
| CGCCTCGTGT | TTCACGGCCT | CAGTTAGTAC | CGTTGTGACC | GCCACCGGCT | TGGCCCTCTC |
| ACTTCTACTC | TTGGCAGCAG | TGGCCAGCTC | ATATGCCGCT | GCACAAAGGA | AACTGCTGAC |
| ACCGGTGACA | GTGCTTACTG | CGGTTGTCAC | TTGTGAGTAC | ACACGCACCA | TTTACAATGC |
| ATGATGTTCG | TGAGATTGAT | CTGTCTCTAA | CAGTTCACTT | CCTCTGCTTT | TCTCCTCAGT |
| CTTTGCAATT | TGCCTAACAT | GGAGGATTGA | GGACCCACCT | TTTAATTCTC | TTCTGTTTGC |
| ATTGCTGGCC | GCAGCTGGCG | GACTACAAGG | CATTTACGGT | TAGTGTGCCT | CTGTTATGAA |
| ATGCAGGTTT | GACTTCATAT | GTATGCCTTG | GCATGACGTC | AACTTTACTT | TTATTTCAGT |
| TCTGGTGATG | CTTGTGCTCC | TGATACTAGC | GTACAGAAGG | AGATGGCGCC | GTTTGACTGT |
| TTGTGGCGGC | ATCATGTTTT | TGGCATGTGT | ACTTGTCCTC | ATCGTCGACG | CTGTTTTGCA |
| GCTGAGTCCC | CTCCTTGGAG | CTGTAACTGT | GGTTTCCATG | ACGCTGCTGC | TACTGGCTTT |
| CGTCCTCTGG | CTCTCTTCGC | CAGGGGGCCT | AGGTACTCTT | GGTGCAGCCC | TTTTAACATT |
| GGCAGCAGGT | AAGCCACACG | TGTGACATTG | CTTGCCTTTT | TGCCACATGT | TTTCTGGACA |
| CAGGACTAAC | CATGCCATCT | CTGATTATAG | CTCTGGCACT | GCTAGCGTCA | CTGATTTTGG |
| GCACACTTAA | CTTGACTACA | ATGTTCCTTC | TCATGCTCCT | ATGGACACTT | GGTAAGTTTT |
| CCCTTCCTTT | AACTCATTAC | TTGTTCTTTT | GTAATCGCAG | CTCTAACTTG | GCATCTCTTT |
| TACAGTGGTT | CTCCTGATTT | GCTCTTCGTG | CTCTTCATGT | CCACTGAGCA | AGATCCTTCT |
| GGCACGACTG | TTCCTATATG | CTCTCGCACT | CTTGTTGCTA | GCCTCCGCGC | TAATCGCTGG |
| TGGCAGTATT | TTGCAAACAA | ACTTCAAGAG | TTTAAGCAGC | ACTGAATTTA | TACCCAGTGA |

properties of the sequence. Hence, we do not want to focus on only one scaling. Instead, the focus should be on finding all possible scalings that bring out all of the interesting features in the data. Rather than choose values arbitrarily, the spectral envelope approach selects scales that help emphasize any periodic feature that exists in a categorical time series of virtually any length in a quick and automated fashion. In addition, the technique can help in determining whether a sequence is merely a random assignment of categories.

### The Spectral Envelope for Categorical Time Series

As a general description, the spectral envelope is a frequency-based, principal components technique applied to a multivariate time series. First, we will focus on the basic concept and its use in the analysis of categorical time series. Technical details can be found in Stoffer et al. (1993).

Briefly, in establishing the spectral envelope for categorical time series, the basic question of how to efficiently discover periodic components in categorical time series was addressed. This, was accomplished via nonparametric spectral analysis as follows. Let $x_t$, $t = 0, \pm 1, \pm 2, \ldots$, be a categorical-valued time series with finite state-space $\mathcal{C} = \{c_1, c_2, \ldots, c_k\}$. Assume $x_t$ is stationary and $p_j = \Pr\{x_t = c_j\} > 0$ for $j = 1, 2, \ldots, k$. For $\boldsymbol{\beta} = (\beta_1, \beta_2, \ldots, \beta_k)' \in \mathbf{R}^k$, denote by $x_t(\boldsymbol{\beta})$ the real-valued stationary time series corresponding to the scaling that assigns the category $c_j$ the numerical value $\beta_j$, $j = 1, 2, \ldots, k$. The spectral density of $x_t(\boldsymbol{\beta})$ will be denoted by $f_x(\nu; \boldsymbol{\beta})$. The goal is to find scalings $\boldsymbol{\beta}$, so the spectral density is in some sense interesting, and to summarize the spectral information by what is called the spectral envelope.

In particular, $\boldsymbol{\beta}$ is chosen to maximize the power at each frequency, $\nu$, of interest, relative to the total power $\sigma^2(\boldsymbol{\beta}) = \text{var}\{x_t(\boldsymbol{\beta})\}$. That is, we chose $\boldsymbol{\beta}(\nu)$, at each $\nu$ of interest, so

$$\lambda(\nu) = \max_{\boldsymbol{\beta}} \left\{ \frac{f_x(\nu; \boldsymbol{\beta})}{\sigma^2(\boldsymbol{\beta})} \right\}, \tag{5.186}$$

over all $\boldsymbol{\beta}$ not proportional to $\mathbf{1}_k$, the $k \times 1$ vector of ones. Note, $\lambda(\nu)$ is not defined if $\boldsymbol{\beta} = a\mathbf{1}_k$ for $a \in \mathbf{R}$ because such a scaling corresponds to assigning each category the same value $a$; in this case, $f_x(\nu\,; \boldsymbol{\beta}) \equiv 0$ and $\sigma^2(\boldsymbol{\beta}) = 0$. The optimality criterion $\lambda(\nu)$ possesses the desirable property of being invariant under location and scale changes of $\boldsymbol{\beta}$.

As in most scaling problems for categorical data, it is useful to represent the categories in terms of the unit vectors $\boldsymbol{u}_1, \boldsymbol{u}_2, ..., \boldsymbol{u}_k$, where $\boldsymbol{u}_j$ represents the $k \times 1$ vector with a one in the $j$-th row, and zeros elsewhere. We then define a $k$-dimensional stationary time series $\boldsymbol{y}_t$ by $\boldsymbol{y}_t = \boldsymbol{u}_j$ when $x_t = c_j$. The time series $x_t(\boldsymbol{\beta})$ can be obtained from the $\boldsymbol{y}_t$ time series by the relationship $x_t(\boldsymbol{\beta}) = \boldsymbol{\beta}'\boldsymbol{y}_t$. Assume the vector process $\boldsymbol{y}_t$ has a continuous spectral density denoted by $f_y(\nu)$. For each $\nu$, $f_y(\nu)$ is, of course, a $k \times k$ complex-valued Hermitian matrix. The relationship $x_t(\boldsymbol{\beta}) = \boldsymbol{\beta}'\boldsymbol{y}_t$ implies $f_y(\nu; \boldsymbol{\beta}) = \boldsymbol{\beta}' f_y(\nu)\boldsymbol{\beta} = \boldsymbol{\beta}' f_y^{re}(\nu)\boldsymbol{\beta}$, where $f_y^{re}(\nu)$ denotes the real part[1] of $f_y(\nu)$. The imaginary part disappears from the expression because it is skew-symmetric, that is, $f_y^{im}(\nu)' = -f_y^{im}(\nu)$. The optimality criterion can thus be expressed as

$$\lambda(\nu) = \max_{\boldsymbol{\beta}} \left\{ \frac{\boldsymbol{\beta}' f_y^{re}(\nu)\boldsymbol{\beta}}{\boldsymbol{\beta}' V \boldsymbol{\beta}} \right\}, \tag{5.187}$$

where $V$ is the variance–covariance matrix of $\boldsymbol{y}_t$. The resulting scaling $\boldsymbol{\beta}(\nu)$ is called the optimal scaling.

The $\boldsymbol{y}_t$ process is a multivariate point process, and any particular component of $\boldsymbol{y}_t$ is the individual point process for the corresponding state (for example, the first component of $\boldsymbol{y}_t$ indicates whether the process is in state $c_1$ at time $t$). For any fixed $t$, $\boldsymbol{y}_t$ represents a single observation from a simple multinomial sampling scheme. It readily follows that $V = D - p\, p'$, where $p = (p_1, ..., p_k)'$, and $D$ is the $k \times k$ diagonal matrix $D = \text{diag}\{p_1, ..., p_k\}$. Because, by assumption, $p_j > 0$ for $j = 1, 2, ..., k$, it follows that $\text{rank}(V) = k - 1$ with the null space of $V$ being spanned by $\mathbf{1}_k$. For any $k \times (k-1)$ full rank matrix $Q$ whose columns are linearly independent of $\mathbf{1}_k$, $Q'VQ$ is a $(k-1) \times (k-1)$ positive-definite symmetric matrix.

With the matrix $Q$ as previously defined, define $\lambda(\nu)$ to be the largest eigenvalue of the determinantal equation

$$|Q' f_y^{re}(\nu) Q - \lambda Q' V Q| = 0,$$

[1]In this section, it is more convenient to write complex values in the form $z = z^{re} + iz^{im}$, which represents a change from previous notation, such as (5.5).

and let $\boldsymbol{b}(\nu) \in \mathbf{R}^{k-1}$ be any corresponding eigenvector, that is,

$$Q' f_y^{re}(\nu) Q \boldsymbol{b}(\nu) = \lambda(\nu) Q' V Q \boldsymbol{b}(\nu).$$

The eigenvalue $\lambda(\nu) \geq 0$ does not depend on the choice of $Q$. Although the eigenvector $\boldsymbol{b}(\nu)$ depends on the particular choice of $Q$, the equivalence class of scalings associated with $\boldsymbol{\beta}(\nu) = Q\boldsymbol{b}(\nu)$ does not depend on $Q$. A convenient choice of $Q$ is $Q = [I_{k-1} \mid \mathbf{0}\,]'$, where $I_{k-1}$ is the $(k-1) \times (k-1)$ identity matrix and $\mathbf{0}$ is the $(k-1) \times 1$ vector of zeros . For this choice, $Q' f_y^{re}(\nu) Q$ and $Q'VQ$ are the upper $(k-1) \times (k-1)$ blocks of $f_y^{re}(\nu)$ and $V$, respectively. This choice corresponds to setting the last component of $\boldsymbol{\beta}(\nu)$ to zero.

The value $\lambda(\nu)$ itself has a useful interpretation; specifically, $\lambda(\nu)d\nu$ represents the largest proportion of the total power that can be attributed to the frequencies $(\nu, \nu + d\nu)$ for any particular scaled process $x_t(\boldsymbol{\beta})$, with the maximum being achieved by the scaling $\boldsymbol{\beta}(\nu)$. Because of its central role, $\lambda(\nu)$ is defined to be the ***spectral envelope of a stationary categorical time series.***

The name spectral envelope is appropriate since $\lambda(\nu)$ envelopes the standardized spectrum of any scaled process. That is, given any $\boldsymbol{\beta}$ normalized so that $x_t(\boldsymbol{\beta})$ has total power one, $f_x(\nu\,;\,\boldsymbol{\beta}) \leq \lambda(\nu)$ with equality if and only if $\boldsymbol{\beta}$ is proportional to $\boldsymbol{\beta}(\nu)$.

Given observations $x_t$, for $t = 1, ..., n$, on a categorical time series, we form the multinomial point process $\boldsymbol{y}_t$, for $t = 1, ..., n$. Then, the theory for estimating the spectral density of a multivariate, real-valued time series can be applied to estimating $f_y(\nu)$, the $k \times k$ spectral density of $\boldsymbol{y}_t$. Given an estimate $\widehat{f}_y(\nu)$ of $f_y(\nu)$, estimates $\widehat{\lambda}(\nu)$ and $\widehat{\boldsymbol{\beta}}(\nu)$ of the spectral envelope, $\lambda(\nu)$, and the corresponding scalings, $\boldsymbol{\beta}(\nu)$, can then be obtained. Details on estimation and inference for the sample spectral envelope and the optimal scalings can be found in Stoffer et al (1993), but the main result of that paper is as follows: If $\widehat{f}_y(\nu)$ is a consistent spectral estimator and if for each $j = 1, ..., J$, the largest root of $f_y^{re}(\nu_j)$ is distinct, then

$$\left\{\eta_n[\widehat{\lambda}(\nu_j) - \lambda(\nu_j)]/\lambda(\nu_j),\ \eta_n[\widehat{\boldsymbol{\beta}}(\nu_j) - \boldsymbol{\beta}(\nu_j)];\ j = 1, ..., J\right\} \tag{5.188}$$

converges $(n \to \infty)$ jointly in distribution to independent zero-mean, normal, distributions, the first of which is standard normal; the asymptotic covariance structure of $\widehat{\boldsymbol{\beta}}(\nu_j)$ is discussed in Stoffer et al (1993). Result (5.188) is similar to (5.151), but in this case, $\boldsymbol{\beta}(\nu)$ and $\widehat{\boldsymbol{\beta}}(\nu)$ are real. The term $\eta_n$ is the same as in (5.188), and its value depends on the type of estimator being used. Based on these results, asymptotic normal confidence intervals and tests for $\lambda(\nu)$ can be readily constructed. Similarly, for $\boldsymbol{\beta}(\nu)$, asymptotic confidence ellipsoids and chi-square tests can be constructed; details can be found in Stoffer et al (1993, Theorems 3.1 – 3.3).

Peak searching for the smoothed spectral envelope estimate can be aided using the following approximations. Using a first-order Taylor expansion, we have

$$\log \widehat{\lambda}(\nu) \approx \log \lambda(\nu) + \frac{\widehat{\lambda}(\nu) - \lambda(\nu)}{\lambda(\nu)}, \tag{5.189}$$

so $\eta_n[\log \widehat{\lambda}(\nu) - \log \lambda(\nu)]$ is approximately standard normal. It follows that $E[\log \widehat{\lambda}(\nu)] \approx \log \lambda(\nu)$ and $\text{var}[\log \widehat{\lambda}(\nu)] \approx \eta_n^{-2}$. If no signal is present in a sequence of length $n$, we expect $\lambda(j/n) \approx 2/n$ for $1 < j < n/2$, and hence approximately $(1-\alpha)\times 100\%$ of the time, $\log \widehat{\lambda}(\nu)$ will be less than $\log(2/n)+(z_\alpha/\eta_n)$, where $z_\alpha$ is the $(1-\alpha)$ upper tail cutoff of the standard normal distribution. Exponentiating, the $\alpha$ critical value for $\widehat{\lambda}(\nu)$ becomes $(2/n)\exp(z_\alpha/\nu_n)$. Useful values of $z_\alpha$ are $z_{.001} = 3.09$, $z_{.0001} = 3.71$, and $z_{.00001} = 4.26$, and from our experience, thresholding at these levels works well.

**Example 5.17 Spectral Analysis of DNA Sequences**

We give explicit instructions for the calculations involved in estimating the spectral envelope of a DNA sequence, $x_t$, for $t = 1, ..., n$, using the nucleotide alphabet.

- In this example, we hold the scale for T fixed at zero. In this case, we form the $3 \times 1$ data vectors $\boldsymbol{y}_t$:

$$\boldsymbol{y}_t = (1,0,0)' \text{ if } x_t = \texttt{A}; \qquad \boldsymbol{y}_t = (0,1,0)' \text{ if } x_t = \texttt{C};$$
$$\boldsymbol{y}_t = (0,0,1)' \text{ if } x_t = \texttt{G}; \qquad \boldsymbol{y}_t = (0,0,0)' \text{ if } x_t = \texttt{T}.$$

The scaling vector is $\boldsymbol{\beta} = (\beta_1, \beta_2, \beta_3)'$, and the scaled process is $x_t(\boldsymbol{\beta}) = \boldsymbol{\beta}'\boldsymbol{y}_t$.

- Calculate the DFT of the data

$$\boldsymbol{Y}(j/n) = n^{-1/2} \sum_{t=1}^{n} \boldsymbol{y}_t \exp(-2\pi i t j/n).$$

Note $\boldsymbol{Y}(j/n)$ is a $3\times 1$ complex-valued vector. Calculate the periodogram, $I(j/n) = \boldsymbol{Y}(j/n)\boldsymbol{Y}^*(j/n)$, for $j = 1, ..., [n/2]$, and retain only the real part, say, $I^{re}(j/n)$.

- Smooth the $I^{re}(j/n)$ to obtain an estimate of $f_y^{re}(j/n)$. For example, using (5.150) with $L = 3$ and triangular weighting, we would calculate

$$\widehat{f}_y^{re}(j/n) = \frac{1}{4} I^{re}\left(\frac{j-1}{n}\right) + \frac{1}{2} I^{re}\left(\frac{j}{n}\right) + \frac{1}{4} I^{re}\left(\frac{j+1}{n}\right).$$

- Calculate the $3 \times 3$ sample variance–covariance matrix,

$$S_y = n^{-1} \sum_{t=1}^{n} (\boldsymbol{y}_t - \overline{\boldsymbol{y}})(\boldsymbol{y}_t - \overline{\boldsymbol{y}})',$$

where $\overline{\boldsymbol{y}} = n^{-1}\sum_{t=1}^{n} \boldsymbol{y}_t$ is the sample mean of the data.

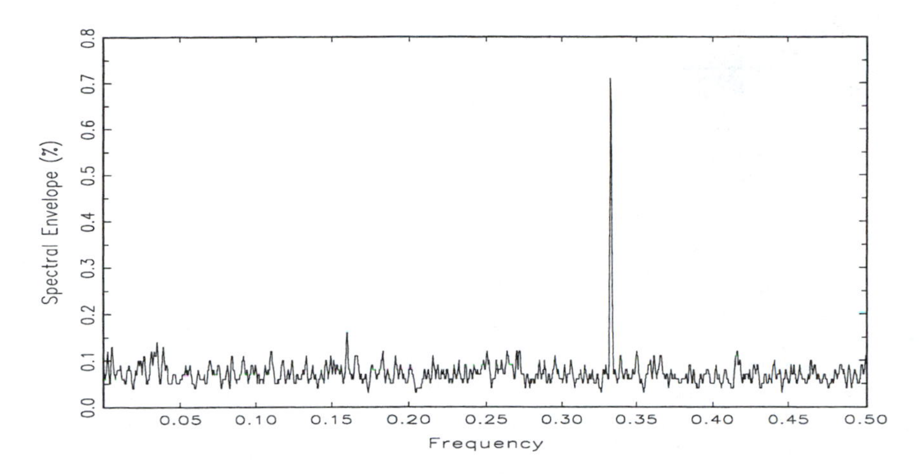


**Figure 5.22:** Smoothed sample spectral envelope of the BNRF1 gene from the Epstein–Barr virus.

- For each $\nu_j = j/n$, $j = 0, 1, ..., [n/2]$, determine the largest eigenvalue and the corresponding eigenvector of the matrix $2n^{-1} S_y^{-1/2} \widehat{f}_y^{re}(\nu_j) S_y^{-1/2}$. Note, $S_y^{1/2}$ is the unique square root matrix of $S_y$.
- The sample spectral envelope $\widehat{\lambda}(\nu_j)$ is the eigenvalue obtained in the previous step. If $\boldsymbol{b}(\nu_j)$ denotes the eigenvector obtained in the previous step, the optimal sample scaling is $\widehat{\boldsymbol{\beta}}(\nu_j) = S_y^{-1/2} \boldsymbol{b}(\omega_j)$; this will result in three values, the value corresponding to the fourth category, T being held fixed at zero.

**Example 5.18 Dynamic Analysis of the Gene Labeled BNRF1 of the Epstein–Barr Virus**

In this example, we focus on a dynamic (or sliding-window) analysis of the gene labeled BNRF1 (bp 1736-5689) of Epstein–Barr. Figure 5.22 shows the spectral envelope, using (5.150) with $L = 11$ and $h_0 = 6/36, h_1 = 5/36, ..., h_5 = 1/36$, of the entire coding sequence (3954 bp long). The figure also shows a strong signal at frequency 1/3; the corresponding optimal scaling was $\texttt{A} = 0.04, \texttt{C} = 0.71, \texttt{G} = 0.70, \texttt{T} = 0$, which indicates the signal is in the strong–weak bonding alphabet, $S = \{\texttt{C}, \texttt{G}\}$ and $W = \{\texttt{A}, \texttt{T}\}$.

Figure 5.23 shows the result of computing the spectral envelope over three nonoverlapping 1000-bp windows and one window of 954 bp, across the CDS, namely, the first, second, third, and fourth quarters of BNRF1.

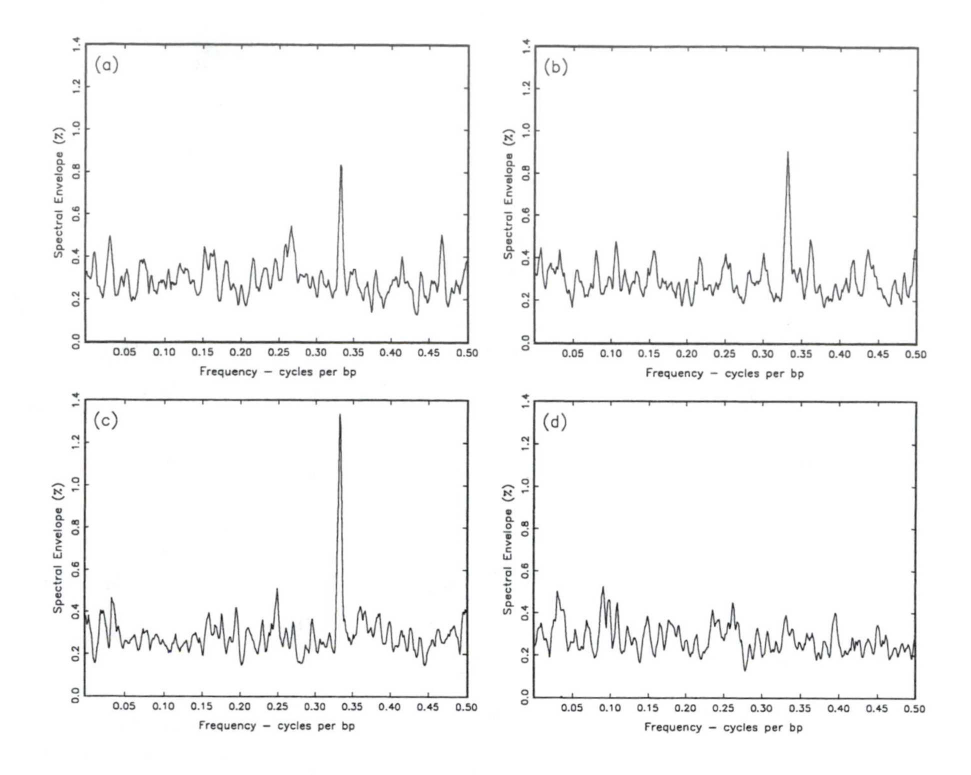


**Figure 5.23:** Smoothed sample spectral envelope of the BNRF1 gene from the Epstein–Barr virus: (a) first 1000 bp, (b) second 1000 bp, (c) third 1000 bp, and (d) last 954 bp.

An approximate 0.001 significance threshold is .69%. The first three quarters contain the signal at the frequency 1/3 (Figure 5.23a-c); the corresponding sample optimal scalings for the first three windows were (a) $\texttt{A} = 0.06, \texttt{C} = 0.69, \texttt{G} = 0.72, \texttt{T} = 0$; (b) $\texttt{A} = 0.09, \texttt{C} = 0.70, \texttt{G} = 0.71, \texttt{T} = 0$; (c) $\texttt{A} = 0.18, \texttt{C} = 0.59, \texttt{G} = 0.77, \texttt{T} = 0$. The first two windows are consistent with the overall analysis. The third section, however, shows some minor departure from the strong-weak bonding alphabet. The most interesting outcome is that the fourth window shows that no signal is present. This leads to the conjecture that the fourth quarter of BNRF1 of Epstein–Barr is actually noncoding.

### The Spectral Envelope for Real-Valued Time Series

The concept of the spectral envelope for categorical time series was extended to real-valued time series, $\{x_t; t = 0, \pm 1, \pm 2, ..., \}$, in McDougall et al (1997). The process $x_t$ can be vector-valued, but here we will concentrate on the univariate case. Further details can be found in McDougall et al (1997). The concept is similar to projection pursuit (Friedman and Stuetzle, 1981). Let $\mathcal{G}$ denote a $k$-dimensional vector space of continuous real-valued transformations with $\{g_1, ..., g_k\}$ being a set of basis functions satisfying $E[g_i(x_t)^2] < \infty$, $i = 1, ..., k$. Analogous to the categorical time series case, define the scaled time series with respect to the set $\mathcal{G}$, to be the real-valued process

$$x_t(\boldsymbol{\beta}) = \boldsymbol{\beta}' \boldsymbol{y}_t = \beta_1 g_1(x_t) + \cdots + \beta_k g_k(x_t)$$

obtained from the vector process

$$\boldsymbol{y}_t = \Big( g_1(X_t), ..., g_k(X_t) \Big)',$$

where $\boldsymbol{\beta} = (\beta_1, ..., \beta_k)' \in \mathbf{R}^k$. If the vector process, $\boldsymbol{y}_t$, is assumed to have a continuous spectral density, say, $f_y(\nu)$, then $x_t(\boldsymbol{\beta})$ will have a continuous spectral density $f_x(\nu; \boldsymbol{\beta})$ for all $\boldsymbol{\beta} \neq \mathbf{0}$. Noting, $f_x(\nu; \boldsymbol{\beta}) = \boldsymbol{\beta}' f_y(\nu) \boldsymbol{\beta} = \boldsymbol{\beta}' f_y^{re}(\nu) \boldsymbol{\beta}$, and $\sigma^2(\boldsymbol{\beta}) = \text{var}[x_t(\boldsymbol{\beta})] = \boldsymbol{\beta}' V \boldsymbol{\beta}$, where $V = \text{var}(\boldsymbol{y}_t)$ is assumed to be positive definite, the optimality criterion

$$\lambda(\nu) = \sup_{\boldsymbol{\beta} \neq \mathbf{0}} \left\{ \frac{\boldsymbol{\beta}' f_y^{re}(\nu) \boldsymbol{\beta}}{\boldsymbol{\beta}' V \boldsymbol{\beta}} \right\}, \tag{5.190}$$

is well defined and represents the largest proportion of the total power that can be attributed to the frequency $\nu$ for any particular scaled process $x_t(\boldsymbol{\beta})$. This interpretation of $\lambda(\nu)$ is consistent with the notion of the spectral envelope introduced in the previous section and provides the following working definition: *The spectral envelope of a time series with respect to the space $\mathcal{G}$ is defined to be $\lambda(\nu)$.*

The solution to this problem, as in the categorical case, is attained by finding the largest scalar $\lambda(\nu)$ such that

$$f_y^{re}(\nu) \boldsymbol{\beta}(\nu) = \lambda(\nu) V \boldsymbol{\beta}(\nu) \tag{5.191}$$

for $\boldsymbol{\beta}(\nu) \neq \mathbf{0}$. That is, $\lambda(\nu)$ is the largest eigenvalue of $f_y^{re}(\nu)$ in the metric of $V$, and the optimal scaling, $\boldsymbol{\beta}(\nu)$, is the corresponding eigenvector.

If $x_t$ is a categorical time series taking values in the finite state-space $\mathcal{S} = \{c_1, c_2, ..., c_k\}$, where $c_j$ represents a particular category, an appropriate choice for $\mathcal{G}$ is the set of indicator functions $g_j(x_t) = I(x_t = c_j)$. Hence, this is a natural generalization of the categorical case. In the categorical case, $\mathcal{G}$ does not consist of linearly independent $g$'s, but it was easy to overcome this problem by reducing the dimension by one. In the vector-valued case, $\boldsymbol{x}_t = (x_{1t}, ..., x_{pt})'$, we consider $\mathcal{G}$ to be the class of transformations from $\mathbf{R}^p$ into $\mathbf{R}$ such that the spectral density of $g(\boldsymbol{x}_t)$ exists. One class of transformations of interest are linear combinations of $\boldsymbol{x}_t$. In Tiao et al (1993), for example, linear transformations of this type are used in a time domain approach to investigate contemporaneous relationships among the components of multivariate time series. Estimation and inference for the real-valued case are analogous to the methods described in the previous section for the categorical case. We focus on two examples here; numerous other examples can be found in McDougall et al (1997).

**Example 5.19 Residual Analysis**

A relevant situation may be when $x_t$ is the residual process obtained from some modeling procedure. If the fitted model is appropriate, the residuals should exhibit properties similar to an iid sequence. Departures of the data from the fitted model may suggest model misspecification, non-Gaussian data, or the existence of a nonlinear structure, and the spectral envelope would provide a simple diagnostic tool to aid in a residual analysis.

The series considered here is the quarterly U.S. real GNP which was analyzed in Chapter 2, Examples 2.32 and 2.33. Recall an MA(2) model was fit to the growth rate, and the residuals from this fit are plotted in Figure 2.16. As discussed in Example 2.33, the residuals from the model fit appear to be uncorrelated; there appears to be one or two outliers, but their magnitudes are not that extreme. In addition, the standard residual analyses showed no obvious structure among the residuals.

Although the MA(2) model appears to be appropriate, Tiao and Tsay (1994) investigated the possibility of nonlinearities in GNP growth rate. Their overall conclusion was that there is subtle nonlinear behavior in the data because the economy behaves differently during expansion periods than during recession periods.

The spectral envelope, used as a diagnostic tool on the residuals, clearly indicates the MA(2) model is not adequate, and that further analysis is warranted. Here, the generating set $\mathcal{G} = \{x, |x|, x^2\}$—which seems natural for a residual analysis—was used to estimate the spectral envelope for the residuals from the MA(2) fit, and the result is plotted in Figure 5.24. A smoothed periodogram estimate was obtained using $L = 21$ and triangular weighting, $h_0 = 11/121, h_{\pm1} = 10/121, ..., h_{\pm10} = 1/121$ in (5.150). Clearly, the residuals are not iid, and considerable power is present at the low frequencies. The presence of spectral power at very low frequencies in detrended economic series has been frequently reported and is typically associated with long-range dependence. In fact, our choice of $\mathcal{G}$ was partly influenced by the work of Ding et al (1993) who applied transformations of the form $|x_t|^d$, for $d \in (0, 3]$, to the S&P 500 stock market series. The estimated optimal transformation at the first nonzero

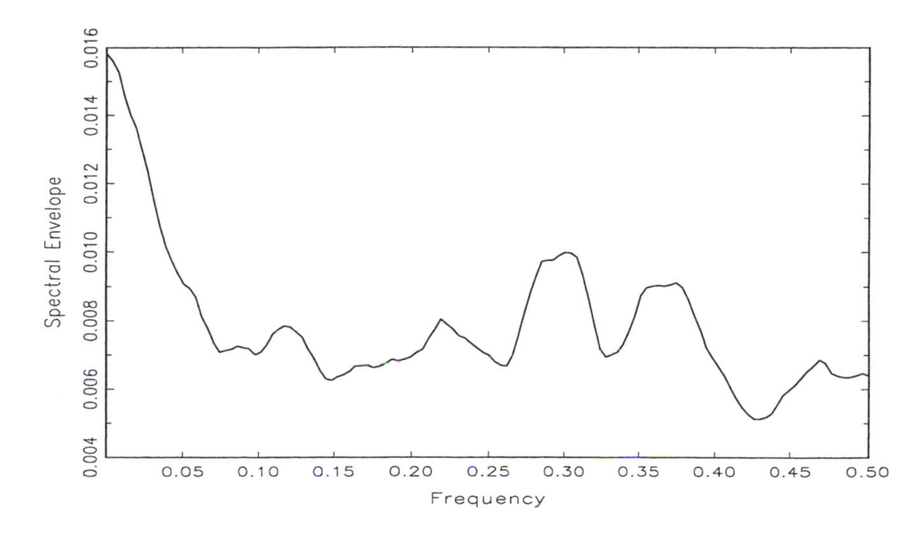


**Figure 5.24:** Spectral envelope with respect to $\mathcal{G} = \{x, |x|, x^2\}$ of the residuals from an MA(2) fit to the U.S. GNP growth rate data.

frequency, $\nu = 0.006$, was $\widehat{\boldsymbol{\beta}}(0.006) = (1, 20, -2916)'$, which leads to the transformation

$$y = x + 20|x| - 2916x^2. \tag{5.192}$$

This transformation is plotted in Figure 5.25. The transformation, (5.192), is basically the absolute value (with some slight curvature and asymmetry) for most of the residual values, but the effect of extreme-valued residuals (outliers) is dampened.

### Example 5.20 Optimal Transformations

In this example, we consider a contrived data set, in which we know the optimal transformation, say, $g_0$, and we determine whether the technology can find the transformation when $g_0$ is not in $\mathcal{G}$. The data, $x_t$, are generated by the nonlinear model

$$x_t = \exp\{3\sin(2\pi t\nu_0) + \epsilon_t\}, \quad t = 1, ..., 512, \tag{5.193}$$

where $\nu_0 = 51/512$ and $\epsilon_t$ is white Gaussian noise with a variance of 16. This example is adapted from Breiman and Friedman (1985), where the ACE algorithm is introduced. The optimal transformation in this case is $g_0(x_t) = \ln(x_t)$, wherein the data are generated from a sinusoid plus

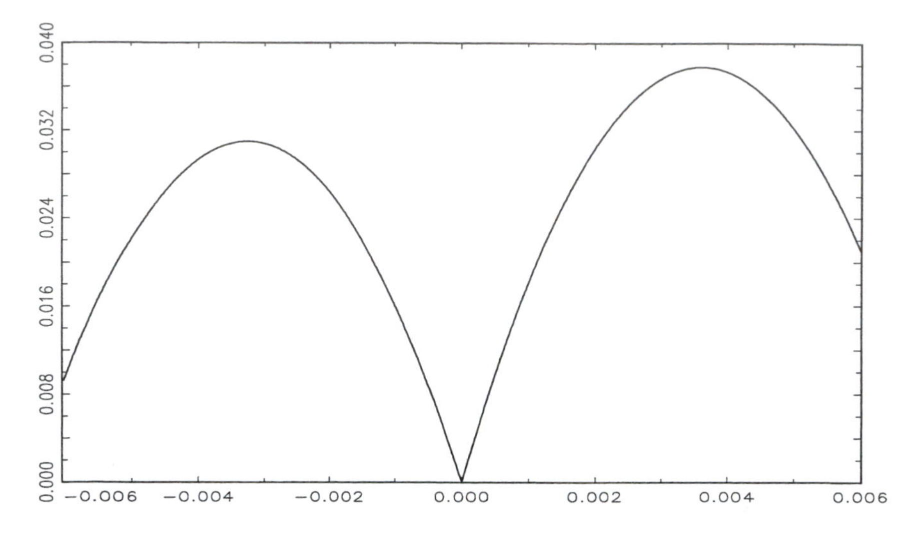


**Figure 5.25:** Estimated optimal transformation, (5.192), for the GNP residuals at $\nu = 0.006$.

noise. Of the 512 generated data, about 98% were less than 4000. Occasionally, the data values were extremely large (the data exceeded 100,000 about four times). The periodogram, in decibels $[10\log_{10} X(\nu_j)]$, of the standardized and tapered (by a cosine bell) data is shown in Figure 5.26 and provides no evidence of any dominant frequency, including $\nu_0$.

In contrast, the sample spectral envelope (Figure 5.27) computed with respect to $\mathcal{G} = \{x, \sqrt{x}, \sqrt[3]{x}\}$ has no difficulty in isolating $\nu_0$. No smoothing was used here; so, based on Stoffer et al (1993, Theorem 3.2), an approximate 0.0001 null significance threshold for the spectral envelope is 4.84% (the null hypothesis being that $x_t$ is iid).

Figure 5.28 compares the estimated optimal transformation with respect to $\mathcal{G}$ with the log transformation for values less than 4000. The estimated transformation at $\nu_0$ is given by

$$y = -.6 + 0.0003x - 0.3638\sqrt{x} + 1.9304\sqrt[3]{x}; \tag{5.194}$$

that is, $\widehat{\beta}(\nu_0) = (0.0003, -0.3638, 1.9304)'$ after rescaling so (5.194) can be compared directly with $y = \ln(x)$.

Finally, it is worth mentioning the result obtained when the rather inappropriate basis, $\{x, x^2, x^3\}$, was used. Surprisingly, the spectral envelope in this case (Figure 5.29) looks similar to that of Figure 5.27. Also, the resulting estimated optimal transformation at $\nu_0$, is close to the log

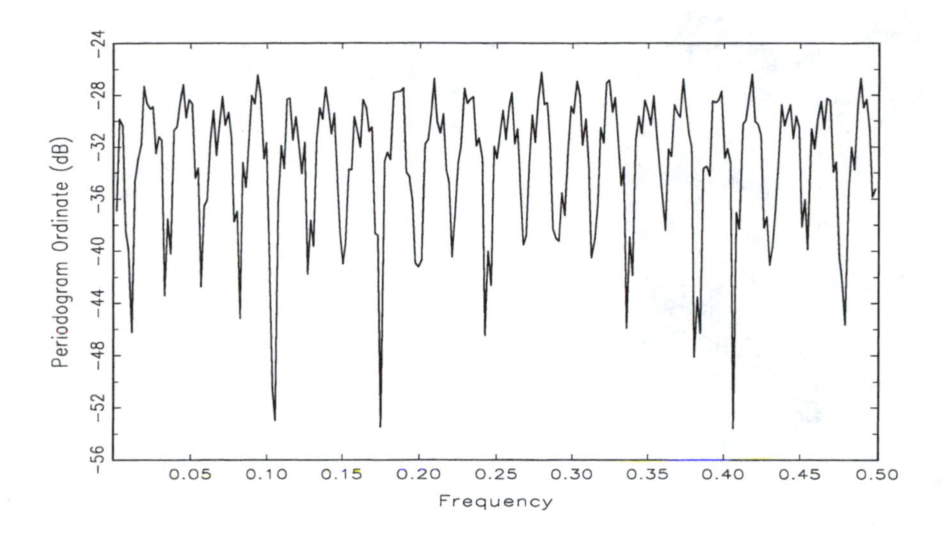


**Figure 5.26:** Periodogram, in decibels, of the data generated from (5.193) after tapering by a cosine bell.

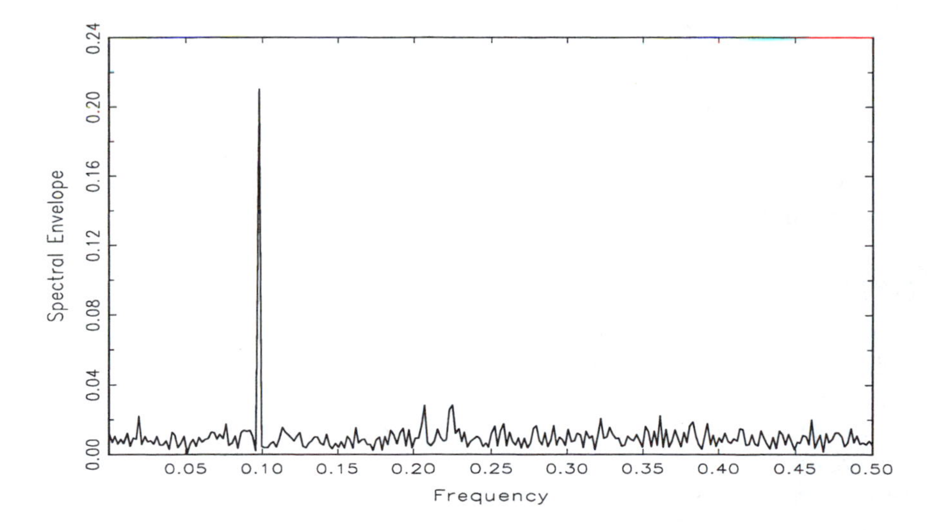


**Figure 5.27:** Spectral envelope with respect to $\mathcal{G} = \{x, \sqrt{x}, \sqrt[3]{x}\}$ of data generated from (5.193).

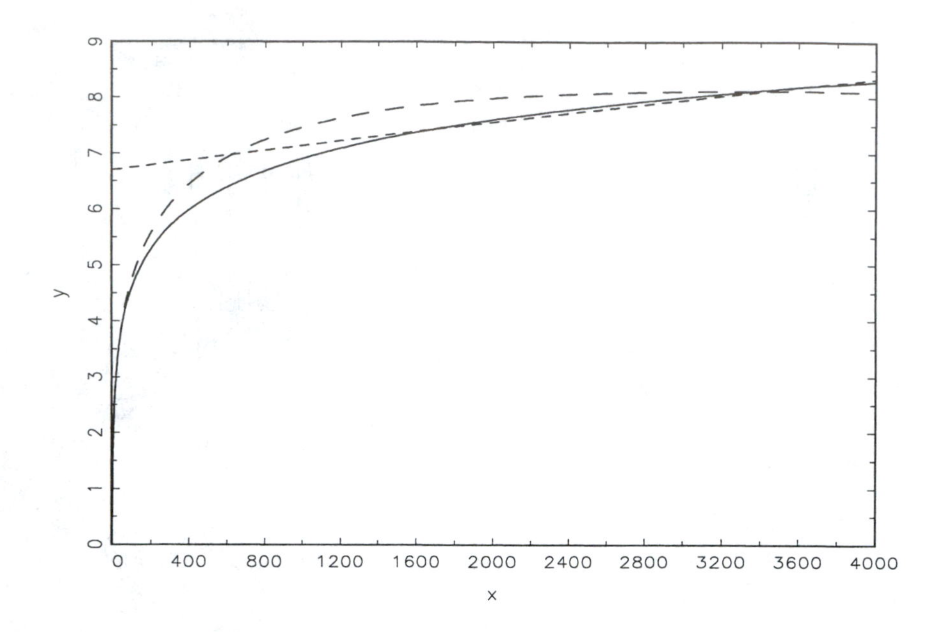


**Figure 5.28:** Log transformation, $y = \ln(x)$ (solid line), the estimated optimal transformation at $\nu_0$ as given in (5.194) (dashed line), and the estimated optimal transformation at $\nu_0$ using the inappropriate basis $\{x, x^2, x^3\}$ (short-dashed line).

transformation. In fact, as seen in Figure 5.28, it looks like what we would imagine as a linear approximation to $y = \ln(x)$ within the range of most of the data.

### Matching Sequences

Here, we consider the problem of quantifying the degree to which two categorical time series are coherent. The goal is to discover whether the sequences contain similar patterns and the problem is motivated by the matching of two DNA sequences. This approach builds on canonical analysis (Section 5.8) and the ideas used in defining the spectral envelope for a qualitative-valued time series; technical details can be found in Stoffer and Tyler (1998).

*The General Problem*

In the general case, $x_{1t}$ and $x_{2t}$, $t = 0, \pm1, \pm2, \ldots$, are categorical time series taking values in possibly different state spaces of dimensions $k_1 + 1$ and $k_2 + 1$, respectively. Consider two nonconstant transformations $g$ and $h$, with $g(x_{1t})$ and $h(x_{2t})$ being real-valued time series such that $g(x_{1t})$ has continuous

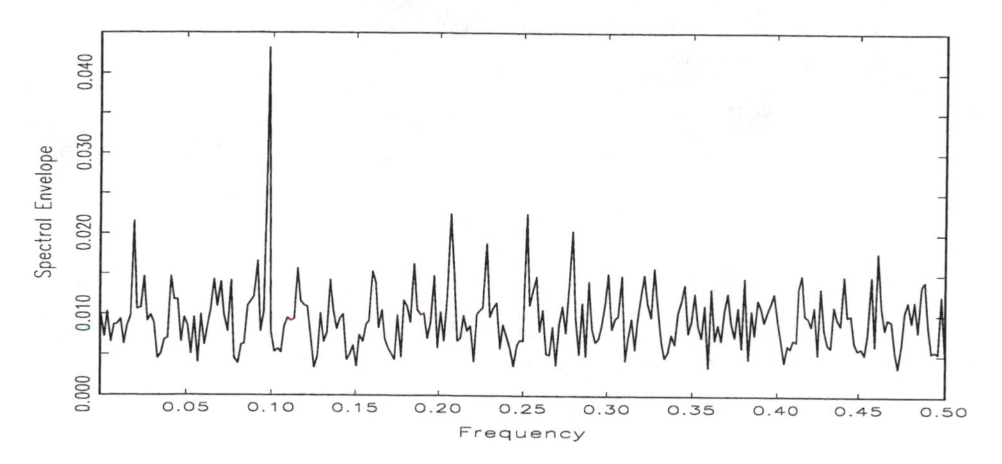


**Figure 5.29:** Spectral envelope with respect to $\mathcal{G} = \{x, x^2, x^3\}$ of data generated from (5.193).

spectral density $f_{gg}(\nu)$ and $h(x_{2t})$ has continuous spectral density $f_{hh}(\nu)$. We denote the complex-valued cross-spectral density of the two series $g(x_{1t})$ and $h(x_{2t})$ by $f_{gh}(\nu)$. A measure of the degree of similarity between the sequences $g(x_{1t})$ and $h(x_{2t})$ at frequency $\nu$ is the squared coherency

$$\rho^2_{gh}(\nu) = \frac{|f_{gh}(\nu)|^2}{f_{gg}(\nu)f_{hh}(\nu)}. \tag{5.195}$$

Of course, the value of $\rho^2_{gh}(\nu)$ will depend on the choices of the transformations $g$ and $h$. If $x_{1t}$ and $x_{2t}$ are independent, then so are $g(x_{1t})$ and $h(x_{2t})$, for any $g$ and $h$. In this case, $\rho^2_{gh}(\nu) = 0$ for all $\nu$. The main goal here is to find $g$ and $h$, under various constraints, to maximize the squared coherency $\rho^2_{gh}(\nu)$. If the maximized value of $\rho^2_{gh}(\nu)$ is small, we can say the two sequences $x_{1t}$ and $x_{2t}$ do not match at frequency $\nu$. If the maximized value of $\rho^2_{gh}(\nu)$ is large, the resulting transformations $g$ and $h$ can help in understanding the nature of the similarity between the two sequences.

As before, we identify the categorical sequence $x_{1t}$ with the multiple indicator process $\boldsymbol{y}_{1t}$. Recall $\boldsymbol{y}_{1t}$ is a $k_1 \times 1$ vector with a one in the $j$-th position if $x_{1t}$ is in state $j$ $(j = 1, ..., k_1)$ at time $t$ and zeros elsewhere. If $x_{1t}$ is in state $k_1 + 1$, then $\boldsymbol{y}_{1t}$ is the zero vector. Similarly, we identify $x_{2t}$ with the $k_2 \times 1$ multiple indicator processes $\boldsymbol{y}_{2t}$. We assume the existence of the $k_i \times k_i$ $(i = 1, 2)$, nonsingular spectral density matrices $f_{11}(\nu)$ and $f_{22}(\nu)$ of $\boldsymbol{y}_{1t}$ and $\boldsymbol{y}_{2t}$, respectively, and denote the $k_1 \times k_2$ cross-spectral matrix between $\boldsymbol{y}_{1t}$ and $\boldsymbol{y}_{2t}$ by $f_{12}(\nu)$.

To describe the problem in terms of scaling categorical time series, let

$\boldsymbol{\alpha} = (\alpha_1, ..., \alpha_{k_1})' \in \mathbf{R}^{k_1}$, $\boldsymbol{\alpha} \neq \mathbf{0}$, be a vector of scalings associated with the categories of the first series, $x_{1t}$, and let $\boldsymbol{\beta} = (\beta_1, ..., \beta_{k_2})' \in \mathbf{R}^{k_2}$, $\boldsymbol{\beta} \neq \mathbf{0}$, be a vector of scalings associated with the categories of the second series, $x_{2t}$. That is, define the real-valued series

$$\begin{aligned} x_{1t}(\boldsymbol{\alpha}) &= \alpha_j \quad \text{if } x_{1t} \text{ is in state } j \text{ for } j = 1, ..., k_1, \\ x_{2t}(\boldsymbol{\beta}) &= \beta_j \quad \text{if } x_{2t} \text{ is in state } j \text{ for } j = 1, ..., k_2, \end{aligned} \tag{5.196}$$

where, in addition, $x_{1t}(\boldsymbol{\alpha}) = 0$ if $x_{1t}$ is in state $k_1 + 1$, and $x_{2t}(\boldsymbol{\beta}) = 0$ if $x_{2t}$ is in state $k_2 + 1$.

Because the scaled series can be written as $x_{1t}(\boldsymbol{\alpha}) = \boldsymbol{\alpha}'\boldsymbol{y}_{1t}$ and $x_{2t}(\boldsymbol{\beta}) = \boldsymbol{\beta}'\boldsymbol{y}_{2t}$, the squared coherency between $x_{1t}(\boldsymbol{\alpha})$ and $x_{2t}(\boldsymbol{\beta})$ can be written as

$$\rho_{12}^2(\nu; \boldsymbol{\alpha}, \boldsymbol{\beta}) = \frac{|\boldsymbol{\alpha}' f_{12}(\nu)\boldsymbol{\beta}|^2}{[\boldsymbol{\alpha}' f_{11}^{re}(\nu)\boldsymbol{\alpha}]\ [\boldsymbol{\beta}' f_{22}^{re}(\nu)\boldsymbol{\beta}]}. \tag{5.197}$$

Setting $\boldsymbol{a} = f_{11}^{re}(\nu)^{1/2}\boldsymbol{\alpha}$ and $\boldsymbol{b} = f_{22}^{re}(\nu)^{1/2}\boldsymbol{\beta}$, subject to $\boldsymbol{a}'\boldsymbol{a} = 1$ and $\boldsymbol{b}'\boldsymbol{b} = 1$, define

$$Q(\nu) = f_{11}^{re}(\nu)^{-1/2} f_{12}(\nu) f_{22}^{re}(\nu)^{-1/2} = Q^{re}(\nu) + i\ Q^{im}(\nu) \tag{5.198}$$

and write (5.197) as

$$\rho_{12}^2(\nu; \boldsymbol{a}, \boldsymbol{b}) = [\boldsymbol{a}'Q^{re}(\nu)\boldsymbol{b}]^2 + [\boldsymbol{a}'Q^{im}(\nu)\boldsymbol{b}]^2. \tag{5.199}$$

The goal is to find $\boldsymbol{a}$ and $\boldsymbol{b}$ to maximize (5.199) for each $\nu$ of interest. Several approaches to the maximization are available; one approach is based on the following property.

***Property 5.1: Maximization of (5.199)***
*Fix $\nu$, and drop it from the notation. Then,* (5.199) *can be written as*

$$\begin{aligned} \rho_{12}^2(\boldsymbol{a}, \boldsymbol{b}) &= \boldsymbol{a}'(Q^{re}\boldsymbol{b}\boldsymbol{b}'Q^{re} + Q^{im}\boldsymbol{b}\boldsymbol{b}'Q^{im})\boldsymbol{a} \\ &= \boldsymbol{b}'(Q^{re}\boldsymbol{a}\boldsymbol{a}'Q^{re} + Q^{im}\boldsymbol{a}\boldsymbol{a}'Q^{im})\boldsymbol{b}. \end{aligned} \tag{5.200}$$

*Let $\boldsymbol{b}_0$ be an arbitrary, real-valued, $k_2 \times 1$ unit length vector. Define the sequence of vectors $\boldsymbol{a}_j$ to be the eigenvector corresponding to the largest root of the at most rank* 2*, nonnegative-definite matrix*

$$Q^{re}\boldsymbol{b}_{j-1}\boldsymbol{b}_{j-1}'Q^{re'} + Q^{im}\boldsymbol{b}_{j-1}\boldsymbol{b}_{j-1}'Q^{im'} \tag{5.201}$$

*and the sequence $\boldsymbol{b}_j$ to be the eigenvector corresponding to the largest root of the at most rank* 2*, nonnegative-definite matrix*

$$Q^{re'}\boldsymbol{a}_j\boldsymbol{a}_j'Q^{re} + Q^{im'}\boldsymbol{a}_j\boldsymbol{a}_j'Q^{im}, \tag{5.202}$$

*for $j = 1, 2, \ldots$ . Then, from the first part of* (5.200), $\rho_{12}^2(\boldsymbol{a}_{j+1}, \boldsymbol{b}_j) \geq \rho_{12}^2(\boldsymbol{a}, \boldsymbol{b}_j)$ *for any* $\boldsymbol{a}$ *of unit length, and from the second part of* (5.200), $\rho_{12}^2(\boldsymbol{a}_{j+1}, \boldsymbol{b}_{j+1}) \geq \rho_{12}^2(\boldsymbol{a}_{j+1}, \boldsymbol{b})$ *for any* $\boldsymbol{b}$ *of unit length. Thus,*

$$\rho_{12}^2(\boldsymbol{a}_{j+1}, \boldsymbol{b}_{j+1}) \geq \rho_{12}^2(\boldsymbol{a}_{j+1}, \boldsymbol{b}_j) \geq \rho_{12}^2(\boldsymbol{a}_j, \boldsymbol{b}_j). \tag{5.203}$$

The algorithm described by Property 5.1 can be used to find the optimal scalings at each frequency, $\nu$, of interest. The algorithm is initialized by setting $\boldsymbol{b}_0$ equal to either $\mathcal{E}_1[Q^{re}(\nu)'Q^{re}(\nu)]$ or $\mathcal{E}_1[Q^{im}(\nu)'Q^{im}(\nu)]$, depending on which vector [we denote the eigenvector corresponding to the largest eigenvalue of matrix $A$ by $\mathcal{E}_1(A)$] produces the larger value of (5.199) for arbitrary $\boldsymbol{a}$. In turn, $\boldsymbol{\alpha}(\nu)$ and $\boldsymbol{\beta}(\nu)$ can be taken proportional to $f_{11}^{re}(\nu)^{-1/2}\boldsymbol{a}(\nu)$ and $f_{22}^{re}(\nu)^{-1/2}\boldsymbol{b}(\nu)$, respectively, where $\boldsymbol{a}(\nu)$ and $\boldsymbol{b}(\nu)$ maximize (5.199). The algorithm requires only the computation of latent roots and vectors of at most rank 2, nonnegative-definite matrices, regardless of the dimension of the state spaces. Moreover, by (5.203), the objective function increases with each step. Unfortunately, it does not guarantee convergence to the global maximum. From simulations, however, it is our experience that the algorithm usually converges; Stoffer and Tyler (1998) also provide tight bounds for the maximum of (5.199).

*Common Scalings*

In many cases, the processes $x_{1t}$ and $x_{2t}$ are defined on the same state-space, $\mathcal{S} = \{c_1, \ldots, c_{k+1}\}$, for example, DNA sequences. To enhance the interpretation in such cases, it would be appropriate to choose ***common scalings***. Henceforth, set $k_1 = k_2 = k$, and assume $\boldsymbol{y}_{1t}$ and $\boldsymbol{y}_{2t}$ have the same spectra; that is, $f_{11}(\nu) = f_{22}(\nu) = f(\nu)$, for at least all $\nu$ of interest. Realistic models that satisfy these conditions will be discussed later.

Let $\boldsymbol{\beta} = (\beta_1, \ldots, \beta_k)' \in \mathbf{R}^k$, $\boldsymbol{\beta} \neq \mathbf{0}$, be a vector of scalings common to the categories of both series; that is, the real-valued series are

$$x_{1t}(\boldsymbol{\beta}) = \beta_j \quad \text{if} \quad x_{1t} = c_j,$$
$$x_{2t}(\boldsymbol{\beta}) = \beta_j \quad \text{if} \quad x_{2t} = c_j,$$

for $j = 1, \ldots, k$. The scale associated with category $c_{k+1}$ is held fixed at zero for both sequences. We restrict attention to the frequencies $\nu$ for which $f_{11}(\nu) = f_{22}(\nu) = f(\nu)$. because the scaled series are $x_{it}(\boldsymbol{\beta}) = \boldsymbol{\beta}'\boldsymbol{y}_{it}$, for $i = 1, 2$, the squared coherency between $x_{1t}(\boldsymbol{\beta})$ and $x_{2t}(\boldsymbol{\beta})$ can be written as

$$\rho_{12}^2(\nu; \boldsymbol{\beta}) = \frac{|\boldsymbol{\beta}' f_{12}(\nu)\boldsymbol{\beta}|^2}{[\boldsymbol{\beta}' f^{re}(\nu)\boldsymbol{\beta}]^2}. \tag{5.204}$$

Setting $\boldsymbol{b} = f^{re}(\nu)^{1/2}\boldsymbol{\beta}$, subject to the standardization $\boldsymbol{b}'\boldsymbol{b} = 1$, and writing

$$Q(\nu) = f^{re}(\nu)^{-1/2} f_{12}(\nu) f^{re}(\nu)^{-1/2} = Q^{re}(\nu) + i\, Q^{im}(\nu), \tag{5.205}$$

we may write (5.204) as

$$\rho_{12}^2(\nu; \boldsymbol{b}) = [\boldsymbol{b}' Q^{re}(\nu)\boldsymbol{b}]^2 + [\boldsymbol{b}' Q^{im}(\nu)\boldsymbol{b}]^2. \tag{5.206}$$

Although $Q^{re}(\nu)$ and $Q^{im}(\nu)$ in (5.206) are not necessarily symmetric, we may assume, without loss of generality, they are because

$$\rho_{12}^2(\nu; \boldsymbol{b}) = [\boldsymbol{b}' Q^{re}(\nu)\boldsymbol{b}]^2 + [\boldsymbol{b}' Q^{im}(\nu)\boldsymbol{b}]^2 = [\boldsymbol{b}' Q_s^{re}(\nu)\boldsymbol{b}]^2 + [\boldsymbol{b}' Q_s^{im}(\nu)\boldsymbol{b}]^2, \tag{5.207}$$

where

$$Q_s^{re}(\nu) = [Q^{re}(\nu) + Q^{re}(\nu)']/2 \tag{5.208}$$

and

$$Q_s^{im}(\nu) = [Q^{im}(\nu) + Q^{im}(\nu)']/2. \tag{5.209}$$

Our goal is to find $\boldsymbol{b}$ to maximize (5.207) for each $\nu$ of interest. The maximization can still be accomplished iteratively via the algorithm (5.201)-(5.202) in conjunction with the following property.

***Property 5.2: Maximization of (5.207)***
*Under the model conditions, if in Property 5.1, $k_1 = k_2 = k$ and the matrices $Q^{re}$ and $Q^{im}$ are symmetric, the maximum value of $\rho_{12}^2(\boldsymbol{a}, \boldsymbol{b})$ is attained when $\boldsymbol{a} = \boldsymbol{b}$.*

Because $Q_s^{re}(\nu)$ and $Q_s^{im}(\nu)$ are symmetric, Property 5.2 can be used to maximize (5.207), initializing the algorithm by setting $\boldsymbol{b}_0$ equal to either $\mathcal{E}_1[Q_s^{re}(\nu)^2]$ or $\mathcal{E}_1[Q_s^{im}(\nu)^2]$, depending on which vector produces the larger value of $\rho_{12}^2(\nu; \boldsymbol{b}_0)$. The sequence

$$\boldsymbol{b}_j = \mathcal{E}_1[Q_s^{re}(\nu)\boldsymbol{b}_{j-1}\boldsymbol{b}_{j-1}' Q_s^{re}(\nu) + Q_s^{im}(\nu)\boldsymbol{b}_{j-1}\boldsymbol{b}_{j-1}' Q_s^{im}(\nu)], \tag{5.210}$$

for $j = 1, 2, \ldots$, replaces the alternating sequences defined in (5.201)-(5.202). Note, $\rho_{12}^2(\nu; \boldsymbol{b}_j) \geq \rho_{12}^2(\nu; \boldsymbol{b}_{j-1})$. The optimal scaling, $\boldsymbol{\beta}(\nu)$, is chosen proportional to $f^{re}(\nu)^{-1/2}\boldsymbol{b}(\nu)$, where $\boldsymbol{b}(\nu)$ maximizes (5.207). *Another important consequence of Property 5.2 is that it gives sufficient conditions under which choosing common scales is not only parsimonious, but also optimal. Specifically, if $Q^{re}(\nu)$ and $Q^{im}(\nu)$ are both symmetric, the maximum of $\rho_{12}^2(\nu; \boldsymbol{a}, \boldsymbol{b})$* [see (5.199)] *is achieved when $\boldsymbol{a} = \boldsymbol{b}$.*

*Models and Applications*
For practical applications of the theory, we address two problems. First is the case in which the two sequences under investigation are in phase and contain at most one common pattern. They may be subsequences of larger sequences. This situation will be termed ***local alignment***. The case of ***global alignment***, in which we do not assume the sequences are in phase, will be discussed next. The local model is

$$\boldsymbol{y}_{it} = \boldsymbol{p}_i + \boldsymbol{s}_t + \boldsymbol{e}_{it}, \tag{5.211}$$

where $\boldsymbol{p}_i = (p_{i1}, ..., p_{ik})'$ is the vector of positive probabilities $p_{ij} = \Pr(x_{it} = c_j)$, for $i = 1, 2$ and $j = 1, ..., k$. In addition, $\boldsymbol{s}_t$ is a realization of a stationary $k \times 1$ vector-valued time series that is uncorrelated with the stationary $k \times 1$ vector-valued series $\boldsymbol{e}_{it}$, for $i = 1, 2$. There may be some dependence structure between $\boldsymbol{s}_t$ and $\boldsymbol{e}_{it}$; refer to Stoffer (1987) for details. Furthermore, $\boldsymbol{s}_t$ has $k \times k$ spectral density matrix $f_{ss}(\nu)$, and $\boldsymbol{e}_{it}$, for $i = 1, 2$, have common $k \times k$ spectra denoted by $f_{ee}(\nu)$. It is hypothesized that the process $\boldsymbol{s}_t$ is common to both sequences.

Let $\boldsymbol{\beta} = (\beta_1, ..., \beta_k)' \in \mathbf{R}^k$, $\boldsymbol{\beta} \neq \mathbf{0}$, be a vector of scalings associated with the categories $\{c_1, ..., c_k\}$. As before, define the real-valued series $x_i(t, \boldsymbol{\beta}) = \beta_j$ if $x_{it} = c_j$, $j = 1, ..., k$, and $x_i(t, \beta) = 0$ if $x_{it} = c_{k+1}$, for $i = 1, 2$. In this case, the conditions of Property 5.2 are met, and hence, *the optimal strategy is to select the common scales for the sequences $x_{1t}$ and $x_{2t}$* .

Note, $x_{it}(\boldsymbol{\beta}) = \boldsymbol{\beta}'\boldsymbol{y}_{it} = \boldsymbol{\beta}'\boldsymbol{p}_i + \boldsymbol{\beta}'\boldsymbol{s}_t + \boldsymbol{\beta}'\boldsymbol{e}_{it}$, for $i = 1, 2$. Let $f_{11}(\nu; \boldsymbol{\beta})$ be the spectrum of scaled process $x_{1t}(\boldsymbol{\beta})$; similarly, let $f_{22}(\nu; \boldsymbol{\beta})$ denote the spectrum of $x_{2t}(\boldsymbol{\beta})$ and let $f_{12}(\nu; \boldsymbol{\beta})$, denote the cross-spectrum between $x_{1t}(\boldsymbol{\beta})$ and $x_{2t}(\boldsymbol{\beta})$. The following conditions hold:

$$\begin{aligned} f_{ii}(\nu; \boldsymbol{\beta}) &= \boldsymbol{\beta}'\{f_{ss}^{re}(\nu) + f_{ee}^{re}(\nu)\}\boldsymbol{\beta}, \quad i = 1, 2, \\ f_{12}(\nu; \boldsymbol{\beta}) &= \boldsymbol{\beta}' f_{ss}^{re}(\nu)\boldsymbol{\beta}. \end{aligned} \tag{5.212}$$

The coherence between $x_{1t}(\boldsymbol{\beta})$ and $x_{2t}(\boldsymbol{\beta})$ is seen to be

$$\rho_{12}(\nu; \boldsymbol{\beta}) = \frac{\boldsymbol{\beta}' f_{ss}^{re}(\nu)\boldsymbol{\beta}}{\boldsymbol{\beta}'[f_{ss}^{re}(\nu) + f_{ee}^{re}(\nu)]\boldsymbol{\beta}}. \tag{5.213}$$

If $f_{ss}(\nu) = 0$, then $\rho_{12}(\nu; \boldsymbol{\beta}) = 0$ for any scaling $\boldsymbol{\beta}$. Thus, the detection of a common signal can be achieved by considering the maximal coherency under the model conditions. Setting $\boldsymbol{b} = [f_{ss}^{re}(\nu) + f_{ee}^{re}(\nu)]^{1/2}\boldsymbol{\beta}$, subject to $\boldsymbol{b}'\boldsymbol{b} = 1$, write (5.213) as

$$\rho_{12}(\nu; \boldsymbol{b}) = \boldsymbol{b}'[f_{ss}^{re}(\nu) + f_{ee}^{re}(\nu)]^{-1/2}\ f_{ss}^{re}(\nu)\ [f_{ss}^{re}(\nu) + f_{ee}^{re}(\nu)]^{-1/2}\boldsymbol{b}. \tag{5.214}$$

Hence, the problem is again an eigenvalue problem, and the maximum value of (5.214) is the largest scalar $\lambda(\nu)$ such that

$$[f_{ss}^{re}(\nu) + f_{ee}^{re}(\nu)]^{-1/2}\ f_{ss}^{re}(\nu)\ [f_{ss}^{re}(\nu) + f_{ee}^{re}(\nu)]^{-1/2}\boldsymbol{b}(\nu) = \lambda(\nu)\boldsymbol{b}(\nu). \tag{5.215}$$

The optimal scaling, $\boldsymbol{\beta}(\nu)$, is taken proportional to $[f_{ss}^{re}(\nu) + f_{ee}^{re}(\nu)]^{-1/2}\boldsymbol{b}(\nu)$. This value will maximize the coherency at frequency $\nu$ between the two sequences, with the maximum value being $\lambda(\nu)$. That is, $\rho_{12}(\nu; \boldsymbol{\beta}) \leq \rho_{12}(\nu; \boldsymbol{\beta}(\nu)) = \lambda(\nu)$, with equality only when $\boldsymbol{\beta}$ is proportional to $\boldsymbol{\beta}(\nu)$. Estimation proceeds in an obvious way: Given consistent estimates $\widehat{f}_{ij}(\nu)$, for $i, j = 1, 2$, put

$$\widehat{f}_{ss}^{re}(\nu) = [\widehat{f}_{12}^{re}(\nu) + \widehat{f}_{21}^{re}(\nu)]/2 \quad \text{and} \quad \widehat{f}_{ss}^{re}(\nu) + \widehat{f}_{ee}^{re}(\nu) = [\widehat{f}_{11}^{re}(\nu) + \widehat{f}_{22}^{re}(\nu)]/2. \tag{5.216}$$

A frequency-based test for a common signal in the scaled sequences $x_{1t}(\boldsymbol{\beta})$ and $x_{2t}(\boldsymbol{\beta})$ is described in Stoffer and Tyler (1998), the null hypothesis being that $f_{ss}(\nu) = 0$. The basic requirement is that we smooth the periodograms by simple averaging; that is, the weights in (5.150) are all equal to $1/L$. In this case it was shown that the estimated coherence based on (5.216) is (we use a bar over the estimates to indicate simple averaging):

$$\overline{\rho}_{12}(\nu_j;\boldsymbol{\beta}) = \frac{\boldsymbol{\beta}'\overline{f}_{ss}^{re}(\nu_j)\boldsymbol{\beta}}{\boldsymbol{\beta}'\overline{f}_{ss}^{re}(\nu_j)\boldsymbol{\beta} + \boldsymbol{\beta}'\overline{f}_{ee}^{re}(\nu_j)\boldsymbol{\beta}} = \frac{F(\nu_j;\boldsymbol{\beta}) - 1}{F(\nu_j;\boldsymbol{\beta}) + 1}, \tag{5.217}$$

provided $\overline{\rho}_{12}(\nu_j;\boldsymbol{\beta}) \neq 1$. Here, $\nu_j$ is a fundamental frequency, and for a fixed value of $\nu_j$ and $\boldsymbol{\beta}$, $F(\nu_j;\boldsymbol{\beta})$ has an asymptotic ($n \to \infty$) $F$-distribution with $2L$ numerator and denominator df. It follows that the scaling, say, $\overline{\boldsymbol{\beta}}(\nu_j)$, that maximizes (5.217) also maximizes $F(\nu_j;\boldsymbol{\beta})$. Moreover, the maximum value of $F(\nu_j;\boldsymbol{\beta})$, under model (5.211), is $\lambda_F(\nu_j) = [1 + \overline{\lambda}(\nu_j)]/[1 - \overline{\lambda}(\nu_j)]$, where $\overline{\lambda}(\nu_j)$ denotes the sample spectral envelope for this problem based on simple averaging. Note, $\lambda_F(\nu_j) = \sup F(\nu_j;\boldsymbol{\beta})$, over $\boldsymbol{\beta} \neq \mathbf{0}$. Under the assumption $\boldsymbol{y}_{1t}$ and $\boldsymbol{y}_{2t}$ are mixing, the asymptotic ($n \to \infty$) null distribution of $\lambda_F(\nu_j)$ is that of Roy's largest root. Finite-sample null distributions under the additional model assumption that $\boldsymbol{e}_{1t}$ and $\boldsymbol{e}_{2t}$ are both white noise can be obtained by direct simulation. Details can be found in Stoffer and Tyler (1998).

The model can be extended to include the possibility more than one signal is common to each sequence, and the sequences are not necessarily aligned. The ***global model*** is

$$\boldsymbol{y}_{1t} = \boldsymbol{p}_1 + \sum_{j=1}^{q} \boldsymbol{s}_{jt} + \boldsymbol{e}_{1t} \quad \text{and} \quad \boldsymbol{y}_{2t} = \boldsymbol{p}_2 + \sum_{j=1}^{q} \boldsymbol{s}_{j,t-\tau_j} + \boldsymbol{e}_{2t}, \tag{5.218}$$

where $\boldsymbol{s}_{jt}$, $j = 1,\ldots, q$, are zero-mean realizations of mutually uncorrelated, stationary, $k \times 1$ vector-valued time series that are uncorrelated with the zero-mean, stationary $k \times 1$ vector-valued series $\boldsymbol{e}_{1t}$ and $\boldsymbol{e}_{2t}$. Furthermore, $\boldsymbol{s}_{jt}$ has $k \times k$ spectral density matrix $f_{s_j}(\nu)$, $j = 1,\ldots, q$, and $\boldsymbol{e}_{it}$, $i = 1, 2$, have common $k \times k$ spectra denoted by $f_{ee}(\nu)$. It is hypothesized that the processes $\boldsymbol{s}_{jt}$ are (stochastic) signals that are common to both time series $x_{1t}$ and $x_{2t}$, or equivalently, $\boldsymbol{y}_{1t}$ and $\boldsymbol{y}_{2t}$.

There is no need to specify the phase shifts, $\tau_1,\ldots,\tau_q$, or the integer $q \geq 0$, however, the problem of their estimation is interesting. We consider the following method to help decide whether $q = 0$. Using the notation established in this section,

$$f_{11}(\nu) = f_{22}(\nu) = \sum_{j=1}^{q} f_{s_j}(\nu) + f_{ee}(\nu) \tag{5.219}$$

and

$$f_{12}(\nu) = \sum_{j=1}^{q} f_{s_j}(\nu)\exp(2\pi i\nu\tau_j). \tag{5.220}$$

Let $\boldsymbol{\beta} = (\beta_1, ..., \beta_k)' \in \mathbf{R}^k$, $\boldsymbol{\beta} \neq 0$, be a vector of scalings, and write $x_{it}(\boldsymbol{\beta}) = \boldsymbol{\beta}' \boldsymbol{y}_{it}$, for $i = 1, 2$, so the squared coherency between $x_{1t}(\boldsymbol{\beta})$ and $x_{2t}(\boldsymbol{\beta})$ is

$$\rho_{12}^2(\nu; \boldsymbol{\beta}) = \frac{\left| \sum_{j=1}^{q} \boldsymbol{\beta}' f_{s_j}^{re}(\nu) \boldsymbol{\beta} \, \exp(2\pi i \nu \tau_j) \right|^2}{\left| \boldsymbol{\beta}' f^{re}(\nu) \boldsymbol{\beta} \right|^2}, \tag{5.221}$$

where $f(\nu) = f_{11}(\nu) = f_{22}(\nu)$. Setting $\boldsymbol{b} = f^{re}(\nu)^{1/2} \boldsymbol{\beta}$, with the constraint $\boldsymbol{b}'\boldsymbol{b} = 1$, write (5.221) as

$$\rho_{12}^2(\nu; \boldsymbol{b}) = \left| \boldsymbol{b}' \left\{ \sum_{j=1}^{q} f^{re}(\nu)^{-1/2} f_{s_j}^{re}(\nu) f^{re}(\nu)^{-1/2} \exp(2\pi i \nu \tau_j) \right\} \boldsymbol{b} \right|^2. \tag{5.222}$$

Define the complex-valued matrix $Q(\nu)$ as

$$Q(\nu) = \sum_{j=1}^{q} f^{re}(\nu)^{-1/2} f_{s_j}^{re}(\nu) f^{re}(\nu)^{-1/2} \exp(2\pi i \nu \tau_j) = Q^{re}(\nu) + i\, Q^{im}(\nu), \tag{5.223}$$

and note both $Q^{re}(\nu)$ and $Q^{im}(\nu)$ are symmetric matrices (but not necessarily positive definite). As noted in Property 5.2, *the optimal strategy is to select the scalings to be the same for both sequences.* Now, write (5.222) as

$$\rho_{12}^2(\nu; \boldsymbol{b}) = [\boldsymbol{b}' Q^{re}(\nu) \boldsymbol{b}]^2 + [\boldsymbol{b}' Q^{im}(\nu) \boldsymbol{b}]^2. \tag{5.224}$$

Given consistent spectral estimates $\widehat{f}_{ij}(\nu)$, we can estimate $f(\nu)$ by $\widehat{f}(\nu) = \frac{1}{2}[\widehat{f}_{11}(\nu) + \widehat{f}_{22}(\nu)]$ so consistent estimates of $Q^{re}(\nu)$ and $Q^{im}(\nu)$ are, respectively,

$$\widehat{Q}^{re}(\nu) = [\widehat{f}_{11}^{re}(\nu) + \widehat{f}_{22}^{re}(\nu)]^{-1/2} \, [\widehat{f}_{12}^{re}(\nu) + \widehat{f}_{21}^{re}(\nu)] \, [\widehat{f}_{11}^{re}(\nu) + \widehat{f}_{22}^{re}(\nu)]^{-1/2}, \tag{5.225}$$

$$\widehat{Q}^{im}(\nu) = [\widehat{f}_{11}^{re}(\nu) + \widehat{f}_{22}^{re}(\nu)]^{-1/2} \, [\widehat{f}_{12}^{im}(\nu) - \widehat{f}_{21}^{im}(\nu)] \, [\widehat{f}_{11}^{re}(\nu) + \widehat{f}_{22}^{re}(\nu)]^{-1/2}. \tag{5.226}$$

The estimated squared coherency can be maximized via Property 5.2 with $Q^{re}(\nu)$ and $Q^{im}(\nu)$ in (5.224) replaced by their estimates (5.225) and (5.226), respectively. In particular, the recursion (5.210) with $Q_s^{re}(\nu)$ and $Q_s^{im}(\nu)$ replaced by (5.225) and (5.226) can be employed. The estimated optimal scaling vector at any particular frequency, $\widehat{\boldsymbol{\beta}}(\nu)$, is taken proportional to $\widehat{f}^{re}(\nu)^{-1/2} \widehat{\boldsymbol{b}}(\nu)$, where $\widehat{\boldsymbol{b}}(\nu)$ is the maximizing vector. Some discussion of the finite sample null behavior in this case is given in Stoffer and Tyler (1998).

### Example 5.21 Matching DNA Sequences

In Example 5.18, we saw a rather strange result about the gene BNRF1 of the Epstein–Barr virus (EBV). There, it was found that, although a cycle of 1/3 could be found in most of the gene, the last 1000 bp

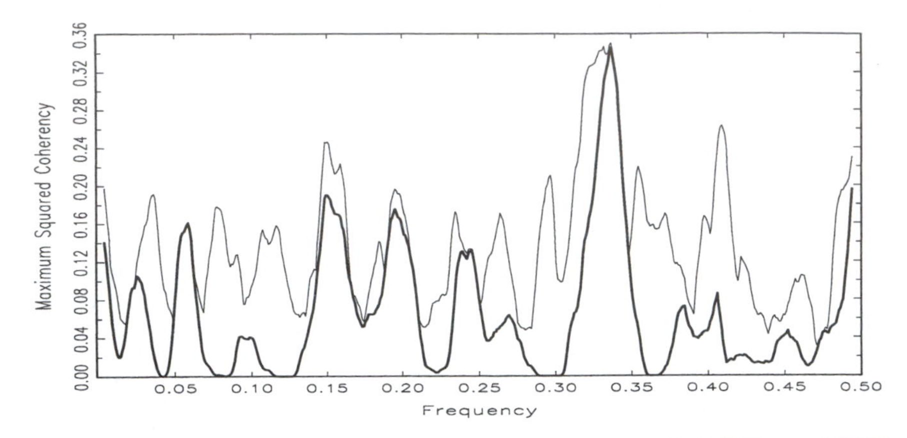


**Figure 5.30:** Maximum squared coherency between EBV-BNRF1 and HVS-BNRF1 using two models, the local model [thick line], (5.211), and the global model [thin line], (5.218).

appeared to contain no cyclic behavior and might be considered to be non-coding; see Figures 5.22 and 5.23. Herpesvirus saimiri (HVS) also contains a gene labeled BNRF1 because similarities between the two have been noted by molecular biologists. The spectral envelope of the entire HVS–BNRF1 gene looks similar to Figure 5.22, but, unlike Figure 5.23, HVS–BNRF1 has considerable power at frequency 1/3 in the final 1000 bp. It is of interest to know if the two genes match in the final 1000 bp, even though no evidence exists that the last part of EBV–BNRF1 is actually coding. Figure 5.30 shows the maximum squared coherency using two models, the local model [thick line], (5.211), and the global model [thin line], (5.218). Because the local model is contained in the global model, it will always be the case that the result from the global model will envelope the result from the local fit assuming the spectra are estimated in the same way (that is, in Figure 5.30, the thick line is never above the thin line). In both cases, triangular smoothing with $L = 31$ was used. The two methods are in agreement, but the evidence that the series match at $\nu = 1/3$ appears stronger in the local case. In fact, a significant peak occurs at $\nu = 1/3$ based on the 1% level-of-significance when using the maximum $F$-statistic approach—this is detailed in Stoffer and Tyler, 1998. Thus, using the local model, we are lead to conclude there is a significant match between the two genes in the final 1000 bp. The estimated optimal common scaling at $\nu = 1/3$ for the local model was $\texttt{A} = 59.4, \texttt{C} = 0.8, \texttt{G} = 64.9, \texttt{T} = 0$ (the global model had $\texttt{A} = 60.8, \texttt{C} = 5.6, \texttt{G} = 67.1, \texttt{T} = 0$), which indicates the match is in the purine–pyrimidine ($\texttt{A} = \texttt{G}$, $\texttt{C} = \texttt{T}$) alphabet.

## 5.10 Dynamic Fourier Analysis and Wavelets

If a time series, $x_t$, is stationary, its second-order behavior remains the same, regardless of the time $t$. It makes sense to match a stationary time series with sines and cosines because, they too, behave the same forever. Indeed, based on the Spectral Representation Theorem (see Section T3.11), we may regard a stationary series as the superposition of sines and cosines that oscillate at various frequencies. As seen in this text, however, many time series are not stationary. Typically, the data are coerced into stationarity via transformations, or we restrict attention to parts of the data where stationarity appears to adhere. In some cases, the nonstationarity of a time series is of interest. That is to say, it is the local behavior of the process, and not the global behavior of the process, that is of concern to the investigator. As a case in point, we mention the explosion and earthquake series first presented in Example 1.6 (see Figure 1.6) and subsequently analyzed using Fourier methods in Chapter 3, Example 3.14. The following example emphasizes the importance of dynamic (or time-frequency) Fourier analysis.

**Example 5.22 Dynamic Fourier Analysis of the Explosion and Earthquake series**

Consider the earthquake and explosion series displayed in Figure 1.6. As a summary of the behavior of these series, the estimated spectra of the P and S waves in Example 3.14 leave a lot to be desired. Figures 5.31 and 5.32 show the time-frequency analysis of the earthquake and explosion series, respectively. First, a Fourier analysis is performed on a short section of the data. Then, the section is shifted, and a Fourier analysis is performed on the new section. This process is repeated until the end of the data, and the results are plotted as in Figures 5.31 and 5.32. Specifically, in this example, let $x_t$, for $t = 1, ..., 2048$, represent the series of interest. Then, the sections of the data that were analyzed were $\{x_{t_k+1}, ...., x_{t_k+256}\}$, for $t_k = 128k$, and $k = 0, 1, ..., 14$. Each section was tapered using a cosine bell, and spectral estimation was performed using a triangular set of $L = 5$ weights. The sections overlap each other.

The results of the dynamic analysis are shown as the estimated spectra (for frequencies up to $\nu = .25$) for each starting location (time), $t_k = 128k$, with $k = 0, 1, ..., 14$. The S component for the earthquake shows power at the low frequencies only, and the power remains strong for a long time. In contrast, the explosion shows power at higher frequencies than the earthquake, and the power of the signals (P and S wave) do not last as long as in the case of the earthquake.

One way to view the time-frequency analysis of Example 5.22 is to consider

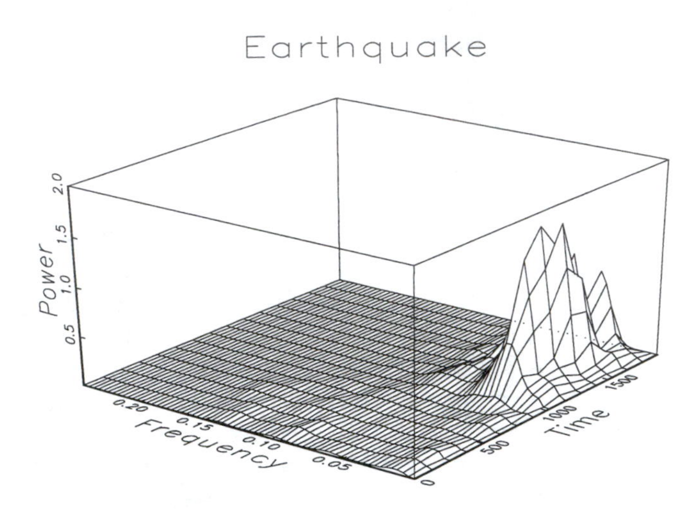


**Figure 5.31:** Time-frequency plot for the dynamic Fourier analysis of the earthquake series shown in Figure 1.6.

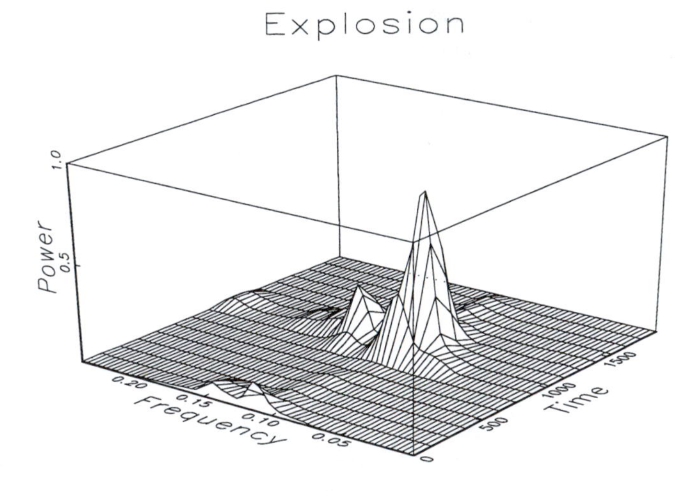


**Figure 5.32:** Time-frequency plot for the dynamic Fourier analysis of the explosion series shown in Figure 1.6.

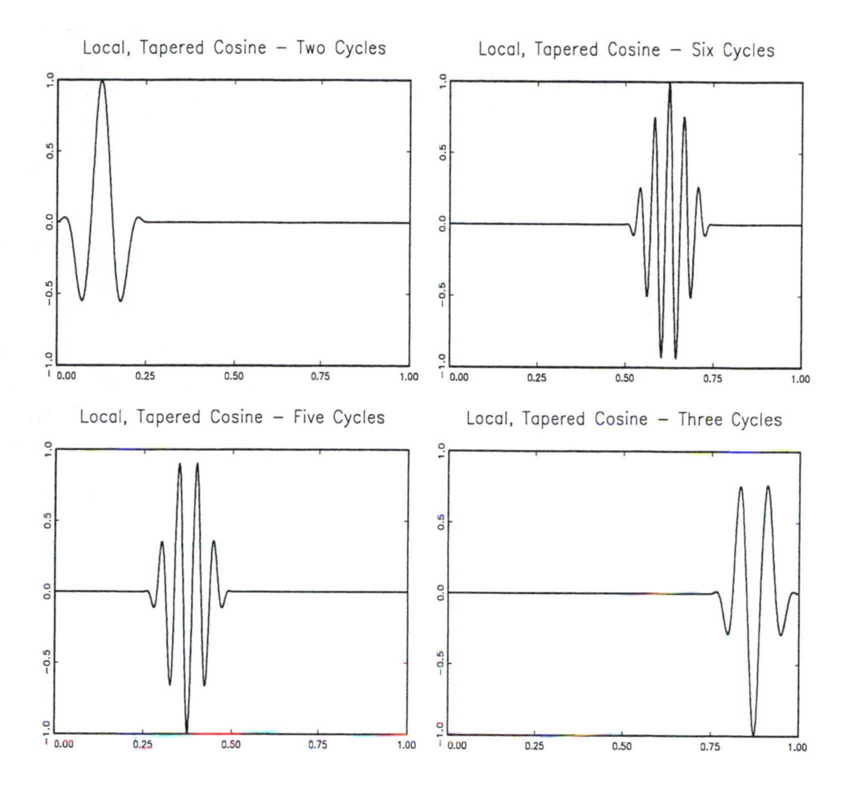


**Figure 5.33:** Local, tapered cosines at various frequencies.

it as being based on local transforms of the data $x_t$ of the form

$$d_{j,k} = n^{-1/2} \sum_{t=1}^{n} x_t \psi_{j,k}(t), \tag{5.227}$$

where

$$\psi_{j,k}(t) = \begin{cases} (n/m)^{1/2} h_t \exp(-2\pi i t j/m), & t \in [t_k + 1, t_k + m], \\ 0, & \text{otherwise}, \end{cases} \tag{5.228}$$

where $h_t$ is a taper and $m$ is some fraction of $n$. In Example 5.22, $n = 2048$, $m = 256$, $t_k = 128k$, for $k = 0, 1, ..., 14$, and $h_t$ was a cosine bell taper over 256 points. In (5.227) and (5.228), $j$ indexes frequency, $\nu_j = j/m$, for $j = 1, 2, ..., [m/2]$, and $k$ indexes the location, or time shift, of the transform. In this case, the transforms are based on tapered cosines and sines that have been zeroed out over various regions in time. The key point here is that the transforms are based on *local* sinusoids. Figure 5.33 shows an example of four local, tapered cosine functions at various frequencies. In that figure, the length of the data is considered to be one, and the cosines are localized to a fourth of the data length.

In addition to dynamic Fourier analysis as a method to overcome the restriction of stationarity, researchers have sought various alternative methods. A recent, and successful, alternative is ***wavelet analysis***. A website `http://www.wavelet.org` is devoted to wavelets, which includes a monthly newsletter, information about books, technical papers, software, and links to other sites. Because the field is a rapidly changing one, the web site is a good source for current information. In addition, we mention the monograph on wavelets by Daubechies (1992), and note that many statistical software manufacturers have wavelet modules that sit on top of their base package. In this section, we rely on the S-plus wavelets module (with a manual written by Bruce and Gao, 1996). The basic idea of wavelet analysis is to imitate dynamic Fourier analysis, but with functions (wavelets) that may be better suited to capture the local behavior of nonstationary time series.

Wavelets come in families generated by a ***father*** wavelet, $\phi$, and a ***mother*** wavelet, $\psi$. The father wavelets are used to capture the smooth, low-frequency nature of the data, whereas the mother wavelets are used to capture the detailed, and high-frequency nature of the data. The father wavelet integrates to one, and the mother wavelet integrates to zero

$$\int \phi(t)dt = 1 \quad \text{and} \quad \int \psi(t)dt = 0. \tag{5.229}$$

For a simple example, consider the Haar function,

$$\psi(t) = \begin{cases} 1, & 0 \le t < 1/2, \\ -1, & 1/2 \le t < 1, \\ 0, & \text{otherwise.} \end{cases} \tag{5.230}$$

The father in this case is $\phi(t) = 1$ for $t \in [0, 1)$ and zero otherwise. The Haar functions are useful for demonstrating properties of wavelets, but they do not have good time-frequency localization properties. Figure 5.34 displays two of the more commonly used wavelets that are available with the S-plus wavelets module, the ***daublet4*** and ***symmlet8*** wavelets, which are described in Daubechies (1992). The number after the name refers to the width and smoothness of the wavelet; for example, the symmlet10 wavelet is wider and smoother than the symmlet8 wavelet. Daublets are one of the first type of continuous orthogonal wavelets with compact support, and symmlets were constructed to be closer to symmetry than daublets. In general, wavelets do not have an analytical form, but instead they are generated using numerical methods.

When we depart from periodic functions, such as sines and cosines, the precise meaning of frequency, or cycles per unit time, is lost. When using

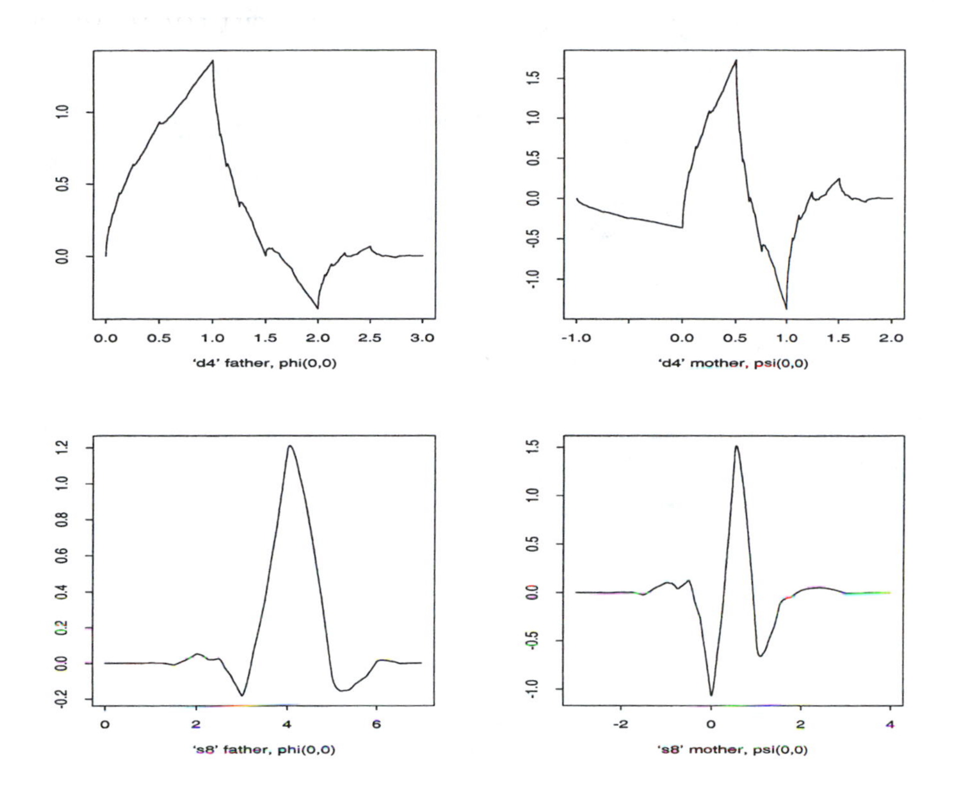


**Figure 5.34:** Father and mother daublet4 wavelets (top row); father and mother symmlet8 wavelets (bottom row).

wavelets, we typically refer to ***scale*** rather than frequency. The orthogonal wavelet decomposition of a time series, $x_t$, for $t = 1, ..., n$ is

$$\begin{aligned} x_t &= \sum_k s_{J,k}\phi_{J,k}(t) + \sum_k d_{J,k}\psi_{J,k}(t) \\ &\quad + \sum_k d_{J-1,k}\psi_{J-1,k}(t) + \cdots + \sum_k d_{1,k}\psi_{1,k}(t), \end{aligned} \tag{5.231}$$

where $J$ is the number of scales, and $k$ ranges from one to the number of coefficients associated with the specified component (see Example 5.23). In (5.231), the wavelet functions $\phi_{J,k}(t), \psi_{J,k}(t), \psi_{J-1,k}(t), ..., \psi_{1,k}(t)$ are generated from the father wavelet, $\phi(t)$, and the mother wavelet, $\psi(t)$, by ***translation*** (shift) and ***scaling***:

$$\phi_{J,k}(t) = 2^{-J/2}\phi\left(\frac{t - 2^J k}{2^J}\right), \tag{5.232}$$

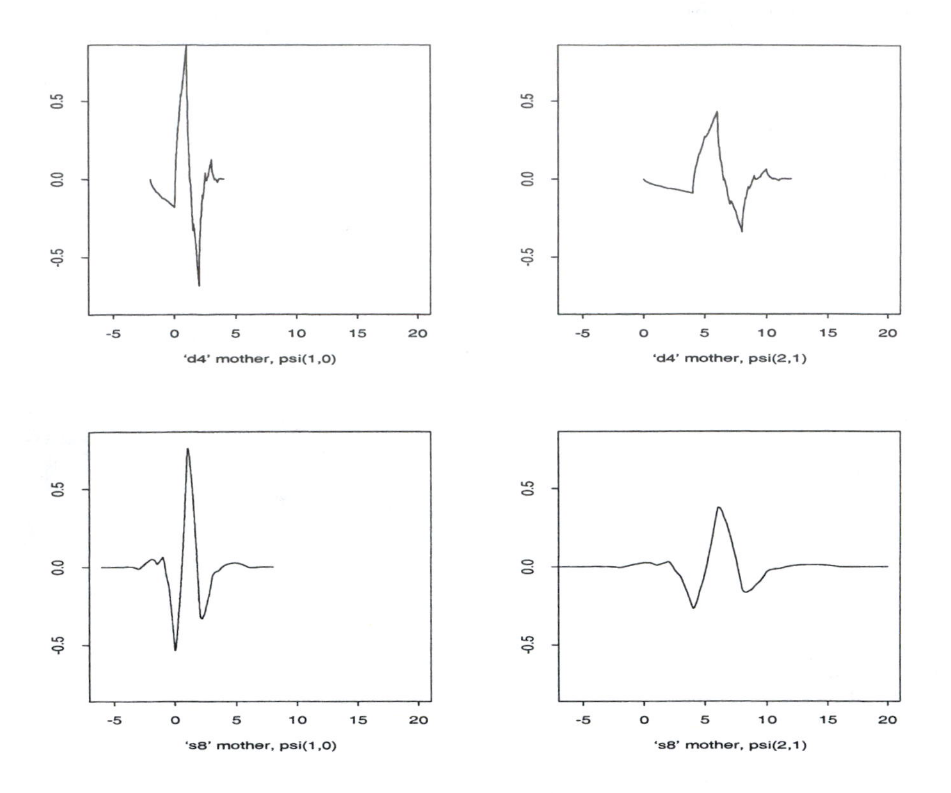


**Figure 5.35:** Scaled and translated daublet4 wavelets, $\psi_{1,0}(t)$ and $\psi_{2,1}(t)$ (top row); scaled and translated symmlet8 wavelets, $\psi_{1,0}(t)$ and $\psi_{2,1}(t)$ (bottom row).

$$\psi_{j,k}(t) \quad = \quad 2^{-j/2}\psi\left(\frac{t-2^jk}{2^j}\right), \quad j=1,...,J. \tag{5.233}$$

The choice of dyadic shifts and scales is arbitrary but convenient. The shift or ***translation parameter*** is $2^jk$, and ***scale parameter*** is $2^j$. The wavelet functions are spread out and shorter for larger values of $j$ (or scale parameter $2^j$) and tall and narrow for small values of the scale. Figure 5.35 shows $\psi_{1,0}(t)$ and $\psi_{2,1}(t)$ generated from the daublet4 (top row), and the symmlet8 (bottom row) mother wavelets. We may think of $1/2^j$ (or 1/scale) in wavelet analysis as being the analog of frequency ($\nu_j = j/n$) in Fourier analysis. For example, when $j=1$, the scale parameter of two is akin to the Nyquist frequency of 1/2, and when $j=6$, the scale parameter of $2^6$ is akin to a low frequency ($1/2^6 \approx 0.016$). In other words, larger values of the scale refer to slower, smoother (or coarser) movements of the signal, and smaller values of the scale refer to faster, choppier (or finer) movements of the signal.

The ***discrete wavelet transform (DWT)*** of the data $x_t$ are the coefficients $s_{J,k}$ and $d_{j,k}$ for $j = J, J-1, ..., 1$, in (5.231). They are given by

$$s_{J,k} = n^{-1/2} \sum_{t=1}^{n} x_t \phi_{J,k}(t), \tag{5.234}$$

$$d_{j,k} = n^{-1/2} \sum_{t=1}^{n} x_t \psi_{j,k}(t) \quad j = J, J-1, ..., 1. \tag{5.235}$$

It is the magnitudes of the coefficients that measure the importance of the corresponding wavelet term in describing the behavior of $x_t$. As in Fourier analysis, the DWT is not computed as shown, but is calculated using a fast algorithm. The $s_{J,k}$ are called the ***smooth*** coefficients because they represent the smooth behavior of the data. The $d_{j,k}$ are called the ***detail*** coefficients because they tend to represent the finer, more high-frequency nature, of the data.

**Example 5.23 Wavelet Analysis of the Explosion and Earthquake Series**

Figures 5.36 and 5.37 show the DWTs, based on the symmlet8 wavelet basis, for the earthquake and explosion series, respectively. Each series is of length $n = 2^{11} = 2048$, and in this example, the DWTs are calculated using $J = 6$ levels. In this case, $n/2 = 2^{10} = 1024$ values are in $d1 = \{d_{1,k};\ k = 1, ..., 2^{10}\}$, $n/2^2 = 2^9 = 512$ values are in $d2 = \{d_{2,k};\ k = 1, ..., 2^9\}$, and so on, until finally, $n/2^6 = 2^5 = 32$ values are in $d6$ and in $s6$. The detail values $d_{1,k}, ..., d_{6,k}$ are plotted at the same scale, and hence, the relative importance of each value can be seen from the graph. The smooth values $s_{6,k}$ are typically larger than the detail values and plotted on a different scale. The top of Figures 5.36 and 5.37 show the inverse DWT (IDWT) computed from all of the coefficients. Because $2^{10} + 2^9 + 2^8 + 2^7 + 2^6 + 2^5 + 2^5 = 2^{11}$ values are in the DWT, the IDWT reproduces the data.

Comparing the DWTs, the earthquake is best represented by wavelets with larger scale than the explosion. One way to measure the importance of each level, $d1, d2, ..., d6, s6$, is to evaluate the proportion of the total power (or energy) explained by each. The total power of a time series $x_t$, for $t = 1, ..., n$, is $TP = \sum_{t=1}^{n} x_t^2$. The total power associated with each level of scale is (recall $n = 2^{11}$),

$$TP_6^s = \sum_{k=1}^{n/2^6} s_{6,k}^2 \quad \text{and} \quad TP_j^d = \sum_{k=1}^{n/2^j} d_{j,k}^2, \quad j = 1, ..., 6.$$

Because we are working with an orthogonal basis, we have

$$TP = TP_6^s + \sum_{j=1}^{6} TP_j^d,$$

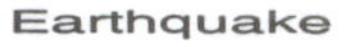


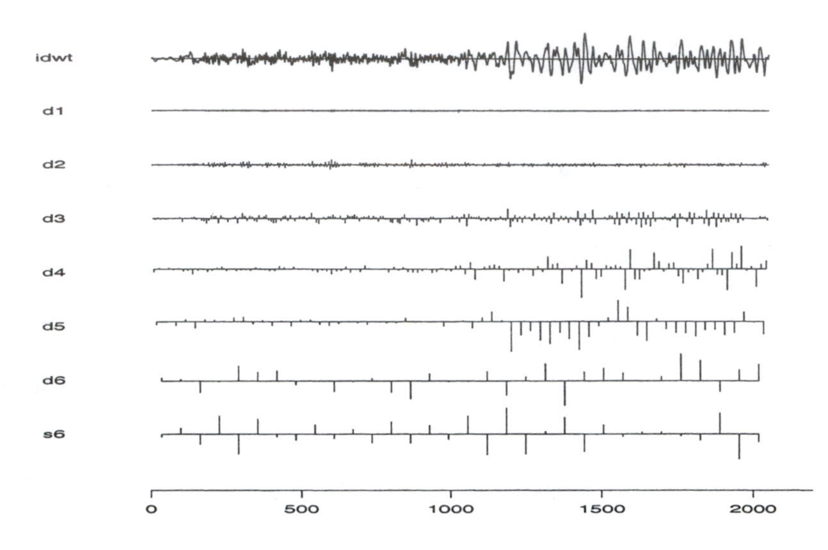


**Figure 5.36:** Discrete wavelet transform of the earthquake series using the symmlet8 wavelets, and $J = 6$ levels of scale.

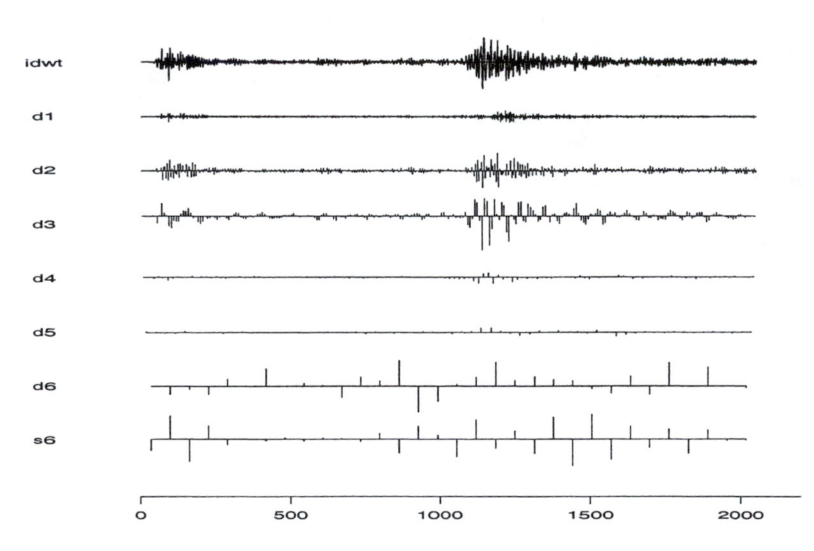


**Figure 5.37:** Discrete wavelet transform of the explosion series using the symmlet8 wavelets, and $J = 6$ levels of scale.

**Table 5.12:** Fraction of the Total Power for the DWTs of the Earthquake and the Explosion

| Component | Earthquake | Explosion |
|---|---|---|
| s6 | 0.009 | 0.002 |
| d6 | 0.043 | 0.002 |
| d5 | 0.377 | 0.007 |
| d4 | 0.367 | 0.015 |
| d3 | 0.160 | 0.559 |
| d2 | 0.040 | 0.349 |
| d1 | 0.003 | 0.066 |

and the proportion of the total power explained by each level of detail would be the ratios $TP_j^d/TP$ for $j = 1, ..., 6$, and for the smooth level, it would be $TP^s/TP$. These values are listed in Table 5.12. From that table nearly 80% of the total power of the earthquake series is explained by the higher scale details $d4$ and $d5$, whereas 90% of the total power is explained by the smaller scale details $d2$ and $d3$ for the explosion.

Figures 5.38 and 5.39 show the time-scale plots based on the DWT, of the earthquake series and the explosion series, respectively. These figures are the wavelet analog of the time-frequency plots shown in Figures 5.31 and 5.32. The power axis represents the magnitude of each value $d_{jk}$ or $s_{6,k}$. The time axis matches the time axis in the DWTs shown in Figures 5.36 and 5.37, and the scale axis is plotted as 1/scale, listed from the coarsest scale to the finest scale. On the 1/scale axis, the coarsest scale values, represented by the smooth coefficients $s6$, are plotted over the range $[0, 2^{-6})$, the coarsest detail values, $d6$, are plotted over $[2^{-6}, 2^{-5})$, and so on. In these figures, we did not plot the finest scale values, $d1$, so the finest scale values exhibited in Figures 5.38 and 5.39 are in $d2$, which are plotted over the range $[2^{-2}, 2^{-1})$.

The conclusions drawn from these plots are the same as those drawn from Figures 5.31 and 5.32. That is, the S wave for the earthquake shows power at the high scales (or low 1/scale) only, and the power remains strong for a long time. In contrast, the explosion shows power at smaller scales (or higher 1/scale) than the earthquake, and the power of the signals (P and S wave) do not last as long as in the case of the earthquake.

Wavelets can be used to perform nonparametric smoothing along the lines first discussed in Chapter 1, Section 1.8, but with an emphasis on localized behavior. Although a considerable amount of literature exists on this topic, we will present the basic ideas. For further information, we refer the reader to Donoho and Johnstone (1994, 1995). As in Section 1.8, we suppose the data

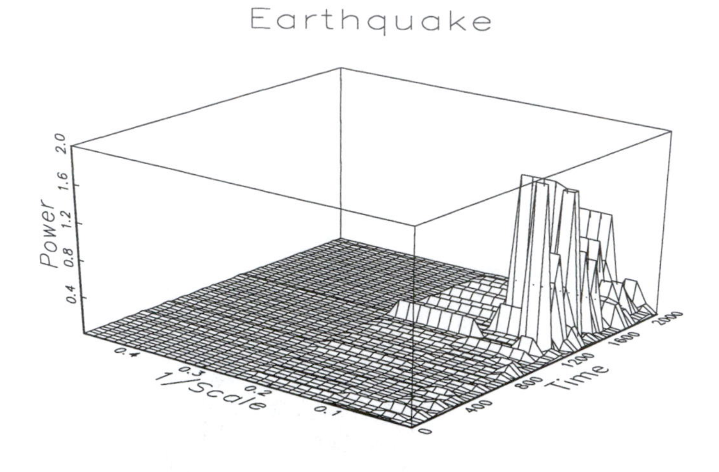


**Figure 5.38:** Time-scale plot of the earthquake series.

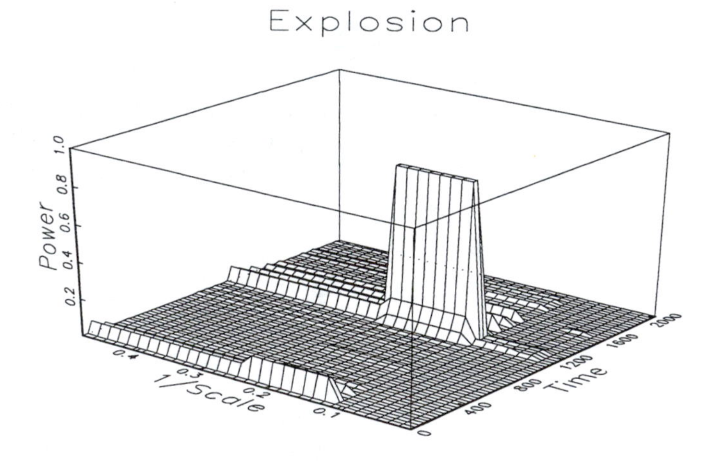


**Figure 5.39:** Time-scale plot of the explosion series.

$x_t$ can be written in terms of a signal plus noise model as

$$x_t = s_t + \epsilon_t. \tag{5.236}$$

The goal here is to remove the noise from the data, and obtain an estimate of the signal, $s_t$, without having to specify a parametric form of the signal. The technique based on wavelets is referred to as ***waveshrink***.

The basic idea behind waveshrink is to shrink the wavelet coefficients in the DWT of $x_t$ toward zero in an attempt to denoise the data, and then to estimate the signal via (5.231) with the new coefficients. One obvious way to shrink the coefficients toward zero is to simply zero out any coefficient smaller in magnitude than some predetermined value, $\lambda$. Such a shrinkage rule is discontinuous, and sometimes it is preferable to use a continuous shrinkage function. One such method, termed ***soft shrinkage*** proceeds as follows. If the value of a coefficient is $a$, we set that coefficient to zero if $|a| \leq \lambda$, and to $\text{sign}(a)(|a| - \lambda)$ if $|a| > \lambda$. The choice of a shrinkage method is based on the goal of the signal extraction. This process entails choosing a value for the shrinkage threshold, $\lambda$, and we may wish to use a different threshold value, say, $\lambda_j$, for each level of scale $j = 1, ..., J$. One particular method that works well if we are interested in a relatively high degree of smoothness in the estimate is to choose $\lambda = \sqrt{2\log(n)}$ for all scale levels. For other thresholding techniques or for a better understanding of waveshrink, see Donoho and Johnstone (1994, 1995), or the S-plus wavelets module manual (Bruce and Gao, 1996, Chapter 6).

**Example 5.24 Waveshrink Analysis of the Explosion and Earthquake Series**

Figure 5.40 shows the results of a waveshrink analysis on the earthquake and explosion series. In this example, soft shrinkage was used with a universal threshold of $\lambda = \sqrt{2\log(n)}$. Figure 5.40 displays the data $x_t$, the estimated signal $\widehat{s}_t$, as well as the residuals $x_t - \widehat{s}_t$. According to this analysis, the earthquake is mostly signal and characterized by prolonged energy, whereas the explosion is comprised of short bursts of energy.

**Example 5.25 The Event at Novaya Zemlya**

In this example, we focus on a wavelet analysis of the event of unknown origin at Novaya Zemlya. The P and S components are displayed in Figure 5.3. Figure 5.41 shows the DWT of the series, and it resembles the DWT of the explosion series shown in Figure 5.37 more than the DWT of the earthquake series shown in Figure 5.36. Table 5.13 lists the power distribution, and like the explosion series, nearly 90% of the total power is explained at the smaller scale details, $d2$ and $d3$. Figure 5.42 shows the time-scale plot for the event, and Figure 5.43 shows the waveshrink estimate of the signal using the universal threshold $\lambda = \sqrt{2\log(n)}$ and

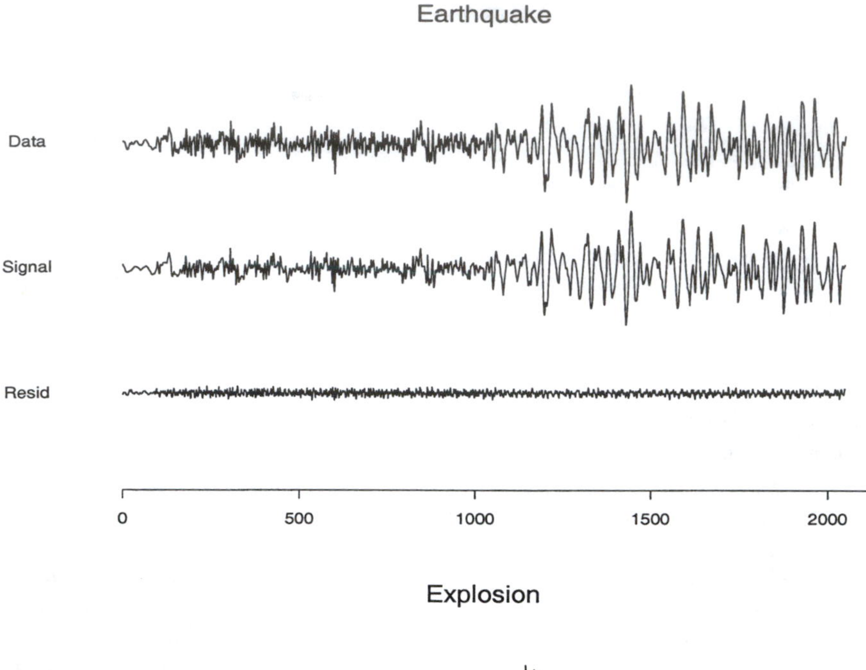


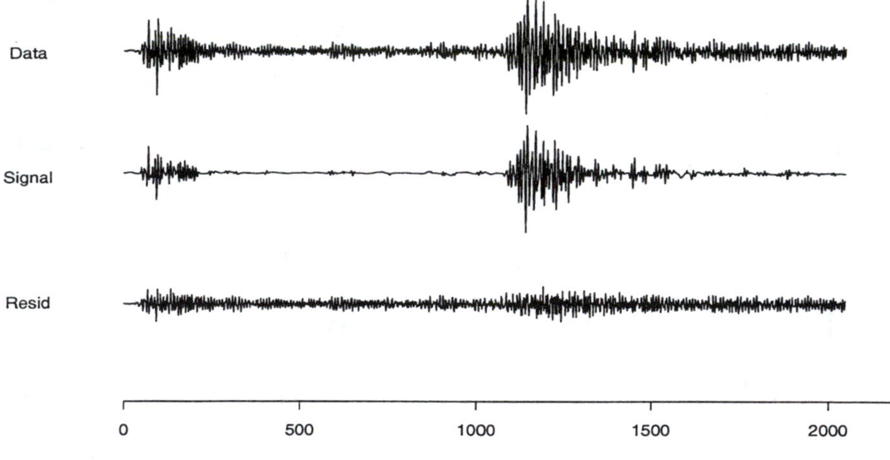


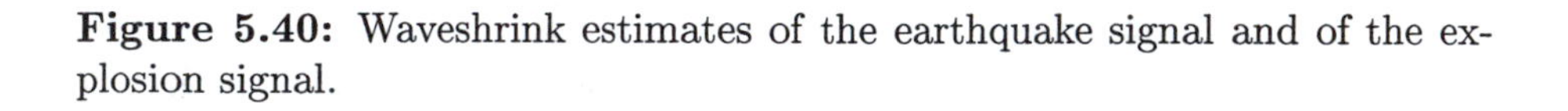

**Figure 5.40:** Waveshrink estimates of the earthquake signal and of the explosion signal.

soft shrinkage. In each case, we note again the similarity to the corresponding exhibits of the explosion series. This event, however, appears to be like many little explosions rather than one big explosion.

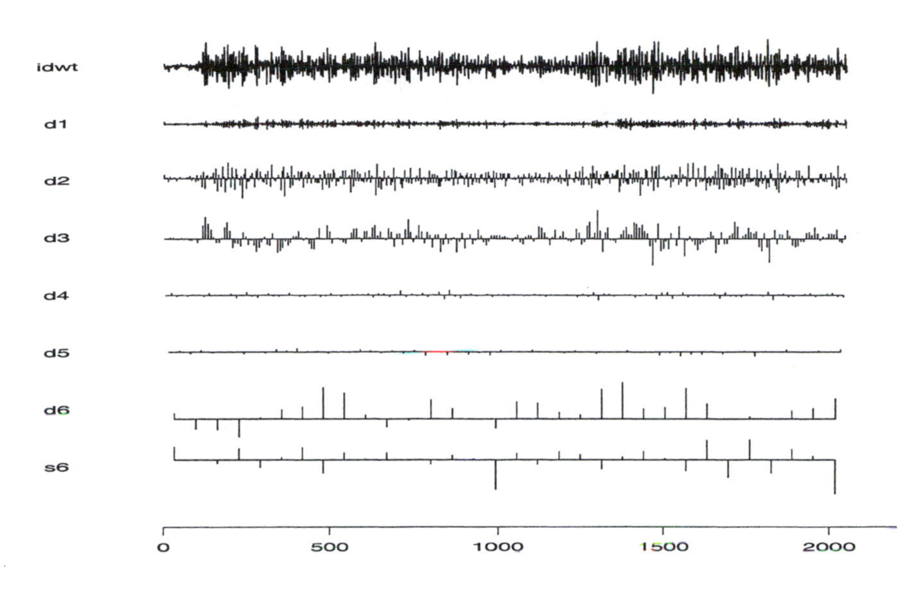


**Figure 5.41:** Discrete wavelet transform of the Novaya Zemlya series using the symmlet8 wavelets, and $J = 6$ levels of scale.

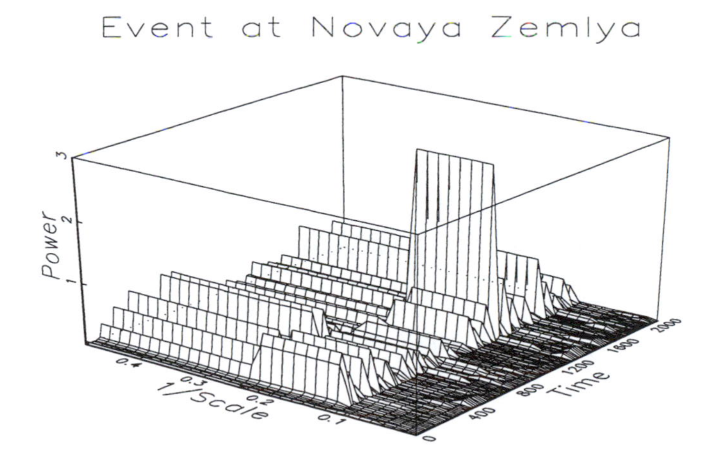


**Figure 5.42:** Time-scale plot of the Novaya Zemlya series.

**Table 5.13:** Fraction of the Total Power for the DWTs of the Event at Novaya Zemlya

| Component | NZ Event |
|---|---|
| s6 | 0.000 |
| d6 | 0.004 |
| d5 | 0.005 |
| d4 | 0.009 |
| d3 | 0.386 |
| d2 | 0.493 |
| d1 | 0.102 |

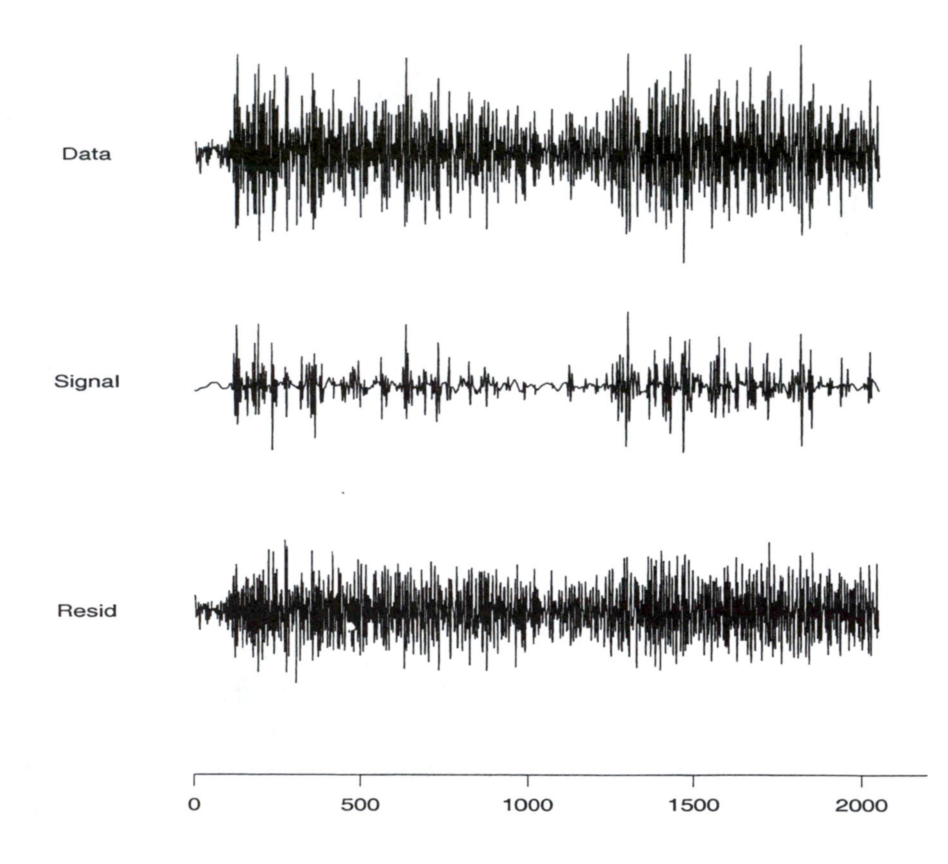


**Figure 5.43:** Waveshrink estimate of the Novaya Zemlya signal.

# Problems

*Section 5.2*

**5.1** Consider the complex Gaussian distribution for the random variable $\boldsymbol{X} = \boldsymbol{X}_c - i\boldsymbol{X}_s$, as defined in (5.1)-(5.3), where the argument $\nu_k$ has been suppressed. Now, the $2p \times 1$ real random variable $\boldsymbol{Z} = (\boldsymbol{X}'_c, \boldsymbol{X}'_s)'$ has a multivariate normal distribution with density

$$p(\boldsymbol{Z}) = (2\pi)^{-p}|\Sigma|^{-1/2} \exp\left\{-\frac{1}{2}(\boldsymbol{Z}-\boldsymbol{\mu})'\Sigma^{-1}(\boldsymbol{Z}-\boldsymbol{\mu})\right\},$$

where $\boldsymbol{\mu} = (\boldsymbol{M}'_c, \boldsymbol{M}'_s)'$ is the mean vector. Prove

$$|\Sigma| = \left(\frac{1}{2}\right)^{2p} |C - iQ|^2,$$

using the result that the eigenvectors and eigenvalues of $\Sigma$ occur in pairs, i.e., $(\boldsymbol{v}'_c, \boldsymbol{v}'_s)'$ and $(\boldsymbol{v}'_s, -\boldsymbol{v}'_c)'$, where $\boldsymbol{v}_c - i\boldsymbol{v}_s$ denotes the eigenvector of $f_x$. Show that

$$\frac{1}{2}(\boldsymbol{Z}-\boldsymbol{\mu})'\Sigma^{-1}(\boldsymbol{Z}-\boldsymbol{\mu})) = (\boldsymbol{X}-\boldsymbol{M})^* f^{-1}(\boldsymbol{X}-\boldsymbol{M})$$

so $p(\boldsymbol{X}) = p(\boldsymbol{Z})$ and we can identify the density of the complex multivariate normal variable $\boldsymbol{X}$ with that of the real multivariate normal $\boldsymbol{Z}$.

**5.2** Prove $\widehat{f}$ in (5.6) maximizes the log likelihood (5.5) by minimizing the negative of the log likelihood

$$L \ln|f| + L \text{ tr } \{\widehat{f} f^{-1}\}$$

in the form

$$L \sum_i \big(\lambda_i - \ln \lambda_i - 1\big) + Lp + L \ln |\widehat{f}|,$$

where the $\lambda_i$ values correspond to the eigenvalues in a simultaneous diagonalization of the matrices $f$ and $\hat{f}$; i.e., there exists a matrix $P$ such that $P^* f P = I$ and $P^* \widehat{f} P = \text{diag}\,(\lambda_1, \ldots, \lambda_p) = \Lambda$. Note, $\lambda_i - \ln \lambda_i - 1 \geq 0$ with equality if and only if $\lambda_i = 1$, implying $\Lambda = I$ maximizes the log likelihood and $f = \widehat{f}$ is the maximimizing value.

*Section 5.3*

**5.3** Verify (5.19) and (5.20) for the mean-squared prediction error MSE in (5.12). Use the orthogonality principle, which implies

$$MSE = E\left[(y_t - \sum_{r=-\infty}^{\infty} \boldsymbol{\beta}'_r \boldsymbol{x}_{t-r}) y_t\right]$$

and gives a set of equations involving the autocovariance functions. Then, use the spectral representations and Fourier transform results to get the final result.

**5.4** Consider the predicted series

$$\widehat{y}_t = \sum_{r=-\infty}^{\infty} \boldsymbol{\beta}_r' \boldsymbol{x}_{t-r},$$

where $\boldsymbol{\beta}_r$ satisfies (5.14). Show the ordinary coherence between $y_t$ and $\widehat{y}_t$ is exactly the multiple coherence (5.21).

**5.5** Consider the complex regression model (5.29) in the form

$$\boldsymbol{Y} = X\mathcal{B} + \boldsymbol{V},$$

where $\boldsymbol{Y} = (Y_1, Y_2, \ldots Y_L)'$ denotes the observed DFTs after they have been re-indexed and $X = (\boldsymbol{X}_1, \boldsymbol{X}_2, \ldots, \boldsymbol{X}_L)'$ is a matrix containing the reindexed input vectors. The model is a complex regression model with $\boldsymbol{Y} = \boldsymbol{Y}_c - i\boldsymbol{Y}_s, X = X_c - iX_s, \mathcal{B} = \mathcal{B}_c - i\mathcal{B}_s$, and $\boldsymbol{V} = \boldsymbol{V}_c - i\boldsymbol{V}_s$ denoting the representation in terms of the usual cosine and sine transforms. Show the partitioned real regression model involving the $2L \times 1$ vector of cosine and sine transforms, say,

$$\begin{pmatrix} \boldsymbol{Y}_c \\ \boldsymbol{Y}_s \end{pmatrix} = \begin{pmatrix} X_c & -X_s \\ X_s & X_c \end{pmatrix} \begin{pmatrix} \mathcal{B}_c \\ \mathcal{B}_s \end{pmatrix} + \begin{pmatrix} \boldsymbol{V}_c \\ \boldsymbol{V}_s \end{pmatrix},$$

is ***isomorphic*** to the complex regression regression model in the sense that the real and imaginary parts of the complex model appear as components of the vectors in the real regression model. Use the usual regression theory to verify (5.28) holds. For example, writing the real regression model as

$$\boldsymbol{y} = x\boldsymbol{b} + \boldsymbol{v},$$

the isomorphism would imply

$$\begin{aligned} L(\widehat{f}_y - \widehat{f}_{xy}^* \widehat{f}_x^{-1} \widehat{f}_{xy}) &= \boldsymbol{Y}^*\boldsymbol{Y} - \boldsymbol{Y}^* X (X^* X)^{-1} X^* \boldsymbol{Y} \\ &= \boldsymbol{y}'\boldsymbol{y} - \boldsymbol{y}' x (x'x)^{-1} x' \boldsymbol{y}. \end{aligned}$$

*Section 5.4*

**5.6** Consider estimating the function

$$\psi_t = \sum_{r=-\infty}^{\infty} \boldsymbol{a}_r' \boldsymbol{\beta}_{t-r}$$

by a linear filter estimator of the form

$$\widehat{\psi}_t = \sum_{r=-\infty}^{\infty} \boldsymbol{a}_r' \widehat{\boldsymbol{\beta}}_{t-r},$$

where $\widehat{\boldsymbol{\beta}}_t$ is defined by (5.43). Show a sufficient condition for $\widehat{\psi}_t$ to be an unbiased estimator; i.e., $E\ \widehat{\psi}_t = \psi_t$, is

$$H(\nu)Z(\nu) = I$$

for all $\nu$. Similarly, show any other unbiased estimator satisfying the above condition has minimum variance (see Shumway and Dean, 1968), so the estimator given is a best linear unbiased (BLUE) estimator.

**5.7** Consider a linear model with mean value function $\mu_t$ and a signal $\alpha_t$ delayed by an amount $\tau_j$ on each sensor, i.e.

$$y_{jt} = \mu_t + \alpha_{t-\tau_j} + v_{jt}$$

Show the estimators (5.43) for the mean and the signal are the Fourier transforms of

$$\widehat{M}(\nu) = \frac{Y_\cdot(\nu) - \phi(\nu)B_w(\nu)}{(1 - |\phi(\nu)|^2)}$$

and

$$\widehat{A}(\nu) = \frac{B_w((\nu) - \phi^*(\nu)Y_\cdot(\nu)}{(1 - |\phi(\nu)|^2)},$$

where

$$\phi(\nu) = \frac{1}{N}\sum_{j=1}^{N} e^{2\pi\nu\tau_j}$$

and $B_w(\nu)$ is defined in (5.65).

*Section 5.5*

**5.8** Consider the estimator (5.68) as applied in the context of the random coefficient model (5.66). Prove the filter coefficients for the minimum mean square estimator can be determined from (5.69) and the mean square covariance is given by (5.72).

**5.9** For the random coefficient model, verify the expected mean square of the regression power component is

$$\begin{aligned} E[SSR(\nu_k)] &= E[Y^*(\nu_k)Z(\nu_k)S_z^{-1}(\nu_k)Z^*(\nu_k)Y(\nu_k)] \\ &= Lf_\beta(\nu_k)\text{tr}\,\{S_z(\nu_k)\} + Lqf_v(\nu_k). \end{aligned}$$

Recall, the underlying frequency domain model is

$$\boldsymbol{Y}(\nu_k) = Z(\nu_k)\mathcal{B}(\nu_k) + \boldsymbol{V}(\nu_k),$$

where $\mathcal{B}(\nu_k)$ has spectrum $f_\beta(\nu)I_q$ and $\boldsymbol{V}(\nu_k)$ has spectrum $f_v(\nu_k)I_N$ and the two processes are uncorrelated.

*Section 5.6*

**5.10** Suppose we have $I = 2$ groups and the models

$$y_{1jt} = \mu_t + \alpha_{1t} + v_{1jt}$$

for the $j = 1, \ldots, N$ observations in group 1 and

$$y_{2jt} = \mu_t + \alpha_{2t} + v_{2jt}$$

for the $j = 1, \ldots, N$ observations in group 2, with $\alpha_{1t} + \alpha_{2t} = 0$. Suppose we want to test equality of the two group means; i.e.,

$$y_{ijt} = \mu_t + v_{ijt}, \quad i = 1, 2.$$

Derive the residual and error power components corresponding to (5.84) and (5.85) for this particular case.

**5.11** Verify the forms of the linear compounds involving the mean given in (5.91) and (5.92), using (5.89) and (5.90).

**5.12** Show the ratio of the two smoothed spectra in (5.104) has the indicated $F$-distribution when $f_1(\nu) = f_2(\nu)$. When the spectra are not equal, show the variable is proportional to an $F$-distribution, where the proportionality constant depends on the ratio of the spectra.

*Section 5.7*

**5.13** The problem of detecting a signal in noise can be considered using the model

$$x_t = s_t + w_t, \quad t = 1, \ldots, n,$$

for $p_1(\boldsymbol{x})$ when a signal is present and the model

$$x_t = w_t, \quad t = 1, \ldots, n,$$

for $p_2(\boldsymbol{x})$ when no signal is present. Under multivariate normality, we might specialize even further by assuming the vector $\boldsymbol{w} = (w_1, \ldots, w_n)'$ has a multivariate normal distribution with mean $\boldsymbol{0}$ and covariance matrix $\Sigma = \sigma_w^2 I_n$, corresponding to white noise. Assuming the signal vector

$\boldsymbol{s} = (s_1, \ldots, s_n)'$ is fixed and known, show the discriminant function (5.113) becomes the ***matched filter***

$$\frac{1}{\sigma_w^2} \sum_{t=1}^{n} s_t x_t - \frac{1}{2} \left( \frac{S}{N} \right),$$

where

$$\left( \frac{S}{N} \right) = \frac{\sum_{t=1}^{n} s_t^2}{\sigma_w^2}$$

denotes the ***signal-to-noise ratio.*** Give the decision criterion if the prior probabilities are assumed to be the same. Express the false alarm and missed signal probabilities in terms of the multivariate normal cdf and the signal-to-noise ratio.

**5.14** Assume the same additive signal plus noise representations as in the previous problem, except, the signal is now a random process with a zero mean and covariance matrix $\sigma_s^2 I$. Derive the comparable version of (5.116) as a ***quadratic detector***, and characterize its performance under both hypotheses in terms of constant multiples of the $F$-distribution.

*Section 5.8*

**5.15** The data set `ch5fmri.dat` contains data from other stimulus conditions in the fMRI experiment, as discussed in Example 5.14 (one location—Caudate—was left out of the analysis for brevity). Perform principal component analyses on the stimulus conditions (i) awake-heat and (ii) awake-shock, and compare your results to the results of Example 5.14.

**5.16** For this problem, consider the first three earthquake series listed in `eq+exp.dat`.

(a) Estimate and compare the spectral density of the P component and then of the S component for each individual earthquake.

(b) Estimate and compare the squared coherency between the P and S components of each individual earthquake. Comment on the strength of the coherence.

(c) Let $x_{ti}$ be the P component of earthquake $i = 1, 2, 3$, and let $\boldsymbol{x}_t = (x_{t1}, x_{t2}, x_{t3})'$ be the $3 \times 1$ vector of P components. Estimate the spectral density, $\lambda_1(\nu)$, of the first principal component series of $\boldsymbol{x}_t$. Compare this to the corresponding spectra calculated in (a).

(d) Analogous to part (c), let $\boldsymbol{y}_t$ denote the $3 \times 1$ vector series of S components of the first three earthquakes. Repeat the analysis of part (c) on $\boldsymbol{y}_t$.

(e) As described in the paragraph containing equation (5.154), let $u_t(\nu)$ and $v_t(\nu)$ be the first canonical variate series at frequency $\nu$ for $\boldsymbol{x}_t$ and $\boldsymbol{y}_t$ defined in parts (c) and (d), respectively. Recall $u_t(\nu)$ and $v_t(\nu)$ are the complex linear combinations of $\boldsymbol{x}_t$ and $\boldsymbol{y}_t$ having maximum squared coherency at frequency $\nu$. Estimate and graph the squared coherency between $u_t(\nu)$ and $v_t(\nu)$, which was called $\lambda_1^2(\nu)$ in (5.155), versus $\nu$. Compare the results with the individual coherencies computed in part (b).

**5.17** In the factor analysis model (5.159), let $p = 3$, $q = 1$, and

$$\Sigma_x = \begin{bmatrix} 1 & .4 & .9 \\ .4 & 1 & .7 \\ .9 & .7 & 1 \end{bmatrix}.$$

Show there is a unique choice for $\mathcal{B}$ and $D$, but $\delta_3^2 < 0$, so the choice is not valid.

**5.18** Extend the EM algorithm for classical factor analysis, (5.165)-(5.170), to the time series case of maximizing $\ln L\big(\mathcal{B}(\nu_j), D_\epsilon(\nu_j)\big)$ in (5.181). Then, for the data used in Example 5.16, find the approximate maximum likelihood estimates of $\mathcal{B}(\nu_j)$ and $D_\epsilon(\nu_j)$, and, consequently, $\Lambda_t$.

*Section 5.9*

**5.19** Verify, as stated in (5.186), the imaginary part of a $k \times k$ spectral matrix, $f^{im}(\nu)$, is skew symmetric, and then show $\boldsymbol{\beta}' f_y^{im}(\nu)\boldsymbol{\beta} = 0$ for a real $k \times 1$ vector, $\boldsymbol{\beta}$.

**5.20** Repeat the analysis of Example 5.18 on BNRF1 of herpesvirus saimiri (the data file is `bnrf1hvs.dat`), and compare the results with the results obtained for Epstein–Barr.

**5.21** For the NYSE returns, say, $r_t$, analyzed in Chapter 4, Example 4.21:

(a) Estimate the spectrum of the $r_t$. Does the spectral estimate appear to support the hypothesis that the returns are white?

(b) Examine the possibility of spectral power near the zero frequency for a transformation of the returns, say, $g(r_t)$, using the spectral envelope with Example 5.19 as your guide. Compare the optimal transformation near or at the zero frequency with the usual transformation $y_t = r_t^2$.

**5.22** In Example 5.18, we investigated the signal components of the EBV–BNRF1 gene (the data are listed in `bnrf1ebv.dat`). Recall no signal was detected in the final 954 bp of the gene, but in Example 5.21, there was evidence that this section matched with a similar region of HVS–BNRF1.

Does evidence exist that the final 954 bp of EBV–BNRF1 matches with any of the other three sections of 1000 bp of EBV–BNRF1 used in Example 5.18?

**5.23** In addition to the result of Property 5.1 on the maximization of (5.199), we can get tight bounds on the maximum squared coherency. Let $A$ and $B$ be real-valued $k_1 \times k_2$ matrices, and let $\boldsymbol{x}$ and $\boldsymbol{y}$ be real-valued unit length vectors of dimensions $k_1$ and $k_2$, respectively. Define

$$u(\boldsymbol{x}, \boldsymbol{y}) = (\boldsymbol{x}'A\boldsymbol{y})^2 + (\boldsymbol{x}'B\boldsymbol{y})^2,$$

which is precisely the form of (5.199) at any specific frequency. Let $\mathcal{L}_1(\cdot)$ and $\boldsymbol{\mathcal{E}}_1(\cdot)$ denote the largest eigenvalue function and corresponding eigenvector function, respectively. Let

$$u_1 = \mathcal{L}_1(A'A) + \{\boldsymbol{\mathcal{E}}_1'(AA')\ B\ \boldsymbol{\mathcal{E}}_1(A'A)\}^2,$$

$$u_2 = \mathcal{L}_1(B'B) + \{\boldsymbol{\mathcal{E}}_1'(BB')\ A\ \boldsymbol{\mathcal{E}}_1(B'B)\}^2,$$

and define

$$u_{min} = \max\{u_1, u_2\} \quad \text{and} \quad u_{max} = \mathcal{L}_1(A'A) + \mathcal{L}_1(B'B).$$

Then, verify the following bounds:

$$u_{min} \le u(\tilde{\boldsymbol{x}}, \tilde{\boldsymbol{y}}) \le \min\{u_{max}, \lambda_c^2\},$$

with $\lambda_c^2$ representing the largest eigenvalue of $C^*C$, where $C$ is the complex matrix given by $C = A + iB$ [see (5.156) and (5.157)], and $\tilde{\boldsymbol{x}}$ and $\tilde{\boldsymbol{y}}$ maximize $u(\boldsymbol{x}, \boldsymbol{y})$.

*Section 5.10*

**5.24** (a) Repeat the dynamic Fourier analysis of Example 5.22 on the remaining seven earthquakes and seven explosions in the data file `eq+exp.dat`. Do the conclusions about the difference between earthquakes and explosions stated in the example still seem valid?

(b) Now repeat the dynamic Fourier analysis on the Novaya Zemlya event, and with justification, state your conclusion about the nature of the event.

**5.25** Repeat the wavelet analyses of Example 5.25 on all earthquake and explosion series in the data file `eq+exp.dat`. Do the conclusions about the difference between earthquakes and explosions stated in Examples 5.23 and 5.24 still seem valid? Compare your wavelet analysis results with the results of Example 5.25, and, with justification, state your conclusion about the nature of the event at Novaya Zemlya.

# REFERENCES


Akaike, H. (1969). Fitting autoregressive models for prediction. *Ann. Inst. Stat. Math.*, 21, 243-247.

Akaike, H. (1973). Information theory and an extension of the maximum likelihood principal. In *2nd Int. Symp. Inform. Theory*, 267-281. B.N. Petrov and F. Csake eds. Budapest: Akademia Kiado.

Akaike, H. (1974). A new look at statistical model identification. *IEEE Trans. Automat. Contr.*, AC-19, 716-723.

Alagón, J. (1989). Spectral discrimination for two groups of time series. *J. Time Series Anal.*, 10, 203-214.

Alspach, D. L. and H. W. Sorensen (1972). Nonlinear Bayesian estimation using Gaussian sum approximations. *IEEE Trans. Automat. Contr.*, AC-17, 439-447.

Anderson, B.D.O. and J.B. Moore (1979). *Optimal Filtering.* Englewood Cliffs, NJ: Prentice-Hall.

Anderson, T.W. (1978). Estimation for autoregressive moving average models in the time and frequency domain. *Ann. Stat.*, 5, 842-865.

Anderson, T.W. (1984). *An Introduction to Multivariate Statistical Analysis, 2nd ed.* New York: Wiley.

Ansley, C.F. and P. Newbold (1980). Finite sample properties of estimators for autoregressive moving average processes. *J. Econ.*, 13, 159-183.

Antognini, J.F., M.H. Buonocore, E.A. Disbrow, and E. Carstens (1997). Isoflurane anesthesia blunts cerebral responses to noxious and innocuous stimuli: a fMRI study. *Life Sci.*, 61, PL349-PL354.

Bandettini, A., A. Jesmanowicz, E.C. Wong, and J.S. Hyde (1993). Processing strategies for time-course data sets in functional MRI of the human brain. *Magnetic Res. Med.*, 30, 161-173.

Bar-Shalom, Y. (1978). Tracking methods in a multi-target environment. *IEEE Trans. Automat. Contr.*, AC-23, 618-626.

Bar-Shalom, Y. and E. Tse (1975). Tracking in a cluttered environment with probabilistic data association. *Automatica*, 11, 4451-4460.

Bazza, M., R.H. Shumway, and D.R. Nielsen (1988). Two-dimensional spectral analysis of soil surface temperatures. *Hilgardia*, 56, 1-28.

Bedrick, E.J. and C.-L. Tsai (1994). Model selection for multivariate regression in small samples. *Biometrics*, 50, 226-231.

Beran, J. (1994). *Statistics for Long Memory Processes.* New York: Chapman and Hall.

Berk, K.N. (1974). Consistent autoregressive spectral estimates. *Ann. Stat.*, 2, 489-502.

Besag, J. (1974). Spatial interaction and the statistical analysis of lattice systems (with discussion). *J. R. Stat. Soc. B*, 36, 192-236.

Bhat, R.R. (1985). *Modern Probability Theory, 2nd ed.* New York: Wiley.

Bhattacharya, A. (1943). On a measure of divergence between two statistical populations. *Bull. Calcutta Math. Soc.*, 35, 99-109.

Blackman, R.B. and J.W. Tukey (1959). *The Measurement of Power Spectra from the Point of View of Communications Engineering.* New York: Dover.

Bloomfield, P. (1976). *Fourier Analysis of Time Series: An Introduction.* New York: Wiley.

Bloomfield, P. and J.M. Davis (1994). Orthogonal rotation of complex principal components. *Int. J. Climatol.*, 14, 759-775.

Bollerslev, T. (1986). Generalized autoregressive conditional heteroscedasticity. *J. Econ.*, 31, 307- 327.

Box, G.E.P., and G.M. Jenkins (1970). *Time Series Analysis, Forecasting, and Control.* Oakland, CA: Holden-Day.

Box, G.E.P., G.M. Jenkins and G.C. Reinsel (1994). *Time Series Analysis, Forecasting, and Control, 3rd ed.* Englewood Cliffs, NJ: Prentice Hall.

Box, G.E.P. and D.A. Pierce (1970). Distributions of residual autocorrelations in autoregressive integrated moving average models. *J. Am. Stat. Assoc.*, 72, 397-402.

Box, G.E.P. and G.C. Tiao (1973). *Bayesian Inference in Statistical Analysis.* New York: Wiley.

Breiman, L. and J. Friedman (1985). Estimating optimal transformations for multiple regression and correlation (with discussion). *J. Am. Stat. Assoc.*, 80, 580-619.

Brillinger, D.R. (1973). The analysis of time series collected in an experimental design. In *Multivariate Analysis-III.*, pp. 241-256. P.R. Krishnaiah ed. New York: Academic Press.

Brillinger, D.R. (1980). Analysis of variance and problems under time series models. In *Handbook of Statistics*, Vol I, pp. 237-278. P.R. Krishnaiah and D.R. Brillinger eds. Amsterdam: North Holland.

Brillinger, D.R. (1981). *Time Series: Data Analysis and Theory, 2nd ed.* San Francisco: Holden-Day.

Brockwell, P.J. and R.A. Davis (1991). *Time Series: Theory and Methods, 2nd ed.* New York: Springer-Verlag,

Bruce, A. and H-Y. Gao (1996). *Applied Wavelet Analysis with S-PLUS.* New York: Springer-Verlag.

Caines, P.E. (1988). *Linear Stochastic Systems.* New York: Wiley.

Carlin, B.P., N.G. Polson, and D.S. Stoffer (1992). A Monte Carlo approach to nonnormal and nonlinear state-space modeling. *J. Am. Stat. Assoc.*, 87, 493-500.

Carter, C. K. and R. Kohn (1994). On Gibbs sampling for state space models. *Biometrika*, 81, 541-553.

Chernoff, H. (1952). A measure of asymptotic efficiency for tests of a hypothesis based on the sum of the observations. *Ann. Math. Stat.*, 25, 573-578.

Cleveland, W.S. (1979). Robust locally weighted regression and smoothing scatterplots. *J. Am. Stat. Assoc.*, 74, 829-836.

Cochrane, D. and G.H. Orcutt (1949). Applications of least squares regression to relationships containing autocorrelated errors. *J. Am. Stat. Assoc.*, 44, 32-61.

Cooley, J.W. and J.W. Tukey (1965). An algorithm for the machine computation of complex Fourier series. *Math. Comput.*, 19, 297-301.

Cressie, N.A.C. (1993). *Statistics for Spatial Data.* New York: Wiley.

Dahlhaus, R. (1989). Efficient parameter estimation for self-similar processes. *Ann. Stat.*, 17, 1749-1766.

Dargahi-Noubary, G.R. and P.J. Laycock (1981). Spectral ratio discriminants and information theory. *J. Time Series Anal.*, 16, 201-219.

Daubechies, I. (1992). *Ten Lectures on Wavelets.* Philadelphia: CBMS-NSF Regional Conference Series in Applied Mathematics.

Davies, N., C.M. Triggs, and P. Newbold (1977). Significance levels of the Box-Pierce portmanteau statistic in finite samples. *Biometrika*, 64, 517-522.

Dent, W., and A.-S. Min. (1978). A Monte Carlo study of autoregressive-integrated-moving average processes. *J. of Econ.*, 7, 23-55.

Dempster, A.P., N.M. Laird and D.B. Rubin (1977). Maximum likelihood from incomplete data via the EM algorithm. *J. R. Stat. Soc. B*, 39, 1-38.

Diggle, P.J., K.-Y. Liang, and S.L. Zeger (1994). *The Analysis of Longitudinal Data.* Oxford: Clarendon Press.

Ding, Z., C.W.J. Granger, and R.F. Engle (1993). A long memory property of stock market returns and a new model. *J. Empirical Finance*, 1, 83-106.

Donoho, D. L. and I. M. Johnstone (1994). Ideal spatial adaptation by wavelet shrinkage. *Biometrika*, 81, 425-455.

Donoho, D. L. and I. M. Johnstone (1995). Adapting to unknown smoothness via wavelet shrinkage. *J. of Am. Stat. Assoc.*, 90, 1200-1224.

Durbin, J. (1960). Estimation of parameters in time series regression models. *J. R. Stat. Soc. B*, 22, 139-153.

Efron, B. and R. Tibshirani (1994). *An Introduction to the Bootstrap.* New York: Chapman and Hall.

Engle, R.F. (1982). Autoregressive conditional heteroscedasticity with estimates of the variance of United Kingdom inflation. *Econometrica*, 50, 987-1007.

Engle, R.F., D. Nelson, and T. Bollerslev (1994). ARCH Models. In *Handbook of Econometrics*, Vol IV, pp. 2959-3038. R. Engle and D. McFadden eds. Amsterdam: North Holland.

Fahrmeir, L. and G. Tutz (1994). *Multivariate Statistical Modelling Based on Generalized Linear Models.* New York: Springer-Verlag.

Fox, R. and M.S. Taqqu (1986). Large sample properties of parameter estimates for strongly dependent stationary Gaussian time series. *Ann. Stat.*, 14, 517-532.

Friedman, J.H. (1984). A Variable Span Smoother. Tech. Rep. No. 5, Lab. for Computational Statistics, Dept. Statistics, Stanford Univ., California.

Friedman, J.H. and W. Stuetzle. (1981). Projection pursuit regression. *J. Am. Stat. Assoc.*, 76, 817-823.

Frühwirth-Schnatter, S. (1994). Data Augmentation and Dynamic Linear Models. *J. Time Series Anal.*, 15, 183–202.

Fuller, W.A. (1995). *Introduction to Statistical Time Series, 2nd ed.* New York: Wiley.

Gabr, M.M. and T. Subba-Rao (1981). The estimation and prediction of subset bilinear time series models with applications. *J. Time Series Anal.*, 2, 155-171.

Gelfand, A.E. and A.F.M. Smith (1990). Sampling-based approaches to calculating marginal densities. *J. Am. Stat. Assoc.*, 85, 398-409.

Gelman, A., J. Carlin, H. Stern, and D. Rubin (1995). *Bayesian Data Analysis.* London: Chapman and Hall.

Geman, S. and D. Geman (1984). Stochastic relaxation, Gibbs distributions, and the Bayesian restoration of images. *IEEE Trans. Pattern Anal. Machine Intell.*, 6, 721-741.

Geweke, J.F. (1977). The dynamic factor analysis of economic time series models. In *Latent Variables in Socio-Economic Models*, pp 365-383. D. Aigner and A. Goldberger eds. Amsterdam: North Holland.

Geweke, J.F. and K.J. Singleton (1981). Latent variable models for time series: A frequency domain approach with an application to the Permanent Income Hypothesis. *J. Econ.*, 17, 287-304.

Geweke, J.F. and S. Porter-Hudak (1983). The estimation and application of long-memory time series models. *J. Time Series Anal.*, 4, 221-238.

Gilks, W.R., S. Richardson, and D.J. Spiegelhalter (Eds.) (1996). *Markov Chain Monte Carlo in Practice.* London: Chapman and Hall.

Giri, N. (1965). On complex analogues of $T^2$ and $R^2$ tests. *Ann. Math. Stat.*, 36, 664-670.

Goldfeld, S.M. and R.E. Quandt (1973). A Markov model for switching regressions. *J. Econ.*, 1, 3-16.

Goodman, N.R. (1963). Statistical analysis based on a certain multivariate complex Gaussian distribution. *Ann. Math. Stat.*, 34, 152-177.

Goodrich, R.L. and P.E. Caines (1979). Linear system identification from nonstationary cross-sectional data. *IEEE Trans. Automat. Contr.*, AC-24, 403-411.

Gordon, K. and A.F.M. Smith (1990). Modeling and monitoring biomedical time series. *J. Am. Stat. Assoc.*, 85, 328-337.

Gouriéroux, C. (1997). *ARCH Models and Financial Applications.* New York: Springer-Verlag.

Granger, C.W. and A.P. Andersen (1978). *Introduction to Bilinear Time Series Models.* Göttingen: Vandengoeck and Ruprecht.

Granger, C.W. and R. Joyeux (1980). An introduction to long-memory time series models and fractional differencing. *J. Time Series Anal.*, 1, 15-29.

Grether, D.M. and M. Nerlove (1970). Some properties of optimal seasonal adjustment. *Econometrica*, 38, 682-703.

Gupta N.K. and R.K. Mehra (1974). Computational aspects of maximum likelihood estimation and reduction in sensitivity function calculations. *IEEE Trans. Automat. Contr.*, AC-19, 774-783.

Hamilton, J.D. (1989). A new approach to the economic analysis of nonstationary time series and the business cycle. *Econometrica*, 57, 357-384.

Hamilton, J.D. and G. Lin (1996). Stock market volatility and the business cycle. *J. App. Econ.*, 11, 573-593.

Hannan, E.J. (1970). *Multiple Time Series.* New York: Wiley.

Hannan, E.J. (1973). The asymptotic theory of linear time series models. *J. Appl. Prob.*, 10, 130-145.

Hannan, E.J. and M. Deistler (1988). *The Statistical Theory of Linear Systems.* New York: Wiley.

Hansen, J. and S. Lebedeff (1987). Global trends of measured surface air temperature. *J. Geophys. Res.*, 92, 1345-1372.

Hansen, J. and S. Lebedeff (1988). Global surface air temperatures: Update through 1987. *J. Geophys. Lett.*, 15, 323-326.

Harrison, P.J. and C.F. Stevens (1976). Bayesian forecasting (with discussion). *J. R. Stat. Soc. B*, 38, 205-247.

Harvey, A.C. and P.H.J. Todd (1983). Forecasting economic time series with structural and Box-Jenkins models: A case study. *J. Bus. Econ. Stat.*, 1, 299-307.

Harvey, A. C. and R. G. Pierse (1984). Estimating missing observations in economic time series. *J. Am. Stat. Assoc.*, 79, 125-131.

Harvey, A.C. (1991). *Forecasting, Structural Time Series Models and the Kalman Filter.* Cambridge: Cambridge University Press.

Harvey, A.C. (1993). *Time Series Models.* Cambridge, MA: MIT Press.

Hastings, W. K. (1970). Monte Carlo sampling methods using Markov chains and their applications. *Biometrika*, 57, 97-109.

Hosking, J.R.M. (1981). Fractional differencing. *Biometrika*, 68, 165-176.

Hurst, H. (1951). Long term storage capacity of reservoirs. *Trans. Am. Soc. Civil Eng.*, 116, 778-808.

Hurvich, C.M. and Zeger, S. (1987). Frequency domain bootstrap methods for time series. *Tech. Report 87-115*, Department of Statistics and Operations Research, Stern School of Business, New York University.

Hurvich, C.M and C.-L. Tsai (1989). Regression and time series model selection in small samples. *Biometrika*, 76, 297-307.

Hurvich, C.M. and K.I. Beltrao (1993). Asymptotics for the low-requency oridnates of the periodogram for a long-memory time series. *J. Time Series Anal.*, 14, 455-472.

Hurvich, C.M., R. Deo and J. Brodsky (1998). The mean squared error of Geweke and Porter-Hudak's estimator of the memory parameter of a long-memory time series. *J. Time Series Anal.*, 19, 19-46.

Jacquier, E., N.G. Polson, and P.E. Rossi (1994). Bayesian analysis of stochastic volatility models. *J. Bus. Econ. Stat.*, 12, 371-417.

Jazwinski, A. H. (1970). *Stochastic Processes and Filtering Theory.* New York: Academic Press.

Jenkins, G.M. and D.G. Watts. (1968). *Spectral Analysis and Its Applications.* San Francisco: Holden-Day.

Johnson, R.A. and D.W. Wichern (1992). *Applied Multivariate Statistical Analysis, 3rd ed..* Englewood Cliffs, NJ: Prentice-Hall.

Jones, P.D. (1994). Hemispheric surface air temperature variations: A reanalysis and an update to 1993. *J. Clim.*, 7, 1794-1802.

Jones, R.H. (1980). Maximum likelihood fitting of ARMA models to time series with missing observations. *Technometrics*, 22, 389-395.

Jones, R.H. (1984). Fitting multivariate models to unequally spaced data. In *Time Series Analysis of Irregularly Observed Data*, pp 158-188. E. Parzen ed. Lecture Notes in Statistics, 25, New York: Springer-Verlag.

Jones, R.H. (1993). *Longitudinal Data With Serial Correlation : A State-Space Approach.* London: Chapman and Hall.

Journel, A.G. and C.H. Huijbregts (1978). *Mining Geostatistics.* New York: Academic Press.

Juang, B.H. and L.R. Rabiner (1985). Mixture autoregressive hidden Markov models for speech signals, *IEEE Trans. Acoust., Speech, Signal Process.*, ASSP-33, 1404-1413.

Kakizawa, Y., R. H. Shumway, and M. Taniguchi (1998). Discrimination and clustering for multivariate time series. *J. Am. Stat. Assoc.*, 93, 328-340.

Kalman, R.E. (1960). A new approach to linear filtering and prediction problems. *Trans ASME J. Basic Eng.*, 82, 35-45.

Kalman, R.E. and R.S. Bucy (1961). New results in filtering and prediction theory. *Trans. ASME J. Basic Eng.*, 83, 95-108.

Kay, S.M. (1988). *Modern Spectral Analysis: Theory and Applications.* Englewood Cliffs, NJ: Prentice-Hall.

Kazakos, D. and P. Papantoni-Kazakos (1980). Spectral distance measuring between Gaussian processes. *IEEE Trans. Automat. Contr.*, AC-25, 950-959.

Khatri, C.G. (1965). Classical statistical analysis based on a certain multivariate complex Gaussian distribution. *Ann. Math. Stat.*, 36, 115-119.

Kitagawa, G. (1987). Non-Gaussian state-space modeling of nonstationary time series (with discussion). *J. Am. Stat. Assoc.*, 82, 1032-1041, (C/R: p1041-1063; C/R: V83 p1231).

Kitagawa, G. and W. Gersch (1984). A smoothness priors modeling of time series with trend and seasonality. *J. Am. Stat. Assoc.*, 79, 378-389.

Kitagawa, G. and W. Gersch (1996). *Smoothness Priors Analysis of Time Series.* New York: Springer-Verlag.

Kolmogorov, A.N. (1941). Interpolation and extrapolation von stationären zufälligen folgen. *Bull. Acad. Sci. U.R.S.S.*, 5, 3-14.

Krishnaiah, P.R., J.C. Lee, and T.C. Chang (1976). The distribution of likelihood ratio statistics for tests of certain covariance structures of complex multivariate normal populations. *Biometrika*, 63, 543-549.

Kullback, S. and R.A. Leibler (1951). On information and sufficiency. *Ann. Math. Stat.*, 22, 79-86.

Kullback, S. (1978). *Information Theory and Statistics, 3rd ed.* Gloucester, MA: Peter Smith.

Lachenbruch, P.A. and M.R. Mickey (1968). Estimation of error rates in discriminant analysis. *Technometrices*, 10, 1-11.

Laird, N. and J. Ware (1982). Random-effects models for longitudinal data. *Biometrics*, 38, 963-974.

Lam, P.S. (1990). The Hamilton model with a general autoregressive component: Estimation and comparison with other models of economic time series. *J. Monetary Econ.*, 26, 409-432.

Lay, T. (1997). Research required to support comprehensive nuclear test ban treaty monitoring. *National Research Council Report, National Academy Press*, 2101 Constitution Ave., Washington, DC 20055.

Levinson, N. (1947). The Wiener (root mean square) error criterion in filter design and prediction. *J. Math. Phys.*, 25, 262-278.

Lindgren, G. (1978). Markov regime models for mixed distributions and switching regressions. *Scand. J. Stat.*, 5, 81-91.

Liu, L.M. (1991). Dynamic relationship analysis of U.S. gasoline and crude oil prices. *J. Forecast.*, 10, 521-547.

Ljung, G.M. and G.E.P. Box (1978). On a measure of lack of fit in time series models. *Biometrika*, 65, 297-303.

Lütkepohl, H. (1985). Comparison of criteria for estimating the order of a vector autoregressive process. *J. Time Series Anal.*, 6, 35-52.

Lütkepohl, H. (1993). *Introduction to Multiple Time Series Analysis, 2nd ed.* Berlin: Springer-Verlag.

McQuarrie, A.D.R. and R.H. Shumway (1994). *ASTSA for Windows.*

McQuarrie, A.D.R. and C-L. Tsai (1998). *Regression and Time Series Model Selection*, Singapore: World Scientific.

Mallows, C.L. (1973). Some comments on $C_p$. *Technometrics*, 15, 661-675.

McBratney, A.B. and R. Webster (1981). Detection of ridge and furrow pattern by spectral analysis of crop yield. *Int. Stat. Rev.*, 49, 45-52.

McCulloch, R.E. and R.S. Tsay (1993). Bayesian inference and prediction for mean and variance shifts in autoregressive time series. *J. Am. Stat. Assoc.*, 88, 968-978.

McDougall, A. J., D.S. Stoffer and D.E. Tyler (1997). Optimal transformations and the spectral envelope for real-valued time series. *J. Stat. Plan. Infer.*, **57**, 195-214.

McLeod A.I. (1978). On the distribution of residual autocorrelations in Box-Jenkins models. *J. R. Stat. Soc. B*, 40, 296-302.

McLeod, A.I. and K.W. Hipel (1978). Preservation of the rescaled adusted range, I. A reassessment of the Hurst phenomenon. *Water Resour. Res.*, 14, 491-508.

Meinhold, R.J. and N.D. Singpurwalla (1983). Understanding the Kalman filter. *Am. Stat.*, 37, 123-127.

Meinhold, R.J. and N.D. Singpurwalla (1989). Robustification of Kalman filter models. *J. Am. Stat. Assoc.*, 84, 479-486.

Meng X.L. and Rubin, D.B. (1991). Using EM to obtain asymptotic variance–covariance matrices: The SEM algorithm. *J. Am. Stat. Assoc.*, 86, 899-909.

Metropolis N., A.W. Rosenbluth, M.N. Rosenbluth, A. H. Teller, and E. Teller (1953). Equations of state calculations by fast computing machines. *J. Chem. Phys.*, 21, 1087-1091.

Mickens, R.E. (1987). *Difference Equations.* New York: Van Nostrand Reinhold.

Newbold, P. and T. Bos (1985). *Stochastic Parameter Regression Models.* Beverly Hills: Sage.

Ogawa, S., T.M. Lee, A. Nayak and P. Glynn (1990). Oxygenation-sensititive contrast in magnetic resonance image of rodent brain at high magnetic fields. *Magn. Reson. Med.*, 14, 68-78.

Palma, W. and N.H. Chan (1997). Estimation and forecasting of long-memory time series with missing values. *J. Forecast.*, 16, 395-410.

Paparoditis, E. and Politis, D.N. (1999). The local bootstrap for periodogram statistics. *J. Time Series Anal.*, 20, 193-222.

Parker, D.E., P.D. Jones, A. Bevan and C.K. Folland (1994). Interdecadal changes of surface temperature since the late 19th century. *J. Geophysical Research*, 90, 14373-14399.

Parker, D.E., C.K. Folland and M. Jackson (1995). Marine surface temperature: observed variations and data requirements. *Climatic Change*, 31, 559-60

Parzen, E. (1961). Mathematical considerations in the estimation of spectra. *Technometrics*, 3, 167-190.

Parzen, E. (1983). Autoregressive spectral estimation. In *Time Series in the Frequency Domain, Handbook of Statistics*, Vol. 3, pp. 211-243. D.R. Brillinger and P.R. Krishnaiah eds. Amsterdam: North Holland.

Pawitan, Y. and R.H. Shumway (1989). Spectral estimation and deconvolution for a linear time series model. *J. Time Series Anal.*, 10, 115-129.

Peña, D. and I. Guttman (1988). A Bayesian approach to robustifying the Kalman filter. In *Bayesian Analysis of Time Series and Dynamic Linear Models*, pp. 227-254. J.C. Spall ed. New York: Marcel Dekker.

Pinsker, M.S. (1964). *Information and Information Stability of Random Variables and Processes*, San Francisco: Holden Day.

Pole, P.J. and M. West (1988). Nonnormal and nonlinear dynamic Bayesian modeling. In *Bayesian Analysis of Time Series and Dynamic Linear Models*, pp. 167-198. J.C. Spall ed. New York: Marcel Dekker.

Press, W.H., S.A. Teukolsky, W. T. Vetterling, and B.P. Flannery (1993). *Numerical Recipes in C : The Art of Scientific Computing, 2nd ed.* Cambridge: Cambridge University Press.

Priestley, M.B., T. Subba-Rao and H. Tong (1974). Applications of principal components analysis and factor analysis in the identification of multivariable systems. *IEEE Trans. Automat. Contr.*, AC-19, 730-734.

Priestley, M.B. and T. Subba-Rao (1975). The estimation of factor scores and Kalman filtering for discrete parameter stationary processes. *Int. J. Contr.*, 21, 971-975.

Priestley, M.B. (1981). *Spectral Analysis and Time Series.* Vol. 1: Univariate Series; Vol 2: Multivariate Series, Prediction and Control. New York: Academic Press.

Priestley, M.B. (1988). *Nonlinear and Nonstationary Time Series Analysis.* London: Academic Press.

Quandt, R.E. (1972). A new approach to estimating switching regressions. *J. Am. Stat. Assoc.*, 67, 306-310.

Rabiner, L.R. and B.H. Juang (1986). An introduction to hidden Markov models, *IEEE Acoust., Speech, Signal Process.*, ASSP-34, 4-16.

Rao, C.R. (1973). *Linear Statistical Inference and Its Applications.* New York: Wiley.

Rauch, H.E., F. Tung, and C.T. Striebel (1965). Maximum likelihood estimation of linear dynamic systems. *J. AIAA*, 3, 1445-1450.

Reinsel, G.C. (1997). *Elements of Multivariate Time Series Analysis, 2nd ed.* New York: Springer-Verlag.

Renyi, A. (1961). On measures of entropy and information. In *Proceedings of 4th Berkeley Symp. Math. Stat. and Probability*, pp. 547-561, Berkeley: Univ. of California Press.

Rissanen, J. (1978). Modeling by shortest data description. *Automatica*, 14, 465-471.

Robinson, P.M. (1995). Gaussian semiparametric estimation of long range dependence. *Ann. Stat.*, 23, 1630-1661.

Rosenblatt, M. (1956). A central limit theorem and a strong mixing condition. *Proc. Nat. Acad. Sci.* , 42, 43-47.

Scheffé, H. (1959). *The Analysis of Variance.* New York: Wiley.

Schuster, A. (1906). On the periodicities of sunspots. *Phil. Trans. R. Soc., Ser. A*, 206, 69-100.

Schwarz, F. (1978). Estimating the dimension of a model. *Ann. Stat.*, 6, 461-464.

Schweppe, F.C. (1965). Evaluation of likelihood functions for Gaussian signals. *IEEE Trans. Inform. Theory*, IT-4, 294-305.

Seber, G.A.G. (1977). *Linear Regression Analysis.* New York: Wiley.

Shepard, N. (1996). Statistical aspects of ARCH and stochastic volatility. In *Time Series Models in Econometrics, Finance and Other Fields* , pp 1-100. D.R. Cox, D.V. Hinkley, and O.E. Barndorff-Nielson eds. London: Chapman and Hall.

Shumway, R.H. and W.C. Dean (1968). Best linear unbiased estimation for multivariate stationary processes. *Technometrics*, 10, 523-534.

Shumway, R.H. (1970). Applied regression and analysis of variance for stationary time series. *J. Am. Stat. Assoc.*, 65, 1527-1546.

Shumway, R.H. (1971). On detecting a signal in $N$ stationarily correlated noise series. *Technometrics*, 10, 523-534.

Shumway, R.H. and A.N. Unger (1974). Linear discriminant functions for stationary time series. *J. Am. Stat. Assoc.*, 69, 948-956.

Shumway, R.H. (1982). Discriminant analysis for time series. In *Classification, Pattern Recognition and Reduction of Dimensionality, Handbook of Statistics Vol. 2*, pp. 1-46. P.R. Krishnaiah and L.N. Kanal eds. Amsterdam: North Holland.

Shumway, R.H. and D.S. Stoffer (1982). An approach to time series smoothing and forecasting using the EM algorithm. *J. Time Series Anal.*, 3, 253-264.

Shumway, R.H. (1983). Replicated time series regression: An approach to signal estimation and detection. In *Time Series in the Frequency Domain, Handbook of Statistics Vol. 3*, pp. 383-408. D.R. Brillinger and P.R. Krishnaiah eds. Amsterdam: North Holland.

Shumway, R.H. (1988). *Applied Statistical Time Series Analysis.* Englewood Cliffs, NJ: Prentice-Hall.

Shumway, R.H., R.S. Azari, and Y. Pawitan (1988). Modeling mortality fluctuations in Los Angeles as functions of pollution and weather effects. *Environ. Res.*, 45, 224-241.

Shumway, R.H. and D.S. Stoffer (1991). Dynamic linear models with switching. *J. Am. Stat. Assoc.*, 86, 763-769, (Correction: V87 p. 913).

Shumway, R.H. and K.L. Verosub (1992). State space modeling of paleoclimatic time series. In *Pro. 5th Int. Meeting Stat. Climatol.*. Toronto, pp. 22-26, June, 1992.

Shumway, R.H. (1996). Statistical approaches to seismic discrimination. In *Monitoring a Comprehensive Test Ban Treaty*, pp. 791-803. A.M. Dainty and E.S. Husebye eds. Doordrecht, The Netherlands: Kluwer Academic

Shumway, R.H., S.E. Kim and R.R. Blandford (1999). Nonlinear estimation for time series observed on arrays. Chapter 7, Ghosh ed. *Asymptotics,*

*Nonparametrics and Time Series*, 227-258. New York: Marcel Dekker.

Small, C.G. and D.L. McLeish (1994). *Hilbert Space Methods in Probability and Statistical Inference.* New York: Wiley.

Smith, A.F.M. and M. West (1983). Monitoring renal transplants: An application of the multiprocess Kalman filter. *Biometrics*, 39, 867-878.

Spliid, H. (1983). A fast estimation method for the vector autoregressive moving average model with exogenous variables. *J. Am. Stat. Assoc.*, 78, 843-849.

Stoffer, D.S. (1982). Estimation of Parameters in a Linear Dynamic System with Missing Observations. Ph.D. Dissertation. Univ. California, Davis.

Stoffer, D.S. (1987). Walsh-Fourier analysis of discrete-valued time series. *J. Time Series Anal.*, 8, 449-467.

Stoffer, D.S., M. Scher, G. Richardson, N. Day, and P. Coble (1988). A Walsh-Fourier analysis of the effects of moderate maternal alcohol consumption on neonatal sleep-state cycling. *J. Am. Stat. Assoc.*, 83, 954-963.

Stoffer, D.S. and K. Wall (1991). Bootstrapping state space models: Gaussian maximum likelihood estimation and the Kalman filter. *J. Am. Stat. Assoc.*, 86, 1024-1033.

Stoffer, D.S., D.E. Tyler, and A.J. McDougall (1993). Spectral analysis for categorical time series: Scaling and the spectral envelope. *Biometrika*, 80, 611-622.

Stoffer, D.S. and D.E. Tyler (1998). Matching sequences: Cross-spectral analysis of categorical time series *Biometrika*, 85, 201-213.

Stoffer, D.S. (1999). Detecting common signals in multiple time series using the spectral envelope. *J. Am. Stat. Assoc.*, 94, in press.

Subba-Rao, T. (1981). On the theory of bilinear time series models. *J. R. Stat. Soc. B*, 43, 244-255.

Sugiura, N. (1978). Further analysis of the data by Akaike's information criterion and the finite corrections, *Commun. in Statist, A, Theory and Methods*, 7, 13-26.

Taniguchi, M., M.L. Puri, and M. Kondo (1994). Nonparametric approach for non-Gaussian vector stationary processes. *J. Mult. Anal.*, 56, 259-283.

Tanner, M. and W.H. Wong (1987). The calculation of posterior distributions by data augmentation (with discussion). *J. Am. Stat. Assoc.*, 82, 528-554.

Tiao, G.C. and R.S. Tsay (1989). Model specification in multivariate time series (with discussion). *J. Roy. Statist. Soc. B*, 51, 157-213.

Tiao, G. C. and R.S. Tsay (1994). Some advances in nonlinear and adaptive modeling in time series analysis. *J. Forecast.*, 13, 109-131.

Tiao, G.C., R.S. Tsay and T .Wang (1993). Usefulness of linear transformations in multivariate time series analysis. *Empir. Econ.*, 18, 567-593.

Tierney, L. (1994). Markov chains for exploring posterior distributions (with discussion). *Ann. Stat.*, 22, 1701-1728.

Tong, H. (1983). *Threshold Models in Nonlinear Time Series Analysis.* Springer Lecture Notes in Statistics, 21. New York: Springer-Verlag.

Tong, H. (1990). *Nonlinear Time Series: A Dynamical System Approach.* Oxford: Oxford Univ. Press.

Tsay, R. (1987). Conditional hetereroscadasticity in time series analysis. *J. Am. Stat. Assoc.*, 82, 590-604.

Venables, W. N. and B.D. Ripley (1994). *Modern Applied Statistics with S-Plus.* New York: Springer-Verlag.

Walker, G. (1931). On periodicity in series of related terms. *Proc. R. Soc. Lond., Ser. A*, 131, 518-532.

Watson, G.S. (1966). Smooth regression analysis. *Sankhya*, 26, 359-378.

Weiss, A.A. (1984). ARMA models with ARCH errors. *J. Time Series Anal.*, 5, 129-143.

West, M. and J. Harrison (1997). *Bayesian Forecasting and Dynamic Models 2nd ed.* New York: Springer-Verlag.

Whittle, P. (1961). Gaussian estimation in stationary time series. *Bull. Int. Stat. Inst.*, 33, 1-26.

Wiener, N. (1949). *The Extrapolation, Interpolation and Smoothing of Stationary Time Series with Engineering Applications.* New York: Wiley.

Wu, C.F. (1983). On the convergence properties of the EM algorithm. *Ann. Stat.* , 11, 95-103.

Young, P.C. and D.J. Pedregal (1998). Macro-economic relativity: Government spending, private investment and unemployment in the USA. Centre for Research on Environmental Systems and Statistics, Lancaster University, U.K.

Yule, G.U. (1927). On a method of investigating periodicities in disturbed series with special reference to Wolfer's Sunspot Numbers. *Phil. Trans. R. Soc. Lond.*, A226, 267-298.

# Index

## Springer Texts in Statistics *(continued from page ii)*

*Nguyen and Rogers:* Fundamentals of Mathematical Statistics: Volume I: Probability for Statistics
*Nguyen and Rogers:* Fundamentals of Mathematical Statistics: Volume II: Statistical Inference
*Noether:* Introduction to Statistics: The Nonparametric Way
*Peters:* Counting for Something: Statistical Principles and Personalities
*Pfeiffer:* Probability for Applications
*Pitman:* Probability
*Rawlings, Pantula and Dickey:* Applied Regression Analysis
*Robert:* The Bayesian Choice: A Decision-Theoretic Motivation
*Robert and Casella:* Monte Carlo Statistical Methods
*Santner and Duffy:* The Statistical Analysis of Discrete Data
*Saville and Wood:* Statistical Methods: The Geometric Approach
*Sen and Srivastava:* Regression Analysis: Theory, Methods, and Applications
*Shao:* Mathematical Statistics
*Shumway and Stoffer:* Time Series Analysis and Its Applications
*Terrell:* Mathematical Statistics: A Unified Introduction
*Whittle:* Probability via Expectation, Third Edition
*Zacks:* Introduction to Reliability Analysis: Probability Models and Statistical Methods